Recent Advances in Geriatric Medicine

Recent Advances in Geriatric Medicine

Editor: Mason Button

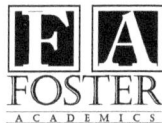

FOSTER
ACADEMICS

www.fosteracademics.com

www.fosteracademics.com

FA
FOSTER
ACADEMICS

Cataloging-in-Publication Data

Recent advances in geriatric medicine / edited by Mason Button.
    p. cm.
Includes bibliographical references and index.
ISBN 978-1-63242-594-2
1. Geriatrics. 2. Aging. 3. Gerontology. 4. Older people--Diseases.
5. Older people--Health and hygiene. I. Button, Mason.
RC952 .R43 2019
618.97--dc23

Foster Academics,
118-35 Queens Blvd., Suite 400,
Forest Hills, NY 11375, USA

ISBN 978-1-63242-594-2 (Hardback)

Contents

Preface IX

Chapter 1   Role of Sociocultural Factors in Depression among Elderly of Twin Cities
(Rawalpindi and Islamabad) of Pakistan 1
Saira Javed

Chapter 2   Unexplained Falls are Frequent in Patients with Fall-Related Injury
Admitted to Orthopaedic Wards: The UFO Study (Unexplained Falls in
Older Patients) 6
Mussi Chiara, Galizia Gianluigi, Abete Pasquale, Morrione Alessandro,
Maraviglia Alice, Noro Gabriele, Cavagnaro Paolo, Ghirelli Loredana,
Tava Giovanni, Rengo Franco, Masotti Giulio, Salvioli Gianfranco,
Marchionni Niccolò and Ungar Andrea

Chapter 3   Intraindividual Variability in Domain-Specific Cognition and Risk of
Mild Cognitive Impairment and Dementia 12
Leslie Vaughan, Iris Leng, Dale Dagenbach, Susan M. Resnick,
Stephen R. Rapp, Janine M. Jennings, Robert L. Brunner, Sean L. Simpson,
Daniel P. Beavers, Laura H. Coker, Sarah A. Gaussoin, Kaycee M. Sink and
Mark A. Espeland

Chapter 4   Prevalence and Determinants of Fall-Related Injuries among Older Adults
in Ecuador 22
Carlos H. Orces

Chapter 5   The Contribution of a "Supportive Community" Program for Older Persons
in Israel to their Offspring who are Primary Caregivers 29
Ahuva Even-Zohar

Chapter 6   It is Always on your Mind: Experiences and Perceptions of Falling of Older
People and their Carers and the Potential of a Mobile Falls Detection Device 39
Veronika Williams, Christina R. Victor and Rachel McCrindle

Chapter 7   The Simplified Acute Physiology Score III is Superior to the Simplified
Acute Physiology Score II and Acute Physiology and Chronic Health
Evaluation II in Predicting Surgical and ICU Mortality in the "Oldest Old" 46
Aftab Haq, Sachin Patil, Alexis Lanteri Parcells and Ronald S. Chamberlain

Chapter 8   Provider Perspectives on the Influence of Family on Nursing Home
Resident Transfers to the Emergency Department: Crises at the End of Life 54
Caroline Stephens, Elizabeth Halifax, Nhat Bui, Sei J. Lee,
Charlene Harrington, Janet Shim and Christine Ritchie

Chapter 9   Relationship-based Care and Behaviours of Residents in Long-Term Care
Facilities 63
Johanne Desrosiers, Anabelle Viau-Guay, Marie Bellemare, Louis Trudel,
Isabelle Feillou and Anne-Céline Guyon

Chapter 10   **Factors Associated with Insomnia among Elderly Patients Attending a
Geriatric Centre in Nigeria** **71**
Adetola M. Ogunbode, Lawrence A. Adebusoye, Olufemi O. Olowookere,
Mayowa Owolabi and Adesola Ogunniyi

Chapter 11   **Factors Influencing Quality of Life for Disabled and Nondisabled Elderly
Population: The Results of a Multiple Correspondence Analysis**.......................... **81**
M. Avolio, S. Montagnoli, M. Marino, D. Basso, G. Furia, W. Ricciardi and
A. G. de Belvis

Chapter 12   **Predicting Delirium Duration in Elderly Hip-Surgery Patients: Does Early
Symptom Profile Matter?** **87**
Chantal J. Slor, Joost Witlox, Dimitrios Adamis, David J. Meagher,
Tjeerd van der Ploeg, Rene W. M. M. Jansen, Mireille F. M. van Stijn,
Alexander P. J. Houdijk, Willem A. van Gool, Piet Eikelenboom and
Jos F. M. de Jonghe

Chapter 13   **Active Aging Promotion: Results from the *Vital Aging* Program** **96**
Mariagiovanna Caprara, María Ángeles Molina, Rocío Schettini,
Marta Santacreu, Teresa Orosa, Víctor Manuel Mendoza-Núñez,
Macarena Rojas and Rocío Fernández-Ballesteros

Chapter 14   **Subjective Memory Complaint and Depressive Symptoms among Older
Adults in Portugal** **110**
Mónica Sousa, Anabela Pereira and Rui Costa

Chapter 15   **Geriatric Hip Fractures and Inpatient Services: Predicting Hospital Charges
Using the ASA Score**.. **116**
Rachel V. Thakore, Young M. Lee, Vasanth Sathiyakumar,
William T. Obremskey and Manish K. Sethi

Chapter 16   **Prevalence and Determinants of Falls among Older Adults in Ecuador:
An Analysis of the SABE I Survey** **124**
Carlos H. Orces

Chapter 17   **Menopausal Symptoms and its Correlates: A Study on Tribe and Caste
Population of East India**... **131**
Doyel Dasgupta, Priyanka Karar, Subha Ray and Nandini Ganguly

Chapter 18   **Anthropometric Measures and Frailty Prediction in the Elderly:
An Easy-to-use Tool** **138**
Vera Elizabeth Closs, Patricia Klarmann Ziegelmann,
João Henrique Ferreira Flores, Irenio Gomes and
Carla Helena Augustin Schwanke

Chapter 19   **Age-Friendliness and Life Satisfaction of Young-Old and Old-Old in
Hong Kong**.. **146**
Alma M. L. Au, Stephen C. Y. Chan, H. M. Yip, Jackie Y. C. Kwok, K. Y. Lai,
K. M. Leung, Anita L. F. Lee, Daniel W. L. Lai, Teresa Tsien and Simon M. K. Lai

Chapter 20   **SABE Colombia: Survey on Health, Well-Being and Aging in Colombia — Study Design and Protocol** 155
Fernando Gomez, Jairo Corchuelo, Carmen-Lucia Curcio,
Maria-Teresa Calzada and Fabian Mendez

Chapter 21   **Physical Activity Scale for the Elderly: Translation, Cultural Adaptation and Validation of the Italian Version** 162
Antonio Covotta, Marco Gagliardi, Anna Berardi, Giuseppe Maggi,
Francesco Pierelli, Roberta Mollica, Julita Sansoni and Giovanni Galeoto

Chapter 22   **Assessment of Osteoporosis in Injured Older Women Admitted to a Safety-Net Level One Trauma Center: A Unique Opportunity to Fulfill an Unmet Need** 169
Elisabeth S. Young, May J. Reed, Tam N. Pham, Joel A. Gross,
Lisa A. Taitsman and Stephen J. Kaplan

Chapter 23   **Investigation of Geriatric Patients with Abdominal Pain Admitted to Emergency Department** 175
Pınar Henden Çam , Ahmet Baydin , Savaş Yürüker, Ali Kemal Erenler and
Erdinç Fengüldür

Chapter 24   **Pancreatic Surgery in the Older Population: A Single Institution's Experience over Two Decades** 183
Bhaumik Brahmbhatt, Abhishek Bhurwal, Frank J. Lukens,
Mauricia A. Buchanan, John A. Stauffer and Horacio J. Asbun

Chapter 25   **Associations of Pet Ownership with Older Adults Eating Patterns and Health** 188
Roschelle Heuberger

Chapter 26   **A Study on Mortality Profile among Fifty Plus- (50+-) Population (FPP) of India: A 5-Year Retrospective Study at New Delhi District** 197
B. L. Chaudhary, Raghvendra K. Vidua, Arvind Kumar and Amrita V. Bajaj

Chapter 27   **Identification of Neuroprotective Factors Associated with Successful Ageing and Risk of Cognitive Impairment among Malaysia Older Adults** 202
Huijin Lau, Arimi Fitri Mat Ludin, Nor Fadilah Rajab and Suzana Shahar

Chapter 28   **Associations between Tactile Sensory Threshold and Postural Performance and Effects of Healthy Aging and Subthreshold Vibrotactile Stimulation on Postural Outcomes in a Simple Dual Task** 209
Marius Dettmer, Amir Pourmoghaddam, Beom-Chan Lee and Charles S. Layne

Chapter 29   **Does Frailty Predict Health Care Utilization in Community-Living Older Romanians?** 220
Marinela Olaroiu, Minerva Ghinescu, Viorica Naumov, Ileana Brinza and
Wim van den Heuvel

Chapter 30   **In their Voices: Client and Staff Perceptions of the Physical and Social Environments of Adult Day Services Centers in Taiwan** 226
Chih-ling Liou and Shannon Jarrott

Chapter 31   **Reaching 100 in the Countryside: Health Profile and Living Circumstances of Portuguese Centenarians from the Beira Interior Region** 235
Rosa Marina Afonso, Oscar Ribeiro, Maria Vaz Patto, Marli Loureiro, Manuel Joaquim Loureiro, Miguel Castelo-Branco, Susana Patrício, Sara Alvarinhas, Tatiana Tomáz, Clara Rocha, Ana Margarida Jerónimo, Fátima Gouveia and Ana Paula Amaral

Chapter 32   **Clinical Screening Tools for Sarcopenia and its Management** 246
Solomon C. Y. Yu, Kareeann S. F. Khow, Agathe D. Jadczak and Renuka Visvanathan

Chapter 33   **Elderly Stroke Rehabilitation: Overcoming the Complications and its Associated Challenges** 256
Siew Kwaon Lui and Minh Ha Nguyen

Chapter 34   **Magnitude of Anemia in Geriatric Population Visiting Outpatient Department at the University of Gondar Referral Hospital, Northwest Ethiopia: Implication for Community-based Screening** 265
Mulugeta Melku, Wondimu Asefa, Ahmed Mohamednur, Tesfahun Getachew, Bayechish Bazezew, Meseret Workineh , Bamlaku Enawgaw, Belete Biadgo, Zegeye Getaneh, Debasu Damtie and Betelihem Terefe

Permissions

List of Contributors

Index

Preface

Geriatric medicine refers to the medical practices and interventions aimed at ensuring quality of life for elderly people along with the prevention and treatment of diseases and conditions that people are prone to as they age. One of the most significant issues in geriatrics is the prevention and treatment of delirium. Promoting interventions that are designed to maintain the physical and cognitive functioning of aged adults, maximizing patients' independence, etc. are some of the ways to manage delirium. Aging may cause changes in the effectiveness of drugs and their side effects. Pharmacological constitution and regimen is another important consideration in geriatric medicine. The elderly are particularly prone to polypharmacy. This happens when a patient suffers from multiple disorders and takes over-the-counter drugs and herbal medications. An important area of study is the efficacy of inappropriate medications and dangerous drug interactions. This book explores all the important aspects of geriatric medicine in the present day scenario. Different approaches, evaluations, methodologies and advanced studies on geriatric medicine have been included herein. The extensive content of this book provides the readers with a thorough understanding of the recent advances in geriatric medicine.

After months of intensive research and writing, this book is the end result of all who devoted their time and efforts in the initiation and progress of this book. It will surely be a source of reference in enhancing the required knowledge of the new developments in the area. During the course of developing this book, certain measures such as accuracy, authenticity and research focused analytical studies were given preference in order to produce a comprehensive book in the area of study.

This book would not have been possible without the efforts of the authors and the publisher. I extend my sincere thanks to them. Secondly, I express my gratitude to my family and well-wishers. And most importantly, I thank my students for constantly expressing their willingness and curiosity in enhancing their knowledge in the field, which encourages me to take up further research projects for the advancement of the area.

Editor

Role of Sociocultural Factors in Depression among Elderly of Twin Cities (Rawalpindi and Islamabad) of Pakistan

Saira Javed

Department of Behavioral Sciences, Fatima Jinnah Women University, The Mall, Rawalpindi 46000, Pakistan

Correspondence should be addressed to Saira Javed; saira.javedbhati@gmail.com

Academic Editor: Moisés Evandro Bauer

This research was conducted to examine the role of sociocultural factors on depression among elderly of twin cities (Rawalpindi and Islamabad) of Pakistan. 310 older adults participated in the present study. Through convenient sampling technique, face to face interview was carried out for data collection. Urdu translated Geriatric Depression Scale Short Form and demographic sheet were used to test hypotheses. Descriptive statistics and t-test were used for data analysis. Results showed significant mean differences among gender, marital status, family system, and status of employment on depression. Financial crisis, feeling of dejection because of isolation, and trend of nuclear family system have been observed as strong predictors of depression in older adults.

1. Introduction/Literature Review

Depression enduring geriatrics was associated with increased medical morbidity, impaired body working, disturbed social functioning, and dementia [1, 2]. Depression is illustrated by insufficient sleeping hours, low or absence of diet, mood swings, glumness or isolation, and suicide ideation [3]. Pathology of depression in older adults has been widely discussed and assessed by researchers in present era. Researchers narrated that comparative to the other age groups elderly experienced elevated prevalence of depression in older people [4] In 2006 more than 400 million sufferers of depression were recorded in the world. Frequency in cases of depression horribly amplified and stood on fourth position according to global burden of diseases. Depression was announced an alarming mental health disorder. In developing countries, it is expected to be on second rank by the year 2020 [5].

Studies conducted by Pakistani researchers revealed that depressive elderly are severely ignored by common population because of lack of awareness. Either they went under or over recognition of depression specifically in developing countries like Pakistan [6, 7]. Though, in 2008 almost 30% incidence of depression has been found in local study conducted on elderly [8].

Biological studies quoted number of times about the physical superiority of women but they lack in reporting the emotional instability of women that leads to mental health issues in later life. A series of studies conducted in 2005 and 2006 demonstrated that female older adults are more vulnerable to later life depression as compared to male older adults [3, 9]. In 2003 a published research study reported the incidence of depression in women is thrice higher than men [10].

In later life females experienced internal marital conflicts that are responsible of marital distress [11]. Result of longitudinal study explains risk of having depressive episodes in later life is directly associated to marital conflicts caused by aging factors [12, 13]. Recently an extensive literature review done in 2011 documented that single elderly, either widowed, divorced, or unmarried are on greater risk of having depression as compared to married and with their siblings and spouse [14].

Family system acts significantly in Asian society. It has been seen that elderly belongs to rural families are less

TABLE 1: Frequency of various demographic variables.

Various demographic variables	f	%
Gender		
Male	158	51
Female	152	152
Marital status		
Married	201	65
Unmarried	109	35.16
Family system		
Nuclear family	190	61.2
Extensive family	120	38.71
Status of employment		
Employed	125	40.32
Unemployed	185	59.68
Source of income		
Self	123	40.32
Siblings/family	146	47.1
Pension	39	12.6
Living in own house?		
Yes	121	39
No	180	58.1
Having peer group		
Yes	220	70.1
No	90	20.03
Any physical aliment?		
Hypertension	52	16.77
Diabetes	67	21.61
Other body complaints	156	50.32
Not as such	37	11.93
Clinically diagnosed with mental ailment?		
Yes	42	13.55
No	268	86.45

depressed than those of urban families [15]. Furthermore, Pakistani researchers examined that the incidence of having depression in older adults living in extensive family system is four times lesser than elderly living in nuclear family system [6].

Like other countries, the common age of retirement in Pakistan is 65 years. After retirement it has been seen that mostly people get relaxed and start doing the things that they missed for so many years. So, according to researchers phase of retirement is not at all depressive stage [11]. Instead they called it honeymoon period. On the other hand elderly who belong to private sector face the black side of later life because of financial issue caused by unemployment [16].

Sociocultural factors consistently have been recognized as chief factor in signifying the unpredictability in the prevalence of depression in elderly. With the advancement in modernization, cases of physical and mental health issues are increasing day by day and society become mechanical [17]. The lust of fame and money makes an individual deprived of sociocultural values. Because of this novel behavior, elderly are significantly affected by health issues including depression. Additionally, stress full life events, ignorance from family members, loss of loved ones, financial crises, phase of retirement, and inter- or intrapersonal conflicts accompanied with other health issues lead to late life depression [11, 18].

1.1. Objective. The main objective of the present study is to see the influence of sociocultural factors on occurrence of depression in older adults.

1.2. Hypotheses. The following hypotheses are presented in the paper.

(1) There exists significant difference in depression between men and women of older adults.
(2) There exists significant difference in depression between married and unmarried older adults.
(3) There exists significant difference in depression between older adults living in nuclear and extensive family system.
(4) There exists significant difference in depression between employed and unemployed older adults.

2. Research Methodology

Data were collected through convenient sampling technique from the twin cities of Pakistan that is, Rawalpindi and Islamabad. Design of the present study was descriptive and quantitative. For data collection face to face survey interview was conducted. 310 elderly were participated in the study by signing written inform consent by significant others on their behalves. Urdu translated 15-item Geriatric Depression Scale (GDS-SF) [6] and demographic profile were used to test hypotheses. 10 to 15 minutes were taken by each individual.

Data of the study was analyzed by using SPSS version 14.0. For elaboration of results tables were used for inclusive view of findings. $P < 0.05$ level of significance was set for each observation. t-test was applied to determine the differences on depression. Where 0.76 cronbach's alpha reliability was recorded of the study.

3. Results

3.1. Characteristics of the Participants. Table 1 of the study shows characteristics of elderly participants of twin cities of Pakistan. Category of unmarried elderly also includes 40 widows and 23 divorced. Likely the category of unemployed contains 42 retired older adults. Most of the geriatrics lie in

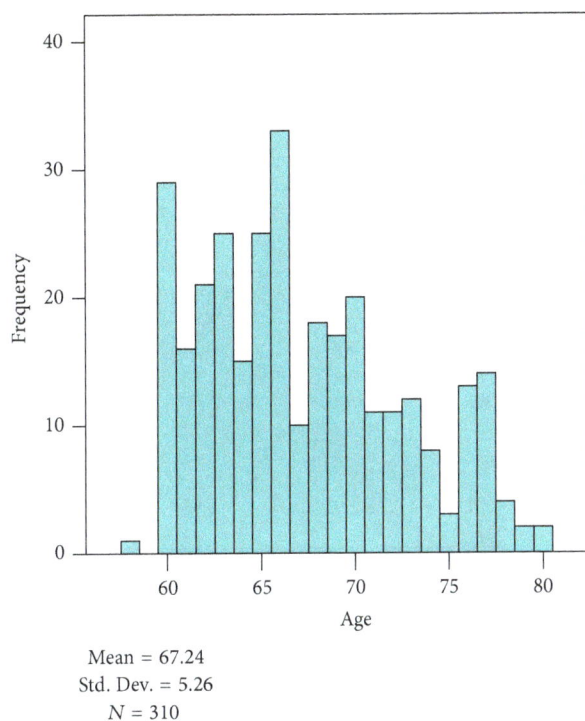

Mean = 67.24
Std. Dev. = 5.26
N = 310

FIGURE 1: Age distribution of older adults who participated in the study.

the category of body complaints experienced muscular pains, digestive problems, and gastric issues.

Figure 1 shows the age distribution of older adults participated in present study. 67.24 mean age is recorded of 310 elderly, where 189 were from Rawalpindi and 121 were from Islamabad.

3.2. Role of Sociocultural Factors in Depression among Elderly. Table 2 indicates the mean differences in various demographic variables among elderly on depression. Results indicate that there are significant mean differences ($P < 0.05$) between men and women, married and unmarried, nuclear family and extensive family system, and employed and unemployed on depression.

4. Discussion

Present survey was conducted to investigate about the role of sociocultural factors on depression among elderly of twin cities of Pakistan. Like previous literature, findings of the study revealed significant mean differences in gender, marital status, family system, and status of employment. So, all hypotheses of the study prove to be true (see Table 2).

Asian women in later life were not able to cope up with daily life issues and house chore as she did before because of the old age factor. On the other way, unlike older women of western world, mostly Pakistani women are not working nor found of social gatherings so they more rapidly get isolated that in short time converted in to depression. It has been observed that elder women get depressed sooner as compared to men. Feeling of dejection and fear of death is very much prominent in older adult women as compare to men [19].

Marital conflicts are also very prominent in later life. Though, it is really hard for single (widow, unmarried, and divorced) women to survive solely in this world. Everyone needs somebody to share last stage of life. To discuss daily life issues to spend time with someone as a partner. It has been observed that married elderly spend healthy life as compared to unmarried. Absence of partner at the last stage of life pushed an individual in to depression. Single/unmarried older adults are more vulnerable to depression as compared to married older adults [10, 20].

Similar to rest of South Asian countries, extensive family system has been practiced in Pakistan by many families [6]. It is assumed that extensive family system is a healthy family system. Number of people was available in joint family system, to play care taker role for their older adults. Love and respect are the main source of happiness for elderly in joint family system. They had been surrounded by their second or third generation and elderly smoothly passed their last stage of life [7]. But in present period several families in Pakistan start adopting nuclear family system because of inflation and growing trend of modernization. They badly indulge in race of mechanical world and forget about the well-being of their assists in the shape of elders of the family. A study conducted Karachi by in Pakistani researchers elaborated that nuclear family system significantly strong predictor of depression for older adults [6, 21].

Findings of the present study and Systematic literature review demonstrated that geriatrics who are financial strong, have source of earning, living in their own house, have no tension of billing, feed by significant others and on pension are less susceptible to depression as compare to elders who are un employed, have no source of income and not supported by the family. Study documented that awfully Pakistan ranked on 9th position in the race of low income holder countries with increasing number of population [22, 23].

5. Conclusion and Recommendation

It is concluded that elderly women undergo late life depression more than men. Widowhood, family conflicts, unsatisfactory family attitude, financial instability, communication gap, death of significant, unfulfilled early life desires, feeling of guilt, and later life general medical condition collectively act as strong predictorsof depression among older adults.

It is highly recommended to future researchers to design qualitative study along with quantitative study for in depth finds. Some questions of the interview would design open ended for comprehensive analysis.

In the beam of the findings of present study, it is immense need in Pakistan to design community support programs, welfare centers, policies for older adults' rights, grants or pensions from government sectors, and medical expense arrangements for older adults.

TABLE 2: Mean differences in various demographic variables among elderly ($N = 310$).

Variables	M	SD	t	P	95% CI		Cohen's d
					LL	UL	
Gender							
Male ($n = 158$)	9.21	2.5	−2.69	0.008	−1.57	−2.44	0.3
Female ($n = 152$)	101.1	3.41					
Marital status							
Married ($n = 201$)	9.25	2.75	−3.24	0.001	−1.83	−0.45	0.4
Unmarried ($n = 109$)	10.4	3.31					
Family system							
Nuclear family ($n = 190$)	10.7	2.3	6.3	0.001	1.14	2.17	0.8
Extensive family ($n = 120$)	9.01	2.20p					
Status of employment							
Employed ($n = 125$)	8.6	1.8	−10.1	0.001	−2.90	−1.95	1.2
Unemployed ($n = 185$)	11	2.3					

$^{*}P < 0.05$, df = 308.

The author declares that there is no conflict of interests regarding the publication of this paper.

Acknowledgments

First of all, the author would like to thank families of older adults for their cooperation and all elderly especially who gave themselves for her study. The author would like to thank her parents for their moral support and friends for helping her in data collection and data entry.

References

[1] D. Satcher, "Mental health: a report of the surgeon general," *Executive Summary*, vol. 31, pp. 15–23, 2000.

[2] D. C. Steffens, E. Otey, G. S. Alexopoulos et al., "Perspectives on depression, mild cognitive impairment, and cognitive decline," *Archives of General Psychiatry*, vol. 63, no. 2, pp. 130–138, 2006.

[3] M. Sherina, L. S. Rampal, M. Aini, and M. H. Norhidayati, "The prevalence of depression among elderly in an urban area of Selangor, Malaysia," *The International Medical Journal*, vol. 4, pp. 57–63, 2005.

[4] C. Ernst, "Epidemiology of depression in late life," *Current Opinion in Psychiatry*, vol. 10, no. 2, pp. 107–112, 1997.

[5] R. Desjarlais, *World Health Report*, World Health Organization, Geneva, Switzerland, 2001.

[6] A. Itrat, A. M. Taqui, F. Qazi, and W. Qidwai, "Family systems: perceptions of elderly patients and their attendents presenting at a university hospital in Karachi, Pakistan," *Journal of the Pakistan Medical Association*, vol. 57, no. 2, pp. 106–110, 2007.

[7] S. N. Zafar, H. A. Ganatra, S. Tehseen, and W. Qidwai, "Health and needs assessment of geriatric patients: results of a survey at a Teaching Hospital in Karachi," *Journal of the Pakistan Medical Association*, vol. 56, no. 10, pp. 470–474, 2006.

[8] H. A. Ganatra, S. N. Zafar, W. Qidwai, and S. Rozi, "Prevalence and predictors of depression among an elderly population of Pakistan," *Aging & Mental Health*, vol. 12, no. 3, pp. 349–356, 2008.

[9] J. K. Djernes, "Prevalence and predictors of depression in populations of elderly: a review," *Acta Psychiatrica Scandinavica*, vol. 113, no. 5, pp. 372–387, 2006.

[10] M. S. Sidi, M. N. A. Zulkefli, and S. A. Shah, "Factors associated with depression among elderly patients in primary health care clinic in Malaysia," *Asia Pacific Family Medicine*, vol. 2, pp. 148–152, 2003.

[11] A. Fiske, J. L. Wetherell, and M. Gatz, "Depression in older adults," *Annual Review of Clinical Psychology*, vol. 5, pp. 362–389, 2009.

[12] N. T. McCall, P. Parks, K. Smith, G. Pope, and M. Griggs, "The prevalence of major depression or dysthymia among aged Medicare Fee-for-Service beneficiaries," *International Journal of Geriatric Psychiatry*, vol. 17, no. 6, pp. 557–565, 2002.

[13] B. Steunenberg, A. T. F. Beekman, D. J. H. Deeg, and A. J. F. M. Kerkhof, "Personality and the onset of depression in late life," *Journal of Affective Disorders*, vol. 92, no. 2-3, pp. 243–251, 2006.

[14] X.-Y. Yan, S.-M. Huang, C.-Q. Huang, W.-H. Wu, and Y. Qin, "Marital status and risk for late life depression: a meta-analysis of the published literature," *The Journal of International Medical Research*, vol. 39, no. 4, pp. 1142–1154, 2011.

[15] M. Gupta, S. S. Lehl, N. S. Boparoy, R. Katyal, and A. Sachdev, "A study of prevalence of depression in elderly with medical disorders," *Journal of the Indian Academy of Geriatrics*, vol. 6, pp. 18–22, 2010.

[16] A. Rashid, A. Manan, and S. Rohana, "Depression among the elderly Malays living in rural Malaysia," *The Internet Journal of Public Health*, vol. 1, no. 2, 2011.

[17] W. Qidwai and T. Ashfaq, "Elderly patients and their health in Pakistan: current status, issues, challenges and opportunities," *Journal of the Liaquat University of Medical and Health Sciences*, vol. 10, no. 3, pp. 100–101, 2011.

[18] S. Zisook and K. S. Kendler, "Is bereavement-related depression different than non-bereavement-related depression?" *Psychological Medicine*, vol. 37, no. 6, pp. 779–794, 2007.

[19] M. S. Sherina, L. Rampal, and A. Mustaqim, "The prevalence of depression among the elderly in Sepang, Selangor," *The Medical Journal of Malaysia*, vol. 59, no. 1, pp. 45–49, 2004.

[20] H. T. Aizan, A. S. Asnarulkhadi, and M. Mazlawati, *A Study on the Perception of Problems and Needs among Elderly in Johor, Malaysia*, University Putra Malaysia, Kuala Lumpur, Malaysia, 2000.

[21] J. T. Cacioppo, M. E. Hughes, L. J. Waite, L. C. Hawkley, and R. A. Thisted, "Loneliness as a specific risk factor for depressive symptoms: cross-sectional and longitudinal analyses," *Psychology and Aging*, vol. 21, no. 1, pp. 140–151, 2006.

[22] N. Akhtar-Danesh and J. Landeen, "Relation between depression and sociodemographic factors," *International Journal of Mental Health Systems*, vol. 1, article 4, 2007.

[23] WHO, *Mental Health Atlas*, World Health Organization, Geneva, Switzerland, 2005.

Unexplained Falls Are Frequent in Patients with Fall-Related Injury Admitted to Orthopaedic Wards: The UFO Study (Unexplained Falls in Older Patients)

Mussi Chiara,[1] Galizia Gianluigi,[2] Abete Pasquale,[2]
Morrione Alessandro,[3] Maraviglia Alice,[3] Noro Gabriele,[4] Cavagnaro Paolo,[5]
Ghirelli Loredana,[6] Tava Giovanni,[4] Rengo Franco,[2] Masotti Giulio,[3] Salvioli Gianfranco,[1]
Marchionni Niccolò,[3] and Ungar Andrea[3]

[1] Geriatric and Gerontology Institute, University of Modena and Reggio Emilia, Modena 41121, Italy
[2] Geriatric Department, Azienda Policlinico Federico II, Naples 80131, Italy
[3] Unit of Gerontology and Geriatric Medicine, Department of Critical Care Medicine and Surgery,
  University of Florence and Azienda Ospedaliero Universitaria Careggi, Florence 50134, Italy
[4] Geriatric Unit, Santa Chiara Hospital, Trento 38122, Italy
[5] Department of Geriatrics, Azienda Sanitaria Locale 4, Chiavari 16043, Italy
[6] Division of Geriatrics, Ospedale S Maria Nuova, Reggio Emilia 42123, Italy

Correspondence should be addressed to Mussi Chiara; cmussi@iol.it

Academic Editor: Arnold B. Mitnitski

To evaluate the incidence of unexplained falls in elderly patients affected by fall-related fractures admitted to orthopaedic wards, we recruited 246 consecutive patients older than 65 (mean age 82 ± 7 years, range 65–101). Falls were defined "accidental" (fall explained by a definite accidental cause), "medical" (fall caused directly by a specific medical disease), "dementia-related" (fall in patients affected by moderate-severe dementia), and "unexplained" (nonaccidental falls, not related to a clear medical or drug-induced cause or with no apparent cause). According to the anamnestic features of the event, older patients had a lower tendency to remember the fall. Patients with accidental fall remember more often the event. Unexplained falls were frequent in both groups of age. Accidental falls were more frequent in younger patients, while dementia-related falls were more common in the older ones. Patients with unexplained falls showed a higher number of depressive symptoms. In a multivariate analysis a higher GDS and syncopal spells were independent predictors of unexplained falls. In conclusion, more than one third of all falls in patients hospitalized in orthopaedic wards were unexplained, particularly in patients with depressive symptoms and syncopal spells. The identification of fall causes must be evaluated in older patients with a fall-related injury.

1. Introduction

Falls in older people are a major public health concern in terms of morbidity, mortality, and health and social services costs [1].

Falls are the leading cause of injury-related visits to emergency department in the United States. Trauma is the fifth leading cause of death in people starting from 65 years,

and falls are responsible for 70% of accidental death in people starting from 75 years.

More than a third of older adults falls each year [2]. About one-third of community-dwelling elderly people and up to 60% of nursing home residents fall each year; one half of these "fallers" have multiple episodes [3]. Nearly all hip fractures occur as a fall result [4]. Fall-related injuries among older adults, especially among older women, are associated with

TABLE 1: Clinical characteristics.

	All ($n = 246$)	65–79 years ($n = 79$)	≥80 years ($n = 167$)	P
Age	82.0 ± 7.0	74.2 ± 4.3	85.7 ± 4.7	0.0001
Sex (males, %)	17.9	21.5	16.2	0.306
Number of drugs	4.2 ± 2.1	4.0 ± 2.2	4.2 ± 2.1	0.569
Use of more than 4 drugs (%)	43.5	43.0	43.7	0.612
CIRS	5.4 ± 4.3	5.1 ± 4.2	5.6 ± 4.4	0.432
Lost BADL	1.6 ± 2.1	0.5 ± 1.3	2.0 ± 2.2	0.0003
Lost IADL	2.5 ± 3.2	1.5 ± 2.5	3.1 ± 3.3	0.001
MMSE	24.6 ± 7.5	27.0 ± 4.4	23.1 ± 8.6	0.003
GDS	4.6 ± 3.3	5.3 ± 3.9	4.0 ± 2.7	0.03
BMI (Kg/m^2)	24.0 ± 4.1	26.0 ± 5.0	23.3 ± 3.6	0.01
Blood glucose (mg/dL)	112.9 ± 31.1	109.0 ± 27.0	114.5 ± 32.6	0.280
Hemoglobin (g/dL)	11.5 ± 1.7	12.1 ± 1.4	11.2 ± 1.7	0.0004
Creatinine (mg/dL)	1.1 ± 0.9	1.2 ± 1.4	1.0 ± 0.4	0.179

Data are expressed as mean ± standard deviation; CIRS: Cumulative Illness Rating Scale; BADL: basal activities of daily living; IADL: instrumental activities of daily living; MMSE: Mini-Mental State Examination; GDS: Geriatric Depression Scale; BMI: body mass index.

substantial economic costs, mostly because of hip fractures and their subsequent disability [5].

Data regarding fall types in patients admitted to orthopaedic wards because of fall-related injury are lacking: the UFO study (Unexplained Falls in Older Patients) was made to assess the incidence and the clinical characteristics of unexplained falls in this specific group of elderly subjects affected by fall-related fractures.

2. Methods

2.1. Definition of Fall. We defined four different types of falls: "accidental" (fall explained by a definite accidental cause), "medical" (fall caused directly by a specific medical disease, e.g., hypoglycemia, drugs, drop and attack, transient ischemic attack, myocardial infarction, arrhythmic drugs, orthostatic hypotension), "dementia-related" (fall in a patient with previous diagnosis of moderate-severe dementia), and "unexplained" (nonaccidental falls, not related to a clear medical or drug-induced cause, where no apparent cause has been found) [6].

2.2. Protocol. All enrolled patients were starting from 65 years and consecutively admitted to orthopaedic wards because of fall-related injury, without any exclusion criteria.

All patients (or relatives if the patient had diagnosis of dementia) gave informed written consent.

Centers involved in the study (the appendix) designated and instructed a trained investigator who used to manage falls and syncope to run the study.

All subjects were asked to complete their clinical history, with a specific questionnaire about fall characteristics, pharmacologic anamnesis considering all drugs taken in the last month, clinical and neurological examination, routine blood chemistry tests, and 12-lead ECG.

Moreover, we performed a multidimensional geriatric evaluation including Mini Mental State Examination- (MMSE) [7] to assess cognitive performance, Geriatric Depression Scale (GDS) [8], to screen the presence of affective disorders, basal (BADL) [9] and instrumental (IADL) activities of daily living [10], to evaluate disability, and

Cumulative Illness Rating Scale to define comorbidity (CIRS) [11].

2.3. Statistical Analysis. Data analysis was performed using SPSS, 14th version (SPSS, Chicago, IL, USA). The χ^2 test was used to compare proportions in univariate analysis of dichotomic variables and to calculate odds ratio and the 95% confidence intervals. Student's t-test for independent samples was used to compare continuous variables. Variables significantly associated with the outcome of interest in univariate analyses were entered into a multivariate logistic regression model (backward stepwise) to assess their independent association with the outcome. A P value <0.05 was considered statistically significant.

3. Results

246 patients (mean age 82.3 ± 7.2 years, 82% females) were submitted to the basal evaluation. We divided patients into two groups, according to age: 65–79 years ($N = 76$), ≥80 ($N = 159$). Most patients ($N = 161$) were admitted because of a fall-related hip fracture.

Clinical characteristics of the studied sample are shown in Table 1.

Patients older than 80 years were more likely to be self-dependent and obtained lower MMSE scores; they were more likely to show depressive symptoms, and they had lower values of BMI. No differences were found in the two groups in terms of biochemical values, except for hemoglobin that was significantly lower in older subjects. 17 patients (8.1%) had syncope as a cause of fall. According to the anamnestic features of the event, older patients had a lower tendency to remember the fall (Table 2).

Data regarding drugs taken in the last 30 days are shown in Table 3: 184 of 246 enrolled patients were taking at least one drug (74.7%). Older patients were more likely to take diuretics, and no other difference was found between the two groups.

4. Fall Types

The different fall types are described in Table 4.

Table 2: Clinical history.

	All ($n = 246$)	65–79 years ($n = 79$)	≥80 years ($n = 167$)	P
Remember the event	78.9	92.2	72.3	0.002
Witness presence	39.4	45.3	36.6	0.244
Syncope	8.1	7.4	8.3	0.967
Fractures	92.6	90.0	93.9	0.300
Prodromes	17.9	17.7	18.0	0.568

Table 3: Drugs taken in the previous month.

	All ($N = 184$)	65–79 years ($N = 60$)	≥80 years ($N = 124$)	P
Antihypertensives (%)	60.1	56.7	62.9	0.416
Antiplatelet agents (%)	35.3	26.7	39.5	0.087
Anticoagulants (%)	9.2	15.0	6.4	0.060
Central nervous system drugs (%)	47.5	40.9	50.8	0.208
Ace inhibitors/AT2 antagonists (%)	38.0	38.3	37.9	0.955
Calcium-channel blockers (%)	16.8	18.3	16.1	0.708
Diuretics	34.2	21.6	40.3	0.02
Beta-blockers	13.1	11.7	13.8	0.685
Alpha-blockers	5.4	6.7	4.8	0.608
Other, n (%)	79.3	80.0	79.0	0.897

Table 4: Different fall types (suggestive diagnosis).

	All ($n = 246$)	65–79 years ($n = 79$)	≥80 years ($n = 167$)	P
Accidental (%)	99 (40.2)	38 (48.1)	61 (36.5)	0.02
Medical (%)	25 (10.2)	7 (8.9)	18 (10.8)	0.323
Dementia-related (%)	31 (12.6)	5 (6.3)	26 (15.6)	0.02
Unexplained (%)	91 (37.0)	29 (36.7)	62 (37.1)	0.475

Data are expressed as number (percentage).

Table 5: Clinical patient features with different fall types.

	Accidental ($N = 99$)	Medical ($N = 25$)	Dementia-related ($N = 31$)	Unexplained ($N = 91$)
Age (years)	80.6 ± 0.7	82.2 ± 1.4	85.9 ± 1.2	82.4 ± 0.7
Sex (males, %)	14.1	24.0	9.7	23.1
Number of falls	1.7 ± 0.3	3.5 ± 0.5	1.6 ± 0.4	1.9 ± 0.3
Number of drugs	3.8 ± 0.2	4.1 ± 0.5	4.6 ± 0.4	4.3 ± 0.2
More than 4 drugs (%)	38.3%	44.0%	51.0%	46.1%
CIRS	4.2 ± 0.5	7.3 ± 1.0	6.9 ± 0.9	5.5 ± 0.6
Lost BADL	0.8 ± 0.2	2.1 ± 0.4	3.7 ± 0.4	1.4 ± 0.2
Lost IADL	1.4 ± 0.4	3.9 ± 0.7	5.7 ± 1.0	2.8 ± 0.4
MMSE	26.1 ± 0.9	20.6 ± 1.8	14.0 ± 3.6	25.0 ± 0.1
GDS	3.8 ± 0.4	4.5 ± 0.9	5.0 ± 2.3	5.3 ± 0.4
BMI (Kg/m^2)	24.2 ± 0.6	26.0 ± 1.3	20.4 ± 1.8	24.0 ± 0.8
Blood glucose (mg/dL)	109.4 ± 3.7	121.3 ± 6.6	108.8 ± 6.5	115.0 ± 3.7
Hemoglobin (g/dL)	11.7 ± 0.2	11.8 ± 0.4	11.1 ± 0.3	11.3 ± 0.2
Creatinine (mg/dL)	0.9 ± 0.1	1.4 ± 0.2	0.9 ± 0.2	1.2 ± 0.1

Data are expressed as mean ± standard error or %; CIRS: Cumulative Illness Rating Scale; BADL: basal activities of daily living; IADL: instrumental activities of daily living; MMSE: Mini-Mental State Examination; GDS: Geriatric Depression Scale; BMI: body mass index.

Younger patients had a higher number of falls documented as accidental (48.1% versus 36.5%, $P = 0.02$), while older patients were more frequently affected by dementia, as expected. No other differences were found for the other fall types (Table 4).

Clinical characteristics of patients with different fall types are shown in Table 5. Patients with dementia-related falls were significantly older than patients with accidental falls (85.9 ± 1.2 versus 80.6 ± 0.7, $P < 0.005$); they were more likely to have a higher degree of comorbidity (CIRS score: 6.9 ± 0.9 versus 4.2 ± 0.5, $P = 0.014$) and of disability (lost BADL: 3.7 ± 0.4 versus 0.8±0.2, $P < 0.001$; lost IADL: 5.7±1.0 versus 1.4 ± 0.4, $P < 0.001$), and, as expected, they obtained lower MMSE scores ($P = 0.001$). Patients with unexplained falls were less self-dependent with respect to patients with medical fall causes (lost BADL: 1.4 ± 0.2 versus 2.1 ± 0.4, $P = 0.016$, lost IADL: 2.8±0.4 versus 3.9±0.7, $P = 0.010$) and to patients with dementia-related falls (lost BADL: 1.4 ± 0.2 versus 3.7±0.4, $P < 0.001$; lost IADL: 2.8±0.4 versus 5.7±1.0, $P = 0.008$).

Patients with falls related to medical causes reached higher levels of comorbidity than patients with accidental

Unexplained Falls Are Frequent in Patients with Fall-Related Injury Admitted to Orthopaedic Wards: The UFO Study...

9

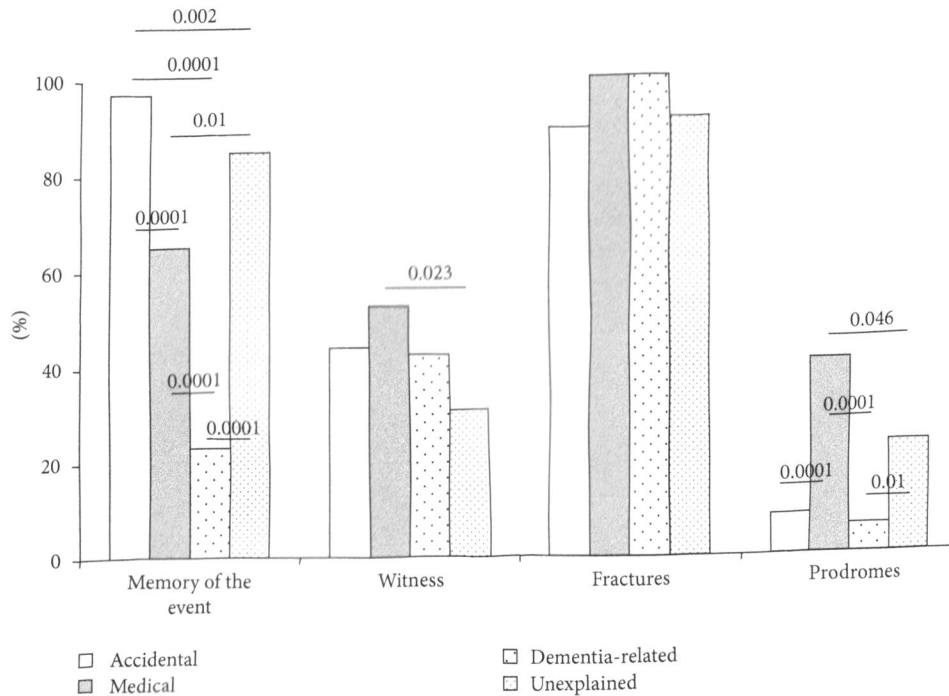

FIGURE 1: History in different syncope types.

falls (CIRS score: 7.3 ± 1.0 versus 4.2 ± 0.5, $P = 0.0007$), and they lost a higher number of BADL (2.1 ± 0.4 versus 0.8 ± 0.2, $P = 0.007$) and IADL (3.9 ± 0.7 versus 1.4 ± 0.4, $P = 0.001$). These latter ones referred to a significantly higher number of anamnestic falls in the last year with respect to patients with accidental ($P = 0.005$), dementia-related ($P = 0.006$), and unexplained ($P = 0.009$) falls. Moreover, they showed worse cognitive performances at MMSE with respect to patients with accidental ($P = 0.006$) and unexplained ($P = 0.030$) falls.

Patients with unexplained falls lost a higher number of IADL with respect to patients with accidental falls (lost IADL: 2.8 ± 0.4 versus 1.4 ± 0.4, $P = 0.006$), and they showed a higher number of depressive symptoms, expressed as GDS score ($P = 0.020$).

No differences were found between the four groups as far as the use of different classes of drugs is concerned.

History in different syncope types is illustrated in Figure 1. Patients with accidental falls remember more often the event, as expected. Witness presence is less than 50% in all the fall types.

5. Multivariate Analysis

We drew four multivariate models (logistic regression, method backward stepwise) separately, considering the four fall types as independent variables. We considered in the models the variables that were significantly different between four groups at the univariate analysis. No predictive factor for medical and dementia-related falls. Younger and no syncopal spells were independent [...]rs (Table 6(A)), while a higher

TABLE 6: Multivariate analysis: types of fall predictors.

	OR	95.0% CI	P
(A) Independent factor: accidental fall			
Age	0.66	0.45–0.98	0.05
GDS	0.63	0.45–0.89	0.01
Syncopal spells (anamnestic)	0.59	0.43–0.83	0.005
(B) Independent factor: unexplained fall			
GDS	1.49	1.06–2.09	0.029
Syncopal spells (anamnestic)	1.49	1.04–2.12	0.036

GDS: Geriatric Depression Scale.

GDS and syncopal spells were independent predictors of unexplained falls (Table 6(B)). Other variables in the multivariate analysis considered in the model, but not significant, were comorbidity (expressed by means of the Cumulative Illness Rating Score) and the number of lost activities and instrumental activities of daily living.

6. Discussion

According to our knowledge, there is no study about causes of falls leading an old patient to an orthopaedic ward in Italy. Our study demonstrates that these patients are very old and frail because of severe comorbidity and polytherapy. The percentage of patients affected by dementia is quite high (12.6%). The majority of our patients were admitted to hospital because of hip fracture. Hip fractures are very common, and their incidence was not reduced in the last ten years [12]. Moreover 14.8% of patients with hip fractures experienced a second hip fracture in a followup of 4.2 years [13]. For all of these reasons it may be very useful to study the fall etiology to reduce recurrence.

Our study found a high number of patients with unexplained falls (37%), when the study of Kenny et al. found a significantly lower number of unexplained falls (15%). This difference is explained by the fact that they also considered younger patients (older than 50) admitted to an emergency department, and not to an orthopaedic ward [14]. Unexplained falls can lead to more serious consequences, like hip fractures. Scuffham et al. demonstrated that unspecified falls, although not so frequent as the accidental ones, lead to a significant higher number of hospital accesses and are responsible for 53% of total costs related to falls [15].

A number of different strategies and interventions for each case are effective, but population-based strategies have not yet been evaluated, particularly in frail old patients, admitted to orthopaedic wards. Multidisciplinary, multifactorial intervention programmes inclusive of risk-factor assessment, screening, cause identification by means of diagnostic flow charts, and appropriate intervention proved to be effective [16], and they are useful to identify the causes of fall in the elderly. This topic is mandatory in older patients in order to abolish risk factors and to build a correct prevention programme. Unfortunately we found that only previous syncope and higher GDS score were predictive factors of unexplained falls. For this reason, all patients with fall-related injury must be evaluated for the possible fall cause. A recent meta-analysis showed that in patients with injury-related falls a multifactorial assessment and a targeted intervention do not reduce fall recurrence, whereas the same programme seems to be effective in patients who fall without getting an injury [17].

In our "faller" cohort, as shown in Table 3, our patients took a great number of antihypertensive drugs (60.1%) which are well-known fall and syncope risk factors [18]. In a multivariate analysis a previous syncope is a predictor of unexplained falls, while it is a negative predictor of accidental falls. We can speculate that unexplained falls may be caused by syncope more often than normally considered in clinical practice.

Our study demonstrates the need to study deeply and correctly patients with falls at the very beginning of the story (e.g., when they are admitted to the orthopaedic ward because of the fall). Unfortunately, at the moment, this is very difficult to achieve because of cultural and organizational problems. Future studies may be conducted to evaluate the correct strategy for patients with unexplained falls, probably in a postacute setting such as a rehabilitation unit.

One limitation to this study is the observational design and the absence of an active "prevention and treatment time." In the literature it is well known that the presence of a team applying comprehensive geriatric assessment and rehabilitation, including prevention, detection, and treatment of fall risk factors, can successfully prevent inpatient falls and injuries, even in those with dementia [19]; this group of old patients is at the highest risk of developing postsurgical complications like delirium [20].

In conclusion, all these data demonstrate that patients admitted to orthopaedic wards after a fall-related injury are frail and affected by severe comorbidity and that unexplained falls are frequent in these patients. These results underline the absolutely relevant role of geriatric evaluation and intervention in older patients admitted to orthopaedic wards. Further studies are necessary to evaluate the impact of diagnostic protocol in patients with unexplained falls.

Appendix

Centers and Investigators Participating to the Study

(1) Florence, Syncope Unit, Department of Geriatric Cardiology, University of Florence and Azienda Ospedaliero Universitaria Careggi. Investigators: Andrea Ungar, Annalisa Landi, Alice Maraviglia, Niccolò Marchionni, Giulio Masotti, Alessandro Morrione, and Martina Rafanelli.

(2) Modena, Chair of Geriatrics, University of Modena and Reggio Emilia: Chiara Mussi, and Gianfranco Salvioli.

(3) Trento, Division of Geriatrics, Santa Chiara Hospital: Gabriele Noro, and Gianni Tava.

(4) Reggio Emilia, Division of Geriatrics, Santa Maria Nuova Hospital: Loredana Ghirelli.

(5) Naples, Department of Geriatrics, Federico II University: Pasquale Abete, Vincenzo Del Villano, Gianluigi Galizia, and Franco Rengo.

(6) Grosseto, Division of Geriatrics, Walter De Alfieri, Fabio Riello.

(7) Chiavari, Department of Geriatrics, Paolo Cavagnaro.

Acknowledgment

This paper is done on behalf of the Italian Group of Syncope in the Elderly of the Italian Society of Gerontology (GIS Group).

References

[1] J. A. Rizzo, R. Friedkin, C. S. Williams, J. Nabors, D. Acampora, and M. E. Tinetti, "Health care utilization and costs in a medicare population by fall status," Medical Care, vol. 36, no. 8, pp. 1174–1188, 1998.

[2] G. F. Fuller, "Falls in the elderly," American Family Physician, vol. 61, no. 7, pp. 2159–2168, 2000.

[3] C. H. Hirsch, L. Sommers, A. Olsen, L. Mullen, and C. H. Winograd, "The natural history of functional morbidity in hospitalized older patients," Journal of the American Geriatrics Society, vol. 38, no. 12, pp. 1296–1303, 1990.

[4] L. Nyberg, Y. Gustafson, D. Berggren, B. Brännström, and G. Bucht, "Falls leading to femoral neck fractures in lucid older people," Journal of the American Geriatrics Society, vol. 44, no. 2, pp. 156–160, 1996.

[5] J. A. Stevens, P. S. Corso, E. A. Finkelstein, and T. R. Miller, "The costs of fatal and non-fatal falls among older adults," Prevention, vol. 12, no. 5, pp. 290–295, 2006.

[6] T. Masud and R. O. Morris, "Epidem..., Ageing, vol. 30, no. 4, pp. 3–7, 20...

[7] M. F. Folstein, S. E. Folstein, and P. R. McHugh, "'Mini mental state'. A practical method for grading the cognitive state of patients for the clinician," *Journal of Psychiatric Research*, vol. 12, no. 3, pp. 189–198, 1975.

[8] J. A. Yesavage, T. L. Brink, T. L. Rose et al., "Development and validation of a geriatric depression screening scale: a preliminary report," *Journal of Psychiatric Research*, vol. 17, no. 1, pp. 37–49, 1982.

[9] S. Katz, A. B. Ford, R. W. Moskowitz, B. A. Jackson, and M. W. Jaffe, "Studies of illness in the aged. The index of ADL: a standardized measure of biological and psychosocial function," *The Journal of the American Medical Association*, vol. 185, pp. 914–919, 1963.

[10] M. P. Lawton and E. M. Brody, "Assessment of older people: self-maintaining and instrumental activities of daily living," *Gerontologist*, vol. 9, no. 3, pp. 179–186, 1969.

[11] Y. Conwell, N. T. Forbes, C. Cox, and E. D. Caine, "Validation of a measure of physical illness burden at autopsy: the cumulative illness rating scale," *Journal of the American Geriatrics Society*, vol. 41, no. 1, pp. 38–41, 1993.

[12] M. Piirtola, T. Vahlberg, R. Isoaho, P. Aarnio, and S. L. Kivelä, "Incidence of fractures and changes over time among the aged in a Finnish municipality: a population-based 12-year follow-up," *Aging—Clinical and Experimental Research*, vol. 19, no. 4, pp. 269–276, 2007.

[13] S. D. Berry, E. J. Samelson, M. T. Hannan et al., "Second hip fracture in older men and women: the framingham study," *Archives of Internal Medicine*, vol. 167, no. 18, pp. 1971–1976, 2007.

[14] R. A. M. Kenny, D. A. Richardson, N. Steen, R. S. Bexton, F. E. Shaw, and J. Bond, "Carotid sinus syndrome: a modifiable risk factor for nonaccidental falls in older adults (SAFE PACE)," *Journal of the American College of Cardiology*, vol. 38, no. 5, pp. 1491–1496, 2001.

[15] P. Scuffham, S. Chaplin, and R. Legood, "Incidence and costs of unintentional falls in older people in the United Kingdom," *Journal of Epidemiology and Community Health*, vol. 57, no. 9, pp. 740–744, 2003.

[16] D. A. Skelton and C. J. Todd, "Thoughts on effective falls prevention intervention on a population basis," *Journal of Public Health*, vol. 13, no. 4, pp. 196–202, 2005.

[17] S. Gates, J. D. Fisher, M. W. Cooke, Y. H. Carter, and S. E. Lamb, "Multifactorial assessment and targeted intervention for preventing falls and injuries among older people in community and emergency care settings: systematic review and meta-analysis," *The British Medical Journal*, vol. 336, no. 7636, pp. 130–133, 2008.

[18] S. Mayor, "NICE issues guideline to prevent falls in elderly people," *The British Medical Journal*, vol. 329, no. 7477, article 1258, 2004.

[19] M. Stenvall, B. Olofsson, M. Lundström et al., "A multidisciplinary, multifactorial intervention program reduces postoperative falls and injuries after femoral neck fracture," *Osteoporosis International*, vol. 18, no. 2, pp. 167–175, 2007.

[20] B. D. Robertson and T. J. Robertson, "Current concepts review: postoperative delirium after hip fracture," *Journal of Bone and Joint Surgery Series A*, vol. 88, no. 9, pp. 2060–2068, 2006.

Intraindividual Variability in Domain-Specific Cognition and Risk of Mild Cognitive Impairment and Dementia

Leslie Vaughan,[1] Iris Leng,[1] Dale Dagenbach,[2] Susan M. Resnick,[3] Stephen R. Rapp,[1]
Janine M. Jennings,[2] Robert L. Brunner,[4] Sean L. Simpson,[1] Daniel P. Beavers,[1]
Laura H. Coker,[1] Sarah A. Gaussoin,[1] Kaycee M. Sink,[1] and Mark A. Espeland[1]

[1] Department of Social Sciences and Health Policy, Wake Forest University School of Medicine, Medical Center Boulevard,
  Winston-Salem, NC, USA
[2] Wake Forest University, Winston-Salem, NC, USA
[3] National Institute on Aging, Baltimore, MD, USA
[4] Family and Community Medicine, University of Nevada School of Medicine, Reno, NV, USA

Correspondence should be addressed to Leslie Vaughan; alvaugha@wakehealth.edu

Academic Editor: Arnold B. Mitnitski

Intraindividual variability among cognitive domains may predict dementia independently of interindividual differences in cognition. A multidomain cognitive battery was administered to 2305 older adult women (mean age 74 years) enrolled in an ancillary study of the Women's Health Initiative. Women were evaluated annually for probable dementia and mild cognitive impairment (MCI) for an average of 5.3 years using a standardized protocol. Proportional hazards regression showed that lower baseline domain-specific cognitive scores significantly predicted MCI ($N = 74$), probable dementia ($N = 45$), and MCI or probable dementia combined ($N = 101$) and that verbal and figural memory predicted each outcome independently of all other cognitive domains. The baseline intraindividual standard deviation across test scores (IAV Cognitive Domains) significantly predicted probable dementia and this effect was attenuated by interindividual differences in verbal episodic memory. Slope increases in IAV Cognitive Domains across measurement occasions (IAV Time) explained additional risk for MCI and MCI or probable dementia, beyond that accounted for by interindividual differences in multiple cognitive measures, but risk for probable dementia was attenuated by mean decreases in verbal episodic memory slope. These findings demonstrate that within-person variability across cognitive domains both at baseline and longitudinally independently accounts for risk of cognitive impairment and dementia in support of the predictive utility of within-person variability.

1. Introduction

There is continued interest in identifying optimal and novel cognitive predictors of dementia of Alzheimer's type (AD) as both diagnostic and predictive entities [1–5]. Although it may be difficult to discriminate AD in its early preclinical stages from normal cognitive aging, it is believed that preclinical markers of AD may be present in older adults for many years before the appearance of clinical symptoms [6, 7]. While neuropsychological tests of both memory and executive function (EF) have been used to discriminate normal cognitive aging from both mild cognitive impairment (MCI) and AD

[8, 9], the role of intraindividual variability among cognitive domains is not well understood.

The preclinical onset of dementia is marked by decreases in both overall global and domain-specific cognition [2, 10–13], in particular episodic memory and executive function (EF). Decrements in verbal episodic memory are generally identified as one of the earliest markers of cognitive decline [14–16], followed by global changes in multiple cognitive domains that occur several years before the onset of dementia [6, 17, 18]. The role of EF is not well characterized as a predictor of dementia, although it has been explored in relation to time of AD onset. Grober et al. [7] examined change points in linear mixed models of cognitive variables over time in persons who later developed AD and found that declines in performance on tests of EF accelerated 2-3 years before diagnosis, whereas declines in performance on tests of verbal episodic memory (sum of immediate recall across 3 learning trials) accelerated 7 years before diagnosis.

Most studies of cognitive predictors of dementia focus on interindividual differences in mean performance, yet increases in within-person intraindividual variability (IAV) also may signal the preclinical onset of dementia. Intra-individual variability refers to changes within persons, and measures of IAV may include across neuropsychological tests of cognitive domains administered on a single occasion (IAV Cognitive Domains), across trials within computerized tasks (IAV Tasks), and longitudinal change in IAV among neuropsychological tests of cognitive domains (IAV Time). The focus of this study is on IAV Cognitive Domains and IAV Time, as described below. For example, Holtzer et al. [19] examined within-person across neuropsychological test variability (IAV Cognitive Domains) of individually admin-istered neuropsychological tests (Free and Cued Selective Reminding Test, Digit Symbol, Vocabulary) and incident dementia and found that a nested Cox proportional hazards model of IAV Cognitive Domains marginally improved the prediction of incident dementia compared to interindividual differences in mean performance on neuropsychological tests and significantly increased the sensitivity for predicting dementia within one year, but the Holtzer et al. study did not address IAV Time. Although IAV Time over the lifespan may be high in normal aging individuals (e.g., [20]), there is little research on how longitudinal changes in within-person variability across neuropsychological tests might predict dementia (although see [21]). Overall, studies of various types of IAV are consistent with the possibility that increased IAV in cognition, independent of interindividual differences in mean performance, may reflect a breakdown in attentional control and memory systems [22–24]. Therefore, IAV Cognitive Domains and IAV Time may improve the preclinical or early detection of incident dementia.

We examined data from the Women's Health Initiative Study of Cognitive Aging (WHISCA) [16, 25, 26] to deter-mine if IAV Cognitive Domains and IAV Time predict risk of MCI and incident dementia, addressing two main questions. First, we examined whether IAV Cognitive Domains predicts risk of MCI and dementia above and beyond mean overall and domain-specific interindividual differences in cognition. Using a similar strategy, we next examined if IAV Time predicts risk of MCI and dementia. We hypothesized that IAV Cognitive Domains should predict risk of MCI and incident dementia above and beyond interindividual differ-ences in cognition, in-line with other studies that have found increased IAV among cognitive domains in persons with dementia [19, 22], with the expectation that verbal episodic memory might partially account for this result. Additionally, we predicted that IAV Time should predict risk of MCI and dementia above and beyond baseline interindividual differences in cognition [21] and baseline intraindividual differences in cognition.

2. Methods

The Women's Health Initiative Memory Study (WHIMS) [27] began enrolling its 7,479 participants from the parent Women's Health Initiative hormone therapy (HT) trials [28] in May, 1996. These women were between 65 and 79 years of age at initial screening, were appropriate candidates for postmenopausal HT, and were free of dementia as assessed with a standard protocol. Women without a uterus were randomly assigned with equal probability to take one daily tablet that contained either 0.625 mg of conjugated equine estrogens (CEE: Premarin, Wyeth-Ayerst Philadelphia, PA) or a matching oral placebo in the WHI CEE-Alone trial. In a similar manner, women with a uterus were randomly assigned to take one daily tablet that contained either 0.625 mg of CEE with 2.5 mg medroxyprogesterone acetate (MPA: PremPro, Wyeth-Ayerst Philadelphia, PA) or placebo in the WHI CEE+MPA trial.

The Women's Health Initiative Study of Cognitive Aging (WHISCA) enrolled 2,304 of these participants from 14 of the WHIMS clinical sites beginning in September, 1999 [16]. These women had been randomly assigned to WHI treatments for a mean (standard deviation) of 3.0 (0.7) years prior to enrollment in WHISCA and were free of probable dementia and mild cognitive impairment (MCI) at baseline according to standardized assessments, as described below. Participants were administered a cognitive battery and 3MSE [29] screening annually for a mean (range) of 5.3 (0.7 to 8.4) years through September, 2007. The National Institutes of Health and Institutional Review Boards for all participating institutions approved protocols and consent forms. Informed written consent was obtained from all participants.

The WHI CEE+MPA trial ended in July, 2002 [30] and the CEE-Alone trial ended in February, 2004 [31]; however, WHIMS annual follow-up, with reconsenting, continued until September, 2007. Results from all cognitive assessments that occurred to the end of this extended follow-up are presented in this paper.

2.1. Cognitive Assessments. A battery of cognitive measures was administered annually to WHISCA participants by trained administrators [16]. It included the primary mental abilities vocabulary test of verbal knowledge (PMA Vocab-ulary) [32], the Benton Visual Retention Test of short-term figural memory (BVRT) [33], a modified version of the California Verbal Learning Test of verbal memory (CVLT) [16, 34, 35], the digit span forward and backward tests of attention and working memory [36], the card rotations test of spatial ability [37], and the letter and semantic fluency tests of verbal fluency [38, 39]. Fluency tasks, widely used to test executive function, are thought to depend on strategic retrieval, initiation of action, inhibition of previously domi-nant responses, and ability to switch search strategies [40, 41]. Additionally, a finger tapping test was administered to assess fine motor speed [42].

The cognitive battery was administered in face-to-face interviews by certified test administrators. Quality control was maintained through recertification of test administrators twice during the first year and annually thereafter.

2.2. Classification of Probable Dementia. Detailed descriptions of the WHIMS protocol for detecting MCI and probable dementia has been published [13, 27, 43]. All WHIMS participants were administered the (3MSE) [29] annually. If women scored below preset standard cut-points based on education level (≤88 for ≥9 years of education; ≤80 for ≤8 years) on the 3MSE, they were given a complete neuropsychiatric evaluation that included the Consortium for the Establishment of a Registry for Alzheimer's Disease (CERAD) [44, 45] battery of neuropsychological tests and standardized questions about acquired cognitive and functional impairments to participants and a knowledgeable friend or family member. Using a standardized protocol developed by the WHIMS Clinical Coordinating Center, a boardcertified local dementia specialist (i.e., neurologist, geropsychiatrist, or geriatrician) reviewed all available data and administered a clinical evaluation. The local dementia specialists then classified each woman into 1 of 3 groups: probable dementia based on clinical diagnostic criteria for Alzheimer's disease from the Diagnostic and Statistical Manual of Mental Disorders, Fourth Edition (DSM-IV) [17], WHIMS MCI, or no impairment. Criteria for WHIMS MCI were based on accepted criteria at the time of WHIMS initiation. This was defined operationally as poor performance (10th or lower percentile on the CERAD norms on at least 1 CERAD test), a report from the designated informant of some functional impairment, no evidence of a psychiatric disorder or medical condition that could account for the decline in cognitive function, and an absence of adjudicated dementia. Those suspected of having probable dementia underwent a noncontrast CT brain scan and laboratory blood tests to rule out possible reversible causes of cognitive decline, and local dementia specialists were required to provide the most probable etiology. All data on the WHIMS participants except the local dementia expert's classification were then submitted to a centralized adjudication committee consisting of dementia experts at the WHIMS coordinating center at Wake Forest University School of Medicine for final classification of no impairment, MCI, or probable dementia. The committee reviewed all the probable dementia cases and a random sample of nonprobable dementia cases without knowledge of the local dementia expert's diagnosis and achieved high reliability with the latter. Our analyses focus on the WHISCA cohort, a subset of the WHIMS participants, who were all cognitively normal at baseline and include all cases of adjudicated dementia that were triggered by clinic-based 3MSE testing during follow-up.

2.3. Statistical Analyses. All analyses were performed using SAS 9.3 (SAS Institute Inc., Cary, NC, USA). The significance level for all tests was set at 0.05. The results of multiple analyses are presented. Because the primary predictors were IAV Cognitive Domains and IAV Time, we considered other predictors exploratory, and no further multiple comparison corrections were made. Test scores from each of the cognitive domains were standardized by converting them to z-scores, using the means and standard deviations (SDs) at WHISCA enrollment. An average of the z-scores from the seven tests

was used as an overall measure of global cognitive function. We also created two composite scores to test the independent contributions of EF and verbal episodic memory: EF was calculated as the average of the z-scores of verbal fluency (letter and semantic fluency tests of verbal fluency [38, 39]) and working memory (the digit span forward and backward tests of attention and working memory [36]); verbal episodic memory was calculated as the average of the z-scores of learning/immediate recall, short-delay free recall, and long-delay free recall subscales from the CVLT [34]. Cronbach's alpha was calculated for the EF and verbal episodic memory composites. The measure of intraindividual variability (IAV Cognitive Domains) was the standard deviation (SD) among the seven cognitive tests at baseline. The longitudinal measure of intraindividual variability (IAV Time) was calculated as follows. First, a regression function of each cognitive test against time was calculated for each woman. Then, the SD of the seven slopes of the cognitive tests was calculated as IAV Time for that woman. In a similar fashion, slopes of overall cognitive function, EF, and verbal episodic memory were calculated.

Cox proportional hazards models were used to evaluate the relative risk of each predictor. The person time at risk was defined as the time since the WHISCA baseline cognitive function evaluation to the time of diagnosis of MCI, probable dementia, and MCI or probable dementia combined. All models were adjusted for age, education, and WHI treatment assignment. The first set of Cox models examined whether interindividual differences in mean performance on overall, composite, and domain-specific test scores predicted MCI, probable dementia, and MCI or probable dementia. The second set of Cox models examined the relationship between IAV Cognitive Domains and MCI, probable dementia, and MCI or probable dementia. The third set of Cox models examined the relationship between IAV Time and MCI, probable dementia, and MCI or probable dementia combined, by additionally adjusting for confounding cognitive factors as shown in Table 3. In the full model, we tested whether IAV Time still predicts MCI, probable dementia, and MCI or probable dementia, after adjusting for baseline overall cognition, EF, verbal episodic memory, IAV Cognitive Domains, on overall slope, EF slope, and verbal episodic memory slope. We also compared those women who had only baseline cognitive data to those who had at least 2 cognitive assessments on overall cognition, EF, and verbal episodic memory composites.

3. Results

The 2,305 women enrolled in WHISCA were followed with annual 3MSE screening for an average (range) of 5.3 (0.7 to 8.4) years through September, 2007, for an average of 5.6 measurement occasions. At the time of their WHISCA enrollment, women averaged 74.0 (range: 66.9 to 84.5) years of age. The distribution of their education levels was: 5.2% less than high school, 21.4% high school graduates, 41.2% some posthigh school education, and 32.2% college graduates.

The cohort included 6.2% African-American women, 1.3% Hispanic/Latina women, 90.1% Caucasian women, and 2.4% women representing other race/ethnicities. The WHI treatment assignments for these women were 30.0% CEE+MPA, 31.7% CEE+MPA placebo, 18.8% CEE alone, and 19.6% CEE alone placebo. A total of $N = 239$ women were excluded from the analyses ($N = 52$ had a WHISCA visit after a cognitive assessment; $N = 24$ had events before their first WHISCA visit; $N = 13$ had missing values on at least one of the seven cognitive measures; $N = 147$ had only a baseline visit and could not be used to calculate slope; and $N = 3$ had missing values on education), with a final sample size of $N = 2066$. Those women who were lost to follow-up (e.g., those who had only WHISCA baseline data; $N = 147$) had lower cognitive scores on each test (all $P < 0.01$), lower overall cognition ($P < 0.0001$), lower EF ($P = 0.0002$), and lower verbal episodic memory composite scores ($P < 0.0001$), with the exception of fine motor speed and the measure of IAV at baseline, IAV Cognitive Domains (all $P > 0.50$). Of the final sample, $N = 74$ women developed MCI, $N = 45$ developed probable dementia, and $N = 101$ had MCI or probable dementia. None of the groups (MCI; probable dementia; MCI or probable dementia) differed from the final sample on HT Arm (all $P > 0.10$) or education (all $P > 0.10$), but all of the groups had greater frequencies of women 75 years and older (MCI 28% versus 12%; probable dementia 38% versus 12%; MCI or probable dementia 33% versus 12%) (all $P < 0.0001$).

Table 1 shows the raw scores from the tests of cognitive function at the first WHISCA visit, for all women ($N = 2066$), women with no cognitive impairment ($N = 1965$), MCI ($N = 74$), probable dementia ($N = 45$), and MCI or probable dementia ($N = 101$). Raw scores were converted to domain-specific z-scores for the use in subsequent analyses. Standardized total scores for verbal fluency, CVLT, digits forward and backwards, and fine motor speed for each group are also shown. Additionally, composite measures of overall cognition (the average of the z-scores for all cognitive domains), EF (the average of the z-scores for verbal fluency and attention and working memory), and episodic verbal memory (the average of the z-scores for CVLT learning/immediate recall (CVLT no. correct 3 list A trials), CVLT short-delay free recall (CVLT no. correct list A short-delay free recall), and CVLT long-delay free recall (CVLT no. correct list A long-delay free recall) are reported. Cronbach's alpha for EF and verbal episodic memory composites were 0.66 and 0.72, respectively.

Table 1 compares women classified with no impairment to women with MCI, probable dementia, and MCI or probable dementia over a mean follow-up of 5.3 (2.0) years. Group differences between women with no impairment and MCI were significant on all standardized cognitive measures (all $P < 0.05$) with the exception of letter fluency ($P = 0.06$). IAV Cognitive Domains did not differ significantly between women with no impairment (M = 0.80, SD = 0.26) and women with MCI (M = 0.81, SD = 0.27) ($P = 0.82$). However, IAV Time demonstrated significant differences between women with no cognitive impairment (M = −0.009, SD = 0.51) and women with MCI (M = 0.22, SD = 0.60) ($P = 0.002$). In the women with probable dementia, group

differences between women with no impairment and probable dementia were significant on all standardized cognitive measures (all $P < 0.001$), except for digits forward ($P = 0.08$), letter fluency ($P = 0.21$), and finger tapping (all $P > 0.20$). IAV Cognitive Domains differed significantly between women with no impairment (M = 0.80, SD = 0.26) and women with probable dementia (M = 0.92, SD = 0.29) ($P = 0.004$). In addition, IAV Time demonstrated significant differences between women with no cognitive impairment (M = −0.009, SD = 0.51) and women with probable dementia (M = 0.28, SD = 0.59) ($P = 0.0002$). Lastly, group differences between women with no impairment and women with MCI or probable dementia were significant on all standardized cognitive measures (all $P < 0.05$). IAV Cognitive Domains did not differ significantly between women with no impairment (M = 0.80, SD = 0.26) and women with MCI or probable dementia (M = 0.84, SD = 0.27) ($P = 0.15$). However, IAV Time demonstrated significant differences between women with no cognitive impairment (M = −0.009, SD = 0.51) and women with MCI or probable dementia (M = 0.24, SD = 0.60) ($P = 0.0001$).

Interindividual differences in each standardized cognitive domain were significantly related to subsequent risk of MCI (all $P < 0.05$) (Table 2). Controlling for all other cognitive domains, domain-specific scores for verbal memory (HR = 0.32; 95% CI = 0.24, 0.42; $P < 0.0001$) and figural memory (HR = 0.74; 95% CI = 0.58, 0.95; $P = 0.019$) significantly predicted MCI. Overall cognition (the standardized mean of the seven individual tests) was also strongly predictive of dementia (HR = 0.32; 95% CI = 0.25, 0.41; $P < 0.0001$), as were EF (HR = 0.48; 95% CI = 0.37, 0.63; $P < 0.0001$) and verbal episodic memory composites (HR = 0.27; 95% CI = 0.21, 0.35; $P < 0.0001$) (see Table 3). For the probable dementia group, interindividual differences in each standardized cognitive domain were also significantly related to subsequent risk (all $P < 0.001$) with the exception of finger tapping ($P = 0.50$) (Table 2). Controlling for all other cognitive domains, domain-specific scores for verbal memory (HR = 0.26; 95% CI = 0.17, 0.39; $P < 0.0001$) and figural memory (HR = 0.68; 95% CI = 0.50, 0.92; $P = 0.012$) significantly predicted probable dementia, whereas vocabulary ($P = 0.05$) and card rotations were marginal ($P = 0.06$). Overall cognition was also strongly predictive of probable dementia (HR = 0.25; 95% CI = 0.18, 0.35; $P < 0.0001$), as were EF (HR = 0.50; 95% CI = 0.35, 0.70; $P < 0.0001$) and verbal episodic memory composites (HR = 0.22; 95% CI = 0.16, 0.31; $P < 0.0001$) (see Table 3). Lastly, interindividual differences in each standardized cognitive domain were significantly related to the risk of MCI or probable dementia (Table 2) (all $P < 0.01$). Controlling for all other cognitive domains, domain-specific scores for verbal memory (HR = 0.34; 95% CI = 0.27, 0.44; $P < 0.0001$) and figural memory (HR = 0.71; 95% CI = 0.57, 0.87; $P = 0.001$) significantly predicted MCI or probable dementia. Overall cognition was also strongly predictive of MCI or probable dementia (HR = 0.30; 95% CI = 0.24, 0.37; $P < 0.0001$), as were EF (HR = 0.48; 95% CI = 0.38, 0.61; $P < 0.0001$) and verbal episodic memory composites (HR = 0.29; 95% CI = 0.23, 0.36; $P < 0.0001$) (see Table 3). Overall, higher cognitive function was associated

TABLE 1: Means (SDs) of the raw and standardized scores for the cognitive measures at baseline, standardized scores for executive function, verbal episodic memory, overall cognition, IAV Cognitive Domains, and IAV Time for WHISCA participants by group.

Cognitive domain	Means (SDs)							
	All (N = 2066)	No impairment (N = 1965)	MCI	P value	Probable dementia	P value	MCI or probable dementia (N = 101)	P value
PMA vocabulary	36.93 (9.580)	37.24 (9.420)	31.19 (10.56)	<0.0001	31.00 (10.44)	<0.0001	30.86 (10.64)	<0.0001
Letter fluency	40.03 (12.35)	40.18 (12.27)	37.47 (13.57)	0.0639	37.82 (14.50)	0.2050	37.15 (13.51)	0.0162
Category fluency	29.15 (6.215)	29.37 (6.168)	24.07 (4.922)	<0.0001	25.44 (6.298)	<0.0001	24.91 (5.589)	<0.0001
*BVRT	6.915 (3.675)	6.755 (3.579)	9.838 (4.122)	<0.0001	10.36 (4.483)	<0.0001	10.01 (4.151)	<0.0001
CVLT (learning)	29.03 (6.174)	29.34 (6.009)	23.05 (5.527)	<0.0001	22.00 (6.931)	<0.0001	23.03 (6.308)	<0.0001
CVLT (short-delay free recall)	8.587 (3.018)	8.756 (2.925)	5.365 (2.672)	<0.0001	4.822 (3.284)	<0.0001	5.287 (2.923)	<0.0001
CVLT (long-delay free recall)	9.334 (2.975)	9.488 (2.893)	6.203 (2.669)	<0.0001	6.022 (3.583)	<0.0001	6.337 (2.984)	<0.0001
Digits forward	7.484 (2.059)	7.524 (2.066)	6.608 (1.719)	<0.0001	6.978 (1.738)	0.0789	6.713 (1.751)	<0.0001
Digits backward	6.723 (2.022)	6.765 (2.029)	6.041 (1.716)	0.0025	5.867 (1.590)	0.0005	5.891 (1.696)	<0.0001
Card rotations	56.38 (26.94)	57.13 (26.81)	43.78 (24.26)	<0.0001	36.89 (26.25)	<0.0001	41.66 (25.30)	<0.0001
Finger tapping (dominant)	38.57 (7.561)	38.67 (7.566)	36.64 (7.242)	0.0237	38.00 (6.801)	0.5583	36.71 (7.245)	0.0113
Finger tapping (nondominant)	36.46 (6.417)	36.58 (6.419)	34.11 (6.080)	0.0012	35.32 (5.915)	0.1931	34.14 (5.955)	0.0002
Standardized total score (z-scores): verbal fluency, CVLT, digits forward and backward, and fine motor speed								
Verbal fluency	−0.046 (0.952)	−0.019 (0.945)	−0.633 (0.873)	<0.0001	−0.490 (1.009)	0.0010	−0.570 (0.932)	<0.0001
CVLT	0.024 (0.932)	0.076 (0.902)	−1.01 (0.813)	<0.0001	−1.11 (1.104)	<0.0001	−0.988 (0.926)	<0.0001
Digits forward and backward	−0.017 (0.993)	0.006 (0.997)	−0.446 (0.805)	<0.0001	−0.396 (0.718)	0.0006	−0.460 (0.787)	<0.0001
Fine motor speed	−0.102 (1.085)	−0.084 (1.085)	−0.456 (1.037)	0.0038	−0.246 (0.995)	0.3216	−0.449 (1.028)	0.0010
Standardized scores (z-scores): executive function, verbal episodic memory, and overall cognition								
Executive function	−0.038 (0.978)	−0.008 (0.976)	−0.661 (0.816)	<0.0001	−0.544 (0.862)	0.0003	−0.633 (0.839)	<0.0001
Verbal episodic memory	0.024 (0.932)	0.076 (0.902)	−1.01 (0.813)	<0.0001	−1.11 (1.104)	<0.0001	−0.988 (0.926)	<0.0001
Overall cognition	−0.128 (0.962)	−0.077 (0.938)	−1.10 (0.887)	<0.0001	−1.12 (0.906)	<0.0001	−1.11 (0.902)	<0.0001
IAV Cognitive Domains (standard deviation across cognitive domains at baseline)								
SD	0.806 (0.260)	0.804 (0.259)	0.811 (0.272)	0.8182	0.917 (0.288)	0.0042	0.843 (0.269)	0.1475
IAV time (slope of IAV Cognitive Domains across measurement occasions)								
Slope SD	0.003 (0.519)	−0.009 (0.512)	0.221 (0.600)	0.0017	0.281 (0.594)	0.0002	0.237 (0.604)	0.0001

Note. PMA vocabulary: primary mental abilities vocabulary (total correct − 1/3 number incorrect); letter fluency: letter fluency (number correct); category fluency: category fluency (number correct); BVRT: Benton Visual Retention Test (total figures with errors); CVLT (learning): California Verbal Learning Test (number correct 3 list A trials); CVLT (short-delay free-recall): California Verbal Learning Test (number correct list A short-delay free recall); CVLT (long-delay free-recall): California Verbal Learning Test (number correct list A long-delay free-recall); digits forward: digit span forward (number correct); digits backward: digit span backward (number correct); card rotations: card rotations (total correct − total incorrect); finger tapping (dominant): finger tapping test (taps for dominant hand); finger tapping (nondominant): finger tapping test (taps for nondominant hand); *higher scores reflect poorer performance.

with lower risk of MCI, probable dementia combined, and MCI or probable dementia, in particular the verbal and visual memory domains.

The measure of IAV at baseline, IAV Cognitive Domains, was a significant predictor of risk for probable dementia (HR = 4.72; 95% CI = 1.76, 12.70; P = 0.002) but not MCI (HR = 1.07; 95% CI = 0.44, 2.59; P = 0.889) or MCI or probable dementia (HR = 1.71; 95% CI = 0.82, 3.55; P = 0.152) (Table 3). IAV Cognitive Domains predicted incident dementia after controlling separately for overall cognition (HR = 4.15; 95% CI = 1.56, 11.0; P = 0.004) and EF (HR = 6.46; 95% CI = 2.37, 17.60; P = 0.0003) but not verbal episodic memory (HR = 2.19; CI = 0.71, 6.73; P = 0.17). Higher intraindividual variability among the cognitive domains at baseline, partially attributable to verbal episodic memory, increased the risk for probable dementia.

IAV Time significantly predicted risk of MCI (HR = 3.13; 95% CI = 2.05, 4.78; P = 0.0001) (Table 3). In the final model controlling for SD at baseline, EF, verbal episodic memory, overall cognition, EF slope, verbal episodic memory

TABLE 2: Hazard ratios for the cognitive domains (alone and controlling for all other cognitive domains) predicting MCI, probable dementia, and MCI or probable dementia.

Cognitive domains	MCI ($N = 74$)			Probable dementia ($N = 45$)			MCI or probable dementia ($N = 101$)		
	HR	95% CI	P value	HR	95% CI	P value	HR	95% CI	P value
Vocabulary alone	0.58	[0.46, 0.73]	<0.0001	0.46	[0.34, 0.62]	<0.0001	0.53	[0.44, 0.65]	<0.0001
Verbal fluency alone	0.49	[0.37, 0.65]	<0.0001	0.53	[0.37, 0.74]	0.0003	0.52	[0.41, 0.66]	<0.0001
Figural memory alone	0.49	[0.40, 0.61]	<0.0001	0.39	[0.30, 0.51]	<0.0001	0.46	[0.38, 0.55]	<0.0001
Verbal memory alone	0.27	[0.21, 0.35]	<0.0001	0.22	[0.16, 0.31]	<0.0001	0.29	[0.23, 0.36]	<0.0001
Attention/Working memory alone	0.63	[0.48, 0.81]	0.0005	0.61	[0.44, 0.85]	0.0039	0.60	[0.48, 0.75]	<0.0001
Spatial ability alone	0.60	[0.45, 0.79]	0.0003	0.36	[0.24, 0.53]	<0.0001	0.52	[0.40, 0.66]	<0.0001
Fine motor speed alone	0.79	[0.64, 0.98]	0.0306	0.91	[0.69, 1.20]	0.4962	0.79	[0.66, 0.95]	0.0113
Vocabulary | others	0.91	[0.69, 1.18]	0.4655	0.70	[0.49, 1.00]	0.0486	0.82	[0.65, 1.04]	0.0955
Verbal fluency | others	0.87	[0.65, 1.17]	0.3608	1.39	[0.95, 2.03]	0.0899	1.00	[0.78, 1.29]	0.9967
Figural memory |others	0.74	[0.58, 0.95]	0.0186	0.68	[0.50, 0.92]	0.0119	0.71	[0.57, 0.87]	0.0014
Verbal memory | others	0.32	[0.24, 0.42]	<0.0001	0.26	[0.17, 0.39]	<0.0001	0.34	[0.27, 0.44]	<0.0001
Attention/Working memory | others	0.95	[0.70, 1.28]	0.7260	0.99	[0.66, 1.47]	0.9555	0.94	[0.72, 1.22]	0.6186
Spatial ability | others	0.91	[0.67, 1.23]	0.5267	0.66	[0.43, 1.02]	0.0639	0.84	[0.64, 1.10]	0.2003
Fine motor speed | others	0.83	[0.66, 1.04]	0.1039	0.86	[0.63, 1.18]	0.3436	0.83	[0.68, 1.00]	0.0549

TABLE 3: Hazard ratios for IAV Cognitive Domains and IAV time (alone and controlling for baseline and slope overall cognition, EF, and verbal episodic memory) predicting MCI, probable dementia, and MCI or probable dementia.

Parameter	MCI ($N = 74$)			Probable dementia ($N = 45$)			MCI or probable dementia ($N = 101$)		
	HR	95% CI	P value	HR	95% CI	P value	HR	95% CI	P value
Overall cognition	0.32	[0.25, 0.41]	<0.0001	0.25	[0.18, 0.35]	<0.0001	0.30	[0.24, 0.37]	<0.0001
EF	0.48	[0.37, 0.63]	<0.0001	0.50	[0.35, 0.70]	<0.0001	0.48	[0.38, 0.61]	<0.0001
Verbal episodic memory	0.27	[0.21, 0.35]	<0.0001	0.22	[0.16, 0.31]	<0.0001	0.29	[0.23, 0.36]	<0.0001
Standard deviation (SD) (IAV Cognitive Domains)	1.07	[0.44, 2.59]	0.8891	4.72	[1.76, 12.7]	0.0021	1.71	[0.82, 3.55]	0.1525
SD | overall cognition	1.09	[0.44, 2.71]	0.8534	4.15	[1.56, 11.0]	0.0043	1.72	[0.82, 3.61]	0.1543
SD | EF	1.23	[0.50, 3.03]	0.6596	6.46	[2.37, 17.6]	0.0003	2.06	[0.98, 4.34]	0.0567
SD | verbal episodic memory	0.45	[0.18, 1.12]	0.0865	2.19	[0.71, 6.73]	0.1727	0.77	[0.36, 1.66]	0.5011
Slope standard deviation (SD) (IAV Time)	3.13	[2.05, 4.78]	<0.0001	3.80	[2.23, 6.46]	<0.0001	3.05	[2.13, 4.36]	<0.0001
Slope SD | overall cognition	2.99	[1.98, 4.51]	<0.0001	3.96	[2.37, 6.61]	<0.0001	3.10	[2.18, 4.41]	<0.0001
Slope SD | EF	3.03	[2.04, 4.52]	<0.0001	4.27	[2.45, 7.43]	<0.0001	3.07	[2.17, 4.34]	<0.0001
Slope SD | verbal episodic memory	3.27	[2.14, 5.00]	<0.0001	4.87	[2.83, 8.38]	<0.0001	3.35	[2.35, 4.78]	<0.0001
Slope SD | overall cognition, overall slope	2.34	[1.65, 3.31]	<0.0001	2.26	[1.51, 3.38]	<0.0001	2.07	[1.53, 2.80]	<0.0001
Slope SD | EF, EF slope	3.05	[2.04, 4.57]	<0.0001	3.76	[2.37, 5.96]	<0.0001	2.89	[2.11, 3.97]	<0.0001
Slope SD | verbal episodic memory, verbal episodic memory slope	2.05	[1.34, 3.15]	0.0010	1.50	[1.01, 2.23]	0.0433	1.58	[1.16, 2.16]	0.0039
Slope SD | SD, overall cognition, EF, verbal episodic memory, overall slope, EF slope, verbal episodic memory slope	2.32	[1.46, 3.69]	0.0004	1.46	[0.84, 2.55]	0.1842	1.70	[1.16, 2.49]	0.0061

slope, and overall cognition slope, the results were slightly attenuated but still significant (HR = 2.32; 95% CI = 1.46, 3.69; $P = 0.0004$).

IAV Time also predicted the incidence of probable dementia (HR = 3.80; 95% CI = 2.23, 6.46; $P = 0.0001$), but in the final model results were fully attenuated (HR =

1.46; 95% CI = 0.84, 2.55; $P = 0.18$), largely by episodic verbal memory and episodic verbal memory slope. Lastly, IAV Time significantly predicted MCI or probable dementia (HR = 3.05; 95% CI = 2.13, 4.36; $P = 0.0001$). In the final model controlling for SD at baseline, EF, verbal episodic memory, overall cognition, EF slope, verbal episodic memory slope, and overall cognition slope, the results were slightly attenuated but still significant (HR = 1.70; 95% CI = 1.16, 2.49; P = 0.006). Overall, controlling for important cognitive variables, IAV Time predicts risk of MCI and MCI or probable dementia above and beyond baseline inter- and intraindividual differences in cognitive function.

4. Discussion

In a large cohort of older women, higher domain-specific cognitive function was associated with a decreased risk of MCI and a decreased risk of probable dementia. After adjustment for all other cognitive domains, deficits in verbal memory and figural memory remained independently associated with increased risk. Additionally, higher scores on composite measures of overall EF, and episodic verbal memory also predicted a lower risk of MCI and a lower risk of probable dementia. The measure of intraindividual variability (IAV Cognitive Domains) was a predictor of probable dementia (but not MCI or both groups combined) even after adjusting for interindividual differences in overall cognition (similar to [19]) and EF. However, adjusting for interindividual differences in episodic verbal memory attenuated the contribution of IAV Cognitive Domains to dementia risk. This research supports the finding that high variability within individuals among cognitive domains may be a significant predictor of dementia, in addition to the between-person differences in global cognitive ability and episodic memory that are a hallmark of the disease [6, 46].

The longitudinal change in intraindividual variability among cognitive domains (IAV Time) appears to be particularly important and robust in signaling the risk of cognitive impairment and dementia, above and beyond baseline interindividual differences in multiple measures of cognition and IAV cognitive Domains, especially in the early stages. Adjusting for multiple measures (baseline differences in overall cognition, EF, and verbal episodic memory, the standard deviation among the cognitive tests, and longitudinal interindividual changes in overall cognition slope, EF slope, and verbal episodic memory slope) in the model of IAV Time did not decrease the risk of MCI or MCI or probable dementia combined. In contrast (but similar to the baseline model), the contribution of IAV Time to probable dementia risk was attenuated after adjusting for longitudinal interindividual changes in verbal episodic memory slope. One possible explanation for this last finding is that on average (SD), women took 3.7 (2.0) years to progress to probable dementia from the time of their baseline cognitive tests, suggesting that most of the changes in IAV Time had already occurred (perhaps resulting in a slope underestimation for the women with probable dementia). While increasing intraindividual variability within tasks has been observed cross-sectionally in aging and may be an indicator of early cognitive impairment (e.g., [4, 22]), the current study's emphasis on longitudinal within-person variability among multiple cognitive domains in women with MCI and probable dementia is unique and shows that IAV time is also an indicator of risk for dementia, especially in the early stages.

One hypothesis that has been posited to explain normal age-related cognitive changes due to intraindividual variability in domains such as memory and executive function is dedifferentiation [47–49]. An increase in the strength of the correlations between various cognitive processes or abilities has been linked to greater within-person variability as well as higher coactivation of different cognitive processes [50, 51]. For example, Papenberg et al. [49] examined the relationship between intraindividual differences in trial-to-trial variability on a measure of forgetting and dedifferentiated memory functions and found that the correlation between episodic memory and spatial working memory was considerably higher in the high than the low variability group. Along these lines, we found that the correlations between most of the cognitive domains were somewhat higher in the probable dementia than in the nonprobable dementia group (data not shown), with the exception of vocabulary and attention with other domains. Although prior studies have not examined the association between intraindividual variability and dedifferentiation in persons with and without dementia, this study provides some support for the hypothesis. In addition, Magnetic resonance imaging (MRI) studies show structural changes linked to increased performance variability that include frontal gray matter lesions and white matter changes on MRI scans (volumetric decline, demyelination, and hyperintensities) due to age-related changes in cerebral bold flow, vascular injury, or neurological conditions such as AD [4, 52]. In our probable dementia cohort, white matter hyperintensities as well as volumetric decreases likely explain poorer cognitive performance and increased performance variability (e.g., [53]).

This study was limited to the WHISCA cohort, which consists of volunteers who were eligible to participate in a clinical trial of hormone therapy, and is not representative of the general population. The classification of probable dementia included multiple etiologies, and while the pattern of cognitive deficits may vary by etiology, we first ruled out group differences in the baseline model and then included all adjudicated cases of probable dementia due to the small sample size. The WHISCA cognitive battery did not include a measure of cognitive processing speed, which may have provided additional important information about cognitive decline in dementia. While IAV Time may be an important marker of cognitive decline, it may not be as easy to evaluate in the clinic as more traditional cross-sectional types of measures, because it requires multiple cognitive assessments; although increasingly, memory disorders clinics provide this.

Within-person variability across multiple tests and measurement occasions explains additional risk for cognitive impairment and dementia beyond that accounted for by interindividual variation in cognitive function and may contribute to the early prediction of dementia. Greater IAV among cognitive domains represents a 3.6 to 4.4 times increased risk of probable dementia, which was only attenuated by adjusting for mean differences in verbal episodic memory. Greater IAV across time predicts a 2.0 to 3.7 times increased risk for MCI, a 1.5 to 6.4 times increased risk for probable dementia, and a 1.6 to 3.1 times increased risk for both groups combined. Adjusting for mean slope decreases in verbal episodic memory only attenuated the contribution of IAV Time to risk of probable dementia.

By extension, these results may have practical implications at the level of the individual that could be further refined with more research. For example, cognitive test batteries that measure multiple domains are commonly administered in memory disorders and other clinics where within-person across test comparisons over time may easily reveal imbalances in test scores that signal preclinical dementia. Greater knowledge of intraindividual differences in cognitive domains, both cross-sectional as well as longitudinal, could be used for early detection and intervention. In particular, longitudinal change in within-person across domain cognitive test scores (keeping in mind that shifts in within-person variability precede changes in mean performance) could signal the early stages of dementia.

Acknowledgments

The Women's Health Initiative Study of Cognitive Aging was supported by the Department of Health and Human Services and the National Institute on Aging (NO1-AG-1-2106). The Women's Health Initiative program is funded by the National Heart, Lung, and Blood Institute. Wyeth Pharmaceuticals provided the study drug and the placebo to the WHI trial. The Women's Health Initiative Memory Study was funded by Wyeth Pharmaceuticals, Wake Forest University, and the National Heart, Lung, and Blood Institute. This work was supported by the following *NIA Program Office*: National Institute of Aging: Alan Zonderman, Susan M. Resnick WHISCA Central Coordinating Center: Sally Shumaker, Principal Investigator; Stephen Rapp, Mark Espeland, Laura Coker, Deborah Farmer, Anita Hege, Patricia Hogan, Darrin Harris, Cynthia McQuellon, Anne Safrit, Lee Ann Andrews, Candace Warren, Carolyn Bell, and Linda Allred; *WHISCA Clinical Sites*: Women's Health Initiative, Durham, NC, Carol Murphy; Rush Presbyterian-Saint Luke's Medical Center, Chicago, IL, Linda Powell; Ohio State University Medical Center, Columbus, OH, Rebecca Jackson; University of California at Davis, Sacramento, CA, John Robbins; University of Iowa College of Medicine, Des Moines, IA, Robert Wallace; University of Florida, Gainesville/Jacksonville, FL, Marian Limacher; University of California at Los Angeles, Los Angeles, CA, Howard Judd; Medical College of Wisconsin, Milwaukee, WI, Jane Kotchen; The Berman Center for Outcomes and Clinical Research, Minneapolis, and MN, Karen Margolis; University of Nevada School of Medicine, Reno, NV, Robert Brunner; Albert Einstein College of Medicine, Bronx, NY, Sylvia Smoller; The Leland Stanford Junior University, San Jose, CA, Marcia Stefanick; The State University of New York, Stony Brook, NY, Dorothy Lane; University of Massachusetts/Fallon Clinic, Worcester, MA, Judith Ockene. The following investigators were the original investigators for these sites: Mary Haan, Davis; Richard Grimm, Minneapolis; Sandra Daugherty (deceased), Nevada. The paper is also supported by; *WHI Program Office*: National Heart, Lung, and Blood Institute, Bethesda, Maryland: Barbara Alving, Jacques Rossouw, Linda Pottern; *WHI Central Coordinating Center*: Fred Hutchinson Cancer Research Center, Seattle, WA: Deborah Bowen, Gretchen VanLom, Carolyn Burns.

References

[1] M. S. Albert, M. B. Moss, R. Tanzi, and K. Jones, "Preclinical prediction of AD using neuropsychological tests," *Journal of the International Neuropsychological Society*, vol. 7, no. 5, pp. 631–639, 2001.

[2] M. F. Elias, A. Beiser, P. A. Wolf, R. Au, R. F. White, and R. B. D'Agostino, "The preclinical phase of Alzheimer disease: a 22-year prospective study of the Framingham cohort," *Archives of Neurology*, vol. 57, no. 6, pp. 808–813, 2000.

[3] D. F. Hultsch, S. W. S. MacDonald, M. A. Hunter, J. Levy-Bencheton, and E. Strauss, "Intraindividual variability in cognitive performance in older adults: comparison of adults with mild dementia, adults with arthritis, and healthy adults," *Neuropsychology*, vol. 14, no. 4, pp. 588–598, 2000.

[4] S. W. S. MacDonald, S.-C. Li, and L. Bäckman, "Neural underpinnings of within-person variability in cognitive functioning," *Psychology and Aging*, vol. 24, no. 4, pp. 792–808, 2009.

[5] S. Sacuiu, M. Sjögren, B. Johansson, D. Gustafson, and I. Skoog, "Prodromal cognitive signs of dementia in 85-year-olds using four sources of information," *Neurology*, vol. 65, no. 12, pp. 1894–1900, 2005.

[6] L. Bäckman, S. Jones, A.-K. Berger, E. J. Laukka, and B. J. Small, "Cognitive impairment in preclinical Alzheimer's disease: a meta-analysis," *Neuropsychology*, vol. 19, no. 4, pp. 520–531, 2005.

[7] E. Grober, C. B. Hall, R. B. Lipton, A. B. Zonderman, S. M. Resnick, and C. Kawas, "Memory impairment, executive dysfunction, and intellectual decline in preclinical Alzheimer's disease," *Journal of the International Neuropsychological Society*, vol. 14, no. 2, pp. 266–278, 2008.

[8] J. C. Morris, M. Storandt, J. P. Miller et al., "Mild cognitive impairment represents early-stage Alzheimer disease," *Archives of Neurology*, vol. 58, no. 3, pp. 397–405, 2001.

[9] R. C. Petersen and S. Negash, "Mild cognitive impairment: an overview," *CNS Spectrums*, vol. 13, no. 1, pp. 45–53, 2008.

[10] M. A. Espeland, S. R. Rapp, S. A. Shumaker et al., "Conjugated equine estrogens and global cognitive funtion in postmenopausal women: Women's Health Initiative Memory Study," *Journal of the American Medical Association*, vol. 291, no. 24, pp. 2959–2968, 2004.

[11] J. R. Hodges, "Memory in the dementias," in *The Oxford Handbook of Memory*, E. Tulving and F. I. M. Craik, Eds., pp. 441–459, Oxford University Press, New York, NY, USA, 2000.

[12] R. T. Linn, P. A. Wolf, D. L. Bachman et al., "The 'preclinical phase' of probable Alzheimer's disease: a 13-year prospective study of the Framingham cohort," *Archives of Neurology*, vol. 52, no. 5, pp. 485–490, 1995.

[13] S. A. Shumaker, C. Legault, S. R. Rapp et al., "Estrogen plus progestin and the incidence of dementia and mild cognitive impairment in postmenopausal women: the Women's Health Initiative Memory Study: a randomized controlled trial," *Journal of the American Medical Association*, vol. 289, no. 20, pp. 2651–2662, 2003.

[14] E. Grober, R. B. Lipton, C. Hall, and H. Crystal, "Memory impairment on free and cued selective reminding predicts dementia," *Neurology*, vol. 54, no. 4, pp. 827–832, 2000.

[15] D. M. Masur, M. Sliwinski, R. B. Lipton, A. D. Blau, and H. A. Crystal, "Neuropsychological prediction of dementia and the absence of dementia in healthy elderly persons," *Neurology*, vol. 44, no. 8, pp. 1427–1432, 1994.

[16] S. M. Resnick, L. H. Coker, P. M. Maki, S. R. Rapp, M. A. Espeland, and S. A. Shumaker, "The Women's Health Initiative Study of Cognitive Aging (WHISCA): a randomized clinical trial of the effects of hormone therapy on age-associated cognitive decline," *Clinical Trials*, vol. 1, no. 5, pp. 440–450, 2004.

[17] American Psychiatric Association, *Diagnostic and Statistical Manual of Mental Disorders*, American Psychiatric Association, Washington, DC, USA, 4th edition, 1994.

[18] S. Sacuiu, D. Gustafson, B. Johansson et al., "The pattern of cognitive symptoms predicts time to dementia onset," *Alzheimer's and Dementia*, vol. 5, no. 3, pp. 199–206, 2009.

[19] R. Holtzer, J. Verghese, C. Wang, C. B. Hall, and R. B. Lipton, "Within-person across-neuropsychological test variability and incident dementia," *Journal of the American Medical Association*, vol. 300, no. 7, pp. 823–830, 2008.

[20] T. A. Salthouse, "Implications of within-person variability in cognitive and neuropsychological functioning for the interpretation of change," *Neuropsychology*, vol. 21, no. 4, pp. 401–411, 2007.

[21] D. F. Hultsch, E. Strauss, M. A. Hunter, and S. W. S. MacDonald, "Intra-individual variability, cognition, and aging," in *The Handbook of Aging and Cognition*, F. I. M. Craik and T. A. Salthouse, Eds., pp. 491–556, Psychology Press, New York, NY, USA, 3rd edition, 2008.

[22] J. M. Duchek, D. A. Balota, C.-S. Tse, D. M. Holtzman, A. M. Fagan, and A. M. Goate, "The utility of intra-individual variability in selective attention tasks as an early marker for Alzheimer's disease," *Neuropsychology*, vol. 23, no. 6, pp. 746–758, 2009.

[23] S. W. S. MacDonald, L. Nyberg, and L. Bäckman, "Intra-individual variability in behavior: links to brain structure, neurotransmission and neuronal activity," *Trends in Neurosciences*, vol. 29, no. 8, pp. 474–480, 2006.

[24] D. J. Schretlen, C. A. Munro, J. C. Anthony, and G. D. Pearlson, "Examining the range of normal intraindividual variability in neuropsychological test performance," *Journal of the International Neuropsychological Society*, vol. 9, no. 6, pp. 864–870, 2003.

[25] S. M. Resnick, P. M. Maki, S. R. Rapp et al., "Effects of combination estrogen plus progestin hormone treatment on cognition and affect," *Journal of Clinical Endocrinology and Metabolism*, vol. 91, no. 5, pp. 1802–1810, 2006.

[26] S. M. Resnick, M. A. Espeland, Y. An et al., "Effects of conjugated equine estrogens on cognition and affect in postmenopausal women with prior hysterectomy," *Journal of Clinical Endocrinology and Metabolism*, vol. 94, no. 11, pp. 4152–4161, 2009.

[27] S. A. Shumaker, B. A. Reboussin, M. A. Espeland et al., "The Women's Health Initiative Memory Study (WHIMS): a trial of the effect of estrogen therapy in preventing and slowing the progression of dementia," *Controlled Clinical Trials*, vol. 19, no. 6, pp. 604–621, 1998.

[28] The Women's Health Initiative Study Group, "Design of the Women's Health Initiative clinical trial and observational study," *Controlled Clinical Trials*, vol. 19, no. 1, pp. 61–109, 1998.

[29] E. L. Teng and H. C. Chui, "The modified mini mental state (3MS) examination," *Journal of Clinical Psychiatry*, vol. 48, pp. 314–318, 1987.

[30] J. E. Rossouw, G. L. Anderson, R. L. Prentice et al., "Risks and benefits of estrogen plus progestin in healthy postmenopausal women: principal results from the Women's Health Initiative randomized controlled trial," *Journal of the American Medical Association*, vol. 288, no. 3, pp. 321–333, 2006.

[31] G. L. Anderson and M. Limacher, "Effects of conjugated equine estrogens in postmenopausal women with hysterectomy: the Women's Health Initiative randomized controlled trial," *Journal of the American Medical Association*, vol. 291, no. 14, pp. 1701–1712, 2004.

[32] A. R. Kuse, *Familial resemblances for cognitive abilities from two test batteries in Hawaii [Unpublished doctoral dissertation]*, University of Colorado, Boulder, 1977.

[33] A. L. Benton, *Revised Visual Retention Test*, Psychological Corporation, New York, NY, USA, 1974.

[34] D. C. Delis, J. H. Kramer, E. Kaplan, and B. A. Ober, *California Verbal Learning Test*, The Psychological Corporation, New York, NY, USA, Research edition, 1987.

[35] C. Legault, P. M. Maki, S. M. Resnick et al., "Effects of tamoxifen and raloxifene on memory and other cognitive abilities: cognition in the study of tamoxifen and raloxifene," *Journal of Clinical Oncology*, vol. 27, no. 31, pp. 5144–5152, 2009.

[36] D. Wechsler, *Manual for the Wechsler Adult Intelligence Scale*, The Psychological Corporation, New York, NY, USA, 1955.

[37] R. B. Ekstrom, J. W. French, and H. H. Harman, *Manual for Kit of Factor-Referenced Cognitive Tests*, Educational Testing Service, Princeton, NJ, USA, 1976.

[38] A. L. Benton, "Differential behavioral effects in frontal lobe disease," *Neuropsychologia*, vol. 6, no. 1, pp. 53–60, 1968.

[39] F. Newcombe, *Missile Wounds of the Brain. A Study of Psychological Deficits*, Oxford University Press, London, UK, 1969.

[40] R. L. C. Mitchell and L. H. Phillips, "The psychological, neurochemical and functional neuroanatomical mediators of the effects of positive and negative mood on executive functions," *Neuropsychologia*, vol. 45, no. 4, pp. 617–629, 2007.

[41] L. H. Phillips, R. Bull, E. Adams, and L. Fraser, "Positive mood and executive function. Evidence from stroop and fluency tasks," *Emotion*, vol. 2, no. 1, pp. 12–22, 2002.

[42] W. C. Halstead, *Brain and Intelligence*, University of Chicago Press, Chicago, Ill, USA, 1947.

[43] S. A. Shumaker, C. Legault, L. Kuller et al., "Conjugated equine estrogens and incidence of probable dementia and mild cognitive impairment in postmenopausal women: Women's Health Initiative Memory Study," *Journal of the American Medical Association*, vol. 291, no. 24, pp. 2947–2958, 2004.

[44] J. C. Morris, D. W. McKeel Jr., K. Fulling, R. M. Torack, and L. Berg, "Validation of clinical diagnostic criteria for Alzheimer's disease," *Annals of Neurology*, vol. 24, no. 1, pp. 17–22, 1988.

[45] K. A. Welsh, N. Butters, R. C. Mohs et al., "The consortium to establish a registry for Alzheimer's disease (CERAD). Part V. A normative study of the neuropsychological battery," *Neurology*, vol. 44, no. 4, pp. 609–614, 1994.

[46] L. Bäckman, S. Jones, A.-K. Berger, E. J. Laukka, and B. J. Small, "Multiple cognitive deficits during the transition to Alzheimer's disease," *Journal of Internal Medicine*, vol. 256, no. 3, pp. 195–204, 2004.

[47] R. Cabeza, "Cognitive neuroscience of aging: contributions of functional neuroimaging," *Scandinavian Journal of Psychology*, vol. 42, no. 3, pp. 277–286, 2001.

[48] E. M. Tucker-Drob, "Differentiation of cognitive abilities across the life span," *Developmental Psychology*, vol. 45, no. 4, pp. 1097–1118, 2009.

[49] G. Papenberg, L. Bäckman, C. Chicherio et al., "Higher intraindividual variability is associated with more forgetting and dedifferentiated memory functions in old age," *Neuropsychologia*, vol. 49, no. 7, pp. 1879–1888, 2011.

[50] S.-C. Li and S. Sikström, "Integrative neurocomputational perspectives on cognitive aging, neuromodulation, and representation," *Neuroscience and Biobehavioral Reviews*, vol. 26, no. 7, pp. 795–808, 2002.

[51] S.-C. Li, U. Lindenberger, and S. Sikström, "Aging cognition: from neuromodulation to representation," *Trends in Cognitive Sciences*, vol. 5, no. 11, pp. 479–486, 2001.

[52] D. Bunce, K. J. Anstey, H. Christensen, K. Dear, W. Wen, and P. Sachdev, "White matter hyperintensities and within-person variability in community-dwelling adults aged 60–64 years," *Neuropsychologia*, vol. 45, no. 9, pp. 2009–2015, 2007.

[53] L. H. Coker, P. E. Hogan, N. R. Bryan et al., "Postmenopausal hormone therapy and subclinical cerebrovascular disease: the WHIMS-MRI Study," *Neurology*, vol. 72, no. 2, pp. 125–134, 2009.

4

Prevalence and Determinants of Fall-Related Injuries among Older Adults in Ecuador

Carlos H. Orces

Department of Medicine, Laredo Medical Center, 1700 East Saunders, Laredo, TX 78041, USA

Correspondence should be addressed to Carlos H. Orces; corces07@yahoo.com

Academic Editor: Tomasz Kostka

Objectives. To estimate the prevalence and determinants of fall-related injuries in the previous year among adults aged 60 years or older in Ecuador. *Methods.* The prevalence of fall-related injuries was estimated using cross-sectional data from the first national survey of Health, Wellbeing, and Aging study. Logistic regression models were used to examine the associations between participants' demographic characteristics and fall-related injuries. *Results.* Of 5,227 participants with a mean age of 72.6 years, 11.4% (95% CI, 10.3%–12.7%) reported a fall-related injury in Ecuador, representing an estimated 136,000 adults aged 60 years or older. Fall-related injuries were more frequently reported among older adults residing in the most urbanized and populated provinces of the country. After controlling for potential confounders, self-reported race as Indigenous (OR 2.2; 95% CI, 2.11–2.31), drinking alcohol regularly (OR 2.54; 95% CI, 2.46–2.63), subjects with greater number of comorbid conditions (OR 2.03; 95% CI, 1.97–2.08), and urinary incontinence (OR 1.83; 95% CI, 1.79–1.87) were factors independently associated with increased odds of sustaining fall-related injuries. *Conclusions.* Fall-related injuries represent a considerable burden for older adults in Ecuador. The present findings may assist public health authorities to implement fall prevention programs among subjects at higher risk for this type of injury.

1. Introduction

Falls among older adults represent a major public health problem associated with increased morbidity, mortality, and health care costs [1, 2]. Approximately 10% of falls result in a major injury such as a fracture, serious soft tissue injury, or traumatic brain injury [3]. Previous studies have demonstrated that fall-related fractures treated in hospital emergency departments and hospitalizations for fall-related injuries are increasing among older adults in developed countries [4–6]. Overall, 44.2% of adults aged 65 years or older with fall-related fractures require hospitalization and hip fractures account for 48% of the hospitalizations for fall-related injuries among women [4, 6]. Although there is scarce data about the epidemiology of fall-related injuries among older Ecuadorians, a previous study suggested that the incidence of hip fracture increased annually by 3.9% in Ecuador between 1999 and 2008 [7]. Moreover, assuming that the average annual percentage change in hip fracture rates remains unchanged, the number of hip fractures in the country is projected to rise to 8,900 and 47,000 by the years 2030 and 2050, respectively [7]. Recently, a study using data from the first

national survey of Health, Wellbeing, and Aging described that 37.4% of older Ecuadorians sustain a fall each year. Moreover, recurrent falls occurred in 23.0% of the subjects and among fallers 30.6% reported a fall-related injury [8].

In Ecuador, the proportion of adults aged 60 years or older was 8.6% in 2010 and it is projected to increase to 14.4% by 2030. Similarly, current life expectancy is 75.5 years and it may reach 79.2 years by 2030 [9]. These demographic changes alone may increase considerably the number of fall-related injuries among older adults. Therefore, the present study extends previous research and aims to estimate the prevalence of and characteristics associated with fall-related injuries among adults aged 60 years or older residing in the coastal and mountains regions of Ecuador.

2. Materials and Methods

The present population-based study was based on cross-sectional data from the first national survey of Health, Wellbeing, and Aging (Encuesta de Salud, Bienestar y Envejecimiento, SABE I), conducted by trained interviewers between

June and August of 2009. The SABE I survey is a probability sample of households with at least one person aged 60 years or older residing in the Andes Mountains and coastal regions of Ecuador. In the primary sampling stage, a total of 317 sectors from the rural areas (<2,000 inhabitants) and 547 sectors from the urban areas of the country were selected from the 2001 population Census cartography. In the secondary sampling stage, 18 households within each sector were randomly selected based on the assumption that at least one person aged 60 years or older lives in 24% and 23% of the households in the coastal and Andes Mountains regions, respectively. Survey data, including operation manuals, are publicly available [10].

2.1. Fall-Related Injury Ascertainment. A fall-related injury was assessed by the following question: "Did you need medical attention after sustaining a fall?" Subjects who answered affirmatively to the question were considered to have developed a fall-related injury in the previous year.

2.2. Demographic and Health Characteristics. Age and sex were self-reported. The race of participants was classified according to the following question: "Do you consider yourself to be white, black, Mestizo, Mulatto, or Indigenous?" Body height in centimeters and weight in kilograms were measured and the body mass index was calculated (Kg/cm^2). Participants were asked about their living status (alone versus living with others) and area of residence (urban versus rural). The average use of alcohol per week during the previous three months was classified as none, one day, or two or more days per week.

Self-reported general health was grouped as excellent to good or fair to poor. The number of comorbidities (0, 1, ≥2) was assessed by asking participants if they had been diagnosed by a physician with the following conditions: diabetes mellitus, chronic obstructive pulmonary disease, arthritis, stroke, coronary artery disease, or cancer. Urinary incontinence was defined as having involuntary incontinence of urine that occurred at least once during the previous year.

Cognitive status was evaluated by the abbreviated Mini Mental State Examination (MMSE). This modified MMSE was developed by Icaza and Albala to identify the MMSE questions that could best explain cognitive deterioration. The abbreviated MMSE was developed with nine variables instead of the 19 original MMSE variables. A cutoff point of 12 or less was defined to identify people with cognitive impairment [11]. The Geriatric Depression Scale was used to evaluate the presence of depressive symptoms. This 15-item scale has been validated in Spanish populations with a sensitivity of 81% and a specificity of 76%. Respondents with a score of 6 or more were considered to have symptoms of depression [12, 13]. The following activities of daily living (ADLs) were included in the present study: walking across a room, dressing, bathing, eating, getting in and out of bed, and using the toilet. Those participants who needed help or were unable to perform one or more of the ADLs were considered functionally impaired. Physical activity was evaluated by the question "Do you regularly exercise such as jogging, dance, or perform rigorous physical activity at least three times weekly for the past year?" Subjects who responded affirmatively were considered to engage in regular physical exercise.

Grip strength was evaluated using a standard hand-held dynamometer. Participants used their dominant hand and the average result of two trials was reported in Kg/sec. The chair stand test was used to assess lower-limb muscle strength. This test was considered successfully completed if participants were able to stand up five times from a chair with their arms folded within 60 seconds [14]. The results of the muscle strength measures were grouped into quartiles to examine the association between grip strength and lower-limb muscle strength and fall-related injuries. Balance was evaluated by the single leg stance test. Subjects who were able to stand in one foot for 10 seconds completed successfully the test.

2.3. Statistical Analysis. Categorical variables were compared using the chi-squared test. Those variables statistically significant (P value < 0.05) in the univariate analyses were entered into a multivariate regression model adjusted for age, gender, and body mass index to evaluate the independent associations between fall-related injuries and demographic and health characteristics of the participants. Results of the logistic regression model are presented as odds ratios (OR) with their 95% confidence intervals (95% CI). To compare the geographic distribution of this injury across the country, the age-specific proportions of fall-related injuries by provinces were age-adjusted by the direct method using the 2010 Census population of Ecuador as the standard. All analyses were weighted to account for the multistage sampling design of the SABE I survey. Statistical analyses were performed using SPSS, version 17 software (SPSS Inc., Chicago, IL).

3. Results

Of 5,227 participants with a mean age of 72.6 years (8.9 years), 11.4% (95% CI, 10.3%–12.7%) reported a fall-related injury in the previous year, representing an estimated 136,000 adults aged 60 years and older in Ecuador. As shown in Figure 1, the prevalence of fall-related injuries varied across regions of the country. After age adjustment, higher fall-related injury rates were predominantly found among subjects residing in the provinces of Guayas and Pichincha, which are the most populated and urbanized provinces of the country.

As shown in Table 1, fall-related injury rates were considerably higher among Indigenous, those living alone, older adults who drink alcohol regularly, and participants with cognitive impairment and symptoms of depression. Moreover, subjects with symptoms of urinary incontinence or greater number of chronic comorbidities reported more frequently fall-related injuries as compared to those who did not. Of relevance, among subjects who completed the physical performance tests, fall-related injury rates progressively increased as the muscle strength decreased in both the grip-strength and chair stand tests.

As shown in Table 2, the results of the multivariate model indicate that after adjusting for age, sex, and BMI, Indigenous older adults, regular use of alcohol, self-reported health as

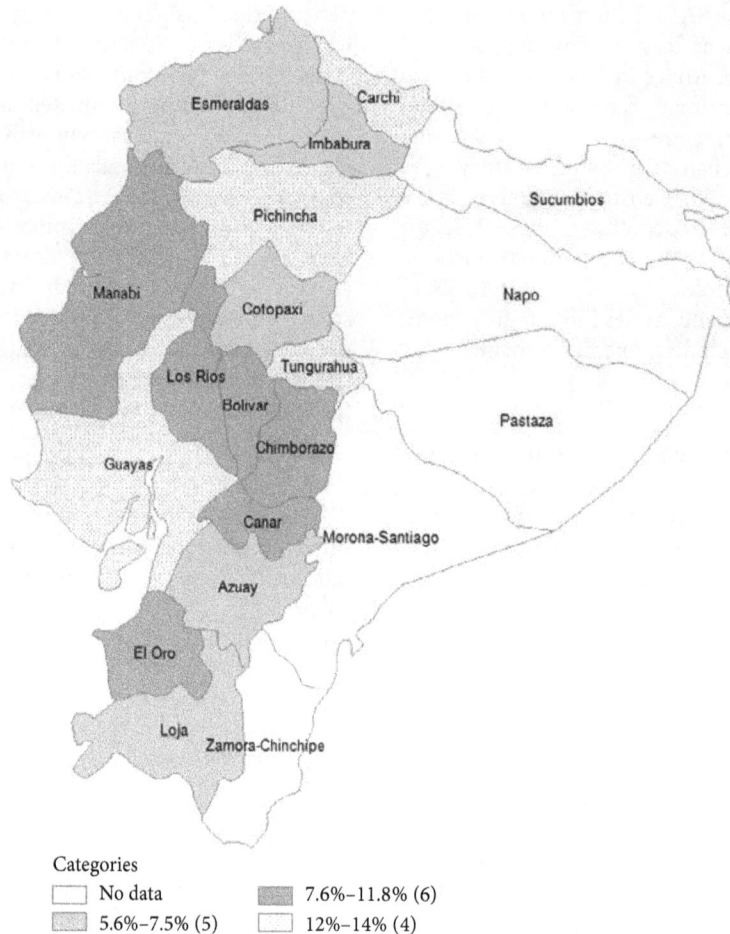

FIGURE 1: Fall-related injury prevalence rates by provinces in Ecuador.

fair to poor, having two or more chronic comorbidities, and symptoms of urinary incontinence were characteristics significantly associated with increased fall-related injury prevalence in Ecuador. Moreover, among subjects who completed the physical performance tests, those with the best scores on the grip strength test, chair-stand test, and single leg stance had 25%, 20%, and 13% lower risk of sustaining fall-related injuries as compared with subjects who performed worse on these tests, respectively.

4. Discussion

The results of the present study indicate that 11.4% of community-dwelling adults aged 60 years or older sustain a fall-related injury each year in Ecuador. In general, fall-related injury rates varied across the country. However, these injuries occurred predominantly among residents from the most populated and urbanized provinces of the country. Overall, the geographic distribution of fall-related injuries among older adults in Ecuador contrasts with results from a recent investigation that demonstrated higher fall prevalence rates among older subjects residing in the rural Andes Mountains of the country [8]. Similarly, previous studies have

demonstrated higher incidence of fall-related injury rates among subjects residing in rural areas [15, 16].

Of relevance, a marked racial disparity in fall-related injuries was seen among older Ecuadorians. For instance, self-reported race as Indigenous was a variable associated with 1.8-fold increased odds of sustaining fall-related injuries as compared with the White. The reasons for higher fall-related injury prevalence rates among this minority ethnic group in Ecuador are unknown. However, high risk occupations among Indigenous people such as farming and construction may partly explain the present findings.

The higher prevalence of fall-related injuries with increasing age and among women found in the present study is consistent with results from previous investigations [17, 18]. Previous studies also have reported that gender differences in fall-related injuries may be attributed to 2- to 3-fold higher fractures rates among women [4, 17–19]. Moreover, gender differences in fall-related injuries have been related to higher prevalence of osteoporosis, frailty, muscle strength, and willingness to seek medical attention among women [20–23].

Self-reported health status as fair to poor and greater number of comorbidities were variables associated with increased odds of sustaining fall-related injuries among older adults in Ecuador. The present findings are consistent with

TABLE 1: Prevalence of fall-related injuries among older adults in Ecuador.

Characteristics	Number of subjects	% (95% CI)
Gender		
Women	2,766	13.9 (12.2–15.8)
Men	2,466	8.5 (7.2–10.0)
Age groups, yrs		
60–69	2,441	9.5 (8.0–11.3)
70–79	1,645	12.7 (10.7–15.2)
≥80	926	14.4 (11.7–17.7)
Area of residence		
Rural	2,354	9.8 (8.4–11.4)
Urban	2,878	12.3 (10.7–14.0)
Race		
Indian	530	15.0 (11.6–19.2)
Black	169	9.4 (5.6–15.5)
Mestizo	3,349	11.7 (11.2–13.4)
Mulatto	179	8.7 (4.8–15.0)
White	670	8.9 (6.7–11.8)
Living arrangements		
Alone	547	15.4 (11.1–20.9)
Accompanied	4,684	11.0 (9.8–12.2)
BMI (Kg/m^2)		
Underweight	163	10.9 (6.4–17.9)
Normal weight	2,045	10.4 (8.7–12.4)
Overweight	1,892	10.6 (8.8–12.6)
Obese	843	12.0 (9.2–15.5)
Alcohol use		
None	4,167	12.2 (10.9–13.6)
1 day	939	7.2 (5.5–9.4)
≥2 days	123	19.3 (9.9–34.2)
Regular physical activity		
No	3,573	12.1 (10.7–13.6)
Yes	1,657	10.1 (8.1–12.5)
GDS ≥ 6		
No	2,633	9.6 (8.1–11.4)
Yes	1,153	14.5 (12.2–17.1)
Cognitive impairment		
No	3,719	9.6 (8.4–10.9)
Yes	1,079	15.9 (13.0–19.2)
ADL's limitations		
No	3,771	9.9 (8.6–11.3)
Yes	1,454	15.6 (13.3–18.1)
Self-reported health		
Excellent to good	1,197	8.1 (6.2–10.5)
Fair to poor	4,027	12.6 (11.2–14.1)
Urinary incontinence		
No	4,041	9.5 (8.4–10.7)
Yes	1,169	17.7 (14.7–21.1)
Comorbidities		
0	2,442	7.8 (6.5–9.4)
1	1,763	13.3 (11.3–15.6)
≥2	860	17.2 (14.1–20.8)

TABLE 1: Continued.

Characteristics	Number of subjects	% (95% CI)
Grip strength (Kg/sec)		
Q1 (1 to 15)	1,301	16.5 (14.0–19.3)
Q2 (16 to 20)	1,205	10.7 (8.5–13.4)
Q3 (21 to 27)	1,198	8.7 (6.9–11.0)
Q4 (28 to 97)	1,214	8.1 (6.1–10.7)
Chair stand test (sec)		
Q1 (4 to 9)	1,187	9.8 (7.6–12.5)
Q2 (10 to 11)	1,041	8.4 (6.3–11.1)
Q3 (12 to 14)	1,073	7.7 (6.0–9.8)
Q4 (≥15)	919	14.0 (11.1–17.7)
Single leg stance (sec)		
0 to 9 sec	2,147	10.1 (8.7–11.9)
10 sec	1,947	8.0 (6.5–9.8)

GDS: Geriatric Depression Scale; BMI: body mass index.

results from a recent study reporting that fair to poor health among older adults was associated with 3-fold increased risk of sustaining fall-related injuries among people aged 85 years or older in the previous 3 months [24]. Moreover, the number of comorbidities has been associated with increased risk for fall-related injuries [25, 26]. For instance, Tinetti et al. demonstrated that community dwelling persons aged 72 years or older with at least two chronic conditions had 2-fold higher odds of sustaining fall-related injuries, which is similar to the present findings [26].

Interestingly, subjects who reported symptoms of urinary incontinence had 1.7-fold higher odds of sustaining fall-related injuries. In Ecuador, urinary incontinence among older adults also was previously found to be an independent factor associated with increased odds of sustaining a fall in the previous year [8]. Falls related to urine incontinence are generally thought to result from loss of balance when rushing to the toilet. However, it is unclear whether incontinence is a primary cause of falls or it is simply a marker of physical frailty [27].

In Ecuador, fall-related injury rates were 10% higher among older adults who took part in rigorous physical activity at least three times weekly as compared with those who did not. In contrast with the present results, an earlier study reported that vigorous physical activity decreased fall-related fracture risk among older adults with no limitations in ADL [28]. Likewise, Cummings et al. demonstrated that women who walked for exercise had a 30% lower risk of hip fracture as compared with those who did not [29]. The reason for the increased fall-related injury risk associated with intense exercise found in the present study is uncertain. However, consistent with the present findings, a recent cross-sectional study among community-dwelling adults aged 50 years and older showed that the likelihood of falling increased by 5% for each 100 metabolic expenditure (MET-min/week) of vigorous-intensity physical activity [29]. Apparently, changes in standing balance among older adults following moderate physical exercise may be a predisposing factor for fall-related injuries [30].

TABLE 2: Characteristics of participants associated with fall-related injuries.

	Unadjusted OR (95% CI)	Adjusted OR (95% CI)[a]
Age groups, yrs		
60–69	1.00	1.00
70–79	1.39 (1.37–1.40)	1.37 (1.36–1.39)
≥80	1.60 (1.58–1.62)	1.63 (1.60–1.65)
Gender		
Men	1.00	1.00
Women	1.74 (1.72–1.76)	1.79 (1.77–1.82)
BMI (Kg/m^2)		
Underweight	1.00	1.00
Normal	0.95 (0.92–0.99)	0.94 (0.91–0.98)
Overweight	0.97 (0.93–1.00)	0.96 (0.92–0.99)
Obesity	1.11 (1.07–1.16)	1.02 (0.98–1.06)
Area of residence		
Rural	1.00	1.00
Urban	1.29 (1.27–1.30)	1.02 (1.02-1.02)
Race		
Indian	1.79 (1.75–1.84)	1.87 (1.82–1.92)
Black	1.06 (1.02–1.10)	1.35 (1.29–1.41)
Mestizo	1.35 (1.33–1.38)	1.49 (1.46–1.52)
Mulatto	0.96 (0.93–1.00)	0.79 (0.76–0.83)
White	1.00	1.00
Living arrangements		
Alone	1.47 (1.45–1.50)	1.35 (1.33–1.37)
Accompanied	1.00	1.00
Alcohol use		
None	1.00	1.00
1 day	0.56 (0.55-0.56)	0.80 (0.78–0.81)
≥2 days	1.71 (1.66–1.77)	2.54 (2.46–2.63)
Regular physical activity		
No	1.00	1.00
Yes	0.81 (0.80–0.82)	1.10 (1.09–1.12)
GDS ≥ 6		
No	1.00	1.00
Yes	1.58 (1.56–1.61)	1.37 (1.35–1.39)
Cognitive impairment		
No	1.00	1.00
Yes	1.78 (1.75–1.80)	1.49 (1.46–1.51)
ADL's limitations		
No	1.00	1.00
Yes	1.68 (1.66–1.70)	1.33 (0.64–0.68)
Self-reported health		
Excellent to good	1.00	1.00
Fair to poor	1.63 (1.61–1.66)	1.60 (1.57–1.62)
Urinary incontinence		
No	1.00	1.00
Yes	2.05 (2.03–2.08)	1.77 (1.75–1.79)

TABLE 2: Continued.

	Unadjusted OR (95% CI)	Adjusted OR (95% CI)[a]
Comorbidities		
0	1.00	1.00
1	1.81 (1.78–1.83)	1.52 (1.49–1.54)
≥2	2.44 (2.40–2.48)	2.22 (2.19–2.26)
Grip strength (Kg/sec)		
Q1 (1 to 15)	1.00	1.00
Q2 (16 to 20)	0.60 (0.59–0.61)	0.65 (0.64–0.66)
Q3 (21 to 27)	0.48 (0.47–0.49)	0.61 (0.60–0.62)
Q4 (28 to 97)	0.44 (0.43–0.45)	0.75 (0.74–0.77)
Chair stand test (sec)		
Q1 (4 to 9)	0.66 (0.65–0.67)	0.80 (0.78–0.81)
Q2 (10 to 11)	0.56 (0.55–0.57)	0.61 (0.60–0.63)
Q3 (12 to 14)	0.50 (0.49–0.51)	0.53 (0.52–0.54)
Q4 (≥15)	1.00	1.00
Single leg stance (sec)		
0 to 9 sec	1.00	1.00
10 sec	0.76 (0.75–0.77)	0.87 (0.86–0.88)

GDS: Geriatric Depression Scale; [a]adjusted for age, sex, and body mass index.

Regular use of alcohol was a potentially modifiable factor associated with increased prevalence of fall-related injuries among older Ecuadorians. In fact, compared with nondrinkers, older adults who self-reported drinking on average 2 or more days per week during the previous 3 months had 2.5-fold higher odds of sustaining fall-related injuries. Similarly, a previous cross-sectional study among older adults in Cataluña, Spain, demonstrated that subjects who drink alcohol heavily had 1.2-fold higher odds of reporting a fall-related injury during the previous year [31]. On the contrary, a recent analysis from the Behavioral Risk Factor Surveillance System Survey found no statistically significant association between consumption of alcohol and fall-related injuries among older adults aged 85 years or older [24]. A possible explanation for these contradictory results may be related to differences in survey definitions regarding alcohol consumption among older adults.

Participants who scored in the highest quartile on the muscle strength measures had considerably lower odds of sustaining fall-related injuries as compared to those in the lowest quartile. The present findings are consistent with results of a systematic review and meta-analysis, which demonstrated that lower extremity weakness is a clinically significant risk factor for falls and fall-related injuries [32]. Previously, lower extremity weakness evaluated by the chair stand test also was found to be associated with higher prevalence of falls among older adult in Ecuador [8]. Likewise, weak grip strength has been reported to be a significant predictor for recurrent falls and nonsyncopal fall-related injuries among community-dwelling older adults [33, 34].

Several limitations must be mentioned in interpreting the present results. First, participants used self-reports of sociodemographic characteristics, medical diagnoses, and

ADL's limitations, which may be a source of recall bias. Second, the SABE I survey did not collect data on specific types of fall-related injury, such as fracture, contusion, abrasion, and laceration. Likewise, other variables associated with increased risk for fall-related injuries such as orthostatic hypotension, bone mineral density, or use of psychotropic drugs were not investigated. Third, the present results may be only generalized to older adults residing in the coastal and Andes Mountains regions of the country. However, older adults from the Amazon region and the Galapagos Islands represented only 3.3% of the population aged 60 years or older in Ecuador [35]. Despite these limitations, this study is the first to estimate the prevalence of fall-related injuries and to examine characteristics associated with this type of injury among older adults in Ecuador.

In conclusion, fall-related injuries represent a considerable burden for older adults in Ecuador. The present findings may assist public health authorities to implement fall prevention programs among subjects at higher risk for this type of injury.

References

[1] L. Z. Rubenstein and K. R. Josephson, "The epidemiology of falls and syncope," *Clinics in Geriatric Medicine*, vol. 18, no. 2, pp. 141–158, 2002.

[2] A. A. Bohl, P. A. Fishman, M. A. Ciol, B. Williams, J. Logerfo, and E. A. Phelan, "A longitudinal analysis of total 3-year healthcare costs for older adults who experience a fall requiring medical care," *Journal of the American Geriatrics Society*, vol. 58, no. 5, pp. 853–860, 2010.

[3] M. E. Tinetti and C. S. Williams, "Falls, injuries due to falls, and the risk of admission to a nursing home," *The New England Journal of Medicine*, vol. 337, no. 18, pp. 1279–1284, 1997.

[4] C. H. Orces, "Emergency department visits for fall-related fractures among older adults in the USA: a retrospective cross-sectional analysis of the National Electronic Injury Surveillance System All Injury Program, 2001–2008," *BMJ Open*, vol. 3, no. 1, article 26, 2013.

[5] K. A. Hartholt, J. A. Stevens, S. Polinder, T. J. M. van Der Cammen, and P. Patka, "Increase in fall-related hospitalizations in the United States, 2001–2008," *Journal of Trauma—Injury, Infection and Critical Care*, vol. 71, no. 1, pp. 255–258, 2011.

[6] K. A. Hartholt, N. van der Velde, C. W. N. Looman et al., "Trends in fall-related hospital admissions in older persons in the Netherlands," *Archives of Internal Medicine*, vol. 170, no. 10, pp. 905–911, 2010.

[7] C. H. Orces, "Trends in hip fracture rates in ecuador and projections for the future," *Revista Panamericana de Salud Publica*, vol. 29, no. 1, pp. 27–31, 2011.

[8] C. H. Orces, "Prevalence and determinants of falls among older adults in Ecuador: an analysis of the SABE I survey," *Current Gerontology and Geriatrics Research*, vol. 2013, Article ID 495468, 7 pages, 2013.

[9] 2014, http://www.eclac.org/celade/proyecciones/basedatos_BD.htm.

[10] January 2014, http://anda.inec.gob.ec/anda/index.php/catalog/292/download/5317.

[11] M. G. Icaza and C. Albala, "MInimental State Examinaitons (MMSE) del studio de la demencia en Chile: análisis Estadístico—serie investigaciones en Salud Pública-Documentos Técnicos," Coordinación de Investigaciones, División de Salud y Desarrollo Humano, OPS, 1999, http://www.paho.org/.

[12] J. A. Yesavage, T. L. Brink, T. L. Rose et al., "Development and validation of a geriatric depression screening scale: a preliminary report," *Journal of Psychiatric Research*, vol. 17, no. 1, pp. 37–49, 1982.

[13] J. Martínez de la Iglesia, M. C. Onís Vilches, R. Dueñas Herrero, C. Aguado Taberné, C. A. Colomer, and M. C. Arias Blanco, "Abbreviating the brief. Approach to ultra-short versions of the Yesavage questionnaire for the diagnosis of depression," *Atencion Primaria*, vol. 35, no. 1, pp. 14–21, 2005.

[14] A. R. Barbosa, J. M. P. Souza, M. L. Lebrão, R. Laurenti, and M. D. F. N. Marucci, "Functional limitations of Brazilian elderly by age and gender differences: data from SABE Survey," *Cadernos de Saúde Pública/ Ministério da Saúde, Fundação Oswaldo Cruz, Escola Nacional de Saúde Pública*, vol. 21, no. 4, pp. 1177–1185, 2005.

[15] H. Tiesman, C. Zwerling, C. Peek-Asa, N. Sprince, and J. E. Cavanaugh, "Non-fatal injuries among urban and rural residents: the National Health Interview Survey, 1997—2001," *Injury Prevention*, vol. 13, no. 2, pp. 115–119, 2007.

[16] C. Moshiro, I. Heuch, A. N. Åstrøm, P. Setel, Y. Hemed, and G. Kvåle, "Injury morbidity in an urban and a rural area in Tanzania: an epidemiological survey," *BMC Public Health*, vol. 5, article 11, 2005.

[17] J. A. Stevens and E. D. Sogolow, "Gender differences for non-fatal unintentional fall related injuries among older adults," *Injury Prevention*, vol. 11, no. 2, pp. 115–119, 2005.

[18] R. W. Sattin, D. A. Lambert Huber, C. A. DeVito et al., "The incidence of fall injury events among the elderly in a defined population," *The American Journal of Epidemiology*, vol. 131, no. 6, pp. 1028–1037, 1990.

[19] P. Saari, E. Heikkinen, R. Sakari-Rantala, and T. Rantanen, "Fall-related injuries among initially 75- and 80-year old people during a 10-year follow-up," *Archives of Gerontology and Geriatrics*, vol. 45, no. 2, pp. 207–215, 2007.

[20] A. C. Looker, L. J. Melton III, T. B. Harris, and J. A. Shepherd, "Prevalence and trends in low femur bone density among older US adults: NHANES 2005–2006 compared with NHANES III," *Journal of Bone and Mineral Research*, vol. 25, no. 1, pp. 64–71, 2010.

[21] H. Syddall, H. C. Roberts, M. Evandrou, C. Cooper, H. Bergman, and A. A. Sayer, "Prevalence and correlates of frailty among community-dwelling older men and women: findings from the Hertfordshire Cohort Study," *Age and Ageing*, vol. 39, no. 2, Article ID afp204, pp. 197–203, 2010.

[22] A. Katsiaras, A. B. Newman, A. Kriska et al., "Skeletal muscle fatigue, strength, and quality in the elderly: the Health ABC Study," *Journal of Applied Physiology*, vol. 99, no. 1, pp. 210–216, 2005.

[23] J. A. Stevens, M. F. Ballesteros, K. A. Mack, R. A. Rudd, E. DeCaro, and G. Adler, "Gender differences in seeking care for falls in the aged medicare population," *The American Journal of Preventive Medicine*, vol. 43, no. 1, pp. 59–62, 2012.

[24] A. C. Grundstrom, C. E. Guse, and P. M. Layde, "Risk factors for falls and fall-related injuries in adults 85 years of age and older," *Archives of Gerontology and Geriatrics*, vol. 54, no. 3, pp. 421–428, 2012.

[25] J. L. O'Loughlin, Y. Robitaille, J.-F. Boivin, and S. Suissa, "Incidence of and risk factors for falls and injurious falls among the community-dwelling elderly," *The American Journal of Epidemiology*, vol. 137, no. 3, pp. 342–354, 1993.

[26] M. E. Tinetti, J. Doucette, E. Claus, and R. Marottoli, "Risk factors for serious injury during falls by older persons in the community," *Journal of the American Geriatrics Society*, vol. 43, no. 11, pp. 1214–1221, 1995.

[27] S. Lord, C. Sherrington, H. Menz, and J. Close, *Falls in Older People*, Cambridge University Press, Cambridge, UK, 2011.

[28] J. A. Stevens, K. E. Powell, S. M. Smith, P. A. Wingo, and R. W. Sattin, "Physical activity, functional limitations, and the risk of fall-related fractures in community-dwelling elderly," *Annals of Epidemiology*, vol. 7, no. 1, pp. 54–61, 1997.

[29] S. R. Cummings, M. C. Nevitt, W. S. Browner et al., "Risk factors for hip fracture in white women," *New England Journal of Medicine*, vol. 332, no. 12, pp. 767–773, 1995.

[30] T. Egerton, S. G. Brauer, and A. G. Cresswell, "The immediate effect of physical activity on standing balance in healthy and balance-impaired older people," *Australasian Journal on Ageing*, vol. 28, no. 2, pp. 93–96, 2009.

[31] J. M. Suelves, V. Martínez, and A. Medina, "Injuries from falls and associated factors among elderly people in Cataluña, Spain," *Revista Panamericana de Salud Publica*, vol. 27, no. 1, pp. 37–42, 2010.

[32] J. D. Moreland, J. A. Richardson, C. H. Goldsmith, and C. M. Clase, "Muscle weakness and falls in older adults: a systematic review and meta-analysis," *Journal of the American Geriatrics Society*, vol. 52, no. 7, pp. 1121–1129, 2004.

[33] S. M. F. Pluijm, J. H. Smit, E. A. M. Tromp et al., "A risk profile for identifying community-dwelling elderly with a high risk of recurrent falling: results of a 3-year prospective study," *Osteoporosis International*, vol. 17, no. 3, pp. 417–425, 2006.

[34] M. C. Nevitt, S. R. Cummings, and E. S. Hudes, "Risk factors for injurious falls: a prospective study," *Journals of Gerontology*, vol. 46, no. 5, pp. M164–M170, 1991.

[35] http://www.ecuadorencifras.gob.ec/informacion-censal-cantonal/.

5

The Contribution of a "Supportive Community" Program for Older Persons in Israel to Their Offspring Who Are Primary Caregivers

Ahuva Even-Zohar

School of Social Work, Faculty of Social Sciences, Ariel University, 40700 Ariel, Israel

Correspondence should be addressed to Ahuva Even-Zohar; ahuvaez@gmail.com

Academic Editor: Arnold B. Mitnitski

The "supportive community" programs in Israel provide a basket of services for older persons living in their own homes. This study examined the differences between caregiver burden and quality of life of 55 offspring who were the primary caregivers of their older parents who were members of a supportive community, compared to 64 offspring whose parents were nonmembers. The findings showed that the role stress factor of caregiving burden was lower, and the psychological health domain of quality of life was higher among offspring whose parents were members of supportive communities. Some of the predictor variables of burden were income status of caregiver, sharing with others in caregiving, and membership of the parent in a supportive community. The primary predictor variable of the quality of life was caregiving burden. The practical conclusion of this study is to further develop and market supportive community programs in various communities.

1. Introduction

The current trend in recent years for older adults in Israel as well as in other countries is "aging in place," which refers to older adults living independently in their current residence or community for as long as possible [1, 2]. According to surveys conducted by the American Association of Retired Persons [3] most of the 50+ population want to age in their homes and communities. In Israel about 97% of older people live in their homes in the community [4].

In recent decades, different types of specialized residential facilities for the older persons in the US have been developed, such as the "Naturally Occurring Retirement Community" (NORC), "Community Innovation for Aging in Place" (CIAIP), and "Program of All-Inclusive Care for the Elderly" (PACE) [5, 6]. Based on the World Health Organization [7, 8] age-friendly communities have been established in the US [9] and in Canada [10]. Many countries operate similar programs in the community, for example, Sweden [11], Finland, Germany, Japan [12], Spain [13], and UK [12, 14]. These programs are based on a multidisciplinary service team and provide medical and social services for the welfare of their members, such as monitoring health, an alarm button connected to a control center, meal service, shopping and accompaniment service, shuttle service, and legal advice.

A program that has been developed in Israel by Eshel (the association for planning and development of services for the aged in Israel) and the departments for social services is the "supportive community" [15]. The program is intended for the general older population at all levels of functioning who are living in both urban and rural settlements in any of the population sectors (Jewish, Arab, immigrant, etc.). The basket of services include the following: an emergency call-button and a 24-hour call center; medical services: a home visit by a doctor, 24/7 at a nominal fee and ambulance service even without a doctor's referral, also at a nominal fee; and social and cultural activities: lectures, exercise, cultural events, classes, parties, and excursions. The unique feature of the program is the "community parent" service. The community parent is the first contact for members for all their daily needs, from emergency situations to minor household repairs. For example, he offers help at home, such as smaller repairs like replacing a light bulb or moving furniture. For more complex repairs, he brings professionals and supervises their work.

He helps in delivering prepared meals and medicines and in accompanying a member to the clinic/hospital. He also initiates telephone calls and home visits to the members, with the help of volunteers, and, if necessary, he contacts a family member—the caregiver. Currently, there are about 250 supportive communities in Israel with some 44,200 members (about 5.8% of those aged 65+). Every program is based on approximately 200 households. Membership fees are about $35 per month, and the needy older persons receive subsidies. Research results indicated that the program provided a solution for the target population; the majority of members expressed general satisfaction with the program and were satisfied with the services they received. The main reasons for joining the program were as follows: increased feeling of personal security, continued living at home, and relieving the burden of their care from family members [15, 16].

However, the family is still the main factor responsible for the care of older adults [17]. Eeven in large families, one family member, usually the spouse or one of the children, is a caregiver, that is, takes on the responsibility for the older person [17–19]. Primary caregivers are engaged in a variety of areas of assistance, such as personal care, financial assistance, housekeeping, and assistance with activities outside the home [17]. In many cases, there is also a pattern of partnership where most older people have a number of informal caregivers who can replace the primary caregiver when necessary, or a group of offspring divides between them the responsibility of providing practical help for the parent [20]. Szinovacz and Davey [21] found that daughters and children living closer to parents were more likely to remain primary caregivers.

Intensive caring for older parents may cause stress in primary caregivers, expressed in the process of losing their quality of life, causing damage to their physical and psychological health, and difficulties in their social and economic situation [22]. Burden can be caused because the caregiver sometimes has difficulty dealing with the demands of caregiving due to deterioration in the health of the aged parent, specifically care of older persons who suffer from cognitive impairment and behavioral problems burden [23]. Another source of the burden is family commitments. Adult children are called the "sandwich generation" because of the many obligations imposed on them by every generation in their family. Married primary caregivers experience a high sense of burden, especially those who shared a residence with the older parent [24]. Caregiving of older family members actually becomes another "career" among person's roles [25]. The unexpected career may cause difficulties in functioning at work, such as absenteeism, and, in extreme cases, even leaving the job [26]. In addition, caregiver obligations impinge upon the social domain by not enabling the caregiver to go on vacation or have recreation and leisure time [27]. Furthermore, care requirements that include a large number of hours of care and multiple tasks increase the burden [28]. Certain other socioeconomic characteristics of the caregiver have been found to affect the caregiver's burden: *gender*: most primary caregivers are women because of the traditional female role to take care of older parents, and they reported greater feeling of burden than men [29, 30],

age: several studies found that advanced age of the primary caregiver was associated with a sense of burden [31] and other studies found younger primary caregivers reported more burden [32], *education*: whereas some studies reported that there is a connection between level of education and burden [29], others reported there is no such connection [33], and *religiosity*: some studies found that religious belief and religious rituals help to moderate the burden of the caregivers [34]. In contrast, coping strategies related to religiosity were not found to moderate the stress and depression of primary caregivers [35]. In addition, ethnic and cultural factors have been associated with caregivers' burden [28]. Although most of the studies dealt with the negative impact of caregiving on the quality of life of caregivers [36], studies over the past decade have reported the positive aspect in terms of finding meaning in the act of caregiving [37].

There are two main factors that help moderate the burden of primary caregivers. The first one is receiving specific help from another family member [38]. The second one is the assistance of formal systems [18, 39].

As stated, the supportive community program is a formal service and was developed to fill the needs of older adults who continue living in their homes. One of the reasons for joining the program was relieving family members of the burden of their care [15] but, to date, no research has examined whether the program helps reduce the caregivers' burden and whether it contributes to their quality of life. Thus, the aim of this study was to add the perspective of the offspring who are primary caregivers of older parents.

The research hypotheses were as follows.

Hypothesis 1. The caregiver burden of offspring who are the primary caregivers of their older parents who are members of a supportive community will be lower than that of the caregivers whose parents are nonmembers.

Hypothesis 2. The quality of life of offspring who are the primary caregivers of their older parents who are members of a supportive community will be higher than that of the caregivers whose parents are nonmembers.

Hypothesis 3. The extent and frequency of providing assistance will be lower among the offspring caregivers whose parents are members of a supportive community.

Hypothesis 4. In the entire sample an inverse correlation will be found between caregiving burden and quality of life so that the lower the caregiving burden, the higher the quality of life.

2. Method

2.1. The Sample and Procedure: Data Collection. The research sample was a convenience sample of 119 participants. Of these, the research group included 55 offspring of parents who were members of a supportive community, and the comparison group included 64 offspring whose parents were nonmembers. All of the older parents were at a normal level of cognitive functioning. Data collection was conducted after receiving approval by the ethics committee at the School of

Social Work in the university. Participants were given an explanation by means of a phone call about the purpose of the research and were assured that their responses were anonymous and would be used for research purposes only. The criterion for inclusion of participants for the study was offspring of older parents who defined themselves as primary caregivers of their older parents. Participants of the research group were identified through social workers of welfare departments and through community parents. They identified which of the offspring were the primary caregivers as whom they contacted when the involvement of a family member for the older parent was needed. Participants in the comparison group were identified through friends and networking applications of the research assistants. In the study group we succeeded in contacting 60 offspring who met the criteria to participate in the study but only 55 offspring agreed to participate in the study and fully filled out the questionnaire. In the comparison group we succeeded in contacting 70 offspring who met the criteria to participate in the study but only 64 offspring agreed to participate in the study and fully filled out the questionnaire. Those who were not included in the study also met the criteria but were not interested in participating in the study because of lack of time or lack of interest. Those who agreed to participate in the study filled out the questionnaires by themselves. All participants lived in central Israel.

2.2. Measures

2.2.1. The Caregiving Burden Questionnaire.
The short version of the Zarit burden interview [40] includes 12 items in its Hebrew version [41]. The questionnaire consists of two factors: (1) Personal stress factor, which includes nine items, for example, "Do you feel that because of the time you spend with your parent, you do not have enough time for yourself?" (2) Role stress factor, which includes three items, for example, "Do you feel you can take care of your parent in a better way?" Answers to the questions were on a five-point Likert scale: 1: "never" to 5: "almost always." Each score was calculated based on the average of the total items. High score represents a greater feeling of caregiving burden. In our study the reliability for the entire scale was $\alpha = 0.79$, for personal stress was $\alpha = 0.81$, and for role stress was $\alpha = 0.55$.

2.2.2. Quality of Life Questionnaire.
The questionnaire was developed by the World Health Organization Quality of Life Group [42] in its Hebrew version [43] and is a measurement tool for self-reported subjective perception of people about their quality of life. The questionnaire measures four domains: Physical health, for example, "How satisfied are you with your sleep?"; psychological health, for example, "How often do you have negative feelings such as blue mood, despair, anxiety, depression?"; social relationships, for example, "How satisfied are you with your personal relationships?" and the environment, for example, "How satisfied are you with your mode of transportation?" In the current study there were 26 questions, and participants had to answer questions related to their life during the previous two weeks. Answers to

the questions were on a five-point Likert scale, where 1 represents the answers "very poor," "not at all," "not satisfied," and "never" and 5 represents the answers "very good," "largely very," "very satisfied," and "always". Each area score is calculated based on the average of the total items. The higher the score, the higher the respondent's quality of life. The reliability of the questionnaire used in our study was $\alpha = 0.94$. In addition, in this study we used ten expressions of emotions [43]: four positive items, like "excited" and "enthusiastic" and six negative items, like "worried" and "scared". The participants had to answer to what extent the emotions were felt during the previous two weeks. Answers were on a five-point Likert scale when 1 indicates "not at all" and 5 "very great extent." The reliability for positive items was $\alpha = 0.85$ and the reliability for negative items was $\alpha = 0.55$.

2.2.3. Demographic Questionnaire.
The questionnaire includes questions about gender, age, years of education, marital status, religiosity, employment, income status, and number of children. Questions about functional status of the older parents was rated by their offspring in accordance with three levels of Activity Daily Living (ADL) and Instrumental Activity Daily Living (LADL) as follows: independent—do not need help; frail—need partial help; and dependent—need full help. The offspring also answered the question about receiving homecare services under the Long Term Insurance Law (1: "yes" and 2: "no"), in addition, the offspring answered the questions concerning the caregiving of the parent, such as number of years of caregiving (1: "up to one year," 2: "2-3 years," and 3: "above 3 years"), number of days of caregiving per week (1: "every day," 2: "several days a week," and 3: "once a week"), and sharing in caregiving (1: "alone" and 2: "with family member"), and questions about the extent and frequency of caregiving assistance, such as housekeeping, transportation, shopping, financial management, and personal care and recreation and leisure (1: "does not provide assistance at all," 2: "provides nonpermanent assistance," and 3: "provides permanent assistance").

2.3. Data Analysis.
Differences in background characteristics were analyzed using chi-square and t-tests. Next, we analyzed the research hypotheses. t-tests for independent samples were calculated to examine differences between the two groups with regard to the following: (1) The total caregiver burden of offspring (12 items) and with regard to personal stress factor (9 items) and with regard to role stress factor (3 items). (2) The total quality of life (26 questions) of offspring and with regard to the four domains, physical health, psychological health, social relationships, and the environment, and to positive and negative emotions. In addition, Multivariate Analysis with Covariates test was conducted while controlling for age, gender, years of education, and functional status. t-test for independent samples was calculated to examine differences between the two groups with regard to the extent of help and frequency of actual assistance giving by offspring caregivers to their parents. Then, Spearman correlation was conducted to examine the relationship between the caregiver burden and quality of life of the offspring in the entire sample. Finally,

TABLE 1: Study sample.

Variable	Characteristic	Offspring of supportive community members (N = 55)		Offspring of not supportive community members (N = 64)		χ^2	t
		N (%)	M	N (%)	M		
Age (average, SD)			51.2, 7.319		50.1, 11.079		.664
Gender	Men	19 (34.5)		16 (25.0)		1.298	
	Women	36 (65.5)		48 (75.0)			
Marital status	Married	39 (70.9)		48 (75.0)		.252	
	Unmarried	16 (29.1)		16 (25.0)			
Years of education			13.4, 3.035		14.7, 2.561		2.39*
Level of religiosity	Secular	24 (43.6)		34 (53.1)		1.866	
	Traditional	21 (38.2)		17 (26.6)			
	Religious	10 (18.2)		13 (20.3)			
Employment status	Employed	46 (83.6)		59 (92.2)		2.084	
	Unemployed	9 (16.4)		5 (7.8)			
Income	Below average	17 (30.9)		24 (37.5)		4.844	
	Average	25 (45.5)		17 (26.6)			
	Above average	13 (23.6)		23 (35.9)			
Functional status of the parent	Independent	17 (30.9)		30 (46.9)		8.754*	
	Frail	31 (56.4)		19 (29.7)			
	Dependent	7 (12.7)		15 (23.4)			
Number of days of caregiving per week	Every day	6 (10.9)		12 (18.7)		3.021	
	Several days a week	24 (43.6)		19 (29.7)			
	Once a week	25 (45.5)		33 (51.6)			
Number of years of caregiving	Up to one year	14 (25.4)		22 (34.4)		2.163	
	2-3 years	15 (27.3)		11 (17.2)			
	Above 3 years	26 (47.3)		31 (48.4)			
Sharing in caregiving	Alone	19 (34.5)		17 (26.6)		1.147	
	With family member	36 (65.5)		47 (73.4)			
Receiving homecare services under Long Term Insurance Law	Yes	26 (47.3)		21 (32.8)		2.588	
	No	29 (52.7)		43 (67.2)			

*p < .05.

linear regression models were constructed to examine the variables that predict the total caregiver burden variable and its factors and total quality of life and its domains.

3. Results

3.1. Sociodemographic Characteristics of the Sample. Table 1 presents the sociodemographic characteristics of the participants. Marital status groups were combined into two groups, married plus living with a partner and singles plus divorced and widowed, due to the small number of participants.

The data in Table 1 show a significant correlation between the functioning status of the parent with membership in supportive community. Of the 55 members of the supportive

community 17 (30.9%) parents were functioning independently, 31 (56.4%) were frail parents, and 7 (12.7%) were dependent parents. Of the 64 who were not members, 30 (46.9%) parents were functioning independently, 19 (29.7%) were frail parents, and 15 (23.4%) were dependent parents. It should be noted that there is discrepancy between the percentage of those who are defined as frail and dependent and those who actually receive long term care services. The gap stems from the fact that the definition of the functional status of the older parents in our study was rated subjectively by their offspring while the benefits of long term insurance are based on tests. The National Insurance Institute sends professionals—a nurse or a physiotherapist—to examine the older person at home (an older person who is 90 years old

TABLE 2: Differences in burden between offspring of supportive community members ($N = 55$) and nonmembers ($N = 64$).

Variable	Factor	Group (offspring of parents of supportive community)	M	SD	t
Total burden		Members	2.05	.479	−1.46
		Nonmembers	2.18	.537	
Burden	Personal stress	Members	1.89	.427	−.73
		Nonmembers	1.97	.618	
Burden	Role stress	Members	2.50	.693	−2.40*
		Nonmembers	2.82	.724	

*$p < .05$.

TABLE 3: Differences in quality of life between offspring of supportive community members ($N = 55$) and nonmembers ($N = 64$).

Variable	Factor	Group (offspring of parents of supportive community)	Mean	SD	t
Total quality of life		Members	3.84	.450	1.18
		Nonmembers	3.74	.461	
Quality of life	Physical health	Members	3.86	.557	.60
		Nonmembers	3.80	.536	
Quality of life	Psychological health	Members	4.00	.472	2.48*
		Nonmembers	3.78	.487	
Quality of life	Social relationships	Members	3.71	.765	.48
		Nonmembers	3.65	.627	
Quality of life	Environment	Members	3.72	.478	−.07
		Nonmembers	3.73	.642	
Emotions	Positive emotions	Members	2.52	.691	−1.07
		Nonmembers	2.66	.704	
Emotions	Negative emotions	Members	2.07	.771	−2.67**
		Nonmembers	2.45	.786	

*$p < .05$; **$p < .01$.

or over may choose to undergo the functioning capacity examination by a gerontologist). Long term care services are provided only for those who are dependent on another for carrying out daily activities and not for those who only need assistance in managing a household. In addition, the entitlement depends on the income of an older person.

3.2. Caregiving Burden of Offspring, the Primary Caregivers. t-tests for independent samples were calculated to examine differences between the two groups.

Table 2 shows no differences between the groups in total caregiving burden. Examining the two factors of caregiving burden separately, a significant difference in role stress was found. Role stress burden among offspring of members of a supportive community was lower (M = 2.50, N = 55) than among offspring of nonmembers (M = 2.82, N = 64), $t = -2.40$, $p < .05$. In addition, a Multivariate Analysis with Covariates test was conducted while controlling for age, gender, years of education, and functional status. According to this analysis a significant difference was also found only with regard to the role stress burden ($F(1,117) = 4.243$, $p < .05$). Hypothesis 1 was partially confirmed.

3.3. Quality of Life among Offspring, the Primary Caregivers. t-tests for independent samples were calculated to examine differences between the two groups.

Table 3 shows that significant difference was found in the psychological domain of quality of life. Psychological health of offspring of members of a supportive community was higher (M = 4.00, N = 55) compared to offspring of non-members (M = 3.78, N = 64), $t = 2.48$, $p < .05$. With regard to the emotions variable, a significant difference was found in the negative emotions. Negative emotions of offspring of members of a supportive community were lower (M = 2.07, N = 55) compared to offspring of nonmembers (M = 2.45, N = 64), $t = -2.67$, $p < .01$. In addition, a Multivariate Analysis with Covariates test was conducted while controlling for age, gender, years of education, and functional status. According to this analysis a significant difference was also found only with regard to the psychological domain ($F(1,117) = 6.742$, $p < .05$). With regard to the emotions variable, a significant difference was also found only in the negative emotions, although the significance was lower ($F(1,117) = 5.459$, $p < .05$). Hypothesis 2 was confirmed regarding the psychological domain.

3.4. The Extent and Frequency of Caregiving. To examine whether there are differences between the groups in the extent and frequency of providing actual assistance to parents, t-tests for independent samples were calculated.

Table 4 indicates that, contrary to the hypothesis, offspring whose parents were supportive community members

TABLE 4: Differences in the extent and frequency of care between offspring of supportive community members ($N = 55$) and nonmembers ($N = 64$).

Variable	Group (offspring of parents of supportive community)	Mean	SD	t
General assistance	Members	3.17	.693	3.41***
	Nonmembers	2.72	.730	
Number of days per week	Members	2.34	.672	.12
	Nonmembers	2.32	.777	
Household chores	Members	2.60	1.69	.89
	Nonmembers	2.34	1.42	
Transportation and/or shopping	Members	3.43	1.06	1.18
	Nonmembers	3.12	1.37	
Personal care	Members	1.76	.130	.96
	Nonmembers	1.56	.973	
Financial management	Members	3.65	1.39	4.08***
	Nonmembers	2.53	1.58	
Financial assistance	Members	2.41	1.37	1.83
	Nonmembers	1.93	1.46	
Emotional support	Members	4.92	.539	3.50***
	Nonmembers	4.34	1.12	
Leisure activities	Members	4.12	1.07	2.77***
	Nonmembers	3.53	1.24	

*** $p < .001$.

gave them more general assistance and helped them more in financial management and leisure activities and supported them more emotionally than offspring whose parents were nonmembers.

3.5. The Correlation between Burden and Quality of Life.
According to the hypothesis, a negative significant correlation was found between the burden and total quality of life ($r = -.42$, $p < .001$, $N = 119$). The lower the burden was, the higher the offspring caregivers' quality of life was. In addition, a positive significant correlation has been found between the expression of negative emotions and burden ($r = 0.37$, $p < .001$, $N = 119$). The higher the burden was, the higher the expression of negative emotions was.

3.6. The Predictor Variables of Burden.
In order to examine the predictor variables of the burden and each of its factors, Stepwise Regression analysis models were conducted. The regression model introduced sociodemographic characteristics of the offspring, as well as variables related to number of years of caregiving, number of days of care per week, sharing in caregiving, functional status of the parent, receiving homecare services from Long Term Insurance Law, and membership in a supportive community.

Table 5 indicates that the income status of the offspring entered in the first step explained 5.2% of the variance in total burden, and number of days of care per week entered in the second step added 3.6% to the explained variance. The total percentage of explained variance is 8.8%. That is, lower income and more days of care per week contribute to higher total burden of offspring.

The number of days of care per week entered in the first step explained 6.3% of the variance in personal stress factor of the offspring, and income status entered in the second step added 5.8% to the explained variance; religiosity entered in the third step added 3.4% to the explained variance, and receiving homecare services from Long Term Insurance Law entered in the fourth step added 2.9% to the explained variance. The total percentage of explained variance is 18.4%. That is, having lower income, being not religious, and not receiving homecare services for the parent contribute to the higher personal stress of offspring.

In addition, membership in a supportive community was the only variable which was entered to explain role stress, and the percentage of explained variance was 4.7%.

3.7. The Predictor Variables of Quality of Life.
In order to examine the predictor variables of the quality of life and each of its domains, Stepwise Regression analyses models were conducted. The regression model introduced sociodemographic characteristics of the offspring, as well as variables related to burden, number of years of caregiving, number of days of care per week, sharing in caregiving, functional status of the parent, receiving homecare services from Long Term Insurance Law, and membership in supportive community.

Table 6 indicates that burden entered in the first step explained 16.2% of the variance in total quality of life, income status entered in the second step added 7.4% to the explained variance, and receiving homecare services from Long Term Insurance Law entered in the third step added 2.7% to the explained variance. The total percentage of explained variance is 26.3%. That is, low burden, having high income, and the parent receiving homecare services contribute to the total quality of life of offspring. Burden entered also in the

TABLE 5: Stepwise Regression predicting burden.

Model	Variables entered	B	SE	β	t	R^2
Total burden						
Step 1	Income	−.145	.057	−.227	−2.53*	.052
Step 2	Income	−.149	.057	−.234	−2.63*	.088
	Number of days of caregiving per week	−.134	.063	−.189	−2.13*	
Personal stress burden						
Step 1	Number of days of caregiving per week	−.199	.071	−.250	−2.80**	.063
Step 2	Number of days of caregiving per week	−.205	.069	−.259	−2.97**	.121
	Income	−.174	.062	−.242	−2.78**	
Step 3	Number of days of caregiving per week	−.208	.068	−.262	−3.06**	.155
	Income	−.183	.062	−.256	−2.98**	
	Religiosity	−.137	.064	−.183	−2.13*	
Step 4	Number of days of caregiving per week	−.185	.068	−.234	−2.72**	.184
	Income	−.170	.061	−.237	−2.78**	
	Religiosity	−.143	.063	−.192	−2.26*	
	Receiving homecare services	−.205	.102	−.174	−2.02*	
Role stress burden						
Step 1	Membership in supportive community	.314	.131	.217	2.40*	.047

*$p < .05$; **$p < .01$.

TABLE 6: Stepwise Regression predicting quality of life.

Model	Variables entered	B	SE	β	t	R^2
Total QoL						
Step 1	Total burden	−.358	.075	−.402	−4.75***	.162
Step 2	Total burden	−.301	.074	−.339	−4.06***	.236
	Income	.158	.047	.280	3.35***	
Step 3	Total burden	−.331	.075	−.372	−4.44***	.263
	Income	.164	.047	.290	3.52***	
	Receiving homecare services	−.158	.076	−.170	−2.07*	
Physical QoL						
Step 1	Total burden	−.453	.089	−.427	−5.10***	.182
Step 2	Total burden	−.384	.087	−.363	−4.41***	.258
	Income	.191	.055	.282	3.43***	
Step 3	Total burden	−.348	.087	−.329	−3.98***	.286
	Income	.200	.055	.296	3.64***	
	Number of days of caregiving per week	.128	.060	.170	2.12*	
Psychological QoL						
Step 1	Total burden	−.359	.082	−.376	−4.39***	.141
Step 2	Total burden	−.357	.080	−.374	−4.48***	.194
	Age of caregiver	.012	.004	.229	2.74**	
Social relationships QoL						
Step 1	Total burden	−.454	.117	−.337	−3.87***	.114
Step 2	Total burden	−.452	.115	−.336	−3.93***	.153
	Gender of caregiver	.299	.129	.197	2.31*	
Environment QoL						
Step 1	Income	.258	.061	.365	4.23***	.133
Step 2	Income	.257	.060	.363	4.29***	.169
	Sharing in caregiving	.156	.069	.191	2.26*	

Note: QoL = Quality of Life, *$p < .05$, **$p < .01$, and ***$p < .001$.

first step explained 18.2% of the variance in physical quality of life, income status entered in the second step added 7.6% to the explained variance, and number of days of care per week entered in the third step added 2.8% to the explained variance. The total percentage of explained variance is 28.6%. That is, low burden, having high income, and less days of care per week contribute to the physical quality of life of offspring. Burden entered also in the first step explained 14.1% of the variance in psychological quality of life; age of caregiver entered in the second step added 5.3% to the explained variance. The total percentage of explained variance is 19.4%. That is, low burden and being younger contribute to the psychological quality of life of offspring. Burden entered also in the first step explained 11.4% of the variance in social relationships; gender of caregiver entered in the second step added 3.9% to the explained variance. The total percentage of explained variance is 15.3%. That is, low burden and being a women contribute to the social relationships of offspring. The income status of the offspring entered in the first step explained 13.3% of the variance in environment quality of life; sharing in caregiving added 3.6% to the explained variance. The total percentage of explained variance is 16.9%. That is, higher income status and sharing in caregiving contribute to the environment quality of life of offspring.

4. Discussion

This study examined the contribution of membership in a supportive community program to reducing the feeling of burden and increasing the quality life of offspring who are primary caregivers. The results of the study provided partial support for the hypotheses.

4.1. Feeling of Burden by Offspring Caregivers.
The research hypothesis about the lower burden felt by offspring whose parents were members of a supportive community program has been confirmed regarding role stress, which consists of elements relating to the knowledge of how to take care of the older parent. Membership in the program allows offspring access to advice on professional care from a social worker, physician, or nurse whom they can consult regarding care requirements. Often this consultation takes place through the community parent who is usually the central figure in each program, and he is in close contact with the parent and aware of his condition [16]. Such consultation may contribute to reducing burden since these professionals are resources that can help bring relief to the caregiver [44]. Explaining why no significant differences were found between the groups with regard to feeling of total burden can focus on other variables that affect burden. The primary predictor of total burden and personal stress factor was income status, which also affects the total quality of life. This finding is supported by the meta-analysis conducted by Pinquart and Sörensen [22], whereby having higher income was related to better physical health of caregivers. It seems, therefore, that the feeling of burden is caused by pressures on the caregiver. He must fulfill

different roles in stressful situations resulting from conflicts that exist between caregiving duties and the demands of employment [26]. Sharing in caregiving and fewer days of caregiving per week have been also been found to reduce feelings of burden. These findings are supported by previous studies that emphasized the importance of partnership of family members with the caregiver [38]. In addition, some formal community services such as receiving homecare help the caregivers to cope with their roles. In Israel a Long Term Insurance Law was enacted in 1986 to enable older people to age in place and was also intended to help the family members in caregiving. According to this law, frail older persons receive personal care and home help by homecare workers and can also visit in day care centers [1, 18]. In accordance with previous studies [18, 44], our study shows that this variable was a predictor of personal stress; that is, accepting such assistance through a homecare worker or visits in day care centers can reduce caregiver's burden. An additional formal resource is a supportive community program which is a predictor, although in low percentage, of the pressure added by role stress. This finding is similar to the difference found between the groups, and it can be concluded that membership in a supportive community helps reduce the offspring caregivers' burden.

4.2. Quality of Life.
As expected, an inverse correlation has been found between burden and quality of life, so the lower the burden, the higher the quality of life among offspring caregivers. An examination of the differences in quality of life between the two groups found higher psychological quality of life among offspring whose parents were members, and they also expressed less negative emotions. The importance of the caregiver's psychological health was revealed in Pinquart and Sörensen's meta-analysis study [45] on differences between caregivers and noncaregivers. Their findings indicated that the largest difference between these two groups was with regard to depression symptoms while the smallest difference was in the dimension of physical health. That is to say, the burden has a far greater influence on the psychological health than on the physical health of primary caregivers. Our findings were also supported by the previous study which was conducted by Iecovich [18] in Israel. She found that the psychological quality of life of caregivers (e.g., spouses, offspring, daughters-in-law, and sons-in-law) was higher among those who care for an older family member who attended a day care center. Adult day care services center offers additional activities for older adults and interventions that help the caregivers in coping with their role and contribute to their overall well-being [39]. Similarly, a supportive community program which includes activities organized in a social club allows the older parent to participate in activities outside the home, as well as receiving in-home services [15]. These services provide help and partnership to caregivers and contribute especially in raising the psychological quality of life. However, burden linked with a negative perception of the quality of life of offspring who are primary caregivers [36]. Our research showed the same results; the regression analysis showed that burden affects quality of life.

4.3. Help Provided by the Offspring Caregivers to Their Parents.
Contrary to the hypothesis, the extent and frequency of general assistance and some other areas of assistance were higher among offspring whose parents were members of a supportive community. A possible explanation for these results is related to parents' functioning, as most frail parents (31 of 50) were members while a minority (19) were nonmembers. Hence, offspring's assistance reflected the condition of the parents who need help and most of them were members. But, in other areas of assistance such as household chores, transportation, and personal care, no differences were found between the groups. Therefore, we can conclude that the filial obligation of offspring is important in modeling their behavior towards parents even if some assistance is received from formal services. Family members are still considered a primary resource for care of the older persons, and offspring have the opportunity to repay the love they received from their parents and provide them with the assistance they need [46, 47].

However, the main focus of our study results is that membership of older parents in supportive community programs contributed to the quality of life of their offspring who are primary caregivers, mainly psychologically. Membership of older parents in supportive community also reduces the feelings of burden particularly related to role stress burden. Therefore it can be concluded that the supportive community project provides a meaningful contribution to the offspring caregivers.

This study has two main limitations. The first limitation refers to the sampling process. We used a convenience and not a large sample which therefore may not be generalizable to all offspring primary caregivers whose older parents are members of a supportive community program. It is important to further examine the point of view of the offspring primary caregivers of older parents who receive this service. The second limitation is that the study examined the questions at one point of time. It would be worthwhile to expand the research study which will review the contribution of the program to reducing burden and increasing the quality of life of the caregivers offspring at several points in time: before membership in the program, after half a year, and after a year. Also, it would be worthwhile to include more questions eliciting the offspring's opinions about the various services provided by the program and their satisfaction with the degree of connection maintained with them as the primary caregivers.

5. Conclusions

The various services that were developed in the community and available for the older persons do not replace the family members' caregiving but help the caregivers. The findings of the present study indicate some contribution of the supportive community program to the well-being of the offspring primary caregivers. That is, the role stress factor of caregiving burden was lower, and the psychological health domain of quality of life was higher among offspring whose parents were members of supportive communities. Therefore, the practical conclusion of this study is to further develop and market supportive community programs in various communities and to enable the older adults to participate in the program.

References

[1] I. Brick, "Ageing in place in Israel," *International Federation on Ageing*, vol. 7, no. 2, pp. 5–16, 2011.

[2] E. Iecovich and I. Doron, "Migrant workers in eldercare in Israel: social and legal aspects," *European Journal of Social Work*, vol. 15, no. 1, pp. 29–44, 2012.

[3] AARP Public Policy Institute, *What is Livable? Community Preferences of Older Adults*, AARP, Washington, DC, USA, 2014, http://www.aarp.org/content/dam/aarp/research/public_policy_institute/liv_com/2014/what-is-livable-report-AARP-ppi-liv-com.pdf.

[4] Israel Central Bureau of Statistics, "Statistical abstract of Israel," Tech. Rep. 65, 2014, http://www.cbs.gov.il/reader/shnatonenew_site.htm.

[5] K. Black, "Health and aging-in-place: implications for community practice," *Journal of Community Practice*, vol. 16, no. 1, pp. 79–95, 2008.

[6] Administration on Aging (AOA), "Community innovations for aging in place," 2009, http://www.aoa.gov/AoA_Programs/HCLTC/CIAIP/index.aspx#Purpose.

[7] World Health Organization (WHO), *Global Age-Friendly Cities: A Guide*, World Health Organization, Geneva, Switzerland, 2007, http://www.who.int/ageing/publications/Global_age_friendly_cities_Guide_English.pdf.

[8] A. E. Scharlach and A. J. Lehning, "Ageing-friendly communities and social inclusion in the United States of America," *Ageing and Society*, vol. 33, no. 1, pp. 110–136, 2013.

[9] N. Keating, J. Eales, and J. E. Phillips, "Age-friendly rural communities: conceptualizing 'best-fit'," *Canadian Journal on Aging*, vol. 32, no. 4, pp. 319–332, 2013.

[10] C. Paúl, O. Ribeiro, and L. Teixeira, "Active ageing: an empirical approach to the WHO model," *Current Gerontology and Geriatrics Research*, vol. 2012, 10 pages, 2012.

[11] C. Henning, U. Åhnby, and S. Österström, "Senior housing in Sweden: a new concept for aging in place," *Social Work in Public Health*, vol. 24, no. 3, pp. 235–254, 2009.

[12] A. Anttonen, J. Baldock, and J. Sipilä, Eds., *The Young, the Old and the State: Social Care Systems in Five Industrial Nations*, Edward Elgar, Cheltenham, UK, 2003.

[13] J. Costa-Font, D. Elvira, and O. Mascarilla-Miró, "'Ageing in place'? Exploring elderly people's housing preferences in Spain," *Urban Studies*, vol. 46, no. 2, pp. 295–316, 2009.

[14] A. Sixsmith and J. Sixsmith, "Ageing in place in the United Kingdom," *Ageing International*, vol. 32, no. 3, pp. 219–235, 2008.

[15] Eshel, "Supportive Community," 2014, http://www.eshelnet.org.il/files/he/Brochure/JDC-ESHEL-2014-Prospect-English.pdf.

[16] A. Berg-Warman, J. Brodsky, and Z. Gazit, "Supportive community: utilization, needs, satisfaction and contribution to members," *Gerontology*, vol. 38, no. 4, pp. 35–63, 2011.

[17] J. Brodsky, S. Resnizky, and D. Citron, *Issues in Family Care of the Elderly: Characteristics of Care, Burden on Family Members and Support Programs*, Myers-JDC-Brookdale Institute, Jerusalem, Israel, 2011, http://brookdale.jdc.org.il/_Uploads/PublicationsFiles/508-11-Issues-in-Family-Care-ES-ENG.pdf.

[18] E. Iecovich, "Caregiving burden, community services, and

quality of life of primary caregivers of frail elderly persons," *Journal of Applied Gerontology*, vol. 27, no. 3, pp. 309–330, 2008.

[19] K. Schumacher, C. A. Beck, and J. M. Marren, "Family caregivers: caring for older adults, working with their families," *American Journal of Nursing*, vol. 106, no. 8, pp. 40–50, 2006.

[20] M. Silverstein, S. J. Conroy, H. Wang, R. Giarrusso, and V. L. Bengtsor, "Reciprocity in parent-child relations over the adult life course," *Journals of Gerontology—Series B Psychological Sciences and Social Sciences*, vol. 57, no. 1, pp. S3–S13, 2002.

[21] M. E. Szinovacz and A. Davey, "Prevalence and predictors of change in adult-child primary caregivers," *International Journal of Aging and Human Development*, vol. 76, no. 3, pp. 227–249, 2013.

[22] M. Pinquart and S. Sörensen, "Correlates of physical health of informal caregivers: a meta-analysis," *The Journals of Gerontology, Series B: Psychological Sciences and Social Sciences*, vol. 62, no. 2, pp. P126–P137, 2007.

[23] E. Papastavrou, A. Kalokerinou, S. S. Papacostas, H. Tsangari, and P. Sourtzi, "Caring for a relative with dementia: family caregiver burden," *Journal of Advanced Nursing*, vol. 58, no. 5, pp. 446–457, 2007.

[24] V. G. Cicirelli, "Attachment and obligation as daughters' motives for caregiving behavior and subsequent effect on subjective burden," *Psychology & Aging*, vol. 8, no. 2, pp. 144–155, 1993.

[25] C. S. Aneshensel, L. I. Parlin, J. T. Mullan, S. H. Zarit, and C. J. Whitlatch, *Profiles in Caregiving: The Unexpected Career*, Academic Press, San Diego, Calif, USA, 1995.

[26] A. S. Wharton and M. Blair-Loy, "Long work hours and family life. A cross-national study of employees' concerns," *Journal of Family Issues*, vol. 27, no. 3, pp. 415–436, 2006.

[27] C. Bamford, B. Gregson, G. Farrow et al., "Mental and physical frailty in older people: the costs and benefits of informal care," *Ageing and Society*, vol. 18, no. 3, pp. 317–354, 1998.

[28] M. Pinquart and S. Sörensen, "Ethnic differences in stressors, resources, and psychological outcomes of family caregiving: a meta-analysis," *The Gerontologist*, vol. 45, no. 1, pp. 90–106, 2005.

[29] M. Navaie-Waliser, A. Spriggs, and P. H. Feldman, "Informal caregiving: differential experiences by gender," *Medical Care*, vol. 40, no. 12, pp. 1249–1259, 2002.

[30] M. Pinquart and S. Sörensen, "Gender differences in caregiver stressors, social resources, and health: an updated meta-analysis," *Journals of Gerontology—Series B Psychological Sciences and Social Sciences*, vol. 61, no. 1, pp. P33–P45, 2006.

[31] L. Gallicchio, N. Siddiqi, P. Langenberg, and M. Baumgarten, "Gender differences in burden and depression among informal caregivers of demented elders in the community," *International Journal of Geriatric Psychiatry*, vol. 17, no. 2, pp. 154–163, 2002.

[32] O. Gilbar, "Gender as a predictor of burden and psychological distress of elderly husbands and wives of cancer patients," *Psycho-Oncology*, vol. 8, no. 4, pp. 287–294, 1999.

[33] S. R. Beach, R. Schulz, J. L. Yee, and S. Jackson, "Negative and positive health effects of caring for a disabled spouse: longitudinal findings from the caregiver health effects study," *Psychology and Aging*, vol. 15, no. 2, pp. 259–271, 2000.

[34] G. J. Heo and G. Koeske, "The role of religious coping and race in Alzheimer's disease caregiving," *Journal of Applied Gerontology*, vol. 32, no. 5, pp. 582–604, 2013.

[35] L. A. Rathier, J. D. Davis, G. D. Papandonatos, C. Grover, and G. Tremont, "Religious coping in caregivers of family members with dementia," *Journal of Applied Gerontology*, vol. 28, article 24, 2013.

[36] E.-M. Merz, H.-J. Schulze, and C. Schuengel, "Consequences of filial support for two generations: a narrative and quantitative review," *Journal of Family Issues*, vol. 31, no. 11, pp. 1530–1554, 2010.

[37] P. S. Jones, B. W. Winslow, J. W. Lee, M. Burns, and X. E. Zhang, "Development of a caregiver empowerment model to promote positive outcomes," *Journal of Family Nursing*, vol. 17, no. 1, pp. 11–28, 2011.

[38] L. D. Clyburn, M. J. Stones, T. Hadjistavropoulos, and H. Tuokko, "Predicting caregiver burden and depression in Alzheimer's disease," *Journal of Gerontology: Social Sciences*, vol. 55, pp. S1–S13, 2000.

[39] N. L. Fields, K. A. Anderson, and H. Dabelko-Schoeny, "The effectiveness of adult day services for older adults: a review of the literature from 2000 to 2011," *Journal of Applied Gerontology*, vol. 33, no. 2, pp. 130–163, 2014.

[40] M. Bédard, D. W. Molloy, L. Squire, S. Dubois, J. A. Lever, and M. O'Donnell, "The Zarit Burden Interview: a new short version and screening version," *Gerontologist*, vol. 41, no. 5, pp. 652–657, 2001.

[41] Y. G. Bachner and L. Ayalon, "Initial examination of the psychometric properties of the short Hebrew version of the Zarit Burden Interview," *Gerontology & Geriatrics*, vol. 39, no. 4, pp. 15–26, 2012 (Hebrew).

[42] The WHOQOL Group, "Development of the World Health Organization WHOQOL-BREF quality of life assessment," *Psychological Medicine*, vol. 28, no. 3, pp. 551–558, 1998.

[43] Y. Ben Ya'acov and M. Amir, "Subjective quality of life: definition and measurement according to the World Health Organization," *Gerontology*, vol. 28, no. 3-4, pp. 155–168, 2001 (Hebrew).

[44] H. Greenberger and H. Litwin, "Can burdened caregivers be effective facilitators of elder care-recipient health care?" *Journal of Advanced Nursing*, vol. 41, no. 4, pp. 332–341, 2003.

[45] M. Pinquart and S. Sörensen, "Differences between caregivers and noncaregivers in psychological health and physical health: a meta-analysis," *Psychology and Aging*, vol. 18, no. 2, pp. 250–267, 2003.

[46] F. Hoffmann and R. Rodrigues, "Informal carers. Who takes care of them? Policy brief, European Centre for Social Welfare Policy and Research," 2010, http://www.euro.centre.org/data/1274190382_99603.pdf.

[47] E. Grundy and J. C. Henretta, "Between elderly parents and adult children: a new look at the intergenerational care provided by the 'sandwich generation'," *Ageing & Society*, vol. 26, no. 5, pp. 707–722, 2006.

6

It Is Always on Your Mind: Experiences and Perceptions of Falling of Older People and Their Carers and the Potential of a Mobile Falls Detection Device

Veronika Williams,[1] **Christina R. Victor,**[2] **and Rachel McCrindle**[3]

[1] *Primary Care Clinical Trials Unit, Department of Primary Care Health Sciences, 23-38 Hythe Bridge Street, Oxford OX1 2ET, UK*
[2] *Gerontology and Public Health, School of Health Sciences and Social Care, Brunel University, Uxbridge, Middlesex UB8 3PH, UK*
[3] *Computer and Human Interaction, School of Systems Engineering, University of Reading, Reading RG6 6AY, UK*

Correspondence should be addressed to Christina R. Victor; christina.victor@brunel.ac.uk

Academic Editor: Abebaw Yohannes

Background. Falls and fear of falling present a major risk to older people as both can affect their quality of life and independence. Mobile assistive technologies (AT) fall detection devices may maximise the potential for older people to live independently for as long as possible within their own homes by facilitating early detection of falls. *Aims*. To explore the experiences and perceptions of older people and their carers as to the potential of a mobile falls detection AT device. *Methods*. Nine focus groups with 47 participants including both older people with a range of health conditions and their carers. Interviews were audio recorded, transcribed verbatim, and thematically analysed. *Results*. Four key themes were identified relating to participants' experiences and perceptions of falling and the potential impact of a mobile falls detector: cause of falling, falling as everyday vulnerability, the environmental context of falling, and regaining confidence and independence by having a mobile falls detector. *Conclusion*. The perceived benefits of a mobile falls detector may differ between older people and their carers. The experience of falling has to be taken into account when designing mobile assistive technology devices as these may influence perceptions of such devices and how older people utilise them.

1. Introduction

The term assistive technologies (AT) covers a wide range of aids and devices designed to support older people with chronic long-term health conditions, disabilities or cognitive impairments to live at home independently. Included within the remit of AT is a plethora of devices ranging from simple mobility aids to complex computer based medical devices. Contemporary technological developments mean that mobile assistive technology (AT) devices have considerable potential—in theory at least—to contribute to the goal of enabling older people to live independently for as long as possible within their own homes by providing a range of support and alert services such as falls detection [1, 2]. Falls are a major public health problem in terms of their prevalence, morbidity, and mortality: additionally falls and

fear of falling can significantly compromise the independence and quality of life of older people [3, 4]. There are a range of studies examining the detailed epidemiology of falls, potential prevention of falls, and exploring older peoples' views on falls prevention advice [5–7]. In addition, previous research into falling has aimed to develop new interventions to detect those at risk of falling, rehabilitate those who have fallen, and minimise the consequences of falls in terms of both reducing morbidity (by providing hip protectors) or reducing the time that an older person is on floor following a fall and before help arrives [5, 8–10]. In terms of falls prevention activity and interventions we can identify strategies that focus upon primary prevention (preventing falls from happening by addressing key risk factors and identifying those most "at risk"); secondary prevention (detecting falls promptly and reducing resultant injuries and other negative outcomes) and tertiary prevention (reducing the mortality/morbidity resultant from falls by prompt and effective treatment of key injuries such as hip fracture).

We can distinguish two distinct aspects of falls prevention and management where AT has a potential contribution to make: technologies that aim to prevent falls from occurring and those which focus upon the identification and notification of falls in order to reduce negative outcomes. These later devices are commonly termed "falls detectors/falls alarms" and form the focus of this paper. Such devices constitute an established assistive technology focussing upon secondary prevention whereby older people who have fallen can be identified and help summoned quickly to reduce the consequences of "long lies" on the floor [10]. The significance of these consequences should not be underestimated. It is estimated that approximately one-third of older people who fall are undetected for at least an hour [10]; there is a relationship between recovery time and the duration of the undetected lie with one study reporting that half of those who are on the floor for an hour will die within 6 months [11]. Ward et al. [12] distinguish between "generations" of falls detectors based upon the nature of the device (reactive versus proactive) and the degree of embedded intelligence within the system using the typology devised by Martin et al. [13]. First-generation falls detectors are the "traditional" falls alarm which is worn by the user and can be used to summon help in an emergency from a support centre 24 hours a day. However, these devices are entirely "reactive" and older people may not wear them as prescribed or use them in the event of an emergency [14] and many AT devices prescribed to older people or bought for them are often not appropriately used or have a low uptake [15]. In addition, these alarms usually only work within the indoor environment, and as previous research has identified there is a particular risk of older people falling outdoors due to environmental factors such as uneven pavements and weather conditions [16] as well as older peoples' fear of falling outdoors [17, 18]. For these reasons first generation falls alarm systems do not meet the needs of older people.

One response to the problems with first-generation falls monitoring devices has been the development of second-generation falls detection devices which employ embedded triaxial accelerometry to identify a fall. Whilst still reactive in nature, the use of accelerometry means that the older person does not have to activate the device. By combining data on posture, velocity, and impact the device can detect that a fall has occurred and will automatically alert the monitoring station. Such devices carry both technological challenges as well as those of acceptance by older people. Older people fall for many reasons [5], and falls may be of several types such as "heavy" falls (rapid loss of verticality), soft falls (person holds themselves up by a piece of furniture, for example, and syncopal falls (falls associated with or resulting from a loss of full consciousness) [19].

This leads to challenges and debates about the sensitivity/specificity of the different algorithms used to detect falls [20] and associated with this minimisation of the number of false negative and false positive detections. Evaluating both sensitivity and specificity is clearly important as, in order for older people to feel secure when using falls detectors, they need to be assured that they are reliable. However, due to the nature of falls, much of this proof is undertaken within laboratory situations. Illustrative of this approach is the paper by Lee and Carlisle [21] which provides proof of concept for a mobile device based upon accelerometry to detect falls events in a laboratory setting, using "young" volunteers to evaluate the sensitivity and specificity of falls detection. Based upon this evidence Lee and Carlisle then go onto to speculate that such devices are acceptable to older people in both theory and in practice. Yet, the types of device reported by Lee and Carlisle [21] have been primarily tested in laboratories with regard to reliability and performance and often with younger people rather than the intended "end users." The capabilities of these devices for falls detection or vital signs monitoring are usually determined by the identification of the "key threats" to older peoples' independence externally that is by the analysis of epidemiological evidence or the importance of factors such as falls for health service costs rather than identifying firsthand the issues that matter most to older people. Given that use of simple alarm devices is far from universal and has limited evidence for effectiveness, there remains a knowledge deficit with regard to the acceptability of these more complex second-generation fall detection and alarm services to older people and their carers.

In this paper, we report the findings from a series of nine focus groups we conducted to (a) explore the experience and perceptions of falling amongst older people (b) explore their views of a wrist-worn AT device that could detect falls, and (c) raise broader issues about the use of mobile AT for use with older people with a particular focus on falls detection services. Our study formed part of a larger EU Framework 6 project "ENABLE—A Wearable System Supporting Service to Enable Older People to Live Well, Independently and at Ease" [22].

The ENABLE project aimed to design, develop, and test a wrist-worn device which was able to support a range of functions to support older people to live at home independently including event reminders (e.g., to take medication or attend a GP or hospital appointment), navigation and identification of a users location via GPS, control of appliances and other devices around the home, a health monitoring system, and a falls detection function which is the focus of this paper. The wrist-worn device was integrated with a mobile phone, enabling the user to get out and about, for visiting, shopping, recreation, and so forth, whilst maintaining contact for help and services [23].

ENABLE was a collaborative project between universities, voluntary/charitable groups for older people in Greece, Belgium, Czech Republic, and several AT companies. Design and development of the ENABLE device was highly user-centric with older people being involved at all stages of the system lifecycle. Central to the project was the requirement to identify the concerns and needs of older people and their carers during the concept proofing and development phases. This was achieved in two ways. A survey was undertaken across 4 EU countries (Belgium, Czech Republic, Greece, and the UK) to determine the general views of older people and their carers towards a wearable AT device and to determine the functions they would like to see provided in the device [23]. From the survey falls were identified by participants as a major concern and falls detection seen as an important element of any such device. The focus groups described in this paper were then undertaken to explore in more detail issues around falls and if (and how) an AT device could help, as well as to elicit participants' views on the device being worn on the wrist (the most favoured option in the quantitative survey).

2. Methods

2.1. Recruitment. To meet our objectives and generate focus groups who could evaluate the device functions and wearability from their experience, we recruited participants who were vulnerable to falling or the fear of falling. We invited potential participants from a number of settings, such as charity run self-help groups (Parkinson's Disease Society, Local Association for the Blind, Stroke Association), sheltered housing associations where vulnerability to falls would be expected among such groups. In addition, participants from a university research cohort of older adults were recruited in order to gain the views of those who may not currently be vulnerable to falls/fear of falling but may be so in the future. Attendees at these groups/members of the University cohort were provided with an information leaflet and reply slip to respond to the research team directly should they be interested in taking part in the study. We then provided further details and interested participants were invited to the focus groups. At the focus group meetings participants gave written consent to participate and to the recording of the group interview.

2.2. Data Collection. Data were collected between June and August 2008. The focus groups took place in community settings convenient to participants and were formed on the basis of recruitment site; that is, participants recruited from a stroke self-help group formed a focus group; people recruited from a vision impairment group formed another. Keeping our groups homogenous in the shared disability/chronic condition encouraged discussion of benefits and difficulties such a device may have in relation to specific impairments such as stroke or visual impairment, as well as being able to identify general issues relating to using a wearable AT falls detection device.

A prepared interview guide was used to ask participants about the difficulties they faced on a daily basis. They were then introduced to a "mock up" of the mobile AT device which would incorporate falls detection and alert services. Participants were asked about their views on the overall appearance and aesthetics of the device (including weight, size, comfort of wearing it); usability/interface (including size of buttons/screen, font size, and style of text); and overall potential challenges and opportunities such a device might bring. This paper focuses upon the potential benefits or challenges the use of this type of falls detector could bring to the lives of older people rather than on the aesthetics of the device.

Focus group interviews lasted between 35 and 50 minutes. Informed consent was taken from all participants prior to focus groups interviews and all focus groups were audiorecorded.

2.3. Data Analysis. Focus group interviews were transcribed verbatim from audio recordings. The software package Atlas.ti was used to store and organise data as well as facilitate the analytical process. Transcripts were analysed using a thematic analysis approach whereby data were coded into short phrases/codes, encapsulating what a particular section of data conveyed [24]. These codes were then collated to explore themes of importance to participants. Emergent themes and interpretations were discussed between the authors and any differences in interpretation resolved by discussion.

3. Findings

3.1. Participants. We conducted nine focus groups, with a total of 47 individual participants, (27 women and 20 men with an age range of 58–91 years) in the South East of England, UK (see Table 1). These groups included healthy older volunteers, older people with a range of chronic conditions and disabilities and their carers to ensure that the views of a broad range of potential users were captured.

3.2. Experience of Falling: Focus Group Themes. Four key themes were identified relating to participants' experiences and perceptions of falling and the potential impact of a mobile falls detector: (1) cause of falling; (2) falling as an everyday vulnerability; (3) environmental context of falling; and (4) mobile fall detection device: reassurance and independence. These themes are presented in a model to illustrate how a mobile falls detection service may impact on older peoples' experience of falling across a number of different domains (see Figure 1).

3.3. Cause of Falling. If we are to successfully intervene, either by the development of AT devices or other programmes, to reduce falls amongst older people, it is vital that researchers understand how older people experience falls. A key narrative from our focus groups was centred on participants' understanding of the "causes" of falling. There is a consensus in the academic literature that falls are multifactorial in nature and relate to a range of intrinsic and extrinsic risk factors. In this study, participants' views on the potential cause of either their own risk, or someone close to them, falling focussed upon the causes of falling being related to pathology.

This was classified as being related to either the onset of ageing or as part of a specific disease process:

> *Especially for people with Parkinson's, because we do fall and very often (FG9).*

> *One of the problems that as you get older you do fall (FG8).*

Thus, participants in focus groups with no specific chronic illness or disability characterised ageing and/or growing older as the cause of falling. Falls were seen as a normal

TABLE 1: Participant characteristics.

	Age range	Gender	Disability/Chronic illness	Living setup
FG1	55–80 years	1 woman, 3 men	Stroke	All with partner/spouse
FG2	68–89 years	4 women, 2 men	Vision impaired	Unknown
FG3	73–88 years	5 women, 2 men	Mild dementia, vascular disease, Parkinson's disease	On own: 3, with partner/spouse/relative: 4
FG4	64–98 years	2 women, 2 men	Arthritis, Parkinson's disease	On own: 4
FG5	62–85 years	2 women, 3 men	None	On own: 2, with partner/spouse: 3
FG6	65–76 years	4 women, 3 men	Arthritis, hearing impaired	All live with partner/spouse
FG7	54–77 years	4 women, 3 men	Parkinson's Disease, stroke	All live with partner/spouse
FG8	72–84 years	3 women, 1 man	Arthritis	All on own
FG9	63–66 years	2 women, 1 man	Parkinson's disease	On own: 1, with partner/spouse: 2

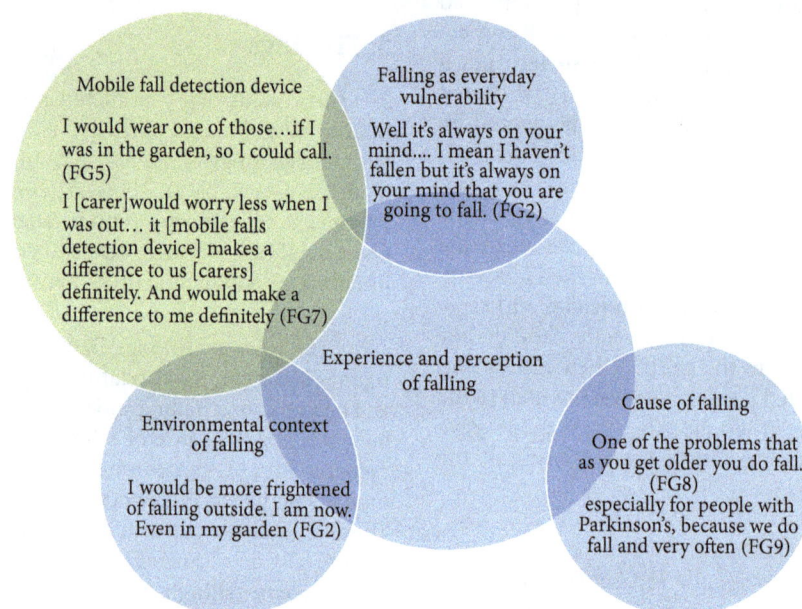

FIGURE 1: Experience of falling amongst older people and potential impact of mobile falls detection device.

consequence of growing old. This contrasts to participants in a predominately "chronic illness/disability" focus group, who related their experience of falling to their specific health condition but not to the more generic process of growing older.

3.4. Falling as Everyday Vulnerability. Participants perceived falling as an "everyday" vulnerability alongside other factors such as living alone or increasing frailty. Falls were seen as especially pernicious in terms of increasing vulnerability reflecting their consequences which were apparent to both "fallers" and those who knew of someone who had experienced a fall. The vulnerability conferred by the real or perceived risk of falling was heightened by the lone living circumstances of many older people, with those who reported living on their own, expressing a fear of falling and this being undetected for long periods of time resulting in "long lies" on the floor. A clear advantage of the AT falls detector was that it could summon help quickly without the need for the older person to activate the system thereby reducing the risk of "long lies" in contrast to the first generation system which required the faller to activate the system:

> I think that's brilliant, no I think that's a good idea, especially for people with Parkinsons because we do fall and very often when we fall we freeze. So we are not going to press any buttons on the phone or anything else (FG9).

> My observation of that system is that when my sister did fall she was so shocked by the fall. She was outside on a frosty night that she forgot to use it (FG5/6).

3.5. Environmental Context of Falling. A key limitation of first-generation falls detectors is that they are limited to the user's home. Similarly the developments of domestic adaptation such as "smart" carpets that can detect falls do not extend beyond the domestic environment. The environmental context of falling was of particular interest as it linked to the previous theme of vulnerability, whilst also being identified as one "threat" that the proposed mobile falls detector could potentially remediate. Whilst the feared consequences of falls inside and outside the home were similar, the incapacity to get back up unassisted and inability to alert a carer or help centre meant that falls outside the home were seen as potentially more problematic as they were beyond the scope of conventional falls detection devices:

> I would wear one of those things, just in case. If I was in the garden, so I could call (FG5/6).

> Something which would tell, feed your location back to wherever, because if you've gone out for a walk and tripped and fallen down it would be useful to presumably the carer would like to know that you have fallen and go and help you. To know where you are to be helped (FG5/6).

3.6. Mobile Fall Detection Device: Reassurance and Independence. With the current state of technology both first- and second-generation falls detectors require the older person to wear them and, in the case of first-generation systems, activate them in the event of a fall. Those participants who had a "traditional" falls alarm reported that they did not always wear it but that they would wear a mobile device since it would work outside as well as within their home. Indeed, when talking about the potential mobile falls detector, participants felt the main benefit of such a device would be its ability to detect falls both inside and outside the home and alert the appropriate person without the faller needing to activate the system which was a disadvantage of first-generation devices:

> Most people who fall over, it can happen you can knock yourself out. It can happen and there is no way round that. Most of the time, nine times out of ten they can press the button (FG7).

> I am sure my wife would appreciate it (the AT falls detection device) . . . Then she would know if I have fallen down like in the area where we are living, you know, she will know that I have fallen down in the garden of the house where I live (FG3).

> . . . two doors away the women there she's fallen getting out of bed and fell against the radiator. It wasn't until a couple of days later that we discovered that she'd fallen. She couldn't activate anything (FG8).

The ability of the Enable device to trigger an automatic alarm when a fall was detected, was perceived as a great benefit by both the older person and carers, and as offering a clear advantage over the tradition falls alarm system, which has to be activated by the older person.

4. Discussion

This exploratory study provides insights into how older people, who are engaged with new technologies, perceive

a wrist-worn AT device for falls detection and its potential benefits and disadvantages. Whilst there are studies looking at AT more generally [25] or at first-generation falls detectors previous studies of second-generation falls detectors have predominantly been undertaken with younger people or, if they have included older people, have not been engaged with the perspectives of their carer(s) [12].

For carers the major advantage of the device was focussed around the notion of reassurance, and this finding is supported by previous research into the perceived benefits of telehealth and assistive technology solutions [26, 27]. Older people living with a chronic illness or disability identified improvements in wellbeing and potential enhanced safety afforded by the emergency and medical functions as the key advantages of the device in early evaluations of telehealth and assistive technological devices [28, 29].

Previous research into a number of assistive technology devices including hearing aids [29], emergency alarm pendants [30], and falls detectors [31] found that participants were reluctant to wear the device during waking hours because of the physical attributes of the devices and perception of social stigmatisation. As one of participants in FG5 stated "*but you see if they have a fall as you say with a pendant, they can always take them off.*" There are other reasons for lack of use of fall detectors including concern for invasion of privacy [32–34]. It has also been reported that some users avoid wearing their fall detector as it is uncomfortable or produces false alarms [15, 35]. Brownsell and Hawley [31] suggested that some older people may not be inclined to adopt a product that would alert their informal and formal carers to falls, fearing institutionalisation. The lack of control over whether an alert is sent has also been postulated to be a factor affecting fall detector use as users do not want to "bother" anyone [15].

Whilst the participants in our study did not voice any concerns regarding being stigmatised when wearing an AT device, they did express issues around vulnerability, when wearing the device in public, which is diametrically opposed to the devices aim of increasing perceived reassurance and safety. Parker et al. [22] also found that older people were concerned about the requirement to wear a sensor at all times and the constant monitoring of their movement, due to anxieties regarding invasion of personal privacy. Our data indicate that older people perceived that the wrist-worn falls detector could address two key deficiencies in traditional falls alarms: overcoming the limitation of devices that only work indoors and the vulnerability resultant from falling and being unable to summon help (which the device can do outside and automatically). However, if the older person does not perceive that they are at risk of falling and, therefore, in need of a fall detector, then, no matter how good the technology is, it will not be adopted. Including potential end users in the development of an AT device and obtaining feedback on the device throughout the development cycle can contribute significantly to ensuring a user-friendly design and the fact that end users' needs and concerns are taken into consideration, thus potentially improving uptake rates and adherence to such devices [36].

5. Conclusion

We fully acknowledge the limitations of our data which were collected as part of a larger project exploring the perceptions and views of older people and their carers on a specific device rather than exploring their attitudes to assistive technology and telehealth in general. Participants were volunteers who were existing mobile phone users and as such may not reflect the use of current technologies amongst the general older population, particularly the oldest old or those with severe disabilities. However, using the example of a falls detection system, we have demonstrated that although laboratory-based evaluations of such devices can be technically successful, the acceptability of such devices to older people cannot simply be extrapolated from such trials. Such technology raises concerns amongst older people, which need to be considered in order to ensure that the objectives of AT devices can be achieved. Furthermore, we have demonstrated that carers and older people articulate different perspectives upon such systems. Carers are seeking reassurance from such devices, but this may be achieved at the cost of increasing the perceived vulnerability and loss of privacy of older people. Further work is required in order to ensure that the voices of older people and their carers are central to the development of technologies to enable older people to live at home independently.

Ethics Approval

The study was approved by the University of Reading Research Ethics Committee (ref no. 07/33).

Acknowledgments

This study (2007–2010) was funded in part by the European Commission in the 6th Framework Programme (Project no.: 045 563). Partners are AT: fortec—Vienna University of Technology—IS, KII—Kompetenznetzwerk Information-stechnologie zur Förderung der Integration von Menschen mit Behinderungen; ES: ARTEC; UK: Docobo Ltd., Cardionetics Ltd., University of Reading; CZ: Zivot 90; SP: Code Factory Ltd.; GR: E-Isotis, BE: Vzw Cassiers Wzc; Website http://www.aat.tuwien.ac.at/enable/index_en.html. The authors would like to thank Julie Barnett for her help with collecting the data and all our participants for taking part in the focus group interviews.

References

[1] M. Brignell, R. Wootton, and L. Gray, "The application of telemedicine to geriatric medicine," Age and Ageing, vol. 36, no. 4, pp. 369–374, 2007.

[2] C. M. Blaschke, P. P. Freddolino, and E. E. Mullen, "Ageing and technology: a review of the research literature," The British Journal of Social Work, vol. 39, no. 4, pp. 641–656, 2009.

[3] N. Noury, P. Rumeau, A. K. Bourke, G. ÓLaighin, and J. E. Lundy, "A proposal for the classification and evaluation of fall detectors," IRBM, vol. 29, no. 6, pp. 340–349, 2008.

[4] N. Deshpande, E. J. Metter, F. Lauretani, S. Bandinelli, J. Guralnik, and L. Ferrucci, "Activity restriction induced by fear of falling and objective and subjective measures of physical function: a prospective cohort study," Journal of the American Geriatrics Society, vol. 56, no. 4, pp. 615–620, 2008.

[5] L. Z. Rubenstein, "Falls in older people: epidemiology, risk factors and strategies for prevention," Age and Ageing, vol. 35, no. 2, pp. ii37–ii41, 2006.

[6] L. Yardley, M. Donovan-Hall, K. Francis, and C. Todd, "Older people's views of advice about falls prevention: a qualitative study," Health Education Research, vol. 21, no. 4, pp. 508–517, 2006.

[7] A. J. Campbell and M. C. Robertson, "Rethinking individual and community fall prevention strategies: a meta-regression comparing single and multifactorial interventions," Age and Ageing, vol. 36, no. 6, pp. 656–662, 2007.

[8] P. Kannus, J. Parkkari, S. Niemi et al., "Prevention of hip fracture in elderly people with use of a hip protector," The New England Journal of Medicine, vol. 343, no. 21, pp. 1506–1513, 2000.

[9] A. Drahota, D. Gal, and J. Windsor, "Flooring as an intervention to reduce injuries from falls in healthcare settings: an overview," Quality in ageing, vol. 8, no. 1, pp. 3–9, 2007.

[10] J. Fleming and C. Brayne, "Inability to get up after falling, subsequent time on floor, and summoning help: prospective cohort study in people over 90," The British Medical Journal, vol. 337, Article ID a2227, 2008.

[11] D. Wild, U. S. L. Nayak, and B. Isaacs, "How dangerous are falls in old people at home?" The British Medical Journal, vol. 282, no. 6260, pp. 266–268, 1981.

[12] G. Ward, N. Holliday, S. Fielden, and S. Williams, "Fall detectors: a review of the literature," Journal of Assistive Technologies, vol. 6, no. 3, pp. 202–215, 2012.

[13] S. Martin, G. Kelly, W. G. Kernohan, B. McCreight, and C. Nugent, Smart Home Technologies for Health and Social Care Support, John Wiley & Sons, Chichester, UK, 2008.

[14] M. Johnson, A. George, and D. T. Tran, "Analysis of falls incidents: nurse and patient preventive behaviours," International Journal of Nursing Practice, vol. 17, no. 1, pp. 60–66, 2011.

[15] K. Horton, "Falls in older people: the place of telemonitoring in rehabilitation," Journal of Rehabilitation Research and Development, vol. 45, no. 8, pp. 1183–1194, 2008.

[16] W. Li, T. H. M. Keegan, B. Sternfeld, S. Sidney, C. P. Quesenberry Jr., and J. L. Kelsey, "Outdoor falls among middle-aged and older adults: a neglected public health problem," The American Journal of Public Health, vol. 96, no. 7, pp. 1192–1200, 2006.

[17] G. J. Wijlhuizen, R. de Jong, and M. Hopman-Rock, "Older persons afraid of falling reduce physical activity to prevent outdoor falls," Preventive Medicine, vol. 44, no. 3, pp. 260–264, 2007.

[18] M. Rantakokko, M. Mänty, S. Iwarsson et al., "Fear of moving outdoors and development of outdoor walking difficulty in older people: clinical Investigations," Journal of the American Geriatrics Society, vol. 57, no. 4, pp. 634–640, 2009.

[19] J. Pigniez, "Fall detection technologies for the elderly," Executive Summary for French National Health at Home Center, 2013, http://www.gerontechnology.com/fall-detection-technologies-for-the-elderly-2/316619.

[20] F. Bagalà, C. Becker, A. Cappello et al., "Evaluation of accelerometer-based fall detection algorithms on real-world falls," *PLoS ONE*, vol. 7, no. 5, Article ID e37062, 2012.

[21] R. Y. W. Lee and A. J. Carlisle, "Detection of falls using accelerometers and mobile phone technology," *Age and Ageing*, vol. 40, no. 6, pp. 690–696, 2011.

[22] S. Parker, G. Nussbaum, H. Sonntag et al., "Computers helping people with special needs: lecture notes in computer science," in *ENABLE—A View on User's Needs*, K. Miesenberger, J. Klaus, W. Zagler, and A. Karshmer, Eds., pp. 1016–1023, Springer, Berlin, Germany, 2008.

[23] R. J. McCrindle, V. M. Williams, C. R. Victor et al., "Wearable device to assist independent living," *International Journal on Disability and Human Development*, vol. 10, no. 4, pp. 349–354, 20112011.

[24] J. Ritchie and J. Lewis, *Qualitative Research Practice*, Sage, Thousand Oaks, Calif, USA, 2006.

[25] A. Tinker, "Assistive technology and its role in housing policies for older people," *Quality in Ageing and Older Adults*, vol. 4, no. 2, pp. 4–12, 2003.

[26] S. Cahill, E. Begley, J. P. Faulkner, and I. Hagen, "'It gives me a sense of independence'—findings from Ireland on the use and usefulness of assistive technology for people with dementia," *Technology and Disability*, vol. 19, no. 2-3, pp. 133–142, 2007.

[27] A. Bowes and G. McColgan, *Smart Technology and Community Care for Older People: Innovation in West Lothian*, Age Concern Scotland, Glasgow, UK, 2006.

[28] N. Goodwin, "The state of telehealth and telecare in the UK: prospects for integrated care," *Journal of Integrated Care*, vol. 18, no. 6, pp. 3–10, 2010.

[29] K. Shinohara and J. Wobbock, "In the shadow of misperception: assistive technology use and social interactions," in *Proceedings of the SIGCHI Conference on Human Factors in Computing Systems (CHI '11)*, Vancouver, Canada, 2011.

[30] A. Dickenson, J. Goodman, A. Syme et al., "Domesticating technology. In-home requirements gathering with frail older people," in *Proceedings of the 10th International Conference on Human-Computer Interaction (HCI '03)*, vol. 4, pp. 827–831, 2003.

[31] S. Brownsell and M. S. Hawley, "Automatic fall detectors and the fear of falling," *Journal of Telemedicine and Telecare*, vol. 10, no. 5, pp. 262–266, 2004.

[32] K. Doughty, K. Cameron, and P. Garner, "Three generations of telecare of the elderly," *Journal of Telemedicine and Telecare*, vol. 2, no. 2, pp. 71–80, 1996.

[33] F. G. Miskelly, "Assistive technology in elderly care," *Age and Ageing*, vol. 30, no. 6, pp. 455–458, 2001.

[34] J. Gatward, "Electronic assistive technology: benefits for all?" *Housing, Care & Support*, vol. 7, no. 4, pp. 13–17, 2004.

[35] G. Williams, K. Doughty, and D. A. Bradley, "Safety and risk issues in using telecare," *Journal of Telemedicine and Telecare*, vol. 6, no. 5, pp. 249–262, 2000.

[36] J. K. Seale, C. McCreadie, A. Turner-Smith, and A. Tinker, "Older people as partners in assistive technology research: the use of focus groups in the design process," *Technology and Disability*, vol. 14, no. 1, pp. 21–29, 2002.

The Simplified Acute Physiology Score III Is Superior to the Simplified Acute Physiology Score II and Acute Physiology and Chronic Health Evaluation II in Predicting Surgical and ICU Mortality in the "Oldest Old"

Aftab Haq,[1] Sachin Patil,[2] Alexis Lanteri Parcells,[1] and Ronald S. Chamberlain[1,2,3]

[1] Saint George's University School of Medicine, West Indies, Grenada
[2] Department of Surgery, Saint Barnabas Medical Center, Livingston, NJ, USA
[3] Department of Surgery, University of Medicine and Dentistry of New Jersey (UMDNJ), 94 Old Short Hills Road Livingston, Newark, NJ 07039, USA

Correspondence should be addressed to Ronald S. Chamberlain; rchamberlain@barnabashealth.org

Academic Editor: Giuseppe Zuccala

Elderly patients in the USA account for 26–50% of all intensive care unit (ICU) admissions. The applicability of validated ICU scoring systems to predict outcomes in the "Oldest Old" is poorly documented. We evaluated the utility of three commonly used ICU scoring systems (SAPS II, SAPS III, and APACHE II) to predict clinical outcomes in patients > 90 years. 1,189 surgical procedures performed upon 951 patients > 90 years (between 2000 and 2010) were analyzed. SAPS II, SAPS III, and Acute APACHE II were calculated for all patients admitted to the SICU. Differences between survivors and nonsurvivors were analyzed using the Student's t-test and binary logistic regression analysis. A receiver operating characteristic (ROC) curve was constructed for each scoring system studied. The area under the ROC curve (aROC) for the SAPS III was 0.81 at a cut-off value of 57, whereas the aROC for SAPS II was 0.75 at a cut-off score of 44 and the aROC for APACHE II was 0.74 at a cut-off score of 13. The SAPS III ROC curve for prediction of hospital mortality exhibited the greatest sensitivity (84%) and specificity (66%) with a score of 57 for the "Oldest Old" population.

1. Introduction

Life expectancy has increased substantially in the past half century due to significant advances in healthcare prevention alongside improvements in diagnosis and treatment approaches. As a result, the most rapidly growing segment of the US population is the elderly, defined as individuals older than 65 years [1]. The "Oldest Old" in the population are those over 85, which currently represents 2% of the US census—a figure, that is, expected to increase over 200% by 2050 [1]. These changing demographics have already had a dramatic effect on ICU admissions, with mean age of patients admitted and total number of ICU admissions increasing faster than healthcare resources can keep pace [2]. Information derivable from validated ICU scales will likely play an increasingly important role in guiding physician decision making and may facilitate evidence-based rationing of limited healthcare resources in the future.

To date, numerous studies have documented the negative impact of advanced age on ICU outcomes [2–7]. Although older age is clearly associated with increased mortality, other age-related factors signifying severity of illness have been shown to be better at predicting ICU outcomes in elderly patients than age alone [8, 9]. These factors include the admitting diagnosis [8, 10–13], comorbidities [14–18], and the functional status of the patient prior to ICU admission [19–22]. Commonly used ICU prognostic scoring models include the Simplified Acute Physiologic Score II (SAPS II), Acute Physiology and Chronic Health Evaluation II (APACHE II), and the newly developed SAPS III. These scoring systems incorporate physiologic parameters, co-morbidities, admitting diagnoses, Glasgow coma scales, and age to provide a numerical score that can in turn predict ICU mortality.

Sakr et al. compared the utility of SAPS III against APACHE II and SAPS II in 1851 surgical ICU patients (mean age of 62 years). They noted that in-hospital mortality was substantially greater in patients with higher SAPS III score, and that a score greater than 80 was associated with a 70% mortality rate whereas a score less than 40 was associated with a less than 3% mortality. The authors concluded that the SAPS II and SAPS III predict mortality better than the APACHE II model in elderly patients [23].

Healthcare advancements in recent decades have permitted more elective surgeries in patients with very advanced age. However, suitable literature documenting the ICU outcomes of this age group is lacking. This study sought to evaluate the utility of the SAPS II, SAPS III, and APACHE II scoring systems in nonagenarians (>90 years) admitted to the surgical ICU.

2. Materials and Methods

A retrospective review of all nonagenarians admitted to Saint Barnabas Medical Center (SBMC) in Livingston, NJ, over a 10-year period (between 2000 and 2010) was performed. 951 unique nonagenarian patients were admitted who underwent 1189 surgical procedures. 117 (9.8%) of those patients were admitted to the Surgical Intensive Care Unit (SICU) postoperatively. Pertinent data was collected using a standard data collection sheet after approval from the institutional review board (IRB: 10–25). Data abstracted included age, gender, comorbidities, procedure type, ASA status, operative time, hospital length of stay, ICU length of stay, ICU admission, and outcome. SAPS II, SAPS III, and APACHE II scores and predicted mortality were calculated by retrospective chart review for 89 patients (28 were excluded due to insufficient chart data). Two study populations were grouped into a mortality group and a survivor group. The mortality group included all patients who died within the SICU and the survivor group consisted of all patients who were discharged. Receiver Operator Characteristic (ROC) Curves were plotted to determine the sensitivity and specificity in the aforementioned ICU scoring models to predict in-hospital mortality in this population.

The outcomes of ICU patients, especially mortality, depend on several factors. Based on these factors, several severity scoring systems have been developed. The severity sores usually comprise two parts: the score itself (higher number indicates higher severity) and a probability model (an equation giving the probability of in-hospital death). The most commonly used severity scoring systems include APACHE II, SAPS II, and SAPS III. The APACHE II was developed by a panel of experts based on their personal opinion whereas SAPS II and SAPS III were developed by prospective multi-institutional studies. Differences between the abovementioned scoring systems are shown in Table 1.

3. Results

See Table 2.

3.1. Age and Sex. The mean overall patient age was 93.2 years (91–100); the mean age among male patients was 92.9 years, while the mean age among female patients was 93.4 years. The M : F ratio was 1 : 1.02. On SICU admission, the survivor group's mean age was 93.2, whereas the mortality group's mean age was 92.8 years, $P < 0.5$.

3.2. Length of Stay and Discharge Status. The mean stay for all patients admitted to the SICU was 6 ± 8 days and the mean hospital stay was 16.6 ± 10 days. The majority of discharged patients were sent to a nursing facility ($N = 30$; 33.7%) or home without assisted living ($N = 29$; 32.6%). The remainder of the patients were discharged to a cancer center ($N = 8$; 9%), or rehabilitation center ($N = 4$; 4.4%), while 14 patients (15.7%) suffered mortality.

3.3. Comorbidities. The co-morbidities most prevalent in our study population were cardiac diseases. These include congestive heart failure (CHF) in 38.2% ($N = 34$) patients, hypertension in 34.8% ($N = 31$) patients, atrial fibrillation in 29.2% ($N = 26$) patients, and coronary artery disease in 21.3% ($N = 19$) patients.

3.4. Anesthesia. The preoperative American Society of Anesthesiologists (ASA) score was available for 64 patients, and the mean ASA score was 3.31 (range: 2–5). The mean ASA score for male patients was 3.33 (range: 2–5) compared to 3.15 (range: 2–4) in female patients, $P = 0.4$. Twenty-eight percent ($N = 18$) of patients had an ASA score of two, 56.2% ($N = 36$) had an ASA score of three, 12.5% ($N = 8$) had an ASA score of four while only 3.1% ($N = 2$) of patients had an ASA score of five. General anesthesia was provided to 74.2% of the patients ($N = 66$), cardiac anesthesia to 10.1% ($N = 9$), and regional anesthesia to 7.9% ($N = 7$). The remaining 7.9% ($N = 7$) of cases were performed under Monitored Anesthesia Care (MAC).

3.5. Surgery. Among the surgical procedures performed 38.2% ($N = 34$) had general surgery, orthopedic surgery 13.5% ($N = 12$), cardiac surgery 10.1% ($N = 9$), urologic surgery 9% ($N = 8$), neurosurgery 7.9% ($N = 7$), vascular surgery 6.7% ($N = 6$), and 14.6% ($N = 13$) of patients had invasive procedures (endoscopy, cystoscopy, and biopsy). The mean operative time was 152 ± 112 minutes.

3.6. SAPS II, SAPS III, and APACHE II Scores. The overall mortality in the studied group was 15.7% (14 of 89). The mean SAPS II, score (predicted mortality) for patients who died was 57.4 ± 20.0 ($55.2\% \pm 29.7\%$) compared to 41.7 ± 14.9 ($30.5\% \pm 23.7\%$) for survivors, $P < 0.001$. The mean SAPS III score (predicted mortality), for patients who died, was 74.6 ± 14.2 ($60.7\% \pm 22.1\%$) compared to 57.8 ± 14.5 ($32.4\% \pm 23.6\%$) for survivors, $P < 0.001$. The mean APACHE II score (predicted mortality), for patients who died, was 23.1 ± 8.7

Table 1: Differences between APACHE II, SAPS II, and SAPS III severity scoring systems.

	APACHE II	SAPS II	SAPS III
Variables	Rectal Temp, MAP, HR, RR, Aa gradient/Po_2, pH/HCO_3, Na, K, creatinine, Hct, WBC, GCS, Age, chronic diagnosis	Age, type of admission, temp, SBP, HR, GCS, UOP, WBC, BUN, K, Na, HCO_3, bilirubin, Pao_2/Fio_2, AIDS, metastatic carcinoma, hematologic malignancy	Age, LOS before ICUA, Intrahospital location (OR, ER, other ICU, other), comorbidities (cancer therapy, cancer, hematologic cancer, AIDS, Chronic HF (NYHA IV), Cirrhosis), Vasoactive drugs before ICUA, ICU admission (planned, unplanned), Reason for Admission (cardiovascular, hepatic, digestive, neurologic), Surgical Status at ICUA (scheduled surgery, emergency surgery, no surgery), site of surgery (transplant, trauma, cardiac surgery, neurosurgery), acute Infection at ICUA (nosocomial, respiratory), GCS, highest Total Bilirubin, highest body temperature, highest creatinine, highest HR, lowest WBC count, lowest pH, lowest platelet, lowest SBP, MV or CPAP PaO_2/FiO_2
Data collection	Within 24 hours of admission to ICU	Within 24 hours of admission to ICU	Within 1 hour of admission to ICU
Major limitation	Not helpful to stratify outcome prediction based on primary diagnosis	May be less accurate for noncardiovascular diseases	

Temp: Temperature, MAP: mean arterial pressure, HR: heart rate, RR: respiratory Rate, Aa: alveolar-arterial, Po_2: partial pressure of oxygen; pH: hydrogen ion concentration, HCO_3: bicarbonate concentration, Na: sodium ion concentration, K: potassium ion concentration, Hct: hematocrit, WBC: white blood cell count, GCS: Glasgow Coma Scale, Temp: temperature, SBP: systolic blood pressure, UOP: urine output, BUN: blood urea nitrogen, Fio_2: fraction of inspired oxygen, AIDS: Acquired Immune Deficiency Syndrome, LOS: length of stay, ICUA: intensive care unit admission, HF: heart failure, NYHA: New York Heart Association, MV: minute ventilation, CPAP: continuous positive pressure ventilation.

($46.4\% \pm 26.4\%$) compared to 16.0 ± 7.0 ($26.8\% \pm 19.1\%$) for survivors, $P < 0.001$ (Table 3).

Using a cut-off score of 44, the SAPS II score predicted hospital mortality with a sensitivity of 77% and a specificity of 65%, with an area under the ROC curve (aROC) of 0.75 (95% CI; 0.60–0.89, $P < 0.004$). With a cut-off score of 57, SAPS III score predicted hospital mortality with a sensitivity of 84% and a specificity of 66%, with an aROC of 0.81 (95% CI; 0.70–0.92, $P < 0.0001$). With a cut-off score of 13, the APACHE II score predicted hospital mortality with a sensitivity of 69% and specificity of 66%, with an aROC of 0.74 (95% CI; 0.59–0.88, $P < 0.006$). The area under the curve for the SAPS III ROC (aROC) curve was 0.81 compared to 0.75 and 0.74 for SAPS II score and APACHE II score, respectively, indicating that the SAPS III score best predicted hospital mortality in this study population (Figures 1, 2, and 3).

4. Discussion

Elderly patients represent nearly 50% of all ICU admissions and account for 60% of ICU days [5]. As the Baby Boomers generation approaches retirement age (65 years), the gap between overall resources and patient needs will rapidly expand exponentially. Advances in healthcare prevention, diagnostics, and treatment modalities have markedly expanded lifespan beyond predicted expectations and a growing body of surgical literature documents improved surgical outcome in the "Oldest Old" is further proof of this fact. Between 1990 and 2000, the total number of abdominal aorta aneurysm (AAA) repairs, coronary artery bypass Graft (CABG), carotid endarterectomy (CEA), colon resections, and lung resections performed on patients older than 80 has increased dramatically with an acceptable 30-day mortality rate of 8.4% [24]. Less commonly, feasible surgical outcomes in nonagenarians and centenarians have also recently been documented [24]. Despite these isolated results, little known questions remain about how we identify "Oldest Old" patients who are likely to do well following surgery versus those who will not. Current economic times have made us all acutely aware that healthcare resources are not intangible, and given the fact that many studies suggest that we spend up to 50% of a patient's entire healthcare expenditure in the last 6 months of their life, viable solutions as who is among likely to

TABLE 2: Demographics and clinical characteristics for 89 nonagenarians admitted to the surgical ICU between 2000 and 2010.

	Overall	Mortality group	Survivor group
Total patients, N (%)	89	14 (16)	75 (84)
Mean age, years (range)	93.2 (91–100)	92.8 (91–96)	93.2 (91–100)
Male : female	1 : 1.02	1 : 1.1	1 : 1.06
Comorbidities, N (%)			
CHF	34 (38)	7 (50)	27 (36)
Hypertension	31 (35)	3 (21)	28 (37)
Atrial fibrillation	26 (29)	4 (29)	22 (29)
CAD	19 (21)	2 (14)	17 (23)
ASA grade, N (%)			
I	0	0	0
II	18 (25)	0 (0.0)	18 (24)
III	36 (49)	3 (21)	33 (44)
IV	18 (25)	2 (14)	16 (21)
V	2 (3)	2 (14)	0
Type of anesthesia, N (%)			
General anesthesia	66 (74)	13 (93)	53 (71)
Cardiac anesthesia	9 (10)	1 (7)	8 (11)
Regional anesthesia	7 (8)	0	7 (9)
MAC	7 (8)	0	7 (9)
Types of procedures, N (%)			
General surgery	34 (38)	10 (71)	24 (32)
Orthopedic surgery	12 (14)	0	12 (16)
Cardiac surgery	9 (10)	1 (7)	8 (11)
Urologic surgery	8 (9)	0	8 (11)
Neurosurgery	7 (8)	1 (7)	6 (8)
Vascular surgery	6 (7)	2 (14)	4 (5)
Invasive procedures*	13 (15)	0	13 (17)
Mean operative time, min ± SD	152 ± 112	152.3 ± 148.0	138.8 ± 103.0
Mean ICU stay, days ± SD	6 ± 8	12.0 ± 6.5	5.0 ± 0.8
Mean length of hospital stay, days ± SD	16.6 ± 15	15.5 ± 14.1	17.4 ± 15.3
Discharge status, N (%)			
Nursing facility	30 (34)	—	30 (40)
Home without assisted living	29 (33)	—	29 (39)
Cancer center	8 (9)	—	8 (11)
Rehabilitation center	4 (4)	—	4 (5)

N: number of patients, CHF: congestive cardiac failure, CAD: coronary artery disease, ASA: American Society of Anesthesiologists, MAC: managed anesthesia care, min: minutes, SD: standard deviation, ICU: intensive care unit.
* Invasive procedures included endoscopy, cystoscopy, and biopsy.

TABLE 3: Comparison of ICU mortality prediction models based on mean score and area under the receiver operator curve for 89 nonagenarians admitted to surgical ICU between 2000 and 2010.

Prediction models	Mortality group scores (mean ± SD) N = 14 (16%)	Survivor group scores (mean ± SD) N = 75 (84%)	Area under ROC curve (95% CI)	P value
SAPS II	57.4 ± 20.0	41.7 ± 14.9	0.75 (0.60, 0.89)	$P < 0.02$
SAPS III	74.7 ± 14.2	57.8 ± 14.5	0.81 (0.70, 0.92)	$P < 0.001$
APACHE II	23.1 ± 8.7	16.0 ± 7.0	0.74 (0.59, 0.88)	$P < 0.02$

SD: Standard deviation, ROC: receiver operator curve, CI: Confidence Interval, N: number of patients, SAPS: standardized Acute Physiology Score, APACHE: Acute Physiology and Chronic Health Evaluation.

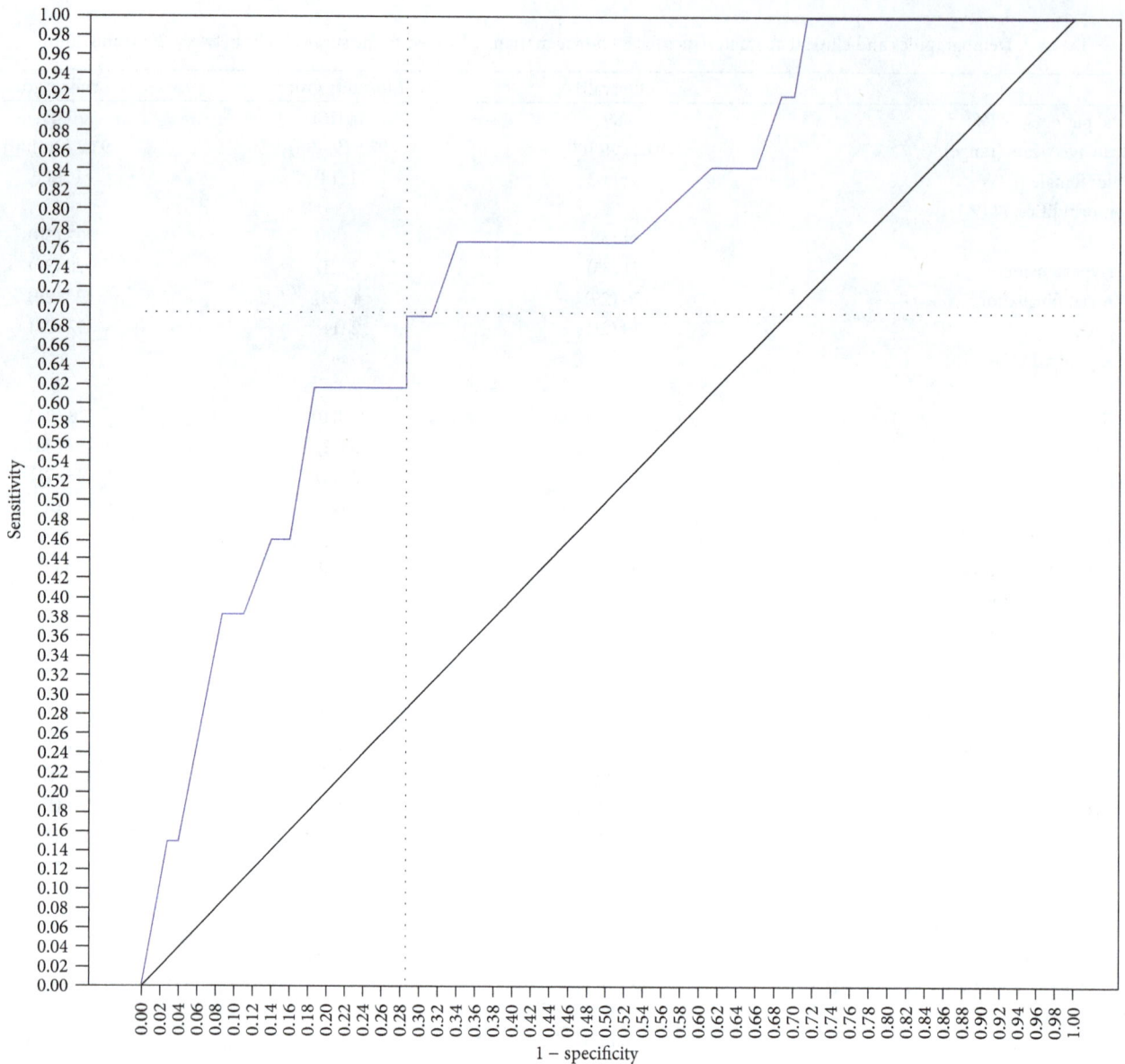

FIGURE 1: SAPS II ROC curve for prediction of hospital mortality. The score of 44 showed better sensitivity (77%) and specificity (65%) for hospital mortality, with an area under the curve of 0.75 (area = 0.5; $P < 0.004$, 95% CI; 0.60–0.89).

benefit from different interventions is vital to future decision making. At present, a number of validated survey systems have been published that can provide some guidance as to how we should ration limited healthcare resources such as surgical intervention and ICU admission in catering younger patient population but whether this applies to "Oldest Old" is unknown.

The SAPS II and APACHE II prognostic models are the most commonly used scoring systems for critically ill patients admitted to the ICU [25–27]. In 2005, the SAPS III model was proposed and differs primarily from the former two models in the fact that data is collected within the first hour following ICU admission rather than within 24 hours [28, 29]. Nearly half of the predictive power of the SAPS III score is based on information available prior to ICU admission, making it

a potential tool for ICU triage as well. Scoring systems that utilize data derived 24 hours after ICU admission obviously have no utility for ICU screening as that data reflects the ICU care provided. Several studies have looked at the utility of SAPS II and APACHE II in surgical patients, but only two studies have described the utility of SAPS III in surgical patients. Furthermore, until now there are no studies that analyze the utility of SAPS III in surgical patients of very advanced age.

All three scoring systems have the ability to predict survivorship (known as discrimination) and to evaluate the predicted mortality against the observed mortality (known as calibration) [30]. This study demonstrates that the SAPS III has slightly better discrimination than the SAPS II and APACHE II in surgical ICU patients over 90-year old.

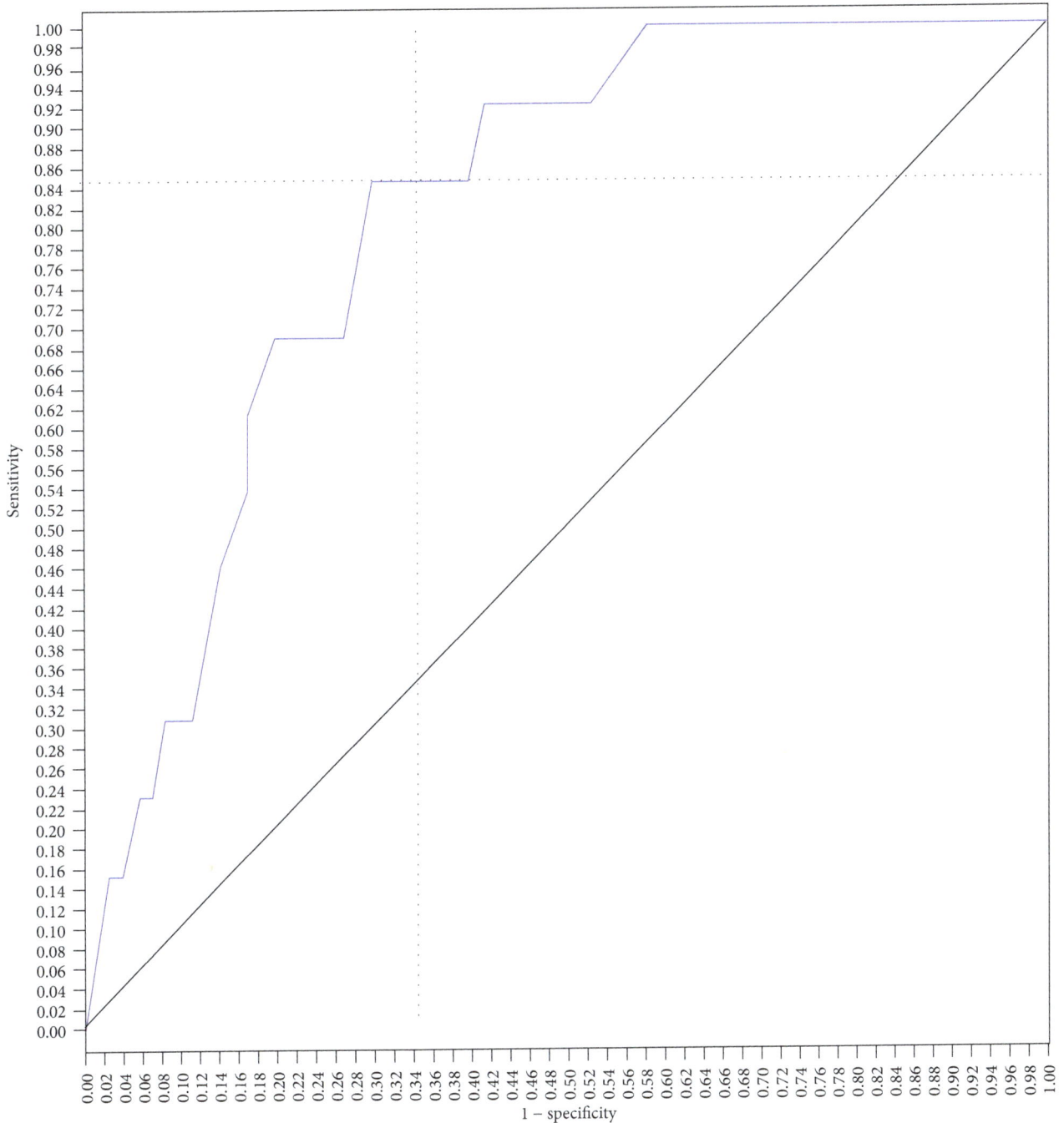

FIGURE 2: SAPS 3 ROC curve for prediction of hospital mortality. The score of 57 showed better sensitivity (84%) and specificity (66%) for hospital mortality, with an area under the curve of 0.81 (area = 0.5; $P < 0.0001$, 95% CI; 0.70–0.92).

These results are consistent with the limited published literature available on the SAPS III scores evidence in surgical patients. Silva et al. studied 1,310 surgical patients with a mean age of 67.1 and found that a SAPS III score of 57 yielded an aROC of 0.86 [31]. Unlike the current study, they did not evaluate the disparity between the various available scoring systems. Sakr et al. evaluated 1851 surgical patients with a mean age of 62 and found that the SAPS III had an aROC of 0.84, which was higher than both the SAPS II and APACHE II of 0.83 and 0.80, respectively [23].

The SAPS III score was developed with data from 303 ICUs and 16,784 patients worldwide [28, 29]. Though comprehensive, the SAPS III data was not representative of all types of patient populations since it was developed using a general ICU population pool. As a result, external validation remains essential before applying this score to any specific patient population, including surgical patients and the elderly. Although our outcomes are similar to those of Sakr et al., our study group consisted only of patients over 90 years of age with the vast majority of patients having

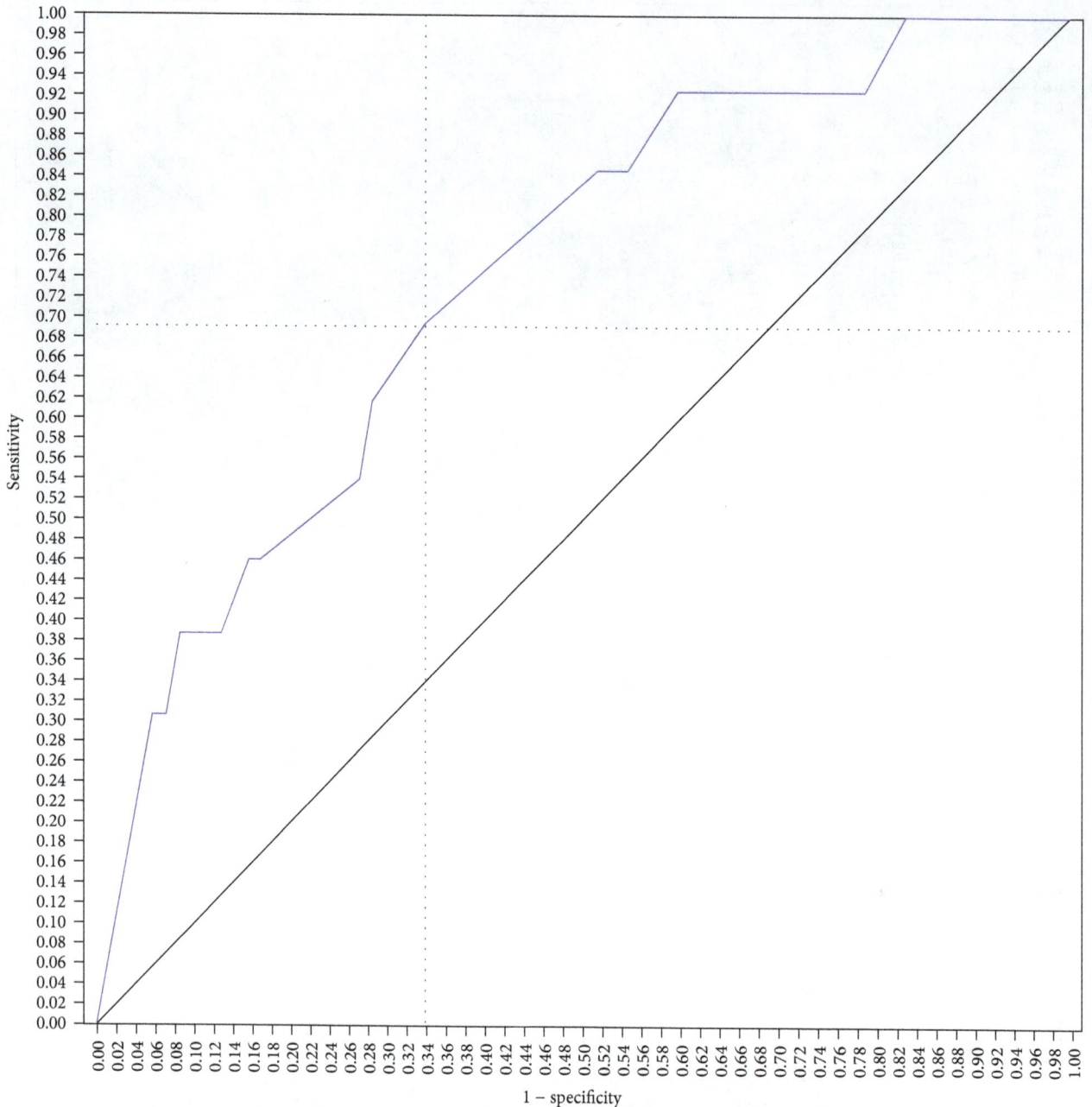

FIGURE 3: APACHE 2 ROC curve for prediction of hospital mortality. The score of 13 showed better sensitivity (69%) and specificity (66%) for hospital mortality, with an area under the curve of 0.74 (area = 0.5; $P < 0.006$, 95% CI; 0.59–0.88).

underwent general surgery. Further, it is difficult to draw specific conclusions about percent increased risk in elderly patients for major or minor procedures from this study set; other studies have clearly documented an increased risk for any invasive procedure in the frail and debilitated elderly patient.

Although the result of this study serves as an external validation for the SAPS III score in nonagenarian surgical ICU patients, this is a retrospective pilot study and as such there are several limitations to the study design. The power of the study is limited by the small number of patients

studied and the fact that the surgical case mix was predominantly in the field of general surgery for gastrointestinal diseases.

In conclusion, the SAPS III is a valuable tool for predicting mortality in surgical ICU patients older than 90 years of age. Given the ease of SAPS III calculations, it may also be a useful tool for ICU triage of "Oldest Old" surgical patients and may assist the physician in making difficult decisions regarding the rationing of healthcare resources and the aggressiveness of initial ICU care.

References

[1] U. S. Census Bureau, "U.S. Interim Projections by Age, Sex, Race, and Hispanic Origin," 3-18-2004. 6-20-2011, 2004.

[2] A. Boumendil, D. Somme, M. Garrouste-Orgeas, and B. Guidet, "Should elderly patients be admitted to the intensive care unit?" *Intensive Care Medicine*, vol. 33, no. 7, pp. 1252–1262, 2007.

[3] S. E. de Rooij, A. Abu-Hanna, M. Levi, and E. de Jonge, "Factors that predict outcome of intensive care treatment in very elderly patients: a review," *Critical Care*, vol. 9, no. 4, pp. R307–R314, 2005.

[4] D. Hennessy, K. Juzwishin, D. Yergens, T. Noseworthy, and C. Doig, "Outcomes of elderly survivors of intensive care: a review of the literature," *Chest*, vol. 127, no. 5, pp. 1764–1774, 2005.

[5] P. E. Marik, "Management of the critically ill geriatric patient," *Critical Care Medicine*, vol. 34, no. 9, pp. S176–S182, 2006.

[6] B. H. Nathanson, T. L. Higgins, M. J. Brennan, A. A. Kramer, M. Stark, and D. Teres, "Do elderly patients fare well in the ICU?" *Chest*, vol. 139, no. 4, pp. 825–831, 2011.

[7] E. Sacanella, J. M. Pérez-Castejón, J. M. Nicolás et al., "Mortality in healthy elderly patients after ICU admission," *Intensive Care Medicine*, vol. 35, no. 3, pp. 550–555, 2009.

[8] E. de Jonge, R. J. Bosman, P. H. J. van der Voort, H. H. M. Korsten, G. J. Scheffer, and N. F. de Keizer, "Intensive care medicine in the Netherlands, 1997–2001. I. Patient population and treatment outcome," *Nederlands Tijdschrift voor Geneeskunde*, vol. 147, no. 21, pp. 1013–1017, 2003.

[9] L. Chelluri, M. R. Pinsky, M. P. Donahoe, and A. Grenvik, "Long-term outcome of critically ill elderly patients requiring intensive care," *Journal of the American Medical Association*, vol. 269, no. 24, pp. 3119–3123, 1993.

[10] I. L. Cohen and J. Lambrinos, "Investigating the impact of age on outcome of mechanical ventilation using a population of 41,848 patients from a statewide database," *Chest*, vol. 107, no. 6, pp. 1673–1680, 1995.

[11] D. G. Jacobs, B. R. Plaisier, P. S. Barie et al., "Practice management guidelines for geriatric trauma: the EAST practice management guidelines work group," *Journal of Trauma*, vol. 54, no. 2, pp. 391–416, 2003.

[12] W. A. Knaus, D. P. Wagner, J. E. Zimmerman, and E. A. Draper, "Variations in mortality and length of stay in intensive care units," *Annals of Internal Medicine*, vol. 118, no. 10, pp. 753–761, 1993.

[13] A. J. Meinders, J. G. van der Hoeven, and A. E. Meinders, "The outcome of prolonged mechanical ventilation in elderly patients: are the efforts worthwhile?" *Age and Ageing*, vol. 25, no. 5, pp. 353–356, 1996.

[14] M. E. Charlson, P. Pompei, K. A. Ales, and C. R. MacKenzie, "A new method of classifying prognostic comorbidity in longitudinal studies: development and validation," *Journal of Chronic Diseases*, vol. 40, no. 5, pp. 373–383, 1987.

[15] S. Greenfield, H. U. Aronow, R. M. Elashoff, and D. Watanabe, "Flaws in mortality data. The hazards of ignoring comorbid disease," *Journal of the American Medical Association*, vol. 260, no. 15, pp. 2253–2255, 1988.

[16] M. H. Kaplan and A. R. Feinstein, "The importance of classifying initial comorbidity in evaluating the outcome of diabetes mellitus," *Journal of Chronic Diseases*, vol. 27, no. 7-8, pp. 387–404, 1974.

[17] W. A. Knaus, E. A. Draper, D. P. Wagner, and J. E. Zimmerman, "APACHE II: a severity of disease classification system," *Critical Care Medicine*, vol. 13, no. 10, pp. 818–829, 1985.

[18] W. A. Knaus, D. P. Wagner, E. A. Draper et al., "The APACHE III prognostic system: risk prediction of hospital mortality for critically III hospitalized adults," *Chest*, vol. 100, no. 6, pp. 1619–1636, 1991.

[19] K. E. Covinsky, A. C. Justice, G. E. Rosenthal, R. M. Palmer, and C. S. Landefeld, "Measuring prognosis and case mix in hospitalized elders: the importance of functional status," *Journal of General Internal Medicine*, vol. 12, no. 4, pp. 203–208, 1997.

[20] S. K. Inouye, P. N. Peduzzi, J. T. Robison, J. S. Hughes, R. I. Horwitz, and J. Concato, "Importance of functional measures in predicting mortality among older hospitalized patients," *Journal of the American Medical Association*, vol. 279, no. 15, pp. 1187–1198, 1998.

[21] S. A. Mayer-Oakes, R. K. Oye, and B. Leake, "Predictors of mortality in older patients following medical intensive care: the importance of functional status," *Journal of the American Geriatrics Society*, vol. 39, no. 9, pp. 862–868, 1991.

[22] D. B. Reuben, L. V. Rubenstein, S. H. Hirsch, and R. D. Hays, "Value of functional status as a predictor of mortality: results of a prospective study," *The American Journal of Medicine*, vol. 93, no. 6, pp. 663–670, 1992.

[23] Y. Sakr, C. Krauss, A. C. K. B. Amaral et al., "Comparison of the performance of SAPS II, SAPS 3, APACHE II, and their customized prognostic models in a surgical intensive care unit," *British Journal of Anaesthesia*, vol. 101, no. 6, pp. 798–803, 2008.

[24] M. P. Hosking, M. A. Warner, C. M. Lobdell, K. P. Offord, and L. J. Melton III, "Outcomes of surgery in patients 90 years of age and older," *Journal of the American Medical Association*, vol. 261, no. 13, pp. 1909–1915, 1989.

[25] W. A. Knaus, J. E. Zimmerman, D. P. Wagner, E. A. Draper, and D. E. Lawrence, "APACHE-acute physiology and chronic health evaluation: a physiologically based classification system," *Critical Care Medicine*, vol. 9, no. 8, pp. 591–597, 1981.

[26] J.-R. le Gall, S. Lemeshow, and F. Saulnier, "A new Simplified Acute Physiology Score (SAPS II) based on a European/North American multicenter study," *Journal of the American Medical Association*, vol. 270, no. 24, pp. 2957–2963, 1993.

[27] M. J. Vassar, F. R. Lewis Jr., J. A. Chambers et al., "Prediction of outcome in intensive care unit trauma patients: a multicenter study of acute physiology and chronic health evaluation (APACHE), trauma and injury severity score (TRISS), and a 24-hour intensive care unit (ICU) point system," *Journal of Trauma*, vol. 47, no. 2, pp. 324–329, 1999.

[28] P. G. H. Metnitz, R. P. Moreno, E. Almeida et al., "SAPS 3—from evaluation of the patient to evaluation of the intensive care unit. Part 1: objectives, methods and cohort description," *Intensive Care Medicine*, vol. 31, no. 10, pp. 1336–1344, 2005.

[29] R. P. Moreno, P. G. H. Metnitz, E. Almeida et al., "SAPS 3—from evaluation of the patient to evaluation of the intensive care unit. Part 2: development of a prognostic model for hospital mortality at ICU admission," *Intensive Care Medicine*, vol. 31, no. 10, pp. 1345–1355, 2005.

[30] D. G. Altman and P. Royston, "What do we mean by validating a prognostic model?" *Statistics in Medicine*, vol. 19, pp. 453–473, 2000.

Provider Perspectives on the Influence of Family on Nursing Home Resident Transfers to the Emergency Department: Crises at the End of Life

Caroline Stephens,[1] Elizabeth Halifax,[1] Nhat Bui,[1] Sei J. Lee,[2] Charlene Harrington,[3] Janet Shim,[3] and Christine Ritchie[4]

[1]Department of Community Health Systems, School of Nursing, University of California, San Francisco, 2 Koret Way, N531E, UCSF Box 0608, San Francisco, CA 94143-0608, USA
[2]Department of Geriatrics, Palliative & Extended Care, San Francisco VA Medical Center, Division of Geriatrics, School of Medicine, University of California, San Francisco, 4150 Clement Street, Building 1, Room 220F, San Francisco, CA 94121, USA
[3]Department of Social & Behavioral Sciences, School of Nursing, University of California, San Francisco, 3333 California Street, Suite 455, UCSF Box 0612, San Francisco, CA 94118, USA
[4]Division of Geriatrics, School of Medicine, University of California, San Francisco, 3333 California Street, Suite 380, San Francisco, CA 94143-1265, USA

Correspondence should be addressed to Caroline Stephens; caroline.stephens@ucsf.edu

Academic Editor: Gilbert B. Zulian

Background. Nursing home (NH) residents often experience burdensome and unnecessary care transitions, especially towards the end of life. This paper explores provider perspectives on the role that families play in the decision to transfer NH residents to the emergency department (ED). *Methods.* Multiple stakeholder focus groups (*n* = 35 participants) were conducted with NH nurses, NH physicians, nurse practitioners, physician assistants, NH administrators, ED nurses, ED physicians, and a hospitalist. Stakeholders described experiences and challenges with NH resident transfers to the ED. Focus group interviews were recorded and transcribed verbatim. Transcripts and field notes were analyzed using a Grounded Theory approach. *Findings.* Providers perceive that families often play a significant role in ED transfer decisions as they frequently react to a resident change of condition as a crisis. This sense of crisis is driven by 4 main influences: insecurities with NH care; families being unprepared for end of life; absent/inadequate advance care planning; and lack of communication and agreement within families regarding goals of care. *Conclusions.* Suboptimal communication and lack of access to appropriate and timely palliative care support and expertise in the NH setting may contribute to frequent ED transfers.

1. Introduction

Transfers of frail nursing home (NH) residents to and from the emergency department (ED) are common and costly and expose vulnerable residents to the well-documented risks associated with care transitions [1–7]. Despite increasing legislation to monitor and enforce NH standards and quality of care over the past decade, the number of ED visits by NH residents has increased 12.8%, from 1.9 million to 2.1 million visits, and there has been no significant change in rates of potentially preventable ED visits [8]. Many of these burdensome care transitions occur in the last 6 months of life [9, 10] or are for symptoms or conditions that can be safely and effectively treated in the NH setting [11–14]. Unfortunately, many NHs not only lack adequate staffing and access to timely on-site medical expertise [6, 15, 16] but also have little to no access to palliative care support and services [17–19].

Experts believe that a key element to preventing avoidable hospitalizations and ED visits is early engagement of families in discussions about advanced care planning (ACP) and reducing nonbeneficial care at the end of life (EOL) [6]. Some have postulated that NH resident families are often poorly informed about their loved one's prognosis as well as treatment options available in the NH setting, therefore opting for a transfer to the hospital as the perceived most reasonable alternative [20]. Several empirical studies suggest that families have a significant influence on hospital transfer decisions [21–25]. However, little is qualitatively known about the nature of this family influence, particularly from the perspective of diverse health care providers across care settings.

The focus of this paper is to describe providers' perspectives on the role that families play in the decision to transfer NH residents to the ED. Findings reported here are part of a larger qualitative study that conducted eight 2-hour focus group interviews to explore diverse stakeholder perspectives on (1) the experiences and challenges they faced with NH resident transfers to the ED and (2) the potential role of technology to help to address those concerns. During the course of data collection for this larger study, the NH and hospital providers consistently spoke about the strong influence family members had on transfer decisions. This emerging concept was included in subsequent iterations of the interview guide and was found to be one of the main themes derived from the data.

2. Methods

2.1. Study Design. This descriptive study employed a qualitative approach using focus group interviews. Focus groups were deemed to be the most efficient method to collect data from this diverse group of individuals that included busy health professionals [26, 27]. In addition, focus groups were considered a useful method for triggering additional stories, examples, and thoughts from participants through the process of listening to one another and being reminded of issues they had not previously considered or remembered [28].

2.2. Sample and Setting. Participants were recruited via multiple methods: in-person meetings and/or emails with NH administrators, medical directors, and/or directors of nursing, as well as hospital/ED administrative leadership; posting of recruitment posters in local facilities and hospitals; emails to local and state-wide NH listservs; and snow ball sampling. Eligible participants were all English-speaking individuals involved in the care of a NH resident transferred to the hospital in the prior 3–6 months.

Table 1 reveals the demographics and characteristics of the 35 provider focus group participants. The sample included 16 NH nurses (including bedside nurses, charge nurses, directors of nursing, minimum data set coordinators, and a director of staff development); 11 primary care providers (including 6 NH physicians, 4 nurse practitioners (NP), and 1 physician assistant); 2 ED physicians; 2 ED nurses; 3 NH administrators; and 1 hospitalist. Forty percent of provider stakeholders were over the age of 46, 60% were female, and

TABLE 1: Demographics and characteristics of provider focus group participants ($N = 35$).

Age (years)	
18–35	6 (17%)
36–40	8 (23%)
41–45	7 (20%)
46–50	3 (9%)
Over 50	11 (31%)
Gender	
Male	14 (40%)
Female	21 (60%)
Race	
American Indian/Alaska Native	1 (3%)
Asian	11 (31%)
Native Hawaiian/other Pacific Islanders	1 (3%)
Black or African American	1 (3%)
White	16 (46%)
More than one race	1 (3%)
Unknown/not reported	4 (11%)
Healthcare role	
NH nurse	16 (46%)
NH physician	6 (17%)
Nurse practitioner/physician assistant	5 (14%)
Emergency department nurse	2 (6%)
Emergency department physician	2 (6%)
NH administrator	3 (9%)
Hospitalist	1 (3%)
Years of experience in clinical practice/NHs	
1–5	8 (23%)
6–10	7 (20%)
10–15	3 (9%)
More than 15	17 (49%)

46% were white. Approximately half of all providers had more than 15 years of clinical experience.

Some of the focus groups included mixed stakeholders (e.g., physician/nurse practitioner), while others were homogenous in membership (e.g., all nurses). No study participant participated in more than one focus group. The majority of groups took place in a private room at a public library in the San Francisco Bay Area.

2.3. Procedures. After informed consent was obtained and prior to the start of the focus group, participants were provided with an iPad to complete a brief web-based survey. This survey asked questions regarding participant sociodemographic characteristics, as well as background, experiences, and opinions about NH resident ED transfers.

Using a semistructured interview guide, the principal investigator (CS) then facilitated the focus group, and the study coordinator (EH) took field notes and made observations. During the first half of the focus groups (the findings of which are the focus of this paper), each participant was asked to describe a recent experience or experiences they had had with a NH resident who became ill and potentially required a transfer to the ED. As described earlier, NH and hospital providers consistently spoke about the strong influence family members had on transfer decisions and this emerging concept guided refinements to the semistructured interview guide. Probes used to elicit more information regarding perceptions of family involvement are shown in the following list:

(i) Please describe what the communication with the family was like during that time.

(ii) How was the family engaged in the decision about the possible care transition?

(iii) Did family engagement occur before or after the decision to transfer had been made?

(iv) Please describe how the resident's goals of care were considered in the care transition?

2.4. Analysis. Data saturation was reached when no new concepts or perspectives were introduced during the focus groups [29, 30]. All interviews were recorded and professionally transcribed verbatim and then checked for accuracy. Using a Grounded Theory approach [29, 30], analysis began with coding immediately after data collection began, including initial coding of text line by line. No a priori codes were used. Categories were created from related codes and themes were developed based on patterns that described the phenomenon of interest. Interview guides for subsequent focus groups were modified to incorporate some of the issues emerging in early analysis. To ensure trustworthiness of this study, several strategies were employed. These included methodological transparency; collection of rich and sufficient data from a wide range of informants; and use of reflexivity by the research team to examine their preconceptions and biases. Approval for this study was obtained from the institutional review board at the authors' university.

3. Findings: Influence of Family

Families were commonly perceived as the major reason NH residents experienced potentially unnecessary transfers to the hospital. Providers reported that families often reacted to resident changes in condition as crises and that this precipitated their efforts to push for hospital transfers. Providers often described family influence as a tension between resident/family autonomy and their own clinical judgment when it came to making transfer decisions. For example, one NH nurse practitioner commented:

> "I think the biggest reason [for NH-ED transfer] is the family piece - because you can know whatever you know, and want to do whatever you want to do, but if mom or brother or sister or DPOA (durable power of attorney), or whatever, doesn't agree with that, it's very difficult to change their mind." [NP]

NH health care providers further related that they often made transfer decisions against their best clinical judgment because of this family influence and for fear of potential repercussions (e.g., complaints, lawsuits, and poor outcomes). An example of this tension is described here by a NH physician:

> "They wanted to take him to the hospital, clearly, but I didn't want that…family has a lot of influence. The family upset at the bedside and pushing for a transfer to the hospital - not doing that is going to lead to more problems in the long run, and the patient is certainly going to end up in the hospital. One way or another, they're going to end up in the hospital with an angry family member rather than a family member who feels like you've addressed their concerns." [physician]

The tensions around transfer between NH staff and families were also recognized by hospital providers who were often on the receiving end of inappropriate NH transfers:

> "So it wasn't necessarily [that] they [NH care team] didn't do the right thing; they tried, but I think they had issues with the patients." [physician]

3.1. Reacting to a Change of Condition as a Crisis. Underpinning this complex phenomenon of family influence on hospital transfer decisions was the perception that families reacted to a resident's change of condition as a crisis. Often this sense of crisis or panic led families to change care decisions resulting in transfers, usually at the EOL.

> "The residents that are long-term residents, some of those, I find, it's a family problem, because they will say "we don't want any heroics. Mom says I never wanted a tube, I never wanted this", and so they fill out the POLST [Physician Orders for Life-Sustaining Treatments]. And then when we call and say—…'their condition has changed a lot', they get panicked… there have been times where the family just panics and goes, 'oh, my God, I didn't mean to do that, let me send her in [to the emergency department (ED)]'." [nurse]

> "I had a lady who just—her heart stopped—and that was it, and there wasn't anything that came before that, and she was totally no code, no anything, but when we called the family to tell the daughter, she said, "no, no, no, start CPR, get that going". So we did, which we hadn't done, because she was a no CPR, so we had nurses in there doing CPR on her." [nurse]

As described in more detail below, this sense of family crisis or panic was driven by 4 main influences, largely stemming from unmet palliative care needs. These 4 dynamic and interdependent influences included insecurities with NH care; being unprepared for EOL; absent or inadequate advance care planning; and lack of communication and agreement within families regarding goals of care.

3.1.1. Insecurities with NH Care.
Providers perceived that families often felt insecure about the care provided in the NH setting and how that frequently seemed to influence family preference for ED transfer. Such insecurities were largely driven by families questioning the quality of NH licensed nurse care and perceiving NH medical capacity and responses as inadequate (e.g., lack of physician support/communication, inability to get timely test results, and failure to provide timely analgesics). For example, NH and hospital providers described that families often insisted on transfer from NH to ED because they felt their loved one's needs were not being met in the NH setting:

> "... patients are brought in [to the ED] because the family is saying, "well, they're not taking care of your pain", or "I'm not getting whatever I need", or conditions are...below their expectations I guess. So that seems to be another challenge." [physician]

Providers further described that this feeling of insecurity and drive for hospital transfer was often exacerbated when families came to visit and perceived that their loved ones were not being sufficiently cared for. For example, one nurse described that transfers were often high on days when families frequently came to visit:

> "Sunday evenings are big for skilled nursing facility transfers, because families come to visit and they don't like what they're seeing." [nurse]

One physician described how these insecurities with NH care would sometimes lead families to change the resident's code status:

> "I'm not quite sure how that happens [hospital DNR patients reverting to full code on return to NH]. I think part of it is that in the hospital, they'll [patient/family] accept a DNR status, because they feel like they're in an acute [care] setting, but that the family members change their mind, because they're afraid that if they're DNR in a nursing home, that not enough will be done. So they make themselves full code while they're in the nursing home, and then with the understanding they'll probably switch back to DNR when they get to the acute." [physician]

3.1.2. Being Unprepared for End of Life.
Many providers perceived that families often seemed emotionally unprepared for their loved one's decline in health and ultimate death. Participants portrayed families who often did not understand or recognize the needs of those at the EOL. Descriptions emerged of family members whose actions were commonly driven by denial about their resident's health status. One nurse described how a resident's sister had an unrealistic understanding of her sister's prognosis:

> "She had pulmonary issues...numerous co-morbidities, so she was constantly going in [to the ED]...She had a sister that took care of her and she was not a do-not-resuscitate. Her sister

wanted everything done for her...she wasn't brain dead, but the sister was insisting that she was able to communicate with her, and she'd talk to her. But there was nothing [she was profoundly demented]...it was kind of sad. We always thought that if she [the resident] could wake up and say, "you know, I don't want this", that she probably would, but her sister was her primary caregiver and wanted everything possible done for her. So we went with her sister's wishes." [nurse]

In describing two terminally ill residents, this nurse tells how the residents did not receive hospice care as recommended but died in the ED, because family were not ready to transition to a symptom-oriented, palliative approach to care:

> "...they [family] were not ready at that time to initiate hospice, so one day he really exacerbated, he went to the hospital, CHF exacerbation, and he expired at the hospital...We have had two of these instances recently: one was metastatic lung cancer, and the other was CHF. And they were both in one month. They [the families] were just not ready at that time for hospice, even though we saw it. We did the consultation, the notes were there from hospice that they're ready physically, however, mentally and psychologically, they were not ready to give up yet." [nurse]

Another nurse described a resident at EOL who had frequent transfers to and from the hospital because the son could not "let her go." This nurse, however, did not blame the resident's son for being unprepared for EOL but rather faulted the lack of good communication and discussion between the physician and the family.

> "...we have one long, long, long, long-term son who sends his mother to the emergency room probably once a month at least, and won't let her go. And the emergency room doctors cannot do anything with him; neither can all the other doctors. So they're used to seeing him, they don't do anything more; it's just a trip back and forth. And some of these things could be, I think, [pause] handled better if the physician who is responsible—the attending physician—had more of a relationship with the family." [nurse]

3.1.3. Absent or Inadequate Advanced Care Planning.
Driving this feeling of panic that influenced families was absent or inadequate advance care planning discussions and decisions. Without medical orders reflecting treatment decisions, providers articulated that the default was to provide all available medical treatment, including ED transfer. The process for making ACP decisions at the NH was described as being centered on the completion of the POLST. However, the process of completing the POLST was described as being largely driven by and completed by admissions coordinators, social services, and/or nursing staff and then the form was

left for the physician to sign. Physicians were perceived to be minimally involved in discussing and completing the POLSTs with residents and families: what one nurse described as simply providing a "*red stamp signature only.*" Several NH nurses described the frustration of taking on responsibility for initiating the POLST forms whilst chasing physicians to help manage residents' and families' expectations and sign off to complete them. Following are a few examples of the process for completing the POLST from the nursing perspective:

> "…*as an IDT [Interdisciplinary team], we work together. And when the doctor is there, we grab the doctor and everything, get him to sign the form right away.*" [nurse]

> "…*we will tell the doctor, you know, doctor, you've got to explain to the family about her condition that this is, you know, what's the goal.*" [nurse]

While lack of physician involvement was implicated as a cause of the absence or inadequate advance care planning, focus group participants also perceived families were frequently reluctant to make what one physician referred to as "hard decisions."

> "…*but a lot of times the families, you're lucky to get them to fill out square one [of the POLST], because they don't want to make that decision. It's like, 'well, call me when that happens'.*" [nurse]

> "*[You] present it [POLST] right to them, okay, now we have a box A, B, and C, can you check one of these and tell us what would be your best answer, or your best directive, and they won't do it.*" [nurse]

Advance care planning was also considered inadequate in situations where POLSTs used were described as "confusing," "incomplete," or "contradictory." The conflict between DNR and full treatment orders caused real frustration for this ED physician:

> "…*[advanced care planning is] a continuous and ongoing issue, not just in terms of patients who don't have POLSTs, but POLSTs that are filled out incorrectly, or POLSTs that are confusing. If you check somebody that is DNR, but then you say full treatment on the second column, that makes no sense.*" [physician]

3.1.4. Lack of Communication and Agreement within Families regarding Goals of Care.

Lack of communication and agreement within families regarding goals of care was another major influence on the decision to transfer a resident to the ED. One nurse stated that family members are often "*not on the same page.*" At times when residents experienced a change of condition, this lack of communication led to disagreements about what treatments/transfers were in the resident's best interests and a disregard for existing advanced care orders. As described in this next quote, this was often exacerbated when

the resident had children locally involved and others engaged at a distance:

> "…*there's a brother [out of state] who wants [ED transfer], and a sister who doesn't…we deal with a tremendous number of family members who are at great odds with each other on end-of-life situations, on transfer to the hospital.*" [nurse]

In a separate example, a nurse described a resident who had become unresponsive. She checked the POLST that stated she had a Do Not Resuscitate (DNR) order. She called the doctor and daughter, but she was unable to reach them.

> "…*she had a son and a daughter, and they were both responsible party. So the son told me, 'oh, it's DNR, keep her there, keep her comfortable'. Okay, so I'm going to follow that…and then I got a call from the doctor who said if they want her out [to the ED], go ahead and send her out…The daughter comes running in…'oh, send her now'. I was like your brother said – 'don't listen to him' (said the daughter) – so it's like communication between the two and it's like something they should have worked…out before, you know, when that actual moment happened. And so yeah, she ended up, a couple days later, passing away [in the hospital], but the communication is horrible.*" [nurse].

Nurses frequently described personal stress and frustration when the resident's family members gave contradictory directions regarding goals of care in times of crisis.

> "*So as far as…[advanced care planning] is concerned, I think that…nurses are…always in, you know, between a rock and a hard place, especially with the families that have the conflict.*" [nurse]

> "*I can think now, probably 5 people with families, that one person has been appointed, the 'primary', or like 'executor person' that will be making the decisions. And then you'll have the other – maybe two other family members coming in at different times during the week, or during the month and it's like 'no one told me about my dad', or 'no one told me this about my mom', and it's just a hard place to be in…it's like well, your sister is the primary decision-maker, and you're not listed here, so that would be up to her to notify you about this. Because then they start in with 'you never called me, you never told me', and it's just a hard place to be as a nurse.*" [nurse].

Many of these family communication challenges and conflicts regarding goals of care were rooted in the complex interplay of the above 4 main influences. The dynamic and interdependent nature of these influences ultimately led to residents and their families having unmet palliative care needs. Such unmet needs included lack of preparation for EOL, inadequate facilitation of goals of care conversations, and lack of advance care planning.

4. Discussion

Providers perceived that families play a significant role in ED transfer decisions as they frequently react to a resident change of condition as a crisis. This sense of crisis was driven by 4 dynamic and interdependent factors: insecurities with NH care; being unprepared for EOL; absent or inadequate advance care planning; and lack of communication and agreement within families regarding goals of care. These findings are congruent with other research citing family insistence [6, 31–34], as well as concerns about advanced care directives [6, 35], as common nonmedical factors associated with hospital transfer decisions. This is the first study to highlight how such family influence on ED transfer decisions is often driven by a sense of crisis and panic, largely stemming from unmet palliative care needs. The lack of access to appropriate and timely palliative care support and expertise in the NH setting may be a contributing factor to frequent and often burdensome ED transfers at the EOL. Many unnecessary transfers could be reduced with improved goals of care discussion, increased sense of security with symptom management, and basic care needs, as well as greater anticipatory guidance regarding what to expect with disease progression, prognosis, and needs at the EOL [36, 37].

Such provision of palliative care, or specialized medical care for people with serious illnesses, has been strongly advocated by experts as a way to enhance the care for vulnerable NH residents with progressive, life-limiting illness and late-life disability [37–40]. Evidence suggests this high risk population has many unmet needs for symptom amelioration, provider communication, emotional support, and being treated with respect, especially near the end of life [9, 10, 39]. As a person-centered model of care that integrates individualized psychosocial and physical care to enhance quality of life for residents and families [40, 41], palliative care may help proactively address the factors identified in this study that precipitated family feelings of crisis. Evidence suggests that NH palliative care is associated with improved care quality and satisfaction, enhanced symptom management, and fewer ED visits [42–45]. Unfortunately, this vulnerable population has historically had little access to formal palliative expertise outside of hospice services [17–19].

Findings further suggest a need to reframe the negatively perceived role of families in hospital transfer decisions. Conceptualizing families as one of the major drivers of inappropriate transfers run the risk of making them adversaries rather than partners in care. Numerous studies underscore the importance and value of eliciting resident perspectives and actively engaging them and their families in shared decision-making [33, 36, 37, 46, 47]. Such "patient-centered care" is a central tenet of the Institute of Medicine (IOM) report, Affordable Care Act and the national NH culture change movement [48–50], and is posited to improve health outcomes and reduce or eliminate any disparities associated with access to needed care and quality [50–52].

Consistent with other studies [32, 53–56], many of the perceived challenges that participants perceived with families often stemmed from limited physician involvement in proactively engaging families in goals of care discussions. A growing body of evidence suggests, however, that there are larger systems issues that inhibit such provider efforts, as well as provision of quality EOL care in general in the NH setting [57]. Moreover, systematic processes to elicit goals of care in NHs are lacking [47, 57, 58]. A recent review article concluded that NH residents wish to be involved in EOL related decisions; however family and staff do not always recognize resident preferences or ability to consent to preferences [59]. Missed opportunities for communication about EOL preferences among NH residents, family, and staff are common [47]. Towsley and colleagues [47] argue that these "missed conversations" occur when no one inquires about EOL preferences; residents, families, or staff assume wishes are known; and resident information is not conveyed due to the lack of a formalized process to converse about or share resident wishes.

Providers in this study highlighted significant challenges with goals of care discussions in general and as documented with the POLST in particular. Some POLST studies indicate that open conversations between NH residents, family members, and medical providers can increase comfort at the EOL, reduce hospitalizations, and increase the likelihood that residents' and families' preferences are solicited, documented, and honored [60–63]. Unfortunately, as this and other studies [64–66] have found, POLST completion often becomes more of an administrative function (e.g., check the boxes and have the doctor sign) versus a platform for providers to engage in an actual discussion regarding goals of care. It is ultimately not about the form but rather the process and it appears that that process may be getting lost in the NH setting.

As Sudore and Fried [67] suggest, ACP needs to occur "upstream," years earlier when individuals have decision-making capacity and are able to voice their wishes to their family. They recommend reframing the purpose of ACP away from having patients and families make premature treatment decisions based on incomplete information; rather ACP should entail "preparing patients and their surrogates for the types of decisions and conflicts they may encounter when they do have to engage in in-the-moment decision-making" [67]. Such ACP discussions are not a one-time occurrence but rather an ongoing process that needs to be frequently revisited and documented as individual preferences and circumstances may change over time.

ACP discussions in the NH setting are increasingly focused on completing the POLST (or related document in other states) [68, 69]. While it is important to have a completed POLST form on the chart and one that accompanies a resident during care transitions, it is only useful and appropriate if it accurately reflects current treatment preferences. More qualitative documentation is needed regarding the nature and content of the ACP discussions as they evolve over time. Greater efforts should be made to move beyond just "checking a box" and properly train all staff on how to engage in these important conversations and appropriately complete POLST forms [70–72]. Staff should think creatively about how to change "missed conversations" into opportunities that involve families, residents, and staff and elicit or account for resident preferences [47]. Since NH residents are in close proximity to other residents and often witness EOL situations first hand, the experience of others could be used as a way to initiate EOL conversations [47, 73]. Involving nurse practitioners in care planning conferences may also represent an excellent opportunity to revisit goals of care with residents and their families in the context of broader interprofessional treatment planning [74].

Limitations. This study has some important limitations worth noting. The goal of the larger study was to better understand the range of challenges our sample of stakeholders experienced in the care of this vulnerable population and how emerging health technologies might help address those concerns. It is therefore not clear how subject preference to participate or not participate in a technology-oriented focus group may have influenced responses received. In addition, the study sample was relatively small and only included perspectives of providers across 3 counties in northern California. Providers in other parts of the state and country might have different experiences and perspectives. Nevertheless, rich qualitative data were obtained from a wide range of providers who worked in diverse settings, including for-profit/not-for-profit and large chain/small chain facilities located in both urban and suburban settings primarily serving ethnically and racially diverse communities.

5. Conclusions

A growing body of evidence suggests that NH residents experience many detrimental and costly care transitions, particularly at the EOL [75–77]. These findings underscore the strong need for greater upstream anticipatory guidance and preparation for "in-the-moment" decision-making to reduce family conflict, crisis, and panic when there is a change in condition. Moreover, study findings further suggest that improved access to timely and appropriate palliative care support and expertise in the NH setting may reduce many of these burdensome and unnecessary transitions at the EOL.

With greater national efforts focused on providing person-centered care, improving care transitions, and reducing health care costs for frail older adults in NHs, policymakers and payers should recognize the value of high quality palliative care in the NH setting. It is also critical to establish appropriate and adequate reimbursement mechanisms for these vital but often time-consuming and sensitive resident and family conversations regarding goals of care [74]. Future research is needed to better understand the specific palliative care needs of nursing home residents and their families. Moreover, as hospitals and NHs work more closely together to reduce inappropriate care transfers and improve value-based care, innovative care strategies that improve access to much needed palliative care services and supports for NH residents need to be evaluated.

Acknowledgments

This work was supported by NIH 8 KL2 TR000143-08 and by the UCSF Pepper Center and Tideswell at UCSF, which promote promising new research aimed at better understanding and addressing late-life disability in vulnerable populations. Findings were presented at the American Geriatrics Society Annual Scientific Meeting May 2015 in Washington, DC.

References

[1] C. Caffrey, "Potentially preventable emergency department visits by nursing home residents: United States, 2004," *National Center for Health Statistics Data Brief*, no. 33, pp. 1–8, 2010.

[2] H. E. Wang, M. N. Shah, R. M. Allman, and M. Kilgore, "Emergency department visits by nursing home residents in the United States," *Journal of the American Geriatrics Society*, vol. 59, no. 10, pp. 1864–1872, 2011.

[3] C. E. Stephens, R. Newcomer, M. Blegen, B. Miller, and C. Harrington, "Emergency Department use by nursing home residents: effect of severity of cognitive impairment," *The Gerontologist*, vol. 52, no. 3, pp. 383–393, 2012.

[4] A. Gruneir, M. J. Silver, and P. A. Rochon, "Emergency department use by older adults: a literature review on trends, appropriateness, and consequences of unmet health care needs," *Medical Care Research and Review*, vol. 68, no. 2, pp. 131–155, 2011.

[5] K. Boockvar, E. Fishman, C. K. Kyriacou, A. Monias, S. Gavi, and T. Cortes, "Adverse events due to discontinuations in drug use and dose changes in patients transferred between acute and long-term care facilities," *Archives of Internal Medicine*, vol. 164, no. 5, pp. 545–550, 2004.

[6] J. G. Ouslander, G. Lamb, M. Perloe et al., "Potentially avoidable hospitalizations of nursing home residents: frequency, causes, and costs," *Journal of the American Geriatrics Society*, vol. 58, no. 4, pp. 627–635, 2010.

[7] D. C. Grabowski, A. J. O'Malley, and N. R. Barhydt, "The costs and potential savings associated with nursing home hospitalizations," *Health Affairs*, vol. 26, no. 6, pp. 1753–1761, 2007.

[8] J. Brownell, J. Wang, A. Smith, C. Stephens, and R. Y. Hsia, "Trends in emergency department visits for ambulatory care sensitive conditions by elderly nursing home residents, 2001 to 2010," *JAMA Internal Medicine*, vol. 174, no. 1, pp. 156–158, 2014.

[9] P. Gozalo, J. M. Teno, S. L. Mitchell et al., "End-of-life transitions among nursing home residents with cognitive issues," *The New England Journal of Medicine*, vol. 365, no. 13, pp. 1212–1221, 2011.

[10] S. C. Miller, J. C. Lima, J. Looze, and S. L. Mitchell, "Dying in U.S. nursing homes with advanced dementia: how does health care use differ for residents with, versus without, end-of-life medicare skilled nursing facility care?" *Journal of Palliative Medicine*, vol. 15, no. 1, pp. 43–50, 2012.

[11] D. B. Reuben, J. F. Schnelle, and J. L. Buchanan, "Primary care of long-stay nursing home residents: a comparison of 3 HMO programs with fee-for-service," *Journal of the American Geriatrics Society*, vol. 47, no. 2, pp. 131–138, 1999.

[12] R. L. Kane, G. Keckhafer, S. Flood, B. Bershadsky, and M. S. Siadaty, "The effect of Evercare on hospital use," *Journal of the American Geriatrics Society*, vol. 51, no. 10, pp. 1427–1434, 2003.

[13] J. G. Ouslander, G. Lamb, R. Tappen et al., "Interventions to reduce hospitalizations from nursing homes: evaluation of

the INTERACT II collaborative quality improvement project," *Journal of the American Geriatrics Society*, vol. 59, no. 4, pp. 745–753, 2011.

[14] M. Loeb, S. C. Carusone, R. Goeree et al., "Effect of a clinical pathway to reduce hospitalizations in nursing home residents with pneumonia: a randomized controlled trial," *The Journal of the American Medical Association*, vol. 295, no. 21, pp. 2503–2510, 2006.

[15] M. Perry and J. Cummings, *To Hospitalize or Not to Hospitalize? Medical Care for Long-Term Care Facility Residents*, The Henry J. Kaiser Family Foundation, 2010.

[16] A. Gruneir, C. M. Bell, S. E. Bronskill, M. Schull, G. M. Anderson, and P. A. Rochon, "Frequency and pattern of emergency department visits by long-term care residents—a population-based study," *Journal of the American Geriatrics Society*, vol. 58, no. 3, pp. 510–517, 2010.

[17] D. Casarett, J. Karlawish, K. Morales, R. Crowley, T. Mirsch, and D. A. Asch, "Improving the use of hospice services in nursing homes: a randomized controlled trial," *The Journal of the American Medical Association*, vol. 294, no. 2, pp. 211–217, 2005.

[18] J. Zerzan, S. Stearns, and L. Hanson, "Access to palliative care and hospice in nursing homes," *Journal of the American Medical Association*, vol. 284, no. 19, pp. 2489–2494, 2000.

[19] M. B. Happ, E. Capezuti, N. E. Strumpf et al., "Advance care planning and end-of-life care for hospitalized nursing home residents," *Journal of the American Geriatrics Society*, vol. 50, no. 5, pp. 829–835, 2002.

[20] D. C. Grabowski, K. A. Stewart, S. M. Broderick, and L. A. Coots, "Predictors of nursing home hospitalization—a review of the literature," *Medical Care Research and Review*, vol. 65, no. 1, pp. 3–39, 2008.

[21] S. F. Simmons, D. W. Durkin, A. N. Rahman, J. F. Schnelle, and L. M. Beuscher, "The value of resident choice during daily care: do staff and families differ?" *Journal of Applied Gerontology*, vol. 33, no. 6, pp. 655–671, 2014.

[22] D. Houttekier, A. Vandervoort, L. Van den Block, J. T. Van der Steen, R. Vander Stichele, and L. Deliens, "Hospitalizations of nursing home residents with dementia in the last month of life: results from a nationwide survey," *Palliative Medicine*, vol. 28, no. 9, pp. 1110–1117, 2014.

[23] G. Lamb, R. Tappen, S. Diaz, L. Herndon, and J. G. Ouslander, "Avoidability of hospital transfers of nursing home residents: perspectives of frontline staff," *Journal of the American Geriatrics Society*, vol. 59, no. 9, pp. 1665–1672, 2011.

[24] K. S. Boockvar and O. R. Burack, "Organizational relationships between nursing homes and hospitals and quality of care during hospital-nursing home patient transfers," *Journal of the American Geriatrics Society*, vol. 55, no. 7, pp. 1078–1084, 2007.

[25] C. A. Robinson, J. L. Bottorff, M. B. Lilly et al., "Stakeholder perspectives on transitions of nursing home residents to hospital emergency departments and back in two Canadian provinces," *Journal of Aging Studies*, vol. 26, no. 4, pp. 419–427, 2012.

[26] M. Sandelowski, "Combining qualitative and quantitative sampling, data collection, and analysis techniques in mixed-method studies," *Research in Nursing & Health*, vol. 23, no. 3, pp. 246–255, 2000.

[27] J. W. Creswell, *Research Design: Qualitative, Quantitative, and Mixed Methods Approaches*, Sage, 4th edition, 2013.

[28] R. S. Jayasekara, "Focus groups in nursing research: methodological perspectives," *Nursing Outlook*, vol. 60, no. 6, pp. 411–416, 2012.

[29] A. Strauss, *Qualitative Analysis for Social Scientists*, Cambridge University Press, 1987.

[30] K. Charmaz, "Premises, principles, and practices in qualitative research: revisiting the foundations," *Qualitative Health Research*, vol. 14, no. 7, pp. 976–993, 2004.

[31] M. Bauer and R. Nay, "Family and staff partnerships in long-term care. A review of the literature," *Journal of Gerontological Nursing*, vol. 29, no. 10, pp. 46–53, 2003.

[32] R. R. Shield, T. Wetle, J. Teno, S. C. Miller, and L. Welch, "Physicians 'missing in action': family perspectives on physician and staffing problems in end-of-life care in the nursing home," *Journal of the American Geriatrics Society*, vol. 53, no. 10, pp. 1651–1657, 2005.

[33] R. M. Tappen, S. M. Worch, D. Elkins, D. J. Hain, C. M. Moffa, and G. Sullivan, "Remaining in the nursing home versus transfer to acute care: resident, family, and staff preferences," *Journal of Gerontological Nursing*, vol. 40, no. 10, pp. 48–57, 2014.

[34] J. L. Buchanan, R. L. Murkofsky, A. J. O'Malley et al., "Nursing home capabilities and decisions to hospitalize: a survey of medical directors and directors of nursing," *Journal of the American Geriatrics Society*, vol. 54, no. 3, pp. 458–465, 2006.

[35] G. Arendts, S. Quine, and K. Howard, "Decision to transfer to an emergency department from residential aged care: a systematic review of qualitative research," *Geriatrics & Gerontology International*, vol. 13, no. 4, pp. 825–833, 2013.

[36] S. Zimmerman, L. Cohen, J. T. van der Steen et al., "Measuring end-of-life care and outcomes in residential care/assisted living and nursing homes," *Journal of Pain and Symptom Management*, vol. 49, no. 4, pp. 666–679, 2015.

[37] M. Ersek and J. G. Carpenter, "Geriatric palliative care in long-term care settings with a focus on nursing homes," *Journal of Palliative Medicine*, vol. 16, no. 10, pp. 1180–1187, 2013.

[38] K. Aragon, K. Covinsky, Y. Miao, W. J. Boscardin, L. Flint, and A. K. Smith, "Use of the medicare posthospitalization skilled nursing benefit in the last 6 months of life," *Archives of Internal Medicine*, vol. 172, no. 20, pp. 1573–1579, 2012.

[39] J. M. Teno, B. R. Clarridge, V. Casey et al., "Family perspectives on end-of-life care at the last place of care," *The Journal of the American Medical Association*, vol. 291, no. 1, pp. 88–93, 2004.

[40] National Consensus Project for Quality Palliative Care, *Clinical Practice Guidelines for Quality Palliative Care*, Hospice & Palliative Association, 3rd edition, 2013.

[41] World Health Organization, *WHO Palliative Care Definition*, 2013, http://www.who.int/cancer/palliative/definition/en/.

[42] D. Casarett, A. Pickard, F. A. Bailey et al., "Do palliative consultations improve patient outcomes?" *Journal of the American Geriatrics Society*, vol. 56, no. 4, pp. 593–599, 2008.

[43] I. G. Finlay, I. J. Higginson, D. M. Goodwin et al., "Palliative care in hospital, hospice, at home: results from a systematic review," *Annals of Oncology*, vol. 13, supplement 4, pp. 257–264, 2002.

[44] S. Hall, A. Kolliakou, H. Petkova, K. Froggatt, and I. J. Higginson, "Interventions for improving palliative care for older people living in nursing care homes," *Cochrane Database of Systematic Reviews*, vol. 3, Article ID CD007132, 2011.

[45] R. E. Berkowitz, R. N. Jones, R. Rieder et al., "Improving disposition outcomes for patients in a geriatric skilled nursing facility," *Journal of the American Geriatrics Society*, vol. 59, no. 6, pp. 1130–1136, 2011.

[46] R. Wetzels, M. Harmsen, C. van Weel, R. Grol, and M. Wensing, "Interventions for improving older patients' involvement in primary care episodes," *Cochrane Database of Systematic Reviews*, no. 1, Article ID CD004273, 2007.

[47] G. L. Towsley, K. B. Hirschman, and C. Madden, "Conversations about end of life: perspectives of nursing home residents, family, and staff," *Journal of Palliative Medicine*, vol. 18, no. 5, pp. 421–428, 2015.

[48] M. J. Koren, "Person-centered care for nursing home residents: the culture-change movement," *Health Affairs*, vol. 29, no. 2, pp. 312–317, 2010.

[49] V. Shier, D. Khodyakov, L. W. Cohen, S. Zimmerman, and D. Saliba, "What does the evidence really say about culture change in nursing homes?" *The Gerontologist*, vol. 54, supplement 1, pp. S6–S16, 2014.

[50] Institute of Medicine, *Crossing the Quality Chasm*, National Academy Press, 2001.

[51] C. Laine and F. Davidoff, "Patient-centered medicine: a professional evolution," *The Journal of the American Medical Association*, vol. 275, no. 2, pp. 152–156, 1996.

[52] S. M. Asch, E. A. Kerr, J. Keesey et al., "Who is at greatest risk for receiving poor-quality health care?" *The New England Journal of Medicine*, vol. 354, no. 11, pp. 1147–1156, 2006.

[53] J. Kayser-Jones, "The experience of dying: an ethnographic nursing home study," *The Gerontologist*, vol. 42, no. 3, pp. 11–19, 2002.

[54] M. Ersek and S. A. Wilson, "The challenges and opportunities in providing end-of-life care in nursing homes," *Journal of Palliative Medicine*, vol. 6, no. 1, pp. 45–57, 2003.

[55] S. J. Farber, T. R. Egnew, J. L. Herman-Bertsch, T. R. Taylor, and G. E. Guldin, "Issues in end-of-life care: patient, caregiver, and clinician perceptions," *Journal of Palliative Medicine*, vol. 6, no. 1, pp. 19–31, 2003.

[56] D. Stillman, N. Strumpf, E. Capezuti, and H. Tuch, "Staff perceptions concerning barriers and facilitators to end-of-life care in the nursing home," *Geriatric Nursing*, vol. 26, no. 4, pp. 259–264, 2005.

[57] D. E. Meier, B. Lim, and M. D. A. Carlson, "Raising the standard: palliative care in nursing homes," *Health Affairs*, vol. 29, no. 1, pp. 136–140, 2010.

[58] C. D. Furman, S. E. Kelly, K. Knapp, R. L. Mowery, and T. Miles, "Eliciting goals of care in a nursing home," *Journal of the American Medical Directors Association*, vol. 8, supplement 2, no. 3, pp. e35–e41, 2007.

[59] A. Fosse, M. A. Schaufel, S. Ruths, and K. Malterud, "End-of-life expectations and experiences among nursing home patients and their relatives-a synthesis of qualitative studies," *Patient Education and Counseling*, vol. 97, no. 1, pp. 3–9, 2014.

[60] S. E. Hickman, C. A. Nelson, A. H. Moss, S. W. Tolle, N. A. Perrin, and B. J. Hammes, "The consistency between treatments provided to nursing facility residents and orders on the physician orders for life-sustaining treatment form," *Journal of the American Geriatrics Society*, vol. 59, no. 11, pp. 2091–2099, 2011.

[61] S. E. Hickman, S. W. Tolle, K. Brummel-Smith, and M. M. Carley, "Use of the physician orders for life-sustaining treatment program in Oregon nursing facilities: beyond resuscitation status," *Journal of the American Geriatrics Society*, vol. 52, no. 9, pp. 1424–1429, 2004.

[62] S. E. Hickman, C. A. Nelson, N. A. Perrin, A. H. Moss, B. J. Hammes, and S. W. Tolle, "A comparison of methods to communicate treatment preferences in nursing facilities: traditional practices versus the physician orders for life-sustaining treatment program," *Journal of the American Geriatrics Society*, vol. 58, no. 7, pp. 1241–1248, 2010.

[63] S. W. Tolle, V. P. Tilden, C. A. Nelson, and P. M. Dunn, "A prospective study of the efficacy of the physician order form for life-sustaining treatment," *Journal of the American Geriatrics Society*, vol. 46, no. 9, pp. 1097–1102, 1998.

[64] S. E. Hickman, E. Keevern, and B. J. Hammes, "Use of the physician orders for life-sustaining treatment program in the clinical setting: a systematic review of the literature," *Journal of the American Geriatrics Society*, vol. 63, no. 2, pp. 341–350, 2015.

[65] S. E. Hickman, C. A. Nelson, E. Smith-Howell, and B. J. Hammes, "Use of the physician orders for life-sustaining treatment program for patients being discharged from the hospital to the nursing facility," *Journal of Palliative Medicine*, vol. 17, no. 1, pp. 43–49, 2014.

[66] T. Sugiyama, D. Zingmond, K. A. Lorenz et al., "Implementing physician orders for life-sustaining treatment in California hospitals: factors associated with adoption," *Journal of the American Geriatrics Society*, vol. 61, no. 8, pp. 1337–1344, 2013.

[67] R. L. Sudore and T. R. Fried, "Redefining the 'planning' in advance care planning: preparing for end-of-life decision making," *Annals of Internal Medicine*, vol. 153, no. 4, pp. 256–261, 2010.

[68] J. L. Meyers, C. Moore, A. McGrory, J. Sparr, and M. Ahern, "Physician orders for life-sustaining treatment form: honoring end-of-life directives for nursing home residents," *Journal of Gerontological Nursing*, vol. 30, no. 9, pp. 37–46, 2004.

[69] N. N. H. McGough, B. Hauschildt, D. Mollon, and W. Fields, "Nurses' knowledge and comfort levels using the Physician Orders for Life-sustaining Treatment (POLST) form in the progressive care unit," *Geriatric Nursing*, vol. 36, no. 1, pp. 21–24, 2015.

[70] E. Whittaker, W. G. Kernohan, F. Hasson, V. Howard, and D. McLaughlin, "The palliative care education needs of nursing home staff," *Nurse Education Today*, vol. 26, no. 6, pp. 501–510, 2006.

[71] L.-L. Dwyer, G. Hansebo, B. Andershed, and B.-M. Ternestedt, "Nursing home residents' views on dying and death: nursing home employee's perspective," *International Journal of Older People Nursing*, vol. 6, no. 4, pp. 251–260, 2011.

[72] S. C. Miller and B. Han, "End-of-life care in U.S. nursing homes: nursing homes with special programs and trained staff for hospice or palliative/end-of-life care," *Journal of Palliative Medicine*, vol. 11, no. 6, pp. 866–877, 2008.

[73] J. C. Munn, D. Dobbs, A. Meier, C. S. Williams, H. Biola, and S. Zimmerman, "The end-of-life experience in long-term care: five themes identified from focus groups with residents, family members, and staff," *The Gerontologist*, vol. 48, no. 4, pp. 485–494, 2008.

[74] G. A. Hartle, D. G. Thimons, and J. Angelelli, "Physician orders for life sustaining treatment in US nursing homes: a case study of CRNP engagement in the care planning process," *Nursing Research and Practice*, vol. 2014, Article ID 761784, 7 pages, 2014.

[75] J. Xing, D. B. Mukamel, and H. Temkin-Greener, "Hospitalizations of nursing home residents in the last year of life: nursing home characteristics and variation in potentially avoidable hospitalizations," *Journal of the American Geriatrics Society*, vol. 61, no. 11, pp. 1900–1908, 2013.

Relationship-Based Care and Behaviours of Residents in Long-Term Care Facilities

Johanne Desrosiers,[1,2] **Anabelle Viau-Guay,**[3,4] **Marie Bellemare,**[5,6]
Louis Trudel,[6,7] **Isabelle Feillou,**[5] **and Anne-Céline Guyon**[7]

[1] *School of Rehabilitation, Faculty of Medicine and Health Sciences, Université de Sherbrooke,*
 3001 12th Avenue North Sherbrooke, Sherbrooke, QC, Canada J1H 5N4
[2] *Research Centre on Aging, CSSS-IUGS, Sherbrooke, QC, Canada*
[3] *Département d'études sur l'Enseignement et l'Apprentissage, Université Laval, QC, Canada*
[4] *Centre de Recherche et d'Intervention sur la Réussite Scolaire (CRIRES), QC, Canada*
[5] *Département des Relations Industrielles, Université Laval, QC, Canada*
[6] *Chaire de Recherche en Gestion de la Santé et de la sécurité du travail, Université Laval, QC, Canada*
[7] *Département de Réadaptation, Université Laval, QC, Canada*

Correspondence should be addressed to Johanne Desrosiers; johanne.desrosiers@usherbrooke.ca

Academic Editor: Jacek Witkowski

Introduction. In long-term care (LTC), person-centred approaches are encouraged. One such approach, relationship-based care (RBC), aims among other things to reduce residents' agitated behaviours. RBC has been used in numerous Quebec LTC facilities over the past decade but it has never been studied. *Objective.* Explore correlations between use of RBC by trained caregivers and the frequency of agitated and positive behaviours of residents with cognitive impairments. *Methods.* Two independent raters observed fourteen caregiver/resident dyads in two LTC facilities during assistance with hygiene and dressing. Checklists were used to quantify caregivers' RBC use and residents' agitated and positive behaviours. *Results.* Scores for RBC use were high, suggesting good application of the approach by caregivers. Correlation analyses showed that offering residents realistic choices and talking to them during care were associated with both positive and agitated behaviours (*P* from 0.03 to 0.003). However, many other components of RBC were not associated with residents' behaviours during care. *Conclusions.* There were only a few quantitative links between the RBC checklist items and the frequency of agitated or positive behaviours. Other studies with a more rigorous research design are needed to better understand the impact of relationship-based care on residents' behaviours.

1. Introduction

1.1. Person-Centred Care: Foundations, Implementation, and Effects. In Quebec, the mission of residential long-term care (LTC) centres is to provide quality care to clients who are severely impaired physically and especially cognitively [1]. Because of cognitive impairments, residents in these centres frequently display problem behaviours [2–4]. These behaviours affect not only the well-being of their formal caregivers (e.g., long-term care staff) [5–7] but also the residents' own quality of life [8].

To meet the needs of clients who present problem or agitated behaviours, new approaches have been developed over the years. Person-centred care is designed to be an alternative to or to complement pharmacotherapy in reducing problem behaviours in individuals with dementia [9]. According to the Committee on Quality of Health Care in America, person-centred care is one of the main areas for improvement that the health care system should address in order to increase the quality of health care, especially long-term care [10]. Such approaches are based on a humanistic concept of health care, where the primary focus must be on the person and his/her life experience and capacities, rather than characterising the person solely by his/her disease [11]. Person-centred care is the opposite of task-centred care. In long-term care, this principle is operationalised in an array of practices aimed at helping residents to establish relationships, be treated as persons with their own life history and interests, and live in an environment that resembles a living environment [12]. From the perspective of long-term care, this conception entails a set of practices aimed at helping the person enter into a relationship (with formal and informal caregivers and other residents) (being in a relationship) and be seen as having a life history and his/her own interests (being in a social world) [11]. The person-centred care approach also implies a favourable context, particularly in terms of the organization of the nursing staff's work (being in place), and a desire to respect the values and preferences of persons when providing care (being with self) [12].

Implementation of person-centred care (PCC) depends not only on the caregivers acquiring skills and knowledge but also on adapting the entire care context (care practices, work organisation, and physical environment) to tailor it to both residents' and caregivers' needs and preferences. This means that there must be flexibility in the organisation, meals, hygiene, and dressing assistance, and so on [13, 14]. Finally, the physical environment must also be adapted to the perspective that it is both a living environment for the residents and a workplace for the caregivers [15].

The results of the research on the effects of implementing PCC are not unanimous about reducing problem behaviours (such as wandering, aggression, and being noisy) or improving well-being during care of residents in long-term care. In 1999, Opie and colleagues [16] conducted a systematic review of studies published in the preceding decade on nonpharmacological strategies to reduce residents' problem behaviours. Despite the methodological limitations of the studies reviewed, 27 of which were described as poor, these researchers concluded that various strategies were effective, including caregiver training and environmental modifications. The literature review published a few years later by Landreville and colleagues [17] reached a similar conclusion: the authors even suggested that caregiver training and environmental modifications are the most effective approaches according to the studies reviewed, the majority of which were quasi-experimental. More recently, however, the meta-analysis done by Kong and colleagues in 2009 [18], which included only randomised clinical trials, maintained that only one nonpharmacological approach (sensory intervention) helped to significantly reduce problem behaviours in dementia. Caregiver training, environmental modifications, and the use of activities, among other things, did not seem to produce any positive outcomes in that regard.

1.2. Context of the Study. One of these approaches was developed in Quebec by the *Association pour la Santé et la Sécurité du Travail, Secteur des Affaires Sociales* (ASSTSAS; Association for Occupational Health and Safety in the Social Affairs Sector). The approach is called *relationship-based care* (RBC) and its objective is to improve both care for residents and occupational health for caregivers. It comprises an array of care practices that help to maintain residents' mobility and function as long as possible. Another aim and expectation

of implementing this approach is a reduction in residents' agitated behaviours.

Relationship-based care (RBC) was developed from a French approach called manutention relationnelle (relationship handling) of Gineste and Pellissier [19] and is based on training tested in and adapted to the situation in Quebec. The goal of the training is not only to acquire skills and knowledge (how to approach residents, interpret their feedback and react in relationship mode, stimulate optimal autonomy based on realistic expectations, and gently ease contractures), but also to develop and maintain humanistic attitudes despite difficulties and constraints.

RBC training is given mostly to patient attendants (orderlies) and, to a lesser extent, other types of workers: nurses, nursing assistants, occupational therapists, physiotherapists, and recreation technicians. The main elements advocated in relationship-based care are outlined in Table 3.

Implementation of RBC in an institution starts with designating a project leader in the institution. Step 1 is a two-day basic group training session for about a dozen caregivers. The next step is a half-day individual session with a peer coach during which each participant delivers two types of care under the supervision of the instructor, who provides personalised feedback. The final step is a half-day consolidation session approximately one month after the training, which brings together all the trainees with their immediate supervisors to review the entire approach and discuss implementation challenges.

1.3. Aim of the Study. Although it has been used in many long-term care institutions in Quebec since 2002, relationship-based care has never been studied with residents or caregivers. The present study focussed specifically on residents. The aim was to explore correlations between Relationship-Based Care (RBC) and the positive and agitation behaviours of residents during assistance with hygiene and dressing. These types of care are some of the interventions with long-term care residents, including individuals with dementia, that trigger the most problem or agitated behaviours since it is impossible at such times to avoid entering their personal space [4]. The working hypothesis was that greater use of RBC by caregivers trained in this approach would be negatively correlated with the frequency of agitated behaviours and positively correlated with the frequency of positive behaviours of residents with cognitive impairment in long-term care facilities.

2. Methods

This exploratory study is part of a larger research project examining the impact of Relationship-Based Care on caregivers and institutions engaged in implementing this approach. The decision to use a correlational cross-sectional observational design for this initial study of RBC and residents was based on practical as well as ethical considerations, which prevented the use of an experimental design. It was both ethically and practically impossible to stop using this humanistic approach with some of the patients since RBC was the foundation of patient care.

2.1. Participants. The participating residents and caregivers were recruited in two Quebec LTC facilities where RBC had been used for a few years. To be eligible for the study, *residents* had to meet the following criteria: (1) have been living in the long-term care facility for at least three months; (2) have presented at least one instance of agitated behaviour or resistance to care in the previous week or presented a clinical profile in which mental impairment or mixed impairment (mental and physical) was predominant. *Caregivers* had to be patient attendants (orderlies) or nursing assistants who had been trained in RBC.

2.2. Data Collection. This study was approved by the Research Ethics Committee of the Centre de Santé et de Services Sociaux, Institut Universitaire de Gériatrie de Sherbrooke (approval number MP-IUGS-09-08). Consent forms were signed by caregivers. Since the majority of the residents were unable to provide informed consent, written consent for them to participate in the study was obtained from their legal representatives. The caregivers also asked residents for their verbal consent before starting the observations. We observed the two members of the dyad (caregiver/resident) during assistance with hygiene and dressing in the early morning or evening, simultaneously by two trained independent observers without any connection to the institution. The observers had received theoretical training on the measuring instruments before administering them to the residents (pretests) with a member of the research team. The results were compared. Any differences were discussed and explained. The frequency of the caregiver's actions, attitudes and behaviours expected when using RBC was scored by one of the two observers using a checklist specifically developed for that purpose (see below). At the same time, the frequency of the resident's positive and agitated behaviours during care was quantified using two instruments (see below) by the other observer. Both observers were in the room but stayed out of the way as much as possible to avoid disturbing the proceedings while being able to observe as well as possible.

2.3. Measuring Instruments. The degree of use of relationship-based care was estimated using the *RBC Use Checklist.* This checklist was initially developed by a member of the research team from (1) components used by ASSTSAS for the instructor's evaluation and feedback during the peer coaching step and (2) an in-house tool from a Quebec LTC facility. The checklist items generated were discussed by the research team, then validated and commented on by ASSTSAS advisors, whose recommendations were incorporated in the checklist. The ASSTSAS advisors are the individuals who developed the RBC training and who trained instructors in the workplace. Finally, a pretest by a team member led to additional modifications to make the instrument realistic and usable in the context of this study. The final checklist consisted of 23 items divided into five categories: *making contact* (6 items), *relationship bubble* (8 items), *general approach*

(5 items), *teamwork* (2 items), and *communication* (2 items) (see Table 3). The observer had to indicate how often the behaviours expected from the caregiver occurred during care. A score was assigned to each item, that is, present (1) or absent (0), for the six items in the *Making contact* category, while a four-level score, that is, always present (3), generally present (2), rarely present (1), or absent (0), was assigned to the items in the other categories. The higher the score is, the better the RBC was correctly used. The observers could also indicate "not applicable" or "not observable."

The resident's behaviours during care were estimated using two instruments, one for agitated behaviours and the other for "positive" behaviours. The frequency of occurrences of physical and verbal agitation during care was quantified using the Cohen-Mansfield Agitation Inventory (CMAI) [20]. The rater uses the inventory to note the frequency of 29 agitated behaviours in real time. At a given time, agitated behaviours are rated on a seven-point scale from 0 (behaviour not observed) to 6 (behaviour observed constantly). A higher score means more agitation of the resident during the care. The internal consistency of the *CMAI* ($\alpha = 0.86$, 0.91, and 0.87 for daytime, evening and nighttime) and its interrater ($r = 0.82$) and test-retest ($r = 0.83$; $P < 0.001$) reliability can be considered good [21–23]. We estimated observable positive behaviours using an instrument developed by the research team and ASSTSAS advisors, called the Positive Behaviour Inventory (PBI), a tool derived from the Geriatric Indices of Positive Behavior [24]. The PBI contains 14 items including 5 verbal and 9 nonverbal indicators, with the same scoring scale as the CMAI. Verbal indicators were as follows: tries to communicate, participates in conversation, initiates conversation, asks to participate actively in own care and thanks the caregiver. Nonverbal indicators were: opens eyes, does not resist care, relaxes muscles, shows affection (e.g., caresses caregiver's arms), makes eye contact, makes appropriate movements during care, smiles, participates in care to the best of his/her ability, and shakes hands. A higher score indicates more frequent positive behaviours during the care. The test-retest reliability of the original version of the Geriatric Indices of Positive Behavior is good ($k = 0.80$) but the reliability of the PBI has not been studied.

The residents' *sociodemographic characteristics* and the caregiver' sociodemographic variables were also collected. In addition, the residents' functional autonomy was measured with the Functional Autonomy Measurement System (SMAF), which is used to estimate functioning in five dimensions: activities of daily living (ADL) (7 items), mobility (6 items), communication (3 items), mental functions (5 items), and instrumental activities of daily living (IADL) (8 items) [25]. In long-term care facilities, IADL are not systematically assessed and were not considered here. The score for each dimension is obtained by adding the item scores, which range from 0 to 3; a higher score indicates a high degree of dependence (maximum of 63). A reliability study showed that the intraclass correlation coefficient for total SMAF scores was 0.95 (95% confidence interval (CI): 0.90 to 0.97) for test-retest and 0.96 (95% CI: 0.93 to 0.98) for interrater reliability [26].

In addition, after-care, caregivers were asked about their perception of their application of RBC during the observed care. We asked them to express their perception as a percentage, with 100% being care that totally adhered to RBC principles as taught during the training and 0% being care that was completely inconsistent with RBC principles. In addition, they were asked about (1) their satisfaction with their care, (2) how they felt during the care (caregiver's feelings), and (3) how they thought the resident felt. For these three questions, the measuring scale consisted of five faces with the expression of the mouth on a continuum from very sad (inverted smile) to very happy (big smile). The caregivers had to indicate which of the faces reflected the situation in question. For each face, a score from −2 to +2 was assigned.

2.4. Data Analyses. The participants' (residents and caregivers) characteristics and the scores obtained on the measuring instruments were first described by mean and standard deviation or frequency and percentage, depending on whether the variable was continuous or categorical. Since some resident/caregiver dyads were observed more than once during assistance with hygiene and dressing, the mean of the scores for each resident was calculated and used for the analyses.

To achieve our objective, correlation analyses, controlled for duration of care, linked the caregivers' scores obtained on each of the RBC checklist items with the scores obtained on the instruments observing residents' behaviours. We also examined correlations between the caregivers' perceptions after-care, the residents' behaviours, and use of RBC (score on the *RBC Use Checklist*).

3. Results

3.1. Participants' Characteristics. A total of 14 residents and 6 caregivers participated in the study. Table 1 presents the residents' characteristics. Some data are missing for two residents from one of the facilities (died shortly after the observations). As expected, the residents were very dependent functionally and their mental functions were very impaired. The majority of the caregivers were women, patient attendants (orderlies), all working full time, mostly on the day shift, with many years of work experience in the institution or on the patient care unit (Table 2). They had all been trained on RBC, some more recently than others, nearly two years before on average.

3.2. Use of RBC by Caregivers. Table 3 presents the mean scores for RBC use, by category and item. On average, the scores suggest that RBC items were applied by the caregivers most of the time when necessary (mean score for checklist items was 2.6 out of a maximum of 3: mean score of 86.6%). In the *Making contact* category, where the rating is based on the presence or absence of the item, only the "touches the resident" item was done less (mean score of 0.66/1). The other desirable actions when initiating care were done most of the time. For the items referring to the relationship with the resident during care (*Relationship bubble*), it was found that in general caregivers looked at the residents, spoke to them, told them what they were going to do, and touched

TABLE 1: Residents' sociodemographic and clinical characteristics (*n* = 14).

Continuous variables	Mean (standard deviation)
Age (*n* = 12)	78.3 (14.4)
Functional autonomy (*n* = 12)	
SMAF ADL (/21)	16.5 (4.3)
SMAF mobility (/18)	8.8 (2.4)
SMAF communication (/9)	1.4 (1.2)
SMAF mental functions (/15)	10.1 (3.4)
SMAF total (/63)	36.8 (8.3)
Categorical variables	Frequency (%)
Sex	
Men	7 (50.0)
Women	7 (50.0)
Language	
French	9 (64.3)
English	4 (28.6)
Other	1 (7.1)
Marital status (*n* = 12)	
Married	2 (14.3)
Widowed	3 (21.4)
Never married	4 (28.6)
Separated/divorced	3 (21.4)

SMAF: functional autonomy measurement system.
ADL: activities of daily living.

TABLE 2: Caregivers' characteristics (*n* = 6).

Continuous variables	Mean (standard deviation)
Age	47.3 (3.4)
Years of experience in the institution	15.8 (6.5)
Years working on the patient care unit	10.5 (8.0)
Number of months since RBC training	22.5 (19.4)
Categorical variables	Frequency (%)
Position	
Patient attendant (orderly)	5 (83.3)
Nursing assistant	1 (16.7)
Sex	
Women	5 (83.3)
Men	1 (16.7)
Work shift	
Day	5 (83.3)
Evening	1 (16.7)

them gently. Massage was rarely used (*n* = 3) since, in RBC, it is recommended for bedridden clients with muscle contractures. Caregivers obtained very high scores for items in the *General approach*, except for "ends the care." *Teamwork* did not often come into play but, when used, was used as expected in RBC. Finally, *Communication* with residents was good (mean scores between 2.71 and 2.90/3).

Following-care, the caregivers' self-rated percentage of application of RBC was high (mean 86%; SD 11.0) (data not shown). Their mean satisfaction can be considered positive

TABLE 3: Mean scores for RBC items obtained by the caregivers when assisting residents ($n = 14$ with some exceptions) with hygiene and dressing.

Items	Mean (standard deviation)
Making contact (score 0 or 1)	
(1) Knocks on the door ($n = 10$)*	0.81 (0.33)
(2) Introduces him-/herself ($n = 13$)*	1.0 (0)
(3) Announces what the care will be	0.90 (0.19)
(4) Looks at the resident	0.98 (0.07)
(5) Speaks to the resident	0.98 (0.07)
(6) Touches the resident	0.66 (0.36)
Total of the RBC Making contact items (/6)	**4.8 (0.7)**
Relationship bubble (/3)	
(7) Looks at the resident during care	2.73 (0.37)
(8) Announces what he/she will do	2.85 (0.35)
(9) Speaks to the resident during care	2.66 (0.79)
(10) Touches, moves the resident gently	2.67 (0.41)
(11) Maintains physical contact	2.02 (0.97)
(12) Announces if leaving	1.94 (0.99)
(13) Uses massage ($n = 3$)*	1.20 (1.69)
(14) Offers realistic choices	2.24 (0.86)
Mean of the RBC Relationship bubble items (/3)	**2.5 (0.5)**
General approach (/3)	
(15) Adapts interventions to feedback	2.53 (0.71)
(16) Ensures comfort (physical and mental)	2.81 (0.33)
(17) Asks resident to participate, allows autonomy	2.84 (0.30)
(18) Prefers standing during care	2.97 (0.09)
(19) Ends the care	1.91 (1.05)
Mean of the RBC General approach items (/3)	**2.6 (0.3)**
Teamwork (/3) ($n = 5$)*	
(20) Does not speak at same time as coworker	2.70 (0.67)
(21) Is client- and task-oriented	2.29 (0.65)
Mean of the RBC Teamwork items (/3)	**2.3 (0.5)**
Communication (/3)	
(22) Gives clear instructions	2.90 (0.27)
(23) Suggests positive ideas/positive reinforcement	2.71 (0.57)
Mean of the RBC Communication items (/3)	**2.8 (0.3)**

*indicates that these items were observed during the care of only some, not all 14, of the residents.

(1.38; SD 0.43; maximum score 2: 69%) and they felt good during the care (1.56; SD 0.39; 75%). Caregivers' perception of how residents felt during care was quite positive but not as good as their perception of their own feelings (mean 1.24; SD 0.62; 62%).

3.3. Residents' Behaviours. The residents' scores on the instruments used to observe agitated and positive behaviours are presented in Table 4. Positive behaviours were observed more often than agitated behaviours.

TABLE 4: Residents' behaviours during care and mean duration of care.

	Mean (standard deviation)
Agitated behaviours	
Cohen-Mansfield Agitation Inventory (/72)	4.9 (6.5)
Positive behaviours	
Verbal (/30)	6.6 (4.8)
Nonverbal (/54)	20.7 (7.3)
Duration of care (minutes)	16.2 (6.0)

The agitated behaviours observed most often during care were negativity, complaining, grabbing, and screaming. Despite a mean score close to 5, it is important to note that the frequency of agitated behaviours varied greatly from one resident to the next (SD 6.5). Sometimes agitated behaviours were rarely observed and although in other cases they were observed at various times during care, the mean duration of care was only 16 minutes, which accounts for their relatively low number.

The positive behaviours observed most often were participating to the best of their ability, making eye contact, and not resisting care. Relatively speaking, positive nonverbal behaviours were observed more often than verbal behaviours.

3.4. Correlations between RBC Use and Residents' Behaviours. Residents' agitated behaviours were significantly and negatively correlated with two RBC checklist items: (1) speaks to the resident during care ($r = -0.75$; $P = 0.003$) and (2) offers realistic choices ($r = -0.62$; $P = 0.03$). Both of these items are in the *Relationship bubble* category.

Residents' positive verbal behaviours were associated with two RBC checklist items: (1) touches the resident when making contact ($r = -0.70$; $P = 0.008$) and (2) offers realistic choices ($r = 0.59$; $P = 0.036$). It is important to note here that the correlation between the presence of touching when making contact and residents' positive verbal behaviours was negative. Positive nonverbal behaviours were also associated with the same two items in the *Relationship bubble* category: (1) speaks to the resident during care ($r = 0.76$; $P = 0.003$), and (2) offers realistic choices ($r = 0.67$; $P = 0.012$).

3.5. Correlations between Caregivers' Perceptions After-Care and Residents' Behaviours. No significant relationship was found between, on the one hand, the caregivers' perception of the percentage application of RBC and, on the other, RBC use observed by the rater or the residents' behaviours. No significant relationship was found either between the caregivers' perception of the percentage of application of RBC and their satisfaction with the care. However, statistically significant correlations were found between caregivers' feelings about the care they gave and residents' positive verbal ($r = 0.57$; $P = 0.04$) and nonverbal ($r = 0.59$; $P = 0.03$) behaviours. Similarly, caregivers' perception of residents' feelings was associated with positive verbal ($r = 0.75$; $P = 0.004$) and nonverbal (0.75; $P = 0.003$) behaviours.

4. Discussion

The objective of this study was to explore for the first time correlations between RBC use and residents' positive and agitated behaviours during assistance with hygiene and dressing. First, the data from the observations of the caregivers show that, generally, RBC items were applied by the caregivers quite often. Second, the data from observations of the residents suggest that agitated behaviours were present but varied from one resident to the next. Positive behaviours were more frequent, particularly nonverbal behaviours, than problem or agitated behaviours. Finally, the correlation analyses show few significant associations between the residents' behaviours and the frequency of use of RBC checklist items.

4.1. Use of Relationship-Based Care. In general, based on external independent observations, caregivers apply RBC well throughout the care, for a general mean use rate of 86.6%. This high percentage of application of the approach is comparable to those obtained in previous studies. For example, in the study by Bourgeois and colleagues [27], the mean of application of communication techniques similar to those encouraged in RBC varied from 50 to 95%, according to the behaviours. Following the training based on a person-centred approach, participants in Hoeffer and colleagues' study [7] applied gentleness during bathing (e.g., spoke quietly) for a percentage of 82.8 to 85.5%. However, in Drach-Zahavy's study [28], the score obtained for their participants' use of patient-centred care was lower (2.08/3), for an application rate of 69.3%.

Even though Epstein and colleagues [29] considered that using measures that are based on caregivers' perceptions to estimate their level of application of a patient-centred approach may be biased, it is very interesting to note that when asked about their personal perception of RBC application, caregivers gave themselves a mean score of 86.3%, which is very similar to the mean rate obtained by the external observer (86.6%). These virtually identical assessments from two different sources support the validity of the RBC checklist developed from various sources. These scores suggest that caregivers are very familiar with RBC and are very aware of whether they are applying it or not. Therefore, the use of caregivers' perceptions might be not so biased. This would be an interesting topic for future research since caregivers' perception could be less complex and less expensive than using external observers.

Although caregivers gave themselves a high score for RBC use, their satisfaction with their care was acceptable but not optimal (mean score of 69%). Nevertheless, they generally felt good during care (mean score of 75%), which was also found in other studies. In the study by Coen and colleagues [30], with a single-group before-after intervention design, even though there was no impact on caregivers' quality of life, burden, or well-being, their satisfaction increased after an education and support program about dementia care. Similarly, the perception of confidence and ease in giving care among Hoeffer's participants [7] increased after training. In another part of our research project carried out with 420 caregivers trained in RBC [31], job satisfaction was among the best perceived positive effects of RBC. However, Boumans and colleagues [32] found that only 3 out of 15 items related to quality of life at work significantly differed between caregivers who applied patient-oriented care after training and a control group.

Satisfaction with care score was significantly associated with residents' positive verbal and nonverbal behaviours but not with problem behaviours during care. Our exploratory cross-sectional study design did not allow us to establish a causal connection but we could hypothesise that the presence of positive behaviours by the residents might have a greater impact on the relationship with caregivers than problem behaviours. Thus, despite the presence of agitated behaviours, when residents present positive behaviours, such as making eye contact, smiling, or participating in their care to the best of their ability, the caregiver can feel good during the care.

4.2. Correlation between RBC Use and Residents' Behaviours. Only a few correlations were identified between RBC use according to the checklist and residents' behaviours. Generally, in our study, applying RBC more or less was not associated with greater or less frequency of residents' behaviours. It is important to reiterate that overall RBC was applied well by the caregivers, which reduces the variability needed to establish significant correlations. However, two items in the *Relationship bubble* category of the RBC Use Checklist, namely speaking to residents and offering them realistic choices, were found to be related to residents' problem as well as positive behaviours. Thus we could hypothesise that the more caregivers speak to residents and the more they allow them to make choices, the more the residents present positive behaviours. Caregivers who participated in the qualitative study by Skovdahl and colleagues [33] noted the importance of empowering residents to make decisions in preventing the occurrence of problem behaviours. However, it is also possible that it was the residents' positive behaviours that induced the caregivers to talk to them more and offer them choices during care. Our research design allowed us only to make a determination regarding the presence of a positive correlation between these variables, not to establish a causal connection.

In RBC, making initial contact with residents is important. One of the elements advocated to establish contact is to touch the resident physically at the beginning of the relationship. A statistically significant correlation was found between the presence of touching when making contact and residents' positive behaviours. According to RBC, this touching helps to reduce agitated behaviours but our study was unable to confirm this correlation. However, our data suggest that touching at the beginning of care is associated with fewer positive verbal behaviours during care. This result is difficult to explain and may be a fluke.

To summarize, the majority of RBC checklist items were not statistically associated with residents' agitated or positive behaviours as measured in this study. These results are similar to those of some studies and contrary to others. Some studies without a control group, like that by Mathews and colleagues [34], concluded that residents' verbal agitation was reduced when implementing a person-centred approach. Similarly, Mickus and colleagues [35], following a short interactive training session with nurses, observed a lessening in the frequency of residents' problem behaviours. Also, some systematic reviews [17, 18] suggest that person-centred approaches are effective in reducing agitated behaviours. However, the meta-analysis of randomised clinical trials by Kong and colleagues [18] showed that those approaches were not effective in that regard. Overall, there is no consensus or conclusive evidence regarding the impact of using person-centred approaches with clients with cognitive impairments on reducing problem behaviours. For example, in their randomised clinical trial with persons with dementia, Beck and colleagues [36] concluded that their person-centred approach did not help to reduce problem behaviours. On the other hand, training certified nurses to use person-centred strategies helped to reduce aggression and agitation in the participants in a study by Sloane and colleagues [37] using a randomised crossover design.

4.3. Strengths and Limitations. The limitations of this exploratory study should be noted. Because of the cross-sectional observational design, it was impossible to establish causal connections or determine the effectiveness of RBC. The sample size was not optimal because in Quebec Bill 21 considerably limits the participation of people with cognitive impairments in research and at the time of this study, only residents with legal representatives could participate in research. Also, the direct observations in residents' rooms could have disturbed the residents and affected the caregivers' work. It would have been interesting to videotape the care from different angles, which might have shed more light on the caregiver/resident relationship. Finally, the checklists used to estimate use of RBC and note positive behaviours were developed specifically for this study and, apart from content validity in their development process, their metrological properties have not been studied.

This study also has some significant strengths. To our knowledge, this is the first time residents' positive behaviours were taken into account and not only agitated behaviours. Also, the degree of use of RBC and occurrence of behaviours were rated by two independent observers not connected to the care facilities, one observer for the resident and the other for the caregiver.

5. Conclusion

In our exploratory study, the caregivers observed applied many of the elements advocated in RBC. As for the residents, problem behaviours were present during assistance with hygiene and dressing, which necessarily involves invading their privacy. Since there was no control group or pretraining measure, we cannot say if the residents' agitated behaviours would have been more frequent if the caregivers had not used RBC. However, we can clearly state that there were only a few quantitative links between the RBC checklist items and the frequency of agitated or positive behaviours.

The desired impact of RBC on reducing the frequency of agitated behaviours is not the only reason to implement this approach in long-term care facilities. In fact, RBC aims to provide quality care to residents, each of whom is unique, to ensure they live their last years in dignity despite disease, by meeting their needs as well as listening to the needs of the family and society and taking a humanistic approach to these individuals.

Acknowledgments

This study was carried out with the financial support of the Institut de Recherche Robert-Sauvé en Santé et en Sécurité du travail (IRSST) and the Canadian Institutes of Health Research under the PHSI Program (funding reference no.: PHE-91295). The authors wish to thank the long-term care institutions that participated in the study, as well as the following individuals: Anne-Sophie Montminy-Roberge and Natacha Savard, Université Laval master's occupational therapy students at the time, and Mylène Trottier, ergonomics student at the time, for observing the residents, and Lise Trottier for her help with the statistical analyses. And last but not least, they wish to salute the huge amount of ethical approval work done by the Research Ethics Board of the CSSS-Institut Universitaire de Gériatrie de Sherbrooke.

References

[1] Ministère de la Santé et des Services Sociaux, *UN Milieu de vie de Qualité Pour les Personnes Hébergees en CHSLD. Orientations Ministérielles*, Ministère de la Santé et des Services Sociaux, Québec, Canada, 2003.

[2] J. Cohen-Mansfield and P. Werner, "The effects of an enhanced environment on nursing home residents who pace," *Gerontologist*, vol. 38, no. 2, pp. 199–208, 1998.

[3] P. Voyer, R. Verreault, G. M. Azizah, J. Desrosiers, N. Champoux, and A. Bédard, "Prevalence of physical and verbal aggressive behaviours and associated factors among older adults in long-term care facilities," *BMC Geriatrics*, vol. 5, article 13, 2005.

[4] A. Zeller, S. Hahn, I. Needham, G. Kok, T. Dassen, and R. J. G. Halfens, "Aggressive behavior of nursing home residents toward caregivers: a systematic literature review," *Geriatric Nursing*, vol. 30, no. 3, pp. 174–187, 2009.

[5] H. Brodaty, B. Draper, and L.-F. Low, "Nursing home staff attitudes towards residents with dementia: strain and satisfaction with work," *Journal of Advanced Nursing*, vol. 44, no. 6, pp. 583–590, 2003.

[6] W. Evers, W. Tomic, and A. Brouwers, "Effects of aggressive behavior and perceived self-efficacy on burnout among staff of homes for the elderly," *Issues in Mental Health Nursing*, vol. 22, no. 4, pp. 439–454, 2000.

[7] B. Hoeffer, K. A. Talerico, J. Rasin et al., "Assisting cognitively impaired nursing home residents with bathing: effects of two bathing interventions on caregiving," *Gerontologist*, vol. 46, no. 4, pp. 524–532, 2006.

[8] G. S. Winzelberg, C. S. Williams, J. S. Preisser, S. Zimmerman, and P. D. Sloane, "Factors associated with nursing assistant quality-of-life ratings for residents with dementia in long-term

care facilities," *Gerontologist*, vol. 45, no. 1, pp. 106–114, 2005.

[9] J. Cohen-Mansfield and J. E. Mintzer, "Time for change: the role of nonpharmacological interventions in treating behavior problems in nursing home residents with dementia," *Alzheimer Disease and Associated Disorders*, vol. 19, no. 1, pp. 37–40, 2005.

[10] Committee on Quality of Health Care in America, "Improving the 21st-century health care system," in *Crossing the Quality Chasm: a New Health System for the 21st Century*, pp. 39–60, CQHCA, Washington, DC.

[11] T. Kitwood, "Towards a theory of dementia care: the interpersonal process," *Ageing and Society*, vol. 13, no. 1, pp. 51–67, 2008.

[12] B. McCormack, "Person-centredness in gerontological nursing: an overview of the literature," *Journal of Clinical Nursing*, vol. 13, no. 3, pp. 31–38, 2004.

[13] J. Cohen-Mansfield and A. Bester, "Flexibility as a management principle in dementia care: the Adards example," *Gerontologist*, vol. 46, no. 4, pp. 540–544, 2006.

[14] J. Cohen-Mansfield and A. Parpura-Gill, "Bathing: a framework for intervention focusing on psychosocial, architectural and human factors considerations," *Archives of Gerontology and Geriatrics*, vol. 45, no. 2, pp. 121–135, 2007.

[15] J. Cohen-Mansfield and P. Werner, "Longitudinal predictors of non-aggressive agitated behaviours in the elderly," *International Journal of Geriatric Psychiatry*, vol. 14, pp. 831–844, 1999.

[16] J. Opie, R. Rosewarne, and D. W. O'Connor, "The efficacy of psychosocial approaches to behaviour disorders in dementia: a systematic literature review," *Australian and New Zealand Journal of Psychiatry*, vol. 33, no. 6, pp. 789–799, 1999.

[17] P. Landreville, A. Bédard, R. Verreault et al., "Non-pharmacological interventions for aggressive behavior in older adults living in long-term care facilities," *International Psychogeriatrics*, vol. 18, no. 1, pp. 47–73, 2006.

[18] E.-H. Kong, L. K. Evans, and J. P. Guevara, "Nonpharmacological intervention for agitation in dementia: a systematic review and meta-analysis," *Aging and Mental Health*, vol. 13, no. 4, pp. 512–520, 2009.

[19] Y. Gineste and J. Pellissier, *Humanitude: Comprendre La Vieillesse, Prendre Soin des Hommes Vieux*, Armand Collin, Paris, France, 2005.

[20] J. Cohen-Mansfield, M. S. Marx, and A. S. Rosenthal, "A description of agitation in a nursing home," *Journals of Gerontology*, vol. 44, no. 3, pp. M77–M84, 1989.

[21] S. I. Finkel, J. S. Lyons, and R. L. Anderson, "Reliability and validity of the Cohen-Mansfield agitation inventory in institutionalized elderly," *International Journal of Geriatric Psychiatry*, vol. 7, no. 7, pp. 487–490, 1992.

[22] R. J. Miller, J. Snowdon, and R. Vaughan, "The use of the Cohen-Mansfield Agitation Inventory in the assessment of behavioral disorders in nursing homes," *Journal of the American Geriatrics Society*, vol. 43, no. 5, pp. 546–549, 1995.

[23] E. Koss, M. Weiner, C. Ernesto et al., "Assessing patterns of agitation in Alzheimer's disease patients with the cohen-mansfield agitation inventory," *Alzheimer Disease and Associated Disorders*, vol. 11, no. 2, pp. S45–S50, 1997.

[24] R. W. Toseland, M. Diehl, K. Freeman, T. Manzanares, M. Naleppa, and P. McCallion, "The impact of validation group therapy on nursing home residents with dementia," *Journal of Applied Gerontology*, vol. 16, no. 1, pp. 31–50, 1997.

[25] R. Hébert, J. Guilbault, J. Desrosiers, and N. Dubuc, "The functional autonomy measurement system (SMAF): a clinical-based instrument for measuring disabilities and handicaps in older people," *Geriatrics Today*, vol. 4, no. 3, pp. 141–147, 2001.

[26] J. Desrosiers, G. Bravo, R. Hebert, and N. Dubuc, "Reliability of the revised functional autonomy measurement system (SMAF) for epidemiological research," *Age and Ageing*, vol. 24, no. 5, pp. 402–406, 1995.

[27] M. S. Bourgeois, K. Dijkstra, L. D. Burgio, and R. S. Allen, "Communication skills training for nursing aides of residents with dementia: the impact of measuring performance," *Clinical Gerontologist*, vol. 27, no. 1-2, pp. 119–138, 2004.

[28] A. Drach-Zahavy, "Patient-centred care and nurses' health: the role of nurses' caring orientation," *Journal of Advanced Nursing*, vol. 65, no. 7, pp. 1463–1474, 2009.

[29] R. M. Epstein, P. Franks, K. Fiscella et al., "Measuring patient-centered communication in Patient-Physician consultations: theoretical and practical issues," *Social Science and Medicine*, vol. 61, no. 7, pp. 1516–1528, 2005.

[30] R. F. Coen, C. A. O'Boyle, D. Coakley, and B. A. Lawlor, "Dementia carer education and patient behaviour disturbance," *International Journal of Geriatrics Psychiatry*, vol. 14, no. 4, pp. 302–306, 1999.

[31] A. Viau-Guay, M. Bellemare, I. Feillou, L. Trudel, J. Desrosiers, and M. J. Robitaille, "Person-centered care training in long-term care settings: usefulness and facility of transfer into practice," *Canadian Journal on Aging*, vol. 32, no. 1, pp. 57–72, 2013.

[32] N. P. G. Boumans, J. A. Landeweerd, and M. Visser, "Differentiated practice, patient-oriented care and quality of work in a hospital in the Netherlands," *Scandinavian Journal of Caring Sciences*, vol. 18, no. 1, pp. 37–48, 2004.

[33] K. Skovdahl, A. L. Kihlgren, and M. Kihlgren, "Different attitudes when handling aggressive behaviour in dementia—narratives from two caregiver groups," *Aging and Mental Health*, vol. 7, no. 4, pp. 277–286, 2003.

[34] E. A. Matthews, G. A. Farrell, and A. M. Blackmore, "Effects of an environmental manipulation emphasizing client-centred care on agitation and sleep in dementia sufferers in a nursing home," *Journal of Advanced Nursing*, vol. 24, no. 3, pp. 439–447, 1996.

[35] M. A. Mickus, D. B. Wagenaar, M. Averill, C. C. Colenda, J. Gardiner, and Z. Luo, "Developing effective bathing strategies for reducing problematic behavior for residents with dementia: the PRIDE approach," *Journal of Mental Health and Aging*, vol. 8, no. 1, pp. 37–43, 2002.

[36] C. K. Beck, T. S. Vogelpohl, J. H. Rasin et al., "Effects of behavioral interventions on disruptive behavior and affect in demented nursing home residents," *Nursing Research*, vol. 51, no. 4, pp. 219–228, 2002.

[37] P. D. Sloane, B. Hoeffer, C. M. Mitchell et al., "Effect of person-centered showering and the towel bath on bathing-associated aggression, agitation, and discomfort in nursing home residents with dementia: a randomized, controlled trial," *Journal of the American Geriatrics Society*, vol. 52, no. 11, pp. 1795–1804, 2004.

Factors Associated with Insomnia among Elderly Patients Attending a Geriatric Centre in Nigeria

Adetola M. Ogunbode,[1] Lawrence A. Adebusoye,[2]
Olufemi O. Olowookere,[1] Mayowa Owolabi,[3] and Adesola Ogunniyi[3]

[1]Department of Family Medicine, University College Hospital, PMB 5116 Agodi, Ibadan 200221, Nigeria
[2]Chief Tony Anenih Geriatric Centre (CTAGC), University College Hospital, Ibadan, Nigeria
[3]Department of Medicine, College of Medicine, University of Ibadan, Nigeria

Correspondence should be addressed to Lawrence A. Adebusoye; larrymacsoye@yahoo.com

Academic Editor: Marco Malavolta

Background. Insomnia is a form of chronic sleep problem of public health importance which impacts the life of elderly people negatively. *Methods*. Cross-sectional study of 843 elderly patients aged 60 years and above who presented consecutively at Geriatric Centre, University College Hospital, Ibadan, Nigeria. The World Health Organization Composite International Diagnostic Interview was used to diagnose insomnia. We assessed the following candidate variables which may be associated with insomnia such as sociodemographic characteristics, morbidities, and lifestyle habits. Statistical analysis was done with SPSS 17. *Results*. The point prevalence of insomnia was 27.5%. Insomnia was significantly associated with being female, not being currently married, having formal education, living below the poverty line, and not being physically active. Health complaints of abdominal pain, generalized body pain, and persistent headaches were significantly associated with insomnia. *Conclusion*. The high prevalence of insomnia among elderly patients in this setting calls for concerted effort by healthcare workers to educate the elderly on lifestyle modification.

1. Introduction

Chronic sleep problem is very common in elderly people [1]. Sufficient total sleep time as well as sleep that is in synchrony with the individual's circadian rhythm is required for a refreshing sleep [1]. More than half of elderly people have at least one chronic sleep problem [1]. In primary care settings, commonly encountered chronic sleep problems are insomnia and excessive daytime sleepiness [1, 2]. Insomnia is defined by the World Health Organization, using the Composite International Diagnostic Interview (CIDI) version 3, as any individual who has one of the following night-time sleep problems: difficulty in initiating sleep (DIS), difficulty in maintaining sleep (DMS), early morning awakening (EMA), and nonrestorative sleep (NRS) almost every night for ≥ 2 weeks [3].

The population of elderly people in Nigeria is increasing and it is expected to reach 15 million by the year 2025 [4].

There are changes in the sleep pattern as people age, with increasing prevalence of insomnia [1, 2, 5]. In Nigeria, the Ibadan Study of Aging (ISA) group reported an incidence of 8.0% and 25.7% for insomnia syndrome and insomnia symptoms, respectively, among the community-dwelling elderly people [3]. Elderly women were twice as likely as men to report difficulty falling asleep [6, 7]. Studies with clinical implications have added to the body of evidence that chronic sleep problems such as insomnia are not benign but rather an important risk marker for mortality in community-dwelling elderly [8]. In Nigeria, the ISA group reported a significant association between insomnia and chronic medical problems such as chronic pain and hypertension [9].

Community-based studies in Nigeria reported high prevalence of chronic sleep problems among the elderly [3, 9]. The paucity of data on the chronic sleep problems and the health implications has created a knowledge gap in its recognition and management by health workers. The main objective of this study was to assess the prevalence of insomnia and associated risk factors in elderly patients in a frontline ambulatory clinic.

2. Methods

2.1. Study Site.
This study was carried out at the Chief Tony Anenih Geriatric Centre (CTAGC) of the University College Hospital (UCH), Ibadan. Ibadan is the capital city of Oyo State in the south-western area of Nigeria and has a population of 3.6 million inhabitants [10]. CTAGC is a purpose-built facility for the care of elderly people and the first in Nigeria. It was commissioned on 17 November 2012 and manages patients both on in- and outpatient basis. The centre has various speciality units such as physiotherapy, dietetics, geriatric lifestyle, ophthalmology, geriatric dentistry, memory, and geriatric psychiatry units. Elderly patients are comprehensively assessed using a checklist while those requiring further specialist care are referred to other specialty clinics within the University College Hospital, Ibadan.

2.2. Study Design.
The cross-sectional design was used for this study.

2.3. Study Population.
All consenting elderly patients (60 years and above) who presented during the period of the study (January 15 to April 30 2013) were recruited. Leslie Kish formula for single proportion was used to calculate the sample size using the best estimate of the prevalence of insomnia in elderly Nigerians [11] and 843 patients were recruited. Those who were too ill to participate in the study and those who did not consent were excluded.

2.4. Sampling Technique.
Respondents were selected consecutively.

2.5. Procedure.
The respondents were interviewed with a semistructured questionnaire which was pretested before use. The World Health Organization Composite International Diagnostic Interview version 3, a fully structured diagnostic interview (CIDI-3) asks questions about difficulty in initiating sleep (DIS), difficulty in maintaining sleep (DMS), early morning awakening (EMA), nonrestorative sleep (NRS), daytime sleepiness, and dissatisfaction with sleep [3]. The CIDI-3 asks questions about difficulty in initiating sleep (DIS), difficulty in maintaining sleep (DMS), early morning awakening (EMA), nonrestorative sleep (NRS), daytime sleepiness, and dissatisfaction with sleep. The CIDI questions have been adapted and used in a previous study on elderly in Ibadan, Nigeria [3]. Insomnia was assigned to respondent who endorsed any one of the four night-time sleep problems (DIS, DMS, EMA, or NRS) almost every night for ≥2 weeks [3].

Detailed history and comprehensive physical examination of the respondents were carried out by the researchers who are physicians. The questionnaire was translated into Yoruba (the local dialect of most respondents) and independently back-translated to English language. It was then field-tested to ensure that the original meaning was retained. The questionnaire took about 40 minutes to be administered.

2.6. Anthropometric Measurements.
Height was recorded to the nearest centimetre with a measurement stand (stadiometer) which was positioned on a flat surface. The respondents were asked to remove their shoes, and their heels were positioned against the stand with their scapula, buttocks, and heels resting against the wall. Weight was recorded to the nearest 0.1 kg. Respondents stood on the weighing scale which was placed on a flat horizontal surface, after removal of their personal effects. The readings were made by the researcher standing in front of the respondents and the zero mark was checked after every reading for accuracy.

The BMI of the patients was calculated by dividing weight (kilogrammes) by height in meters squared and this was graded using the WHO anthropometric classification [12]. Underweight was defined as BMI $< 18.4 \, kg/m^2$ and 18.5–24.9 kg/m^2 was defined as normal. Overweight was BMI 25.0–29.9 kg/m^2; class I obesity was defined as BMI 30.0 to 34.9 kg/m^2, class II obesity was defined as BMI 35.0–39.9 kg/m^2, and Class III obesity, which is morbid obesity, was defined as BMI of greater than 40.0 kg/m^2 [12].

2.7. Waist-Hip Ratio (WHR).
The waist and hip circumferences were measured using a flexible nonelastic measuring tape and these were measured to the nearest 0.1 cm. The hip circumference was measured at a level parallel to the floor, at the largest circumference of the buttocks. The waist circumference was measured at the end of several consecutive natural breaths, at a level parallel to the floor, midpoint between the top of the iliac crest and the lower margin of the last palpable rib in the mid axillary line. The waist circumference was used to identify individuals with increased risks for metabolic complications based upon threshold values of 80 cm or greater for women and 94 cm or greater for men as defined by the World Health Organization (WHO) and International Diabetic Federation (IDF) [13]. Waist to Hip ratio (WHR) was estimated by dividing waist circumference by hip circumference. The WHR threshold used for elderly women was 0.85 or more and for men was 1.00 or more [13, 14].

2.8. Neck Circumference.
It was measured with a flexible inelastic measuring tape and recorded to the nearest 0.1 cm. Neck circumferences greater than 40 cm in women and 43 cm in men correlate strongly with the development of obstructive sleep apnea and have been adopted as the upper limit for both genders [15].

2.9. Throat Examination.
Oropharyngeal crowding was assessed during throat examination using the Mallampati visual assessment classification (see Appendix/Figure 2) [16]. This was classified as follows: class I: tonsils, pillars, and soft palate were clearly visible; class II: the uvula, pillars, and

upper pole were visible; class III: only part of the soft palate was visible; the tonsils, pillars, and base of the uvula could not be seen; and class IV: only the hard palate was visible [16].

3. Ethical Consideration

3.1. Consent for the Study. Ethical approval was received from the University of Ibadan/UCH Institutional Ethical Review Board (NHREC/05/01/2008a). Informed consent of each respondent was obtained before examination and administration of questionnaire.

3.2. Respondent's Follow-Up. All the elderly patients recruited were given health education and counselling on their health complaints. They were treated for their primary complaints and those needing further evaluation were referred to other specialist units within the hospital facility for further management of their conditions.

3.3. Data Analysis. At the end of each day of the study, the administered questionnaires were sorted out, cross-checked after each interview, and coded serially. Data entering, cleaning, and analysis were carried out using SSPS (version 17). Descriptive statistics was used to describe sociodemographic characteristics of the respondents. Appropriate charts were used to illustrate categorical variables. Chi-square statistics was used to assess association between categorical variables and Student's t-test to test association between continuous variables. The values of significance were set at $P \leq 0.05$. Logistic regression analysis was used to explore relationship between significant variables and insomnia.

4. Results

There were 340 (40.3%) male and 503 (59.7%) female respondents. Their mean (SD) age was 69.3 (7.1) with a range of 60–98 years. The modal age group of the males was 65–69 years, while for the females it was 60–64 years. Majority (86.2%) of the men were currently married while half (52.5%) of the women were widowed. The greatest proportion (50.1%) of the women had no formal education, while the highest proportion (27.6%) of the men attained tertiary education. Half (52.1%) of the male respondents had six or more children, while a higher proportion (62.4%) of the female respondents had less than six children; see Table 1.

The point prevalence of insomnia was 27.5%. The prevalence of insomnia was significantly higher among the women compared with the men (30.2% versus 23.5%, $\chi^2 = 4.551$; $P = 0.033$). Respondents who were not currently married (31.7%) had significant higher prevalence of insomnia compared with those who were currently married (24.9%) ($\chi^2 = 4.718$, $P = 0.019$). Significantly, higher proportion of respondents with formal education (32.8%) had insomnia compared with those who had no formal education (24.1%) ($\chi^2 = 7.744$, $P = 0.004$). Respondents who were currently engaged in occupational activities had higher prevalence of insomnia compared with those not currently engaged in occupational activities (30.2%

versus 26.5%) without a statistically significant difference ($\chi^2 = 1.128$, $P = 0.164$). Respondents who were living (28.6%) and depended financially (28.0%) on others such as spouse, children, grandchildren, and relatives had higher prevalence of insomnia compared with those who were self-supporting (25.8%) and who lived alone (19.8%). The prevalence of insomnia was significantly higher among respondents living below the World Bank defined poverty line of $1.25 per day compared with those living above the poverty line (34.7% versus 23.6%) ($\chi^2 = 11.783$, $P < 0.0001$); see Table 2.

The lifestyle habits and hospital care utilization pattern of the respondents were shown in Table 3. Insomnia was more common without statistical difference among respondents who drank alcohol (34.0% versus 27.1%), smoked tobacco (37.5% versus 27.3%), took cannabis (50.0% versus 27.2%), drank coffee (32.3% versus 27.5%), and were not engaged in physical activities (34.8% versus 26.4%) compared with those who did not engage in these lifestyle habits. The proportion of respondents with insomnia decreased significantly with the increased level of reported physical activities from those who were active (35.4%) through those who were moderately active (27.8%) to those who were very active (22.6%) ($\chi^2 = 6.062$; $P = 0.048$). Hospital care utilization pattern showed insomnia to be more common without statistical difference among respondents who visited hospital four or more times (28.1% versus 26.8%), were previously hospitalized (30.1% versus 25.9%), and were first hospitalized after the age of 60 years (32.0% versus 26.4%) compared with those who visited the hospital less than four times, never got hospitalized, and were hospitalized before the age of 60 years.

The prevalence of insomnia was significantly associated with the complaints of abdominal discomfort (OR = 1.83, $P = 0.032$), generalized body pain (OR = 1.72, $P = 0.001$), and persistent headaches (OR = 1.93, $P = 0.040$), see Table 4. The oropharyngeal crowding in the respondents using the Mallampati classification is shown in Figure 1. Mallampati classes 1 and 2 had higher proportions of respondents who had no insomnia compared with those diagnosed with insomnia. Conversely, higher proportions of respondents with insomnia were in classes 3 and 4 when compared with those without insomnia.

The mean time estimated by the respondents to fall asleep was significantly higher in those with insomnia (25.9 ± 9.4 minutes) compared with those without insomnia (12.2 ± 2.4 minutes) ($t = 10.023$; $P < 0.0001$). Significantly, respondents without insomnia had more hours of sleep during the night compared with those with insomnia (6.9 ± 1.6 hours versus 4.7 ± 1.7 hours, $t = 43.316$; $P < 0.0001$). When asked to estimate the total hours of sleep in a day (24 hours), respondents without insomnia enjoyed more total hours of sleep compared with those with insomnia (9.2 ± 2.0 hours versus 9.0 ± 2.2 hours, $t = 60.642$; $P < 0.0001$).

Table 5 shows the anthropometric measurements by the prevalence of insomnia. Among the males, respondents with waist-hip ratio (WHR) of ≥0.90 had higher prevalence of insomnia when compared with those with WHR of <0.90 without significant difference (25.2% versus 13.0%) ($\chi^2 =$

TABLE 1: Sociodemographic characteristics.

	Male = 340 n (%)	Females = 503 n (%)	Total = 843 N (%)
Age groups (years)			
60–64	83 (24.4)	151 (30.0)	234 (27.8)
65–69	98 (28.8)	123 (24.5)	221 (26.2)
70–74	72 (21.2)	119 (23.7)	191 (22.7)
75–79	48 (14.1)	51 (10.1)	99 (11.7)
≥80	39 (11.5)	59 (11.7)	98 (11.6)
Marital status			
Married	293 (86.2)	222 (44.1)	515 (61.1)
Widowed	38 (11.2)	264 (52.5)	302 (35.8)
Separated	5 (1.5)	8 (1.6)	13 (1.5)
Divorced	3 (0.9)	8 (1.6)	11 (1.3)
Single	1 (0.3)	1 (0.2)	2 (0.2)
Formal education			
None	80 (23.5)	252 (50.1)	332 (39.4)
Primary	80 (23.5)	100 (19.9)	180 (21.4)
Secondary	86 (25.3)	70 (13.9)	156 (18.5)
Tertiary	94 (27.6)	81 (16.1)	175 (20.8)
Occupational activities			
Not currently engaged in occupational activities	225 (75.0)	356 (70.8)	611 (72.5)
Currently engaged in occupational activities	85 (25.0)	147 (29.2)	232 (27.5)
Living arrangement			
Alone	41 (12.7)	65 (13.5)	106 (13.2)
With spouse	247 (76.2)	197 (41.0)	444 (55.2)
With children/grandchildren	32 (9.9)	197 (41.0)	229 (28.4)
With relatives/friends	4 (1.2)	22 (4.6)	26 (3.2)
Financial support			
Self	109 (32.3)	85 (17.1)	194 (23.2)
Spouse	8 (2.4)	13 (2.6)	21 (2.5)
Children/grandchildren	210 (62.3)	390 (78.5)	600 (71.9)
Relatives/friends	10 (3.0)	9 (1.8)	19 (2.3)
Number of children			
0–5	163 (47.9)	314 (62.4)	477 (56.6)
≥6	177 (52.1)	189 (37.6)	366 (43.4)
Income			
Below the poverty line (<$1.25 per day)	89 (26.2)	208 (41.4)	297 (35.2)
Above the poverty line (≥$1.25 per day)	251 (73.8)	295 (58.6)	546 (64.8)

3.251; $P = 0.071$). Among the females, respondents with neck circumference of ≥40 cm had higher prevalence of insomnia when compared with those with neck circumference of <40 cm without significant difference (31.6% versus 30.2%) ($\chi^2 = 0.017$; $P = 0.895$). None of the variables found significant in the bivariate analysis remain so in the final multivariate model.

5. Discussion

This hospital-based study was carried out among 843 elderly respondents with a female preponderance. This was comparable to the Ibadan study on ageing by Gureje et al. in 2011 in which there was a higher proportion of female respondents though their study was community based [3]. Globally, life expectancy is more favourable for women than men, 65.9

years for women as compared with 59.4 years for men [17]. We used 60 years as the cut-off for the elderly in this study because of the low life expectancy in the developing countries especially Nigeria which was 51 and 52 years for males and females, respectively [18]. Similarly, the United Nations designated the elderly as people aged 60 years and above [19].

In this study, the point prevalence of insomnia was found to be 27.5%. This was similar to one prospective cohort study in United State of America (USA) that found 23 to 34% of elderly people with insomnia [5]. Similarly, a Chinese study reported a prevalence of chronic insomnia of 4–22% [15]. A study in Nigeria among community-dwelling elderly people indicated an incidence of 25.7% for insomnia symptoms [3].

Female respondents had a significant higher prevalence of insomnia than men. In general, insomnia symptoms are more prevalent in women than in men and tended to increase with

TABLE 2: Sociodemographic characteristics and the prevalence of insomnia.

	Insomnia		
	Yes = 232 n (%)	No = 611 n (%)	
Age groups (years)			
60–64	70 (29.9)	164 (70.1)	
65–69	66 (29.9)	155 (70.1)	$\chi^2 = 4.123$
70–74	47 (24.6)	144 (75.4)	$P = 0.390$
75–79	21 (21.2)	78 (78.8)	
≥80	28 (28.6)	70 (71.4)	
Sex			
Males	80 (23.5)	260 (76.5)	$\chi^2 = 4.551$
Females	152 (30.2)	351 (69.8)	$P = 0.033^*$
Marital status			
Currently married	128 (24.9)	387 (75.1)	$\chi^2 = 4.718$
Not currently married	104 (31.7)	224 (68.3)	$P = 0.019^*$
Education			
None	123 (24.1)	388 (75.9)	$\chi^2 = 7.744$
Had formal education	109 (32.8)	223 (67.2)	$P = 0.004^*$
Occupational activities			
Not currently engaged in occupational activities	162 (26.5)	449 (73.5)	$\chi^2 = 1.128$
Currently engaged in occupational activities	70 (30.2)	162 (69.8)	$P = 0.164$
Living arrangement			
Alone	21 (19.8)	85 (80.2)	$\chi^2 = 3.613$
With others	211 (28.6)	526 (71.4)	$P = 0.057$
Financial support			
Self	50 (25.8)	144 (74.2)	$\chi^2 = 0.386$
Others	182 (28.0)	467 (72.0)	$P = 0.535$
Number of children			
0–5	127 (26.6)	350 (73.4)	$\chi^2 = 0.442$
≥6	105 (28.7)	261 (71.3)	$P = 0.506$
Income			
Below the poverty line (<$1.25 per day)	103 (34.7)	194 (65.3)	$\chi^2 = 11.783$
Above the poverty line (≥$1.25 per day)	129 (23.6)	417 (76.4)	$P < 0.0001^*$

*Significant at 5% level of significance.

age [20]. This was corroborated by the Ibadan study of ageing in Nigeria [3]. Widowhood, depression and vulnerability to chronic physical conditions have been reported in older women [3, 21]. Our study found no association between age and insomnia. This finding is similar to a community-based study in the same location where this study was conducted but was dissimilar to the report of a survey in the USA which reported that the prevalence of insomnia increased with age [3, 5].

Marital status was found to be significantly associated with insomnia in our study as about a third of those who were not currently married had insomnia compared with a quarter of those who were currently married. This was in contrast to Gureje et al. who reported higher levels of insomnia in the married respondents [3]. Those who were classified as not currently married in our study included the widows and those

who were either separated or divorced from their spouses. Studies have shown a relationship between widowhood and insomnia [3, 21].

Occupation played an important role in the prevalence of insomnia as respondents who were employed had a higher prevalence of insomnia. This was corroborated by Abamara in 2012 among low cadre workers in South Eastern Nigeria in which he found that low cadre workers had more insomnia than others. The female workers attributed their insomnia to the domestic chores normally done after closing hours, with the males resorting to drinking alcohol such as beer and smoking cigarettes or Indian hemp which may initiate insomnia [22].

We employed the World Bank definition of the abject poverty and found a strong association between insomnia and living below the poverty line of less than $1.25 per day.

TABLE 3: Lifestyle habits and hospital care utilization by the prevalence of insomnia.

	Insomnia		Total = 843 N (%)
	Yes = 232 n (%)	No = 611 n (%)	
Alcohol			
Yes	18 (34.0)	35 (66.0)	53 (100.0)
No	214 (27.1)	576 (72.9)	790 (100.0)
$\chi^2 = 1.176$, df = 1, $P = 0.278$			
Tobacco			
Yes	6 (37.5)	10 (62.5)	16 (100.0)
No	226 (27.3)	601 (72.7)	827 (100.0)
$\chi^2 = 0.814$, df = 1, $P = 0.367$[†]			
Cannabis			
Yes	4 (50.0)	4 (50.0)	8 (100.0)
No	228 (27.2)	607 (72.8)	835 (100.0)
$\chi^2 = 2.046$, df = 1, $P = 0.153$[†]			
Coffee			
Yes	10 (32.3)	21 (67.7)	31 (100.0)
No	222 (27.5)	590 (72.5)	812 (100.0)
$\chi^2 = 0.362$, df = 1, $P = 0.547$			
Engagement in physical activities			
Yes	193 (26.4)	538 (73.6)	731 (100.0)
No	39 (34.8)	73 (65.2)	112 (100.0)
$\chi^2 = 3.451$, df = 1, $P = 0.632$			
Level of physical activities			
Not active	40 (35.4)	73 (64.6)	113 (100.0)
Moderately active	145 (27.8)	377 (72.2)	522 (100.0)
Very active	47 (22.6)	161 (77.4)	208 (100.0)
$\chi^2 = 6.062$, df = 2, $P = 0.048$[*]			
Hospital visits in the past 12 months			
0–3 times	95 (26.8)	260 (73.2)	355 (100.0)
≥4 times	137 (28.1)	351 (71.9)	488 (100.0)
$\chi^2 = 0.178$, df = 1, $P = 0.673$			
Previous hospital admission			
Yes	99 (30.1)	230 (69.9)	329 (100.0)
No	133 (25.9)	381 (74.1)	514 (100.0)
$\chi^2 = 1.787$, df = 1, $P = 0.181$			
Age at first hospital admission			
Never or before the age of 60 years	178 (26.4)	496 (73.4)	674 (100.0)
After the age of 60 years	54 (32.0)	115 (68.0)	169 (100.0)
$\chi^2 = 2.081$, df = 1, $P = 0.149$			
Has been on regular medications in the past one month			
Yes	106 (27.2)	276 (72.3)	382 (100.0)
No	126 (27.3)	335 (72.7)	461 (100.0)
$\chi^2 = 3.451$, df = 1, $P = 0.063$			

[†]Yates corrected, [*]Significant at 5% level of significance.

TABLE 4: Morbidities by prevalence of insomnia.

Morbidities	Insomnia		Odds ratio	95% CI	P
	Yes = 232 n (%)	No = 611 n (%)			
Abdominal discomfort	22 (40.0)	33 (60.0)	1.83	1.05–3.20	0.032*
Generalized body pain	77 (36.0)	137 (64.0)	1.72	1.23–2.40	0.001*
Breathlessness	7 (33.3)	14 (66.7)	1.33	0.54–3.26	0.546
Chest pain	4 (25.0)	12 (75.0)	0.88	0.29–2.65	0.374
Fever	2 (16.7)	10 (83.3)	0.52	0.12–2.25	0.528
Severe cough	10 (35.7)	18 (64.3)	1.48	0.68–3.22	0.324
Psychosomatic symptoms	10 (40.0)	15 (60.0)	1.79	0.81–3.98	0.156
Diabetes mellitus	17 (24.6)	52 (75.4)	0.85	0.48–1.50	0.531
Lower urinary tract symptoms	11 (34.4)	21 (65.6)	1.40	0.67–2.91	0.376
Generalized body weakness	5 (27.8)	13 (72.2)	1.01	0.37–2.79	0.953
Persistent headaches	17 (41.5)	24 (58.5)	1.93	1.03–3.64	0.040*
Hypertension	49 (25.9)	140 (74.1)	0.90	0.62–1.30	0.577

*Significant at 5% level of significance.

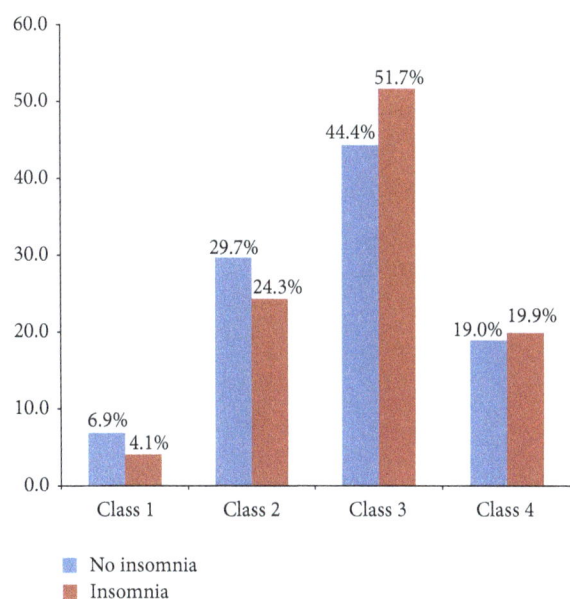

FIGURE 1: Oropharyngeal crowding (Mallampati classification) by prevalence of insomnia.

The Centre for Disease Control and Prevention (CDC) of USA reported higher prevalence of insomnia among adults living below the poverty level (24.8%) compared with those living above the poverty level (15.8%) [23]. Poverty is most likely to be found among low cadre worker who often engage in poor lifestyle habits such as excessive drinking of alcohol and tobacco and cannabis smoking [22].

Insomnia was found to be more common among respondents who consumed alcohol, smoked tobacco, took cannabis, and consumed coffee. This was corroborated by the study which found that substance abuse such as the use of cigarettes, Indian hemp, and alcohol contributed significantly

to the causes of insomnia [22]. Those who lived a sedentary lifestyle were found to have more insomnia in our study as the prevalence of insomnia was inversely associated with the level of physical activities. Excessive daytime sleepiness following insomnia has been found to be strongly associated with reduced physical activities [24].

In elderly people, the problem of comorbidity in insomnia is important [25]. Insomnia is associated with poor health, depression, angina, limitations in activities of daily living, and use of benzodiazepines [7]. Across different populations, several studies have found a significant deleterious effect of sleep disturbances on self-rated health, incidence of cardio-metabolic diseases, quality of life, and mortality [3, 7, 15]. In our study, the prevalence of insomnia was higher in those respondents who had abdominal discomfort, generalized body pain, and continuous headaches. Hospital care utilization pattern demonstrated that insomnia was more among respondents who visited hospital over four times, had been hospitalized in the past, and had their first hospitalization over age of 60 years.

Most studies reported a direct association between insomnia and obesity [24, 26, 27]. But our study found no significant association between the prevalence of insomnia and generalized obesity (BMI) and central obesity (WHR) measures. This could be due to racial and cultural differences in the perception of insomnia and/or the presence of chronic morbidities like diabetes mellitus, hay fever, arthritis, and depression [13, 24].

Oropharyngeal crowding among respondents was graded using the Mallampati classification. Insomnia was more prevalent among respondents in classes 3 and 4. High Mallampati score has been found to be strongly associated with obstructive sleep apnoea which in turn leads to poor sleep [16]. The relative risk of individuals in the Mallampati class 3 or 4 having obstructive sleep apnoea was estimated to be twice those in Mallampati class 1 or 2 [16].

TABLE 5: Anthropometric measurements by prevalence of insomnia.

| | Insomnia | | |
| | Yes = 232 | No = 611 | Total = 843 |
	n (%)	n (%)	N (%)
Waist circumference			
Males			
<94 cm	47 (25.7)	136 (74.6)	183 (100.0)
≥94 cm	33 (21.0)	124 (79.0)	157 (100.0)
$\chi^2 = 1.022$, df = 1, $P = 0.312$			
Females			
<80 cm	15 (32.6)	31 (67.4)	46 (100.0)
≥80 cm	137 (30.0)	320 (70.0)	457 (100.0)
$\chi^2 = 0.137$, df = 1, $P = 0.711$			
Waist-hip ratio (WHR)			
Males			
<0.90	6 (13.0)	40 (87.0)	46 (100.0)
≥0.90	74 (25.2)	220 (74.8)	294 (100.0)
$\chi^2 = 3.251$, df = 1, $P = 0.071$			
Females			
<0.85	15 (32.6)	31 (67.4)	46 (100.0)
≥0.85	137 (30.0)	320 (70.0)	457 (100.0)
$\chi^2 = 0.374$, df = 1, $P = 0.541$			
Neck circumference			
Males			
<43 cm	75 (23.9)	239 (76.1)	314 (100.0)
≥43 cm	5 (19.2)	21 (80.8)	26 (100.0)
$\chi^2 = 0.289$, df = 1, $P = 0.591$			
Females			
<40 cm	146 (30.2)	338 (69.8)	484 (100.0)
≥40 cm	6 (31.6)	13 (68.4)	19 (100.0)
$\chi^2 = 0.017$, df = 1, $P = 0.895$			
Body mass index (BMI)			
Males			
Not obese (<30 kg/m^2)	72 (24.7)	220 (75.3)	292 (100.0)
Obese (≥30 kg/m^2)	8 (16.7)	40 (83.3)	48 (100.0)
$\chi^2 = 1.463$, df = 1, $P = 0.226$			
Females			
Not obese (<30 kg/m^2)	111 (33.0)	225 (67.0)	336 (100.0)
Obese (≥30 kg/m^2)	41 (24.6)	126 (75.4)	167 (100.0)
$\chi^2 = 3.809$, df = 1, $P = 0.051$			

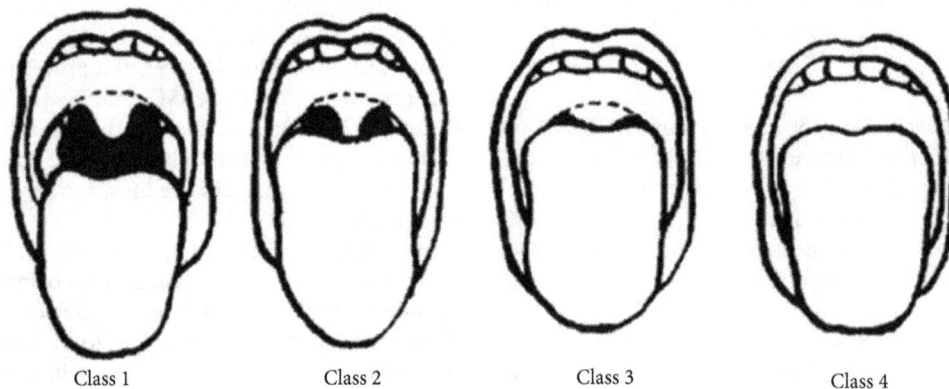

Class 1 Class 2 Class 3 Class 4

FIGURE 2: Oropharyngeal crowding (Mallampati classification).

6. Conclusion

The proportion of elderly patients with insomnia in our setting is high, and in view of the increasing population of the elderly in Nigeria, as well as associated clinical morbidities, it is important to evaluate insomnia during routine clinic consultations. More research on sleep disorders such as insomnia needs to be done among the elderly who are more prone to cardiovascular and other comorbid medical conditions [28].

Appendix

See Figure 2.

Authors' Contribution

Adesola Ogunniyi was the project leader; he was involved in the project design and writing of the paper and he made conceptual contributions. Adetola M. Ogunbode, Lawrence A. Adebusoye, Olufemi O. Olowookere, and Mayowa Owolabi were responsible for the project design, collection of data, analysis, and writing of the paper.

References

[1] D. N. Neubauer, "Sleep problems in the elderly," *American Family Physician*, vol. 59, no. 9, pp. 2551–2558, 1999.

[2] C. A. V. Fragoso and T. M. Gill, "Sleep complaints in community-living older persons: a multifactorial geriatric syndrome," *Journal of the American Geriatrics Society*, vol. 55, no. 11, pp. 1853–1866, 2007.

[3] O. Gureje, B. D. Oladeji, T. Abiona, V. Makanjuola, and O. Esan, "The natural history of insomnia in the Ibadan study of ageing," *Sleep*, vol. 34, no. 7, pp. 965–973, 2011.

[4] L. A. Adebusoye, I. O. Ajayi, M. D. Dairo, and A. O. Ogunniyi, "Nutritional status of older persons presenting in a primary care clinic in Nigeria," *Journal of Nutrition in Gerontology and Geriatrics*, vol. 31, no. 1, pp. 71–85, 2012.

[5] P. Montgomery and J. Lilly, "Insomnia in the elderly," in *Clinical Evidence 2007*, vol. 10, p. 2302, BMJ, 2007.

[6] A. B. Newman, C. F. Spiekerman, P. Enright et al., "Daytime sleepiness predicts mortality and cardiovascular disease in older adults. The Cardiovascular Health Study Research Group," *Journal of the American Geriatrics Society*, vol. 48, no. 2, pp. 115–123, 2000.

[7] A. B. Newman, P. L. Enright, T. A. Manolio, E. F. Haponik, and P. W. Wahl, "Sleep disturbance, psychosocial correlates, and cardiovascular disease in 5201 older adults: the Cardiovascular Health Study," *Journal of the American Geriatrics Society*, vol. 45, no. 1, pp. 1–7, 1997.

[8] European Society of Cardiology, "Daytime Sleepiness Provides Red Flag For Cardiovascular Disease," February 2009, http://www.sciencedaily.com/releases/2009/02/090226160743.htm.

[9] O. Gureje, L. Kola, A. Ademola, and B. O. Olley, "Profile, comorbidity and impact of insomnia in the Ibadan study of ageing," *International Journal of Geriatric Psychiatry*, vol. 24, no. 7, pp. 686–693, 2009.

[10] National Population Commission of Nigeria, *National and States Population and Housing Tables. 2006 Population and Housing Census of the Federal Republic of Nigeria*, National Population Commission of Nigeria, Abuja, Nigeria, 2009, http://www.population.gov.ng.

[11] Population Reference Bureau, "World Population Data Sheet," 2012, http://www.prb.org/pdf12/2012-population-data-sheet_eng.pdf.

[12] World Health Organization, "Physical status: the use and interpretation of anthropometry," Technical Report Series 854, World Health Organization, Geneva, Switzerland, 1995.

[13] World Health Organization, "Waist circumference and waist-hip ratio: report of a WHO expert consultation," Geneva, Switzerland, December 2008, http://whqlibdoc.who.int/publications/2011/9789241501491_eng.pdf.

[14] R. R. Hajjar, H. K. Karmel, and K. Denson, "Malnutrition in aging," *The Internet Journal of Geriatrics and Gerontology*, vol. 1, p. 1, 2004.

[15] N. Haseli-Mashhadi, T. Dadd, A. Pan, Z. Yu, X. Lin, and O. H. Franco, "Sleep quality in middle-aged and elderly Chinese: distribution, associated factors and associations with cardio-metabolic risk factors," *BMC Public Health*, vol. 9, article 130, 2009.

[16] G. Liistro, P. Rombaux, C. Belge, M. Dury, G. Aubert, and D. O. Rodenstein, "High Mallampati score and nasal obstruction are associated risk factors for obstructive sleep apnoea," *European Respiratory Journal*, vol. 21, no. 2, pp. 248–252, 2003.

[17] L. A. Adebusoye, M. M. Ladipo, E. T. Owoaje, and A. M. Ogunbode, "Morbidity pattern amongst elderly patients presenting at a primary care clinic in Nigeria," *African Journal of Primary Health Care & Family Medicine*, vol. 3, no. 1, 6 pages, 2011.

[18] Population Reference Bureau (PRB), "World Population Data sheet," 2013, http://www.prb.org/pdf13/2013-population-data-sheet_eng.pdf.

[19] United Nations Department of Economic and Social Affairs (UNDESA), World Population Ageing and Development 2012, Wall Chart, 2012, http://www.un.org/en/development/desa/population.

[20] X. Liu and L. Liu, "Sleep habits and insomnia in a sample of elderly persons in China," *Sleep*, vol. 28, no. 12, pp. 1579–1587, 2005.

[21] M. LeBlanc, C. Merette, J. Savard, H. Ivers, L. Baillargeon, and C. M. Morrin, "Incidence and risk factors of insomnia in a population-based sample," *Sleep*, vol. 31, pp. 881–886, 2009.

[22] N. C. Abamara, "Factors precipitating insomnia as perceived by low cadre company workers in Nigeria," *Journal of Biology, Agriculture and Healthcare*, vol. 3, no. 16, pp. 31–36, 2013.

[23] Center for Disease Control and Prevention (CDC), "Percentage of men and women who regularly had insomnia or trouble sleeping by family income as a percentage of poverty level," *Morbidity and Mortality Weekly Report*, 2014, http://www.cdc.gov/nchs/nhis.htm.

[24] C. W. Whitney, P. L. Enright, A. B. Newman, W. Bonekat, D. Foley, and S. F. Quan, "Correlates of daytime sleepiness in 4578 elderly persons: the cardiovascular health study," *Sleep*, vol. 21, no. 1, pp. 27–36, 1998.

[25] B. Sivertsen and I. H. Nordhus, "Management of insomnia in older adults," *British Journal of Psychiatry*, vol. 190, pp. 285–286, 2007.

[26] P. G. Kopelman, "Obesity as a medical problem," *Nature*, vol. 404, no. 6778, pp. 635–643, 2000.

[27] I. O. Amole, A. D. OlaOlorun, L. O. Odeigah, and S. A. Adesina, "The prevalence of abdominal obesity and hypertension amongst adults in Ogbomoso, Nigeria," *African Journal of Primary Health Care & Family Medicine*, vol. 3, no. 1, article 188, 2011.

[28] National Institute Of Health (NIH), "Workshop report on effects of sleep disorders and sleep restriction on adherence to cardiovascular and other disease treatment regimens: research needs," NIH Neuroscience Center, March 2003, https://www.nhlbi.nih.gov/meetings/workshops/adherence.pdf.

Factors Influencing Quality of Life for Disabled and Nondisabled Elderly Population: The Results of a Multiple Correspondence Analysis

M. Avolio,[1] S. Montagnoli,[2] M. Marino,[1] D. Basso,[1] G. Furia,[1] W. Ricciardi,[1] and A. G. de Belvis[1]

[1] Institute of Hygiene and Public Health, Università Cattolica del Sacro Cuore, Largo Francesco Vito 1, 00168 Rome, Italy
[2] Dynamic and Clinical Psychology Department, Università "Sapienza", Piazzale Aldo Moro 5, 00185 Rome, Italy

Correspondence should be addressed to G. Furia; giuseppefuria87@libero.it

Academic Editor: Gjumrakch Aliev

Objectives. The aim of our study is to examine the role of some factors (sociodemographic patterns, social relationship support, and trust in healthcare actors) on structure of quality of life among the Italian elderly population, by stratifying according to presence or absence of disability. *Methods.* Using data of the Italian National Institute of Statistics (ISTAT) survey, we obtained a sample of 25,183 Italian people aged 65+ years. Multiple Correspondence Analysis (MCA) was used to test such a relationship. *Results.* By applying the MCA between disabled and nondisabled elderly population, we identified three dimensions: "demographic structure and social contacts," "social relationships," "trust in the Italian National Health Services (INHS)." Furthermore, the difference in trust on the INHS and its actors was seen among disabled and non-disabled elderly population. *Conclusions.* Knowledge on the concept of quality of life and its application to the elderly population either with or without disability should make a difference in both people's life and policies and practices affecting life. New domains, such as information and trusting relationships both within and towards the care network's nodes, are likely to play an important role in this relationship.

1. Introduction

The 20th century has been characterized by a great advance in life expectancy; over the last century, chronic health problems have replaced infectious diseases as the dominant health care burden, and almost all chronic conditions are strongly related to aging. Only in the last few years many health care planners and governments have become aware of this phenomenon and population-based studies regarding age-related chronic diseases have been implemented. Despite the worldwide aging phenomenon, data regarding health and time trends referring to the health of the elderly population are still inadequate [1].

Welfare systems urge to address the social determinants and social gradients of health among the elderly population, for whom social relationships play an important role in access and use of higher quality healthcare services [2].

Among the elderly population, participation in social relationships is likely to be associated with better health status indicators [3–10]. Similarly, poor social relationships are likely to be associated with worse measures of quality of life [11, 12].

Furthermore, the association between social networks and health status is likely to be influenced by social context and therefore by behavioral, cultural, psychological, and physiological condition and material instability [13, 14].

Over the last years, in health and social science fields, growing interest has been devoted to services, programs, and treatments that improve individual quality of life. For this reason perceived well-being of service users is crucial to assess the effects and importance of treatments and services and determining quality of life dimensions. The concept of quality of life for disabled people has different meaning and the improvement of life conditions becomes a shared goal of many programs aimed at these people, acquiring great relevance in outcome analyses.

For this reason, determining and promoting the quality of life of consumers of educational, social, health, and/or healthcare services become a priority [15].

A recent analysis of the literature by Schalock [16] on disabled people about quality of life domains yielded several indicators. The vast majority of these indicators were related to seven core quality of life domains: interpersonal relations, social inclusion, personal development, physical well-being, self-determination, material well-being, and rights.

Following our previous studies [17], we realized that the application of one-dimensional measures in social relationships and the limits of the application of multiple logistic regression models were not exhaustive to fully explore the influence of other linked dimensions (e.g., trust is a basic element in healthcare as well as social care and it is at the same time a difficult phenomenon to conceptualize) and their relationships to quality of life among the elderly population.

The aim of our study is to explore—by stratifying the subjects into disabled and nondisabled elderly population—the influence of the following factors on structure of quality of life: "interpersonal relations," "social inclusion," "physical well-being," "self-determination," "material well-being," and "personal development."

2. Materials and Methods

The study was conducted using data from the last available version of National Survey on "Health conditions and health care services use," a five-year nationwide survey conducted by the Italian National Centre for Statistics (ISTAT) [18]. We focused on a sample of 25,183 elderly population (aged 65+) residing in Italy between 2004 and 2005.

The sample was stratified by the presence or absence of disability:

(i) 2,887 disabled people;

(ii) 22,296 non-disabled people.

We assumed that people with disabilities would perceive their health status and quality of life differently than people without disabilities [19]. ISTAT, according to International Classification of Impairments, Disabilities and Handicaps (WHO 1980), defines disability as impairments, activity limitations, and participation restrictions. "Health conditions and health care services use" survey shows that disability population is 2,6 million, about 4,8% of population older than 6 years old. Data on disabled and non-disabled people were categorized according to the ISTAT classifications [18]. The indicator for disability was built up by ISTAT making refer to Organization for Economic Cooperation and Development (OECD) set of questions about International Classification of Impairments Disabilities and Handicaps (ICIDH) of World Health Organization (WHO) to study specific disability dimensions: physical disability (confinement-troubles in walking, lower yourself, going up/going down, and brush), people care (functional autonomy), and dimension of communication (sight, hearing, and speech).

Statistical weight coefficients were assigned to the data by the carrying rate of the sample size.

According to findings of Schalock [16], the collected data from the survey questions dealing with the social determinants of health were categorized into "interpersonal relations" (interactions, relationships, support-emotional, physical, financial, and feedback), "social inclusion" (community integration and participation, community roles, social support network, and services), "physical well-being" (health, activities of daily living, leisure, and access to health care), "self-determination" (autonomy/personal control, goals and personal values, choices-opportunities, options, and preferences), "material well-being" (financial status, employment, and housing), and "personal development" (education, personal competence, and performance) (Table 1). By considering all Schalock dimensions, all mentioned variables were included in the MCA analyses.

2.1. Statistical Analysis. A preliminary descriptive analysis was carried out to address the modalities of each variable in the same direction, so as to let them occur together. To explore the factors influencing the perceived quality of life among the elderly population, we applied the Multiple Correspondence Analysis (MCA).

MCA is a descriptive/exploratory technique designed to analyze simple two-way and multiway tables containing some measures of correspondence between the rows and columns.

MCA is used to analyze a set of observations described by a set of nominal variables. This is a particular/special technique of Factor Analysis [20] that has been chosen for flexibility and applicability. The results provide information which is similar in nature to those produced by Factor Analysis techniques, allowing to explore the structure of categorical variables included a table. The interpretation of the axes is based upon the contributions of the categories.

The explained inertia (i.e., variance) is therefore severely underestimated, and we used the correct formula that provides a better estimate of the inertia, extracted by each eigenvalue. The correct formula is provided by Benzécri [21]. The interpretation in MCA is often based upon proximities between points in a low-dimensional map (i.e., two or three dimensions). As well as for Correspondence Analysis (CA), proximities are meaningful only between points from the same set (i.e., rows with rows, columns with columns). Since the interpretation of MCA is more delicate than simple CA, several approaches have been suggested to offer the simplicity of interpretation of CA for indicator matrices. When the indicators were a very low frequency (<2%), we randomly (re)assigned this variables, by using SPAD software, to control so-called "rare statistic modality."

By applying MCA, variable numbers were reduced in the latent factors. On each of the factorial axes, we obtained a discrimination measure to represent the intensity with which the variable explained the axis [21]. Moreover, we analyzed the relative contributions of variables and we assessed which modalities are represented on the axes. Each MCA dimension's name was arbitrarily attributed according to the interpretation of its list of variables.

TABLE 1: A framework of determinants on quality of life.

Dimensions	Variables (modalities)
Interpersonal relations (interactions, relationships, support-emotional, physical, financial, feedback)	Living alone (no, yes)
	Marital status (married, unmarried, or not yet married)
	In case of life troubles, my family trust/count on: relatives, friends, neighbors, nonprofit associations, other? (no, yes)
	Home health/social career on behalf of the municipality (no, yes)
	Home worker (no, yes)
	Elderly/handicapped care (no, yes)
Social inclusion (community integration and participation, community roles, social support network, services)	Distance too long between own home and relatives' home (no, yes)
	Do your relatives use a mobile? (yes, no)
	Do you have telephone at home? (yes, no)
Physical well-being (health, activities of daily living, leisure, access to health care)	Physical disability (no, yes)
	Mental disability (no, yes)
	Need to home care services (no, yes)
	Recourse to health-rehabilitation services in the last three months (no, yes)
	Home health career on behalf of local health unit, (no, yes)
	Do you ask someone for important decision on own health? (I ask my GP, I ask a specialist, I ask my private physician, I ask other health professionals, I take final decision by myself)
	Flu vaccination in the last twelve months (yes, no)
	Frequency of blood hypertension check (At least once a year, less than once a year, never)

All analyses were performed using SPSS (Version 17) and SPAD (Version 5).

3. Results

The disabled sample shows that 43.40% of disabled people are married if compared with non-disabled (58.60%) and they live alone more frequently (32.21% versus 27.12%). Above one fifth of the elderly population, with presence or absence of disability, declares to live too far from own relatives' home. "In case of life troubles," 81.29% of the disabled aged 65–74 and 83.86% aged 75 and more can instead count on their relatives; these percentages for non-disabled rise to 83.74% and 87.33%, respectively. Disabled people declared to need homecare services for the 33.91% and home assistance assigned by Local Health Unit (LHU) for the 18.08%; among non-disabled people these percentages decrease to 5.32% and 2.03%, respectively.

In addition, descriptive analysis shows that in the last year, 53.80% of overall sample perceived quality of National Health Service as "the same" or "better." In order to take decision on their own health, more than 87.01% of disabled people used to ask an advice to the health professional if compared to 85.58% in non-disabled sample.

By applying the MCA among the disabled elderly population, we identified three dimensions (axes), which explained a 71.64% improved estimate of the inertia among the ten factors. For the first factorial axis ("demographic structure and social contacts"), the principal discrimination measures are included in "interpersonal relation" and "social inclusion" configured in living alone, marital status and availability, and

mobile for one's own relatives. For the second axis ("social relationships"), the discrimination measures can be mostly associated with "interpersonal relations" (in case of life troubles, my family can trust/count on: friends, neighbors, non-profit associations). The third factorial axis ("trust in the INHS") was made via measures related to trust in the General Practitioner (GP) or specialist. The percentages of total variance explained by each dimension are the following: dimension 1 explained 34.69% of the total variance while dimensions 2 and 3 explained 20.84% and 16.12%, respectively (Table 2).

In the non-disabled sample, we identified three main dimensions which explained 77.38% of the improved estimate of the inertia among the ten factors. The percentages of the variance explained by each dimension are the following: dimension 1 that explained 40.20% of the total variance, and dimensions 2 and 3 that explained 21.44% and 15.74%, respectively. Among the non-disabled elderly population in the first factorial axis ("demographic structure and social contacts"), the principal discrimination measures are associated with "interpersonal relation" and "social inclusion," these including living alone, marital status, and a mobile phone not available for own relatives. The second axis ("social relationships") includes interpersonal relations and the availability of support and advice ("In case of life troubles, my family can trust/count on: friends, neighbors, non-profit associations"). Finally, in the third factorial axis ("trust in the INHS"), there is a relevant influence of "trust on GP" and "trust on specialist", which are classified as "self-determination" according to Schalock's work [16] (Table 3).

TABLE 2: Factor sets of the three main dimensions among the disabled elderly population.

Dimensions	Dimension 1: Demographic structure and social contacts (relative contribution)	Dimension 2: Social relationships (relative contribution)	Dimension 3: Trust in the INHS (relative contribution)
Inertia	34.69%	20.84%	16.12%
Factors	Marital status (unmarried or not yet married = 9.6, married = 13)	My family count on friends (no = 7.4, yes = 11.6)	Trust in GP (no = 14.3, yes = 5.9)
	Living alone (yes = 19.5, no = 9.7)	My family count on neighbors (no = 7.3, yes = 9.9)	Trust in specialist (no = 3.5, yes = 11.0)
	Availability of mobile for own relatives (yes = 6.4, no = 6.6)	My family count on people belonging to voluntary association (no = 2.3, yes = 14.6)	

TABLE 3: Factor sets of the three main dimensions among the non-disabled elderly population.

Dimensions	Dimension 1: Demographic structure and social contacts (relative contribution)	Dimension 2: Social relationships (relative contribution)	Dimension 3: Trust in the INHS (relative contribution)
Inertia	40.20%	21.44%	15.74%
Factors	Marital status (unmarried or not yet married = 14.3, married = 10.0)	My family count on friends (no = 14.8, yes = 15.1)	Trust in GP (no = 18.4, yes = 6.3)
	Living alone (yes = 19.8, no = 7.3)	My family count on neighbors (no = 12.7, yes = 13.2)	Trust in specialist (no = 4.0, yes = 13.3)
	Availability of mobile for own relatives (yes = 5.4, no = 9.5)	My family count on people belonging to voluntary association (no = 1.7, yes = 13.1)	

4. Discussion

In the last years there was an increasing interest in the social and psychological dynamics of the perceived status of well-being, including factors related to social relationships/support, interpersonal trust, internal control, autonomy/independence, self-confidence, aspirations/expectations, and values having to do with family, job, and life in general [16].

Social relationship affiliations and social activity participation could be influenced by the disability [14, 17], and cross-sectional surveys do not provide assistance in the investigation of the strength and direction of such a relationship. Furthermore, being disabled can lead to unfavorable outcomes in both the access and quality of healthcare services, as well as outcomes regarding expectations and trust on its actors [20, 22].

Previous studies explored the influence on self-perceived quality of life of the health status, the social relationships/social inclusion, and the access to healthcare services.

Our study adds new findings on the role of sociodemographic patterns, social relationship support, and trust to healthcare actors on quality of life, among the Italian elderly population by stratifying the sample according to the presence or absence of disability.

In addition, the application of MCA helped to better test the relationship between quality of life and social/health factors in the elderly population.

The MCA analysis confirmed the role of social relationships on the quality of life (first dimension: "structural socio-demographic conditions"). Its role was the most influent, more among disabled than in non-disabled elderly population, respectively, thus confirming previous analysis [7, 10].

Within such dimension, the factor "marital status" is oppositely shaped among the two strata, thus confirming, among the elderly population, not such a positive perception of being married on quality of life (e.g., among women in Italy) [17].

Elderly and disabled people can count on the supportive, active role of their own spouse and of family as a whole, and they are likely to recognize family integration as relevant for the individual inclusion in the community. Such a network would count on availability; that is why disabled people are more likely to recognize the utility of a permanent connection with their own relatives (e.g., by mobile).

Among the disabled elderly population, to count on elective social relationships (i.e., "counting on friends" and "counting on neighbors") is more developed if compared to the overall elderly population. This would be due to the necessity of a supportive network against isolation, exclusion, and other additional negative life occurrences [23]. In addition, among the stratum of the disabled in our sample, a bigger role of voluntary associations in supporting and counseling the disabled on health issues is recorded. Such a role was confirmed by its interaction with structural socio-demographic conditions as well [24].

These findings would be particularly useful in the design of welfare policies towards the disabled elderly population [25]. In particular, the incoming financial constraints are urging the welfare agencies to address the main determinants for social inclusion for the elderly people, and such findings would help them to target the most effective (and cost-effective too) policies and to stratify among disable and not disabled.

Previous studies assessed that access and utilization of social services are also influenced by features of the caregiver, socioeconomic factors, and the available resources. While caregivers' needs influence the services use, the family enabling factors are the most important predictors of the amount of services used [26].

Among the disabled enrolled in the survey, trust in INHS involves mostly GPs, thus confirming that a daily consolidated relationship regarding health issues is likely to be privileged.

As for the non-disabled, the analysis confirmed a protective role of "counting on neighbors" and "counting on friends" on the quality of life. "Counting on people belonging to voluntary associations" is likely to play a relevant role as well.

Furthermore, a role of trust on INHS and its actors emerged, even though with different relative attributes to GP and specialist in the disabled and non-disabled strata, respectively.

In countries like Italy with a socialized health care system, trust might be of two types [27, 28]. The first type is the trust in doctors and nurses we see in GP clinics and hospitals, together with the unspoken trust in all of the unseen support staff in the laboratories and offices. The second type is the trust in systems of the INHS to deliver the health care that people need, at least most of the time.

Our analysis revealed different figures regarding trust in INHS' actors; trust in specialist, rather than in the GP, confirms different attitudes and expectations regarding the health delivery system among the non-disabled, whose satisfaction and trust seems to derive from a more selected demand of specialized services [29].

It should be stated that our analysis contains certain limitations. One limitation derives from our cross-sectional design, which means that temporal directions of associations between reciprocally connected variables could not be defined.

The entire social relationship dimension was not completely explored in the ISTAT questionnaire. A low power of analysis inside the kin or nonkin networks was a limit of such an investigation [30].

Trust regarding care would take into account healthcare as well social care.

As clear questions regarding social supports/services were contained in the multipurpose survey, the social services were found to be inadequately supplied to the disabled, and public financial help to their families was also seen to be inadequate according to our analysis [31].

Unfortunately, the multipurpose survey [18] does not explain which kind of interventions is provided by voluntary associations, so as to disaggregate between the disabled and the non-disabled elderly population.

The comprehensive interactive role of information and trust in relationships and self-perceived health in the elderly population has not been widely investigated, due to the scarcity of information in the ISTAT questionnaire.

A limit of the MCA involves its mainly explorative role [21]. Further analysis is needed to evaluate the role of the key results.

By applying MCA, together with marital status ("unmarried" or "not yet married") and "living alone," we found out

that the most outstanding dimensions in the relationship with quality of life among the elderly population were the use of healthcare services, the trust on own doctors (GP and Specialist), and the availability of a confidant/adviser on health problems.

Knowledge regarding the concept of quality of life and its application to the elderly population either with or without a disability should make a difference in both people's lives and the policies and practices that impact those lives [16].

Social relationships represent an important factor in improving quality of life among the elderly population, and new domains are likely to play an important role in this relationship.

References

[1] A. Marengonia, S. Anglemana, R. Melisa, F. Mangialaschea, A. Karpa, A. Garmena et al., "Aging with multimorbidity: a systematic review of the literature," *Ageing Research Reviews*, vol. 10, pp. 430–439, 2011.

[2] C. E. Sluzki, "Social networks and the elderly: conceptual and clinical issues, and a family consultation," *Family Process*, vol. 39, no. 3, pp. 271–284, 2000.

[3] K. J. Ajrouch, A. Y. Blandon, and T. C. Antonucci, "Social networks among men and women: the effects of age and socioeconomic status," *Journals of Gerontology B*, vol. 60, no. 6, pp. S311–S317, 2005.

[4] L. F. Berkman, "Assessing the physical health effects of social networks and social support," *Annual Review of Public Health*, vol. 5, pp. 413–432, 1984.

[5] J. S. House, K. R. Landis, and D. Umberson, "Social relationships and health," *Science*, vol. 241, no. 4865, pp. 540–545, 1988.

[6] B. H. Kaplan, J. C. Cassel, and S. Gore, "Social support and health," *Medical Care*, vol. 15, no. 5, pp. 47–58, 1977.

[7] L. F. Berkman and T. Glass, "Social integration, social networks, social support, and health," in *Social Epidemiology*, L. F. Berkman and I. Kawachi, Eds., pp. 137–173, Oxford University Press, New York, NY, USA, 2000.

[8] C. McCamish-Svensson, G. Samuelsson, B. Hagberg, T. Svensson, and O. Dehlin, "Social relationships and health as predictors of life satisfaction in advanced old age: results from a Swedish longitudinal study," *International Journal of Aging and Human Development*, vol. 48, no. 4, pp. 301–324, 1999.

[9] A. Rodriguez-Laso, M. V. Zunzunegui, and A. Otero, "The effect of social relationships on survival in elderly residents of a Southern European community: a cohort study," *BMC Geriatrics*, vol. 7, article 19, 2007.

[10] M. Á. E. Bravo, D. Puga, and M. Martín, "Protective effects of social networks on disability among older adults in Madrid and Barcelona, Spain, in 2005," *Revista Espanola de Salud Publica*, vol. 82, no. 6, pp. 637–651, 2008.

[11] B. Ydreborg, K. Ekberg, and A. Nordlund, "Health, quality of life, social network and use of health care: a comparison between those granted and those not granted disability pensions," *Disability and Rehabilitation*, vol. 28, no. 1, pp. 25–32, 2006.

[12] L. Hansson and T. Björkman, "Are factors associated with subjective quality of life in people with severe mental illness consistent over time?: a 6-year follow-up study," *Quality of Life Research*, vol. 16, no. 1, pp. 9–16, 2007.

[13] M. V. Zunzunegui, A. Koné, M. Johri, F. Béland, C. Wolfson, and H. Bergman, "Social networks and self-rated health in two French-speaking Canadian community dwelling populations over 65," *Social Science and Medicine*, vol. 58, no. 10, pp. 2069–2081, 2004.

[14] M. Melchior, L. F. Berkman, I. Niedhammer, M. Chea, and M. Goldberg, "Social relations and self-reported health: a prospective analysis of the French Gazel cohort," *Social Science and Medicine*, vol. 56, no. 8, pp. 1817–1830, 2003.

[15] M. A. Verdugo, G. Prieto, C. Caballo, and A. Peláez, "Factorial structure of the quality of life questionnaire in a Spanish sample of visually disabled adults," *European Journal of Psychological Assessment*, vol. 21, no. 1, pp. 44–55, 2005.

[16] R. L. Schalock, "The concept of quality of life: what we know and do not know," *Journal of Intellectual Disability Research*, vol. 48, no. 3, pp. 203–216, 2004.

[17] A. G. de Belvis, M. Avolio, L. Sicuro et al., "Social relationships and HRQL: a cross-sectional survey among older Italian adults," *BMC Public Health*, vol. 8, article 348, 2008.

[18] The Italian National Institute of Statistics [ISTAT], "Indagine multiscopo annuale sulle famiglie: 'Condizioni di salute e ricorso ai servizi sanitari,'" Anni 2004-2005, 2007, http://www3.istat.it/salastampa/comunicati/non_calendario/20070302_00/testointegrale.pdf.

[19] World Health Organization and World Bank, *World Report on Disability*, WHO Press, Geneva, Switzerland, 2011.

[20] U. Sonn, "Longitudinal studies of dependence in daily life activities among elderly persons," *Scandinavian Journal of Rehabilitation Medicine*, Supplement, no. 34, pp. 1–35, 1996.

[21] J. P. Benzécri, *Correspondenceanalysis Handbook*, Marcel Dekker, New York, NY, USA, 1992.

[22] E. Barba, "Attitudes toward the chronically ill and disabled: implications for the health care systems," *Social Work in Health Care*, vol. 3, no. 2, pp. 199–210, 1977.

[23] F. Dal Sasso and A. Pigatto, "Psychological consulting for the elderly," in *Clinical Psychology Consultancy*, G. Disnan and G. Fava Viziello, Eds., pp. 192–206, Elsevier, Milan, Italy, 2009.

[24] S. Cohen and T. A. Wills, "Stress, social support, and the buffering hypothesis," *Psychological Bulletin*, vol. 98, no. 2, pp. 310–357, 1985.

[25] F. Folgheraiter, *The Social Logic of Aid: Foundations For A relational Theory of Welfare*, Erickson studies centre, Trent, Italy, 2007.

[26] Y.-C. Chou, Y.-C. Lee, L.-C. Lin, A.-N. Chang, and W.-Y. Huang, "Social services utilization by adults with intellectual disabilities and their families," *Social Science and Medicine*, vol. 66, no. 12, pp. 2474–2485, 2008.

[27] M. A. Hall, B. Zheng, E. Dugan et al., "Measuring patients' trust in their primary care providers," *Medical Care Research and Review*, vol. 59, no. 3, pp. 293–318, 2002.

[28] D. H. Thom, R. L. Kravitz, R. A. Bell, E. Krupat, and R. Azari, "Patient trust in the physician: relationship to patient requests," *Family Practice*, vol. 19, no. 5, pp. 476–483, 2002.

[29] S. Sofaer and K. Firminger, "Patient perceptions of the quality of health services," *Annual Review of Public Health*, vol. 26, pp. 513–559, 2005.

[30] G. Costa, T. Spadea, and M. Cardano, "Health inequalities in Italy," *Epidemiologia e prevenzione*, vol. 28, no. 3, pp. 1–162, 2004.

[31] L. C. Giles, G. F. V. Glonek, M. A. Luszcz, and G. R. Andrews, "Effect of social networks on 10 year survival in very old Australians: the Australian longitudinal study of aging," *Journal of Epidemiology and Community Health*, vol. 59, no. 7, pp. 574–579, 2005.

Predicting Delirium Duration in Elderly Hip-Surgery Patients: Does Early Symptom Profile Matter?

Chantal J. Slor,[1] Joost Witlox,[1] Dimitrios Adamis,[2]
David J. Meagher,[3] Tjeerd van der Ploeg,[4] Rene W. M. M. Jansen,[1]
Mireille F. M. van Stijn,[5] Alexander P. J. Houdijk,[5] Willem A. van Gool,[6]
Piet Eikelenboom,[6] and Jos F. M. de Jonghe[1]

[1] Department of Geriatric Medicine, Medical Center Alkmaar, P.O. Box 501, 1800 AM Alkmaar, The Netherlands
[2] Research and Academic Institute of Athens, 27 Themistokleous Street and Akadimias, 106 77 Athens, Greece
[3] University Hospital Limerick and Department of Adult Psychiatry, University of Limerick Medical School, Limerick, Ireland
[4] Medical Center Alkmaar, Pieter van Foreest Institute for Education and Research, 1800 AM Alkmaar, The Netherlands
[5] Department of Surgery, Medical Center Alkmaar, 1800 AM Alkmaar, The Netherlands
[6] Department of Neurology, Academic Medical Center, P.O. Box 22660, 1100 DD Amsterdam, The Netherlands

Correspondence should be addressed to Chantal J. Slor; jjochemina@hotmail.com

Academic Editor: Abebaw Yohannes

Background. Features that may allow early identification of patients at risk of prolonged delirium, and therefore of poorer outcomes, are not well understood. The aim of this study was to determine if preoperative delirium risk factors and delirium symptoms (at onset and clinical symptomatology during the course of delirium) are associated with delirium duration. *Methods.* This study was conducted in prospectively identified cases of incident delirium. We compared patients experiencing delirium of short duration (1 or 2 days) with patients who had more prolonged delirium ($\geq$3 days) with regard to DRS-R-98 (Delirium Rating Scale Revised-98) symptoms on the first delirious day. Delirium symptom profile was evaluated daily during the delirium course. *Results.* In a homogenous population of 51 elderly hip-surgery patients, we found that the severity of individual delirium symptoms on the first day of delirium was not associated with duration of delirium. Preexisting cognitive decline was associated with prolonged delirium. Longitudinal analysis using the generalised estimating equations method (GEE) identified that more severe impairment of long-term memory across the whole delirium episode was associated with longer duration of delirium. *Conclusion.* Preexisting cognitive decline rather than severity of individual delirium symptoms at onset is strongly associated with delirium duration.

1. Introduction

Postoperative delirium is a common complication in elderly hip-fracture patients, that is associated with high mortality, cognitive deterioration, and a high rate of subsequent institutionalization [1–3]. Delirium follows a variable course, ranging from a brief transient state to more persistent illness that can evolve into long-term cognitive impairment [4, 5]. Factors that may allow earlier identification of patients who are at risk of more prolonged delirium are not well understood [6, 7]. Although studies over the past decade have improved our understanding of the phenomenology

of delirium, little is known about the association between specific delirium symptoms and duration of delirium [8].

Few studies have examined delirium symptoms as a risk factor for an extended duration of the delirious episode. Previous studies have used the Delirium Rating Scale (DRS) [9] to measure the severity of delirium symptoms [10, 11]. Rudberg et al. (1997) found that patients experiencing delirium of a single day's duration did not differ from more persistent (multiple days) cases with regard to individual DRS item scores on the first day of delirium [10]. Conversely, Wada and Yamaguchi (1993), who also used the DRS, found that more severe cognitive impairment, sleep-wake cycle disturbances, and mood lability were associated with longer delirium episodes (>1 week versus ≤1 week) [11]. However, these studies used the original DRS which focuses upon a relatively narrow range of delirium symptoms compared to the revised version (DRS-R-98) and/or did not control for factors such as preexisting cognitive problems, including dementia. This is a significant shortcoming of previous research since dementia may be a predictor of illness duration [12, 13], in addition to being an important risk factor for delirium [14].

Most studies that investigated delirium duration restricted delirium monitoring to specific time intervals. The risk of mortality is increased by 11% for every additional 48 hours that delirium persists [15]. This makes it imperative to gain more insight into the determinants of delirium duration. Moreover, frequent (e.g., daily) assessments make it possible to determine that the character of delirium is related to episode duration.

In this prospective observational study we investigated a homogenous cohort of elderly hip-surgery patients aged 75 or older, who were carefully monitored on a daily basis for the occurrence of delirium. The aim of the present study was to identify patient characteristics that are associated with prolonged delirium and explore how delirium symptomatology evolves over time.

2. Methods

2.1. Ethical Considerations. The study was undertaken in accordance with the Declaration of Helsinki and the guidelines on Good Clinical Practice. Approval of the regional research ethics committee was obtained. Patients or their relatives gave fully informed written consent.

2.2. Study Design and Objectives. This was a prospective cohort study in elderly hip-fracture patients. Evaluating the relationship between patient characteristics and delirium was a prespecified aim of this study.

Patient characteristics and risk factors for delirium were assessed preoperatively. Presence and severity of delirium were assessed daily. Since all participants were at high risk for delirium (i.e., age 75 years or older, and acute hospital admission), all patients received routine care with prophylactic treatment of 0.5 mg haloperidol, three times daily, from time of admission until postoperative day three, unless contraindications regarding its use were present [16].

We investigated the association between delirium symptoms on the first delirious day, with subsequent duration of the delirious episode. We compared incident delirium cases experiencing short delirium episodes (1 or 2 days) with patients who experienced more prolonged delirium (≥3 days). Thereafter, we investigated the association between delirium symptom profile over time and duration in days until recovery. For this longitudinal analysis, data on DRS-R-98 item scores gathered over all days of active delirium was included.

2.3. Participants. The study was conducted in a series of consecutively admitted elderly hip-fracture patients to a teaching hospital in Alkmaar, The Netherlands. Eligibility was checked for all patients 75 years and older admitted for primary surgical repair of hip fracture. From March 2008 to March 2009, 192 hip-fracture patients were eligible, and they fulfilled criteria for participation and provided consent. A subgroup of this study cohort, 122 patients, also participated in a clinical trial that compared the effectiveness of taurine versus placebo in reducing morbidity and one-year mortality in elderly hip fracture patients (Clinicaltrials.gov; registration number NCT00497978; this project has been the subject of a previous report [17]). The 122 patients who participated in the RCT were younger compared to the rest of the 192 eligible patients.

Patients were ineligible to participate in the study if they had no surgery, had a malignancy, had a previous hip fracture on the identical side, were in contact isolation, incapable of participating in interviews (language barrier, aphasia, and coma), had no acute trauma, were transferred to another hospital, or received a total hip prosthesis.

For the current analysis we also excluded cases who died during hospitalization, were already delirious before surgery or could not be allocated to one of the duration groups according to the definition of recovery. The people who died during admission were more often male, had a history of previous delirium, and were more dependent in their activities of daily living compared to the rest of the 192 eligible patients. Preoperative delirium cases were excluded because we focused upon a well-defined homogeneous group of incident delirium, and the presence of preoperative delirium includes cases where delirium may have contributed to falls and need for subsequent hip-fracture surgery. Patients with no data available on the two days after the last delirious day could not be allocated to one of the duration groups. In this instance we could not define the exact count of delirious days according to the definition used for recovery.

2.4. Measurements and Procedures

2.4.1. Baseline Assessment. Baseline assessment was completed within 12 hours of admission and prior to surgery. This comprised delirium assessment, patient and proxy interviews and questionnaires, and inspection of the medical record to assess for risk factors for delirium. Preoperative cognitive functioning was assessed with the Mini-Mental State Examination (MMSE) on a scale of 0 to 30 with scores lower than 24 indicating cognitive impairment [18]. Prefracture cognitive decline was estimated with the short version of the Informant Questionnaire on Cognitive Decline in the Elderly (IQCODE-N), scored by a close relative or caregiver. This measures preexisting cognitive decline during the past 10 years on a scale of 16 (improvement) to 70 (decline) [19]. A total score higher than 57 (i.e., a mean item-score higher than 3.6) indicates cognitive decline [20]. For the IQCODE-N proxies were asked to describe the patient's condition a week before the fracture as to determine function unbiased by the event of hip fracture itself or any acute or subacute event leading to hip fracture. Burden of illness included the number and type of medical comorbidities and medications before hospital admission. Demographic factors included age and gender. Data on medication was collected as part of the prospective data collection and checked again afterwards by medical record review. We also reviewed medical records to document the Acute Physiology Age and Chronic Health Examination (APACHE II) score (range of 0 (no acute health problems) to 70 (severe acute health problems)) [21]. Functional status comprised prefracture living arrangement, visual acuity, activities of daily living (ADL), and instrumental activities of daily living (IADL). Visual acuity was assessed with the standardized Snellen test for visual impairment [22], and visual impairment was defined as binocular near vision, after correction, worse than 20/70. Prefracture ADL functioning was determined with the Barthel Index (BI) which is scored by a close relative or caregiver on a scale from 0 (dependence) to 20 (independence) [23]. IADL was also assessed by a close relative or caregiver on the Lawton IADL scale with a range of 8 (no disability) to 31 (severe disability) [24].

2.4.2. Outcome. The primary outcome was duration of delirium. The highly fluctuating nature of delirium makes for problems in reliably defining recovery, and therefore a standard definition is lacking [25]. We followed a conservative approach to define recovery of delirium as two subsequent days without delirium according to the Confusion Assessment Method (CAM) [26]. For some analyses (specified in what follows) delirium duration was used as a continuous variable, whereas we also used a dichotomy with incident cases who were delirious for 1 or 2 days labeled as "short delirium" with the remaining cases who were delirious for three days or more, labeled as prolonged delirium. A single day without delirium but followed by further delirium was considered part of the delirium episode.

Delirium was defined according to the Confusion Assessment Method (CAM) and validated with a diagnosis based on DSM IV criteria [26, 27]. The CAM consists of acute onset and fluctuating course of cognitive function, inattention, and either disorganized thinking and/or altered level of consciousness. Delirium severity was measured using the Delirium Rating Scale Revised-98 (DRS-R-98), a 16-item rating scale comprised of thirteen severity items and 3 diagnostic items. The item scores have range of 0 (no severity) to 3 (maximum severity). Possible total severity scores have range of 0 (no severity) to 39 (maximum severity) [28]. Presence and severity of delirium were assessed within 12 hours after admission and before surgery and continued daily after delirium onset or until the fifth postoperative day for delirium onset. Delirium usually presents itself within the first few days after surgery, if delirium onset is after this time frame it is mostly caused by secondary complications (e.g., urinary tract infection) [29–34]. The CAM and DRS-R-98 rating were based on all available information, collected by trained research assistants, including (i) brief formal cognitive testing with the MMSE, (ii) patient and hospital staff interviews, and (iii) scrutiny of the medical and nursing records.

2.5. Data Analysis. Data analysis was performed using SPSS for Windows, version 19 (SPSS, Inc., Chicago, Il).

Comparisons of group characteristics were made using chi-square or Fisher's exact test for differences in proportions, *t*-testing for differences in means, and nonparametric tests for rank differences.

The univariate significant baseline variables between the short and prolonged delirium group were analyzed with binary logistic regression using the backward Wald method, in order to select the control variables for the first and second part of the research question.

For the first research question (the prediction of short versus prolonged delirium duration by the initial severity of DRS-R-98 items and baseline characteristics) binary logistic regression with the backward Wald method was used. Delirium duration was the binary-dependent variable (short (≤ 2 days) versus long (≥ 3 days)).

At first we applied a logistic regression model with only the scores (range 0 to 3) on the 13 DRS-R-98 severity items on the first day of delirium. Afterwards the same model was repeated but including the covariates: age, sex, and prior cognitive decline (IQCODE > 3.6). The variables were checked for collinearity (collinearity statistics, tolerance, and variance inflation factor (VIF) were performed; all variables entered into the model had a VIF less than 10 and Tolerance more than 0.1).

For the second research question (clinical symptomatology during the course of delirium) a generalised estimating equations model was used to analyze longitudinal data for patterns of individual items from the DRS-R-98 (items 1–13) between cases with different delirium duration until recovery (range from 1 through 9 days). All available DRS-R-98 item scores (1–13) from first day of delirium until the defined end of the delirium episode were included as independent variables. The continuous dependent variable was duration, measured as the sum of the delirium days from the first day of delirium until the end of delirium. Because it is factually a count variable, following a Poisson distribution, we treated this as such. The GEE method takes into account the fact that observations within a subject are correlated and estimates the population average across time. All scale items were included in each analysis although only those that were significantly different are shown in the results tables.

Results were classified as significant if the *P* value was less than 0.05.

3. Results

After excluding ineligible patients ($n = 73$), patients who died in hospital ($n = 12$), and prevalent cases ($n = 23$) there were 57/157 (36.3%) incident delirium cases (Figure 1). Six cases were excluded, since they could not be defined with certainty as belonging to the short or prolonged delirium group because of missing data. The second research question involved exclusion of another 8 cases because of missing data that impeded determining exact duration of delirium according to our definition of recovery. Treatment (taurine or placebo) had no effect on daily CAM diagnosis, DRS-R-98 total scores, and delirium duration, so this was not entered as a control variable in further analysis. Logistic regression

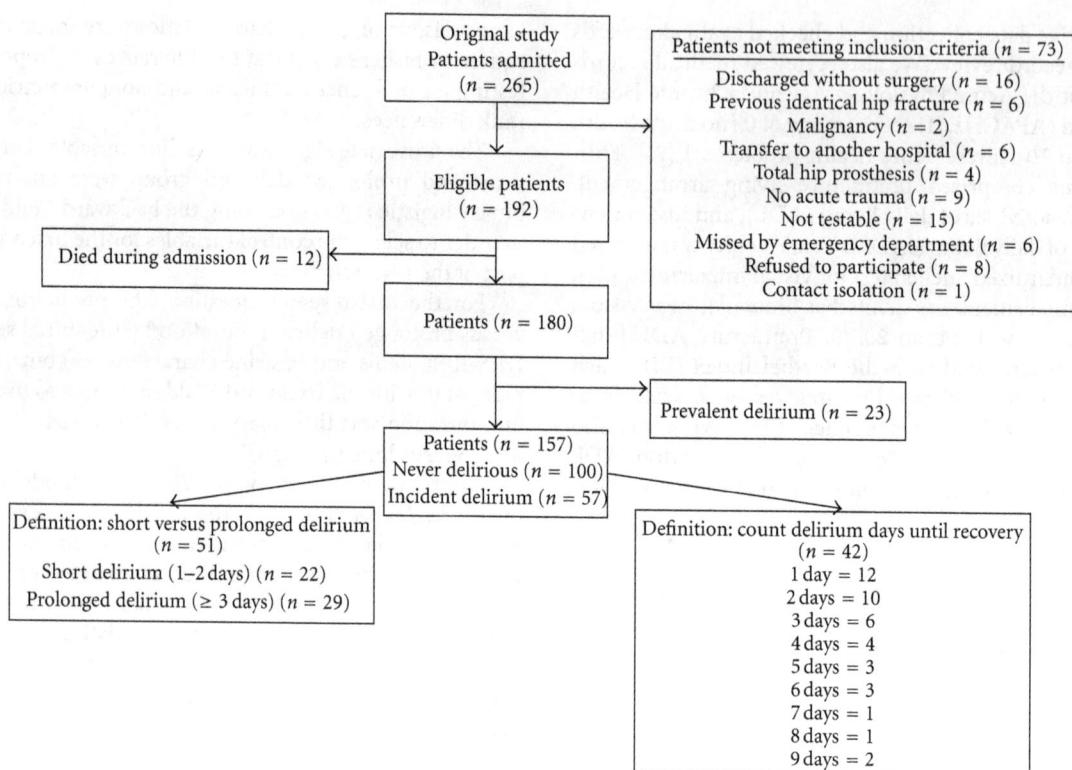

FIGURE 1: Flow diagram of the study.

analysis with baseline characteristics identified IQCODE score > 3.6 as the only significant factor, so this was entered as a control variable in further analysis.

The average age of the 13 male and 38 female patients was 85.1 ± 5.4 (mean ± standard deviation). A total of 22/51 cases (43.1%) had short delirium (1 or 2 days) and 29/51 cases (56.9%) had prolonged delirium (≥3 days). Within the prolonged delirium 20/28 cases could be further defined with regard to exact duration (3 days: $n = 6$; 4 days; $n = 4$; 5 days, $n = 3$; 6 days: $n = 3$; 7 days: $n = 1$; 8 days: $n = 1$ and 9 days: $n = 2$). A significantly greater ($P = 0.003$) proportion of patients within the prolonged delirium group (26/29 cases: 89.7%) compared to the short delirium group 11/22 cases (50%) had an IQCODE > 3.6. A further comparison of the short and prolonged delirium group on other variables is depicted in Table 1. The use (yes or no) of medication classes (sedative hypnotics, antipsychotics, opioids, beta-blocking agents, antidepressants, antihistamines for systemic use, antiparkinson agents, corticosteroids for systemic use, nonsteroidal anti-inflammatory agents, antiepileptics, diuretics, and H_2-antagonists did not differ significantly between the short and prolonged delirium group.

Table 2 shows a descriptive analysis of the presence (score ≥1) of delirium symptoms within the short and prolonged delirium group on the first day. Disturbed orientation and attention were prominent features in both groups. Only visuospatial functioning differed significantly (OR 5.3, 95% CI 1.28–21.57, $P = 0.02$).

Figure 2 displays the mean scores on DRS-R-98 items on the first day of delirium within the short and prolonged

delirium groups. None of the individual item scores differed significantly between the groups.

Logistic regression analysis indicated that more severe motor retardation on the DRS-R-98 was associated with prolonged delirium (OR 1.88, 95% CI 1.03–3.42, $P = 0.04$). The model's R^2 (Nagelkerke) was 0.16, and percentage of correctly classified patients was 61.5% (1-2 days: 0%, ≥3 days: 100%).

After controlling for time-invariant variables (gender, age, and preexistent cognitive decline) none of the DRS-R-98 items on the first day of delirium were associated with delirium duration. Only preexistent cognitive decline (IQCODE > 3.6) was associated with prolonged delirium (OR 0.1, 95% CI 0.02–0.61, $P = 0.01$). The model's R^2 (Nagelkerke) was 0.24, and the overall percentage of correctly classified patients was 74.4% (1-2 days: 46.7%, ≥3 days: 91, 7%).

The longitudinal analysis with data on DRS-R-98 item scores gathered over all the delirium days gave the final most parsimonious GEE model (113 observations, 38 patients included) that is shown in Table 3. A higher score on long-term memory (DRS-R-98 item 12) was associated with a longer duration of delirium until recovery considering all assessments within the delirium episode.

4. Discussion

This study is one of the few to describe the predictive value of delirium symptomatology in the early phase of the delirium episode for subsequent duration. In a homogenous population of elderly hip-surgery patients, we found that the

TABLE 1: Baseline clinical and demographic characteristics of patients in the short and prolonged delirium group.

Characteristic	Short delirium n = 22	Prolonged delirium n = 29	OR (95% CI)	P value
Age*	84.6 ± 4.7	85.6 ± 5.9	1.04 (0.93–1.15)	0.50
Female°	17 (77.3)	21 (72.4)	1.30 (0.36–4.69)	0.69
Mini-Mental State Examination (MMSE) score*¶	23.0 ± 3.1	19.6 ± 5.5	0.84 (0.71–0.99)	0.02
APACHE II score*§	13.3 ± 3.0	13.9 ± 3.1	1.14 (0.87–1.49)	0.34
Snellen test*	31.6 ± 18.1	38.6 ± 35.5	1.01 (0.98–1.04)	0.41
Barthel ADL Index score*△	17.4 ± 3.0	14.0 ± 4.1	0.76 (0.62–0.93)	0.003
Lawton IADL score*≈	14.8 ± 5.8	18.6 ± 8.3	1.08 (0.99–1.17)	0.08
Geriatric Depression Scale-15 score*†	6.4 ± 1.1	6.4 ± 1.7	0.98 (0.61–1.59)	0.95
CRP value*	12.7 ± 25.2	13.4 ± 28.5	1.00 (0.98–1.02)	0.76
History of previous delirium°	0 (0)	12 (46.2)	N.A.	0.001
IQCODE-N > 3.6°	11 (50)	26 (89.7)	8.7 (2.02–37.26)	0.002
Number of concomitant diseases at admission*	2.4 ± 1.5	3.2 ± 2.5	1.20 (0.90–1.60)	0.18
Number of medication at admission*	4.2 ± 2.4	5.6 ± 3.8	1.15 (0.95–1.38)	0.12
MMSE score on the first day of delirium*¶	18.1 ± 6.3	15.1 ± 6.0	0.92 (0.83–1.03)	0.13
¥DRS-R-98 score on the first day of delirium*	18.6 ± 6.4	20.6 ± 6.5	1.05 (0.96–1.15)	0.28

Data are presented as mean ± SD or n (%) unless otherwise indicated.
*Continuous variables, °dichotomous variables.
OR: odds ratio, the chance of developing prolonged delirium, CI: confidence interval.
APACHE II: Acute Physiological and Chronic Health Evaluation II.
IQCODE-N: Informant Questionnaire on Cognitive Decline in the Elderly, >3.6 indicates preexistent cognitive decline.
DRS-R-98: Delirium Rating Scale Revised-98.
¶Range 0 (severe cognitive impairment) to 30 (no cognitive impairment).
§Range 0 (no acute health problems) to 70 (severe acute health problems).
△Range 0 (severe disability) to 20 (no disability).
≈Range 8 (no disability) to 31 (severe disability).
†Range 0 (depression not likely) to 15 (depression very likely).
¥Range 0 (no delirium symptoms) to 39 (maximum severity).

TABLE 2: Presence of individual DRS-R-98 delirium symptoms on first day of delirium.

DRS-R-98 item	Short delirium (n = 22)	Prolonged delirium (n = 29)	P value
(1) Sleep-wake cycle disturbance	21 (95.5%)	29 (100%)	0.43
(2) Perceptual disturbances and hallucinations	8/21 (38.1%)	13/27 (48.1%)	0.49
(3) Delusions	11/21 (52.4%)	14/27 (51.9%)	0.97
(4) Affective lability	15 (68.2%)	15/28 (53.6%)	0.30
(5) Language problems	18 (81.8%)	22 (75.9%)	0.74
(6) Thought process abnormalities	19 (86.4%)	27 (93.1%)	0.64
(7) Motor agitation	14 (63.6%)	20 (69%)	0.69
(8) Motor retardation	11/21 (52.4%)	20 (69%)	0.23
(9) Orientation problems	22 (100%)	28 (96.6%)	1.00
(10) Attention deficits	22 (100%)	28 (96.6%)	1.00
(11) Short-term memory impairment	20/21 (95.2%)	27/28 (96.4%)	1.00
(12) Long-term memory impairment	12/18 (66.7%)	22/28 (78.6%)	0.37
(13) Visuospatial impairment	9/18 (50%)	21/25 (84%)	0.02

Data are presented as n (%) or n/n (%) in case of missing data.

severity of individual delirium symptoms at the first day of delirium was not associated with short or prolonged delirium. Initially motor retardation was identified as a predictor for longer delirium duration (≥3 days), but when controlling for gender, age, and preexisting cognitive decline, only preexisting cognitive impairment was associated with prolonged delirium. In addition more severe impairment of long-term memory (as it was also measured with DRS-98 R item 12) across the whole delirium episode was associated with longer duration of delirium.

Preexisting cognitive impairment is thought to be more common in hypoactive delirium, although there is quite limited data to support this observation [35]. Our data indicate that the observed relationship between relatively

TABLE 3: Generalised equation estimation (GEE) model for DRS items 1–13 for different lengths of delirium episodes until recovery (count of days). $N = 113$ included observations.

	β	SE	df	Wald χ^2	95% CI	P
DRS-R-98 item 6 Thought process abnormalities	$-7.9E-6$	$6.30E-6$	1	1.558	$-2.03E-5, 4.5E-6$	0.21
DRS-R-98 item 9 Orientation	$-6E-6$	$8.88E-6$	1	0.456	$-2.34E-5, 1.14E-5$	0.50
DRS-R-98 item 10 Attention	$-5.17E-6$	$8.83E-6$	1	0.343	$-2.25E-5, 1.21E-5$	0.56
DRS-R-98 item 11 Short-term memory	$-1.08E-6$	$9.67E-6$	1	0.012	$-2.01E-5, 1.79E-5$	0.91
DRS-R-98 item 12 Long-term memory	$1.45E-5$	$7.20E-6$	1	4.044	$3.67E-7, 2.86E-5$	0.04
DRS-R-98 item 13 Visuospatial impairment	$8.86E-6$	$1.16E-5$	1	0.580	$-1.40E-5, 3.17E-5$	0.45
Constant	1.21	0.11	1	119.487	0.99, 1.42	0.000

SE: standard error, C.I.: confidence interval, E with a minus sign signals the number of places the decimal point has to be moved to the left.

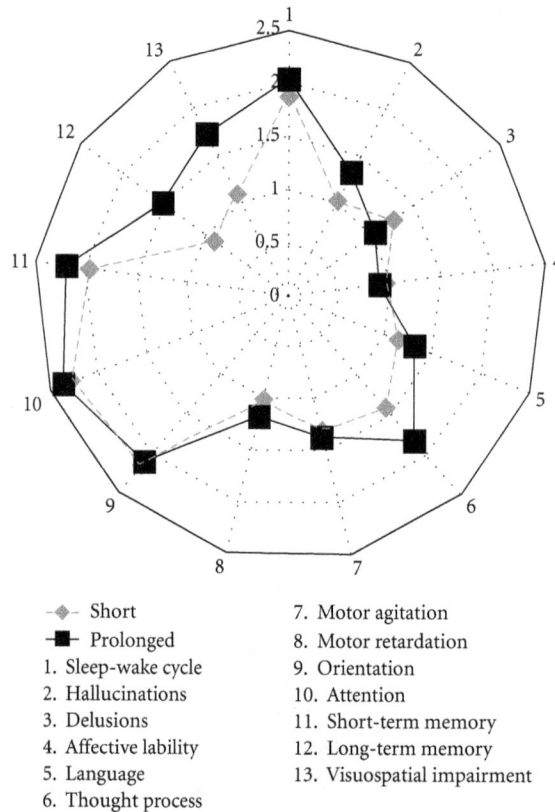

- ◆- Short
- ■- Prolonged
1. Sleep-wake cycle
2. Hallucinations
3. Delusions
4. Affective lability
5. Language
6. Thought process
7. Motor agitation
8. Motor retardation
9. Orientation
10. Attention
11. Short-term memory
12. Long-term memory
13. Visuospatial impairment

FIGURE 2: Mean DRS-R-98 item scores for short (1-2 days) versus prolonged (≥3 days) delirium on the first delirious day.

hypoactive clinical profile (as measured on item 8 of the DRS-R98) and more prolonged delirium is confounded by the relationship between motor retardation and preexisting cognitive impairment. This observation supports clinical experience where delirium superimposed on dementia is more likely to be hypoactive and resolves more slowly.

There have been few studies investigating the predictive value of delirium symptoms on the first day of delirium, and findings have been inconsistent. Rudberg et al. (1997) determined the duration within a mixed sample of 64 general medical and surgical patients who were found to have delirium [10]. Similar to our findings, there was no difference between delirium lasting a single day versus that of more prolonged cases in relation to individual delirium symptoms. They did find that the multiple day cases had higher DRS total scores on the first day. In contrast, Wada and Yamaguchi [11] found that poor cognitive status, sleep-wake cycle disturbances, and mood lability were associated with delirium lasting more than a week. However, in our study item 12 (long term memory) was the only predictive item from DRS-R-98 for delirium duration such that participants with more severe long-term memory problems experienced more prolonged delirium. However, the two previously mentioned studies measured symptoms with the original 10-item DRS, which includes a more restricted range of symptoms than the revised DRS-R-98 which captures a wider range of cognitive and neuropsychiatric disturbances that occur in delirium and is widely used in the assessment of delirium severity and in phenomenological studies. In addition, both patient populations were highly heterogeneous and not only limited to only postoperative delirium and focused only on univariate analysis without controlling for confounding factors, like pre-existing cognitive decline.

The study by Wada and Yamaguchi described delirium duration according to a general category (≤1 week versus >1 week) [11]. However, we found that almost half of the delirious patients experienced a delirium episode of 1 to 2 days. Rudberg et al. also found a high percentage of cases (69%) with a single day of delirium in their sample [10]. Recent work has highlighted the impact of short periods of delirium upon outcomes and emphasises the importance of daily assessments in studies of delirium [15].

Our work includes some significant strengths that include the use of daily measurements with the DRS-R-98. Moreover, given the challenges in longitudinal studies of handling the effects of dropouts, interdependence of ratings across visits within patients, and individual patient variability in delirium severity over time, we used the GEE modeling method because it manages these issues in longitudinal datasets and is therefore particularly suited to investigating the course of delirium, considering its fluctuating nature.

Preexisting cognitive decline is thought to be associated with more prolonged delirium. It has been postulated that this reflects the effects of uncontrolled neuroinflammation contributing to delirium symptoms [36]. Experimental findings and neuropathological observations suggest that activation of microglia is pivotal for mediation of the acute behavioural and cognitive effects of systemic inflammation [36]. A mild systemic inflammatory response suffices to increase the production of proinflammatory cytokines within the brain when microglia are already "primed" by chronic pathologic events as chronic neurodegeneration or advanced age [37]. After hip surgery the release of pro-inflammatory cytokines as a consequence of fracture and surgery induces a systemic inflammatory response. Since inflammatory markers have been shown to be elevated in dementia as well as MCI [38–40], it follows that preexisting cognitive impairment might not only increase the chance of developing delirium but also prolong it.

This work also has some limitations. The present study was naturalistic in design. Patients received optimal care, which incorporates extensive general geriatric care and haloperidol as prophylactic interventions in high risk patients and delirium treatment according to study site protocol. Both are known to impact positively upon the course of delirium.

Although we cannot exclude the effect haloperidol might have had on motor symptom profile in this population, similar longitudinal work in a palliative care setting suggests a limited relationship between motor activity and use of antipsychotic agents [41]. Furthermore, since all patients in our sample were of high risk for delirium and thus all received haloperidol prophylaxis, any likely effects would be likely similar for all the patients in our sample. Although a subsample of the patients participated in a clinical trial, analysis showed that study treatment (taurine/placebo) did not have effect on study outcomes. Also, delirium treatment was delivered according to a standard protocol, and this did not differ between the sample participating in the clinical trial and the naturalistic cohort.

The exclusion of participants who could not be classified regarding the duration of delirium episode might reduce the strength of this study. This study is not the first to define two consecutive negative delirium assessments as resolution of the delirium episode [42]. However, to allow for greater confidence, we repeated the analysis twice. First, the analysis was repeated with the excluded patients added to the short delirium group, because we had data of at least 1 or 2 delirious days. Second, the prolonged delirium group was limited to patients who could be exactly defined according to duration of the delirium episode in exact count of days, similar to the short delirium group. This did not change the results evident in the initial analysis.

This study excluded preoperative delirium cases and focused upon incident delirium cases, a well-defined and homogeneous group of elderly hip-fracture patients. Preoperative delirium cases might have experienced hip fracture because of their confusion and subsequent other causes. Lee et al. (2011) demonstrated that delirium duration can last as long as 4 weeks or longer [13]. The main cause of this prolonged delirium was preoperative delirium. The duration of delirium has been noted to be shorter, suggesting that preoperative delirium may include a different group who warrants separate study.

The sample size was relatively small as it was limited to incident cases of delirium. The main finding that cognition rather than delirium profile is associated with delirium duration was demonstrated by two separate methods. The GEE method is an innovative statistical analysis used for longitudinal data analysis, and the small sample size is less important with this analysis because we have a relative large number of observations due to the use of daily assessments.

In conclusion, this study explores the relationship between baseline status and early symptoms of delirium with delirium duration in a homogenous population using validated measurement scales. Preexisting cognitive decline, a concept intertwined with dementia, rather than specific delirium symptoms, was the principal predictor of delirium duration.

Acknowledgments

The authors would like to thank Gisela Dekker, RN (data acquisition), Ralph Vreeswijk, RN, M.S. (data acquisition), Milko van Langen (data acquisition), and Tjerk Schoemaker, M.S. (data acquisition for their work on the study); trial name: The Effect of Taurine on Morbidity and Mortality in the Elderly Hip Fracture Patient; URL: http://clinicaltrials .gov/ct2/show/NCT00497978?term=taurine+hip+fracture& rank=1; registration no. NCT00497978.

References

[1] S. K. Inouye, C. M. Viscoli, R. I. Horwitz, L. D. Hurst, and M. E. Tinetti, "A predictive model for delirium in hospitalized elderly medical patients based on admission characteristics," *Annals of Internal Medicine*, vol. 119, no. 6, pp. 474–481, 1993.

[2] M. Dasgupta and A. C. Dumbrell, "Preoperative risk assessment for delirium after noncardiac surgery: a systematic review," *Journal of the American Geriatrics Society*, vol. 54, no. 10, pp. 1578–1589, 2006.

[3] J. Witlox, L. S. M. Eurelings, J. F. M. de Jonghe, K. J. Kalisvaart, P. Eikelenboom, and W. A. van Gool, "Delirium in elderly patients and the risk of postdischarge mortality, institutionalization, and dementia: a meta-analysis," *Journal of the American Medical Association*, vol. 304, no. 4, pp. 443–451, 2010.

[4] J. C. Jackson, S. M. Gordon, R. P. Hart, R. O. Hopkins, and E. W. Ely, "The association between delirium and cognitive decline: a review of the empirical literature," *Neuropsychology Review*, vol. 14, no. 2, pp. 87–98, 2004.

[5] A. M. J. MacLullich, A. Beaglehole, R. J. Hall, and D. J. Meagher, "Delirium and long-term cognitive impairment," *International Review of Psychiatry*, vol. 21, no. 1, pp. 30–42, 2009.

[6] D. M. Edelstein, G. B. Aharonoff, A. Karp, E. L. Capla, J. D. Zuckerman, and K. J. Koval, "Effect of postoperative delirium on outcome after hip fracture," *Clinical Orthopaedics and Related Research*, vol. 422, pp. 195–200, 2004.

[7] S. Nightingale, J. Holmes, J. Mason, and A. House, "Psychiatric illness and mortality after hip fracture," *The Lancet*, vol. 357, no. 9264, pp. 1264–1265, 2001.

[8] N. Gupta, J. de Jonghe, J. Schieveld, M. Leonard, and D. Meagher, "Delirium phenomenology: what can we learn from the symptoms of delirium?" *Journal of Psychosomatic Research*, vol. 65, no. 3, pp. 215–222, 2008.

[9] P. T. Trzepacz, R. W. Baker, and J. Greenhouse, "A symptom rating scale for delirium," *Psychiatry Research*, vol. 23, pp. 89–97, 1988.

[10] M. A. Rudberg, P. Pompei, M. D. Foreman, R. E. Ross, and C. K. Cassel, "The natural history of delirium in older hospitalized patients: a syndrome of heterogeneity," *Age and Ageing*, vol. 26, no. 3, pp. 169–174, 1997.

[11] Y. Wada and N. Yamaguchi, "Delirium in the elderly: relationship of clinical symptoms to outcome," *Dementia*, vol. 4, no. 2, pp. 113–116, 1993.

[12] J. McCusker, M. Cole, N. Dendukuri, L. Han, and E. Belzile, "The course of delirium in older medical inpatients: a prospective study," *Journal of General Internal Medicine*, vol. 18, no. 9, pp. 696–704, 2003.

[13] K. H. Lee, Y. C. Ha, Y. K. Lee, H. Kang, and K. H. Koo, "Frequency, risk factors, and prognosis of prolonged delirium in elderly patients after hip fracture surgery," *Clinical Orthopaedics and Related Research*, vol. 469, pp. 2612–2620, 2011.

[14] T. N. Robinson, C. D. Raeburn, Z. V. Tran, E. M. Angles, L. A. Brenner, and M. Moss, "Postoperative delirium in the elderly: risk factors and outcomes," *Annals of Surgery*, vol. 249, no. 1, pp. 173–178, 2009.

[15] M. González, G. Martínez, J. Calderón et al., "Impact of delirium on short-term mortality in elderly inpatients: a prospective cohort study," *Psychosomatics*, vol. 50, no. 3, pp. 234–238, 2009.

[16] K. J. Kalisvaart, J. F. M. de Jonghe, M. J. Bogaards et al., "Haloperidol prophylaxis for elderly hip-surgery patients at risk for delirium: a randomized placebo-controlled study," *Journal of the American Geriatrics Society*, vol. 53, no. 10, pp. 1658–1666, 2005.

[17] J. Witlox, K. J. Kalisvaart, J. F. M. de Jonghe et al., "Cerebrospinal fluid β-amyloid and tau are not associated with risk of delirium: a prospective cohort study in older adults with hip fracture," *Journal of the American Geriatrics Society*, vol. 59, no. 7, pp. 1260–1267, 2011.

[18] M. F. Folstein, S. E. Folstein, and P. R. McHugh, "'Mini mental state'. A practical method for grading the cognitive state of patients for the clinician," *Journal of Psychiatric Research*, vol. 12, no. 3, pp. 189–198, 1975.

[19] A. F. Jorm and P. A. Jacomb, "The Informant Questionnaire on Cognitive Decline in the Elderly (IQCODE): socio-demographic correlates, reliability, validity and some norms," *Psychological Medicine*, vol. 19, no. 4, pp. 1015–1022, 1989.

[20] J. F. de Jonghe, B. Schmand, M. E. Ooms, and M. W. Ribbe, "Abbreviated form of the Informant Questionnaire on cognitive decline in the elderly," *Tijdschrift voor Gerontologie en Geriatrie*, vol. 28, pp. 224–229, 1997.

[21] W. A. Knaus, E. A. Draper, D. P. Wagner, and J. E. Zimmerman, "APACHE II: a severity of disease classification system," *Critical Care Medicine*, vol. 13, pp. 818–829, 1985.

[22] R. Hetherington, "The Shellen chart as a test of visual acuity," *Psychologische Forschung*, vol. 24, no. 4, pp. 349–357, 1954.

[23] F. I. Mahoney and D. W. Barthel, "Functional evaluation: the Barthel index," *Maryland State Medical Journal*, vol. 14, pp. 61–65, 1965.

[24] M. P. Lawton and E. M. Brody, "Assessment of older people: self-maintaining and instrumental activities of daily living," *Gerontologist*, vol. 9, no. 3, pp. 179–186, 1969.

[25] J. W. Devlin, R. J. Roberts, J. J. Fong et al., "Efficacy and safety of quetiapine in critically ill patients with delirium: a prospective, multicenter, randomized, double-blind, placebo-controlled pilot study," *Critical Care Medicine*, vol. 38, no. 2, pp. 419–427, 2010.

[26] S. K. Inouye, C. H. van Dyck, C. A. Alessi, S. Balkin, A. P. Siegal, and R. I. Horwitz, "Clarifying confusion: the confusion assessment method: a new method for detection of delirium," *Annals of Internal Medicine*, vol. 113, no. 12, pp. 941–948, 1990.

[27] American Psychiatric Association, *Diagnostic and Statistical Manual of Mental Disorders*, American Psychiatric Association, Washington, DC, USA, 2000.

[28] P. T. Trzepacz, D. Mittal, R. Torres, K. Kanary, J. Norton, and N. Jimerson, "Validation of the Delirium Rating Scale-revised-98: comparison with the delirium rating scale and the cognitive test for delirium," *Journal of Neuropsychiatry and Clinical Neurosciences*, vol. 13, no. 2, pp. 229–242, 2001.

[29] H. J. Lee, D. S. Hwang, S. K. Wang, I. S. Chee, S. Baeg, and J. L. Kim, "Early assessment of delirium in elderly patients after hip surgery," *Psychiatry Investigation*, vol. 8, pp. 340–347, 2011.

[30] P. Tognoni, A. Simonato, N. Robutti et al., "Preoperative risk factors for postoperative delirium (POD) after urological surgery in the elderly," *Archives of Gerontology and Geriatrics*, vol. 52, no. 3, pp. e166–e169, 2011.

[31] R. Katznelson, G. Djaiani, G. Tait et al., "Hospital administrative database underestimates delirium rate after cardiac surgery," *Canadian Journal of Anesthesia*, vol. 57, no. 10, pp. 898–902, 2010.

[32] A. W. Lemstra, K. J. Kalisvaart, R. Vreeswijk, W. A. van Gool, and P. Eikelenboom, "Pre-operative inflammatory markers and the risk of postoperative delirium in elderly patients," *International Journal of Geriatric Psychiatry*, vol. 23, no. 9, pp. 943–948, 2008.

[33] F. S. Santos, L. O. Wahlund, F. Varli, I. T. Velasco, and M. E. Jönhagen, "Incidence, clinical features and subtypes of delirium in elderly patients treated for hip fractures," *Dementia and Geriatric Cognitive Disorders*, vol. 20, no. 4, pp. 231–237, 2005.

[34] J. F. M. de Jonghe, K. J. Kalisvaart, M. Dijkstra et al., "Early symptoms in the prodromal phase of delirium: a prospective cohort study in elderly patients undergoing hip surgery," *American Journal of Geriatric Psychiatry*, vol. 15, no. 2, pp. 112–121, 2007.

[35] D. Meagher, "Motor subtypes of delirium: past, present and future," *International Review of Psychiatry*, vol. 21, no. 1, pp. 59–73, 2009.

[36] W. A. van Gool, D. van de Beek, and P. Eikelenboom, "Systemic infection and delirium: when cytokines and acetylcholine collide," *The Lancet*, vol. 375, no. 9716, pp. 773–775, 2010.

[37] C. Cunningham, "Systemic inflammation and delirium: important co-factors in the progression of dementia," *Biochemical Society Transactions*, vol. 39, no. 4, pp. 945–953, 2011.

[38] F. Licastro, S. Pedrini, L. Caputo et al., "Increased plasma levels of interleukin-1, interleukin-6 and α-1-antichymotrypsin in patients with Alzheimer's disease: peripheral inflammation or signals from the brain?" *Journal of Neuroimmunology*, vol. 103, no. 1, pp. 97–102, 2000.

[39] A. Álvarez, R. Cacabelos, C. Sanpedro, M. García-Fantini, and M. Aleixandre, "Serum TNF-alpha levels are increased and correlate negatively with free IGF-I in Alzheimer disease," *Neurobiology of Aging*, vol. 28, no. 4, pp. 533–536, 2007.

[40] J. N. Trollor, E. Smith, B. T. Baune et al., "Systemic inflammation is associated with MCI and its subtypes: the Sydney memory and aging study," *Dementia and Geriatric Cognitive Disorders*, vol. 30, no. 6, pp. 569–578, 2010.

[41] D. J. Meagher, M. Leonard, S. Donnelly, M. Conroy, D. Adamis, and P. T. Trzepacz, "A longitudinal study of motor subtypes in delirium: relationship with other phenomenology, etiology, medication exposure and prognosis," *Journal of Psychosomatic Research*, vol. 71, pp. 395–403, 2011.

[42] J. R. Fann, C. M. Alfano, B. E. Burington, S. Roth-Roemer, W. J. Katon, and K. L. Syrjala, "Clinical presentation of delirium in patients undergoing hematopoietic stem cell transplantation: delirium and distress symptoms and time course," *Cancer*, vol. 103, no. 4, pp. 810–820, 2005.

Active Aging Promotion: Results from the *Vital Aging* Program

Mariagiovanna Caprara,[1] **María Ángeles Molina,**[2] **Rocío Schettini,**[3] **Marta Santacreu,**[4] **Teresa Orosa,**[5] **Víctor Manuel Mendoza-Núñez,**[6] **Macarena Rojas,**[7] **and Rocío Fernández-Ballesteros**[4]

[1] *Department of Psychology, Madrid Open University (UDIMA), Collado Villaba, 28400 Madrid, Spain*
[2] *Institute for Advanced Social Studies, Spanish National Research Council, 14004 Córdoba, Spain*
[3] *University Program for Older Adults (PUMA), Autonomous University of Madrid, Cantoblanco Campus, 28049 Madrid, Spain*
[4] *Department of Psychobiology and Health, Autonomous University of Madrid, Cantoblanco Campus, 28049 Madrid, Spain*
[5] *University of La Habana, 11600 La Habana, Cuba*
[6] *Gerontology Research Group, National Autonomous University of Mexico, FES Zaragoza Campus, 09230 Mexico City, DF, Mexico*
[7] *Older Adults Program, Catholic University of Chile, Santiago Metropolitan Region, Santiago, Chile*

Correspondence should be addressed to María Ángeles Molina; mmolina@iesa.csic.es

Academic Editor: Jean Marie Robine

Active aging is one of the terms in the semantic network of aging well, together with others such as successful, productive, competent aging. All allude to the new paradigm in gerontology, whereby aging is considered from a positive perspective. Most authors in the field agree active aging is a multidimensional concept, embracing health, physical and cognitive fitness, positive affect and control, social relationships and engagement. This paper describes *Vital Aging*, an individual active aging promotion program implemented through three modalities: Life, Multimedia, and e-Learning. The program was developed on the basis of extensive evidence about individual determinants of active aging. The different versions of *Vital Aging* are described, and four evaluation studies (both formative and summative) are reported. Formative evaluation reflected participants' satisfaction and expected changes; summative evaluations yielded some quite encouraging results using quasi-experimental designs: those who took part in the programs increased their physical exercise, significantly improved their diet, reported better memory, had better emotional balance, and enjoyed more cultural, intellectual, affective, and social activities than they did before the course, thus increasing their social relationships. These results are discussed in the context of the common literature within the field and, also, taking into account the limitations of the evaluations accomplished.

1. Introduction

The concept of aging well as a scientific field dates back to the early 1960s, within the context of the World Health Organization (WHO), when Roth highlighted the importance of health promotion and illness prevention throughout the life span, and especially in old age [1]. Most importantly, in the 1980s, one of the pioneers in the field of aging well, Fries, would stress the modifiability and plasticity of the human being throughout life and into old age, listing non-modifiable negative conditions associated with age and their correspondence with modifiable preventive factors [2–4]. Recently, Christensen, Doblhammer, Rau, and Vaupel noted how, since the 1950s, mortality after age 80 years has steadily fallen, with life expectancy lengthening almost in parallel with best practices over the last 150 years [5] and they showed evidence that human senescence has been delayed by a decade [6] strongly associated with "healthy best practices."

In fact, the aging revolution is the result of falling mortality rates and the corresponding increase in life expectancy. But, these changes in the population are due not only to biomedical advances, but also to the exponential development of human society across history: compulsory education, economic growth, the extension and democratization of the improvement of life conditions, better healthy practices, extended scientific knowledge, and so forth, have all made their contributions to this revolution. At the same time, we have seen the emergence of the active aging paradigm [7, 8].

In the WHO document *active ageing. A policy framework*, the determinants of active aging posited were mainly population-based: Economic, Social, Environmental, and Health and Social Services, suggesting that the responsibility for active aging lies with the public sector, through public health programs and social policies [9]. The implementation and evaluation of such programs are necessarily long-term, and therefore highly complex. As Christensen et al. show, one way of evaluating "best practice" in health is through the association of such practices with population-based indicators such as mortality, or life expectancy, or even disability-free life expectancy, healthy life expectancy, or quality-adjusted life years [5].

Even so, as stressed elsewhere, not only it is important to promote active aging from a population-based point of view, it is also relevant to do so from an individual perspective. Aging well is not a random phenomenon: the individual is an agent of his/her own aging process, and the capacity for aging actively comes not only from sociopolitical actions, but also through decisions taken by individuals themselves. Thus, among the determinants posited by the WHO, two types of individual-based factors can be found: Behavioral (lifestyles) and Personal (both biogenetic and psychological) [10].

Active aging is a multidisciplinary concept (also called successful, productive, or optimal aging), and cannot simply be reduced to "healthy aging," needing, rather, to take into account protective behavioral determinants (protective life styles and the prevention of risk factors) [10–12]. Moreover, a definition of aging well must include other psychosocial factors, such as cognitive and mental functioning, positive mood, sense of control, active coping styles, and social participation and engagement. Promotion and education in relation to these factors through psychosocial initiatives extending the encouragement of healthy lifestyles (such as physical activity or good nutrition) to other aspects, such as memory training, stress management, self-efficacy coaching, or training in prosocial behavior, would appear to represent a step forward in the promotion of active aging. Supporting literature of those aspects will see shortly listed when our four domains model will be presented.

This paper deals with a set of psychosocial and educational interventions called "*Active Aging*" with various formats (*Life Course, Multimedia*, and e-Learning) for the promotion of active aging at the *individual level*—that is, *without* modifying any of the posited determinants at the population-based level (income, macrosocial and environmental conditions, or health and social services).

Here we consider three programs, all of which have been implemented at the Autonomous University of Madrid (UAM; Spain), and the last one also in other three Latin American Universities: *Vital Aging* life, *Vital Aging* multimedia and *Vital Aging* e-Learning.

2. *Vital Aging* Program

Here we provide a brief presentation of the *Vital Aging* Program summarized from other published materials [10, 12–17].

2.1. Basic Principles. Underlying the *Vital Aging* is a set of theoretical assumptions.

(1) There are major differences in forms of aging (normal, optimal, and pathological), and there is empirically-based knowledge about how to age well [4, 18].

(2) This diversity across the life course is not random. External circumstances are crucial to the aging process, but the individual is also an agent of his or her own aging process [19].

(3) Plasticity is a property of the Central Nervous System, but also of the human organism. Plasticity, though subject to certain limitations, remains throughout the life span and into old age. Over the course of life, plasticity is expressed through learning and modifiability [7, 20, 21].

(4) Selection, Optimization, and Compensation are adaptive mechanisms found within the aging process; knowledge-based pragmatics, high motivation, and technology can compensate decline [7].

2.2. A Four-Domain Model for the Vital Aging Program. Underpinning the content of the *Vital Aging* program is a 4-domain model of aging well posited by Fernández-Ballesteros, [10, 22] whereby active aging is defined as the lifelong adaptation process of maximizing health and independence; physical and cognitive functioning; positive affect and control; and social engagement [10].

As shown in Figure 1, this four-domain model of aging well has recently been tested by Fernández-Ballesteros et al. [23] through Structural Equation Modeling, with data both from our cross-cultural project on lay definitions of aging well provided by older adults from 7 Latin American and 3 European, [24–26] and from the ELEA research project (Longitudinal Study of Active Aging) [27].

As far as the four domains of active aging are concerned, they are not only based on Structural Equation Modeling using empirical data (from lay definitions and research findings), but also strongly supported by the scientific literature. Although, this is not the place to present all such evidence (for a review, see: Fernández-Ballesteros, 2008), [10] let us consider some examples.

(i) Behavioral Lifestyles. (1) Regular physical exercise reduces mortality risk by about 35% (e.g., Healthy Aging Longitudinal European study) [28, 29]. (2) Elders with healthy behavioral life styles show *four times less* disability than those who smoke, drink too much, do not exercise, and are obese. Moreover, in those with good behavioral habits the onset of *initial disability was postponed by 7.75 years* [30]. (3) Netz et al. carried out the most recent meta-analysis of those studies linking physical activity to mental health and well-being.

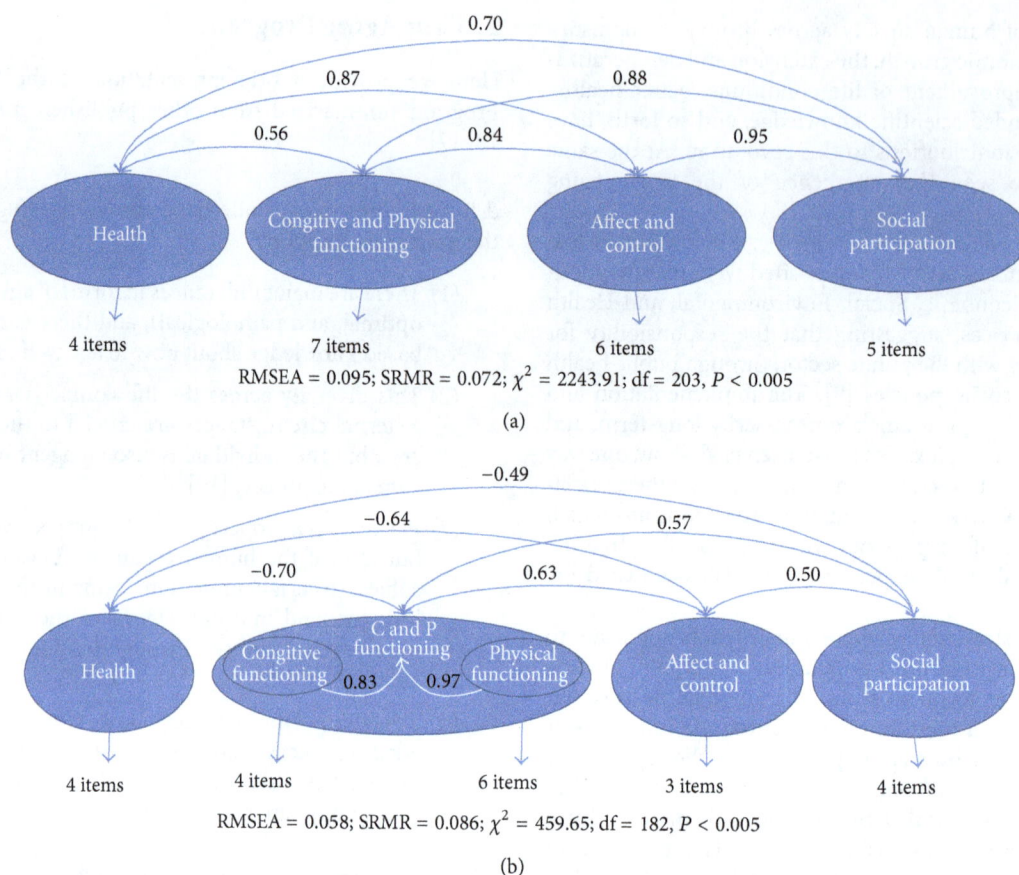

RMSEA = 0.095; SRMR = 0.072; χ^2 = 2243.91; df = 203, $P < 0.005$

(a)

RMSEA = 0.058; SRMR = 0.086; χ^2 = 459.65; df = 182, $P < 0.005$

(b)

FIGURE 1: Structural Equations Modeling of four-domains model of ageing well: (a) from lay conceptalizations ($N = 1,189$), and (b) from ELEA PROJECT multimethod data base ($N = 458$).

Studies with older adults shows that effect sizes for physical exercising treatment groups were almost 3 times as large as the mean for control groups [31]. (4) Mediterranean diet (low intake of saturated and trans fat and high consumption of fruit and vegetable) is stronger related to survival and life expectancy [32–34]. (5) This type of diet decreases coronary mortality about 40% and all causes of mortality about 20% [35, 36].

(ii) Cognitive Activity and Training. (1) More frequent cognitive activity in everyday life is associated with a reduction of approximately 19% in annual rate of cognitive decline, and is also a protective factor against dementia [37, 38]. (2) The effects on cognitive functioning of cognitive training are of a magnitude equivalent to the decline expected in elders without dementia over a period of 7 to 14 years, though longer follow-up study is required [39]. (3) Memory training yields effects sizes of 0.75 SD, by comparison with 0.40 as a practice effect, in both objective memory tests and subjective memory functioning [40, 41]. (4) A meta-analysis carried out by Colcombe and Kramer with 18 intervention studies examining the effects of physical fitness training on cognitive functions yielded robust effects for several measures of cognitive functioning [42]. In sum, all these progresses support not only a more complex view of cognitive functioning across life

span but a new panorama in which effective cognitive trainings and intervention can optimize cognitive functioning, compensate intellectual losses and declines or even palliative cognitive impairment (for a review see: Hertzog et al, 2009) [41].

(iii) Positive Affect, Coping, and Control. (1) *Positive Affect* reduces mortality in older individuals. The benefits of positive affect can be observed in conditions as diverse as stroke, rehospitalization for coronary problems, the common cold, and accidents; highly activated positive emotions were associated with better functioning of cardiovascular, endocrine, and immune systems [43]. A positive attitude towards life may help us avoid becoming frail. For those reporting positive affect 7 years earlier, the chance of becoming frail fell by 3%, while the chances of having better health outcomes, greater functional independence increased, as did survival rates. The authors conclude from these finding that positive affect is protective against functional and physical decline in old age as well as negative affect such anxiety are requiring coping and management [44]. The most important conclusion emerging from coping and aging literature is that although there is a broad evidence about the stability of coping behaviour across life span, authors distinguish specific positive coping skills in old age which can be trained and promoted [45, 46]. (3) Sense

of Control and Self-efficacy. Older adults with a high sense of control are better off on many indicators of health and well-being and those who have a lower sense of control may be at increased risk for a wide range of negative behavioral, affective, and functional outcomes, including higher levels of depression, anxiety, and stress, use of fewer health protective behaviors (e.g., exercise) and compensatory memory strategies (e.g., internal or external memory aids), and have poorer health and memory functioning. Also, the sense of control is a powerful psychosocial factor that influences well-being and it is a good predictor of healthy and active aging; finally, sense of control can be trained as has been largely tested [47–49]. Among control concepts, self-efficacy is perhaps the best well-known construct in successful ageing literature. In the last twenty five years self-efficacy has been searched through cross-sectional, longitudinal and experimental designs [19]. Self-efficacy beliefs are strongly related with successful aging, firstly because they contribute to perceive age related situations not as threats but as challenges; secondly, because they support to individual to remain committed in selected goals and, finally, because self-efficacy perceptions have a synergic power with other factors for enhancing outcomes [10]. (4) Self-stereotypes or self-images about aging reduce the risk ratio of .87 ($P < .001$). Persons with positive images about aging (assessed 25 years earlier) lived 7.5 years more than those reporting poor self-perception of aging at baseline. One aspect of the positive self-perception of aging measure, risk of dying, fell by 13% [50, 51].

(iv) Social Functioning and Participation. (1) The association between social relationships and the prevalence and incidence of and recovery from disability has been well established [52]. (2) Research results have shown a strong and robust cross-sectional association between social engagement and disability, more socially active persons reporting lower levels of disability than their less active counterparts [53]. (3) There is empirical evidence that social activity and participation improve cognitive functioning [54]. (4) Results have shown that the protective effects of social engagement diminish slowly over time [55].

In summary, there is strong support for these four domains of active aging on which the *Vital Aging* Program is based (for a review, see Fernández-Ballesteros, 2008) [10].

2.3. Vital Aging Program Versions. The starting point was the *Vital Aging* course (Vivir con Vitalidad) developed in 1996 at the autonomous university of Madrid (UAM), developed by Fernández-Ballesteros as an open life course. Since 1996, several editions of the *Vital Aging* course have been run; a multimedia version and an e-Learning course have also been developed. Let us now describe these three programs.

(i) Vital Aging L (1996–2003). Organized as a continuing education course at the UAM, it consists of 20 thematic units over 70 hours (3 hours per session, 2 sessions per week). Trainers are experts in a variety of subjects, teaching in highly practical way and supported by a basic text (drawn up by Fernández-Ballesteros) [12]. All sessions have a similar structure: (1) the trainer makes a general presentation of the

content in question, talking about the supporting evidence on each unit; (2) a pretest for the particular behavioral or psychological characteristic (diet, physical exercise, self-efficacy, pleasant activities, etc.) is administered; (3) practical strategies for better aging are described and reviewed, and exercises are performed; (4) at the end of the class a post-test is administered, and the results are discussed; (5) finally, the trainer makes some concluding remarks (for a summary, see Table 1).

(ii) Vital Ageing M. The *Vital Aging*-L was transformed in to the *Vital Aging* multimedia course developed under the auspices of the European Commission, as a Socrates-Minerva Program, by a Consortium made up of UAM (Spain), Nettuno (Italy) and the University of Heidelberg-Institute of Gerontology (Germany), and with the cooperation of the Open University (UK). *Vital Aging*-M consists of 48 hours of video lessons grouped in 20 Thematic Units with supporting materials on the Internet. Each Unit comprises 2 to 4 hours' video-lessons taught by European experts from Germany, Italy, and Spain (so far the program is available only in Spanish). Although, at the very beginning *Vital-Aging*-M program was broadcasted through the Italian TV-Chanel 2, all our evaluation studies were based on the administration of those video-lessons in the class-room by a trained tutor who is in charge of all equipments, the distribution among participants of the supporting materials, and the assessment instruments for each video-lesson. Participants follow all sessions of each lesson, fill out the instruments, and work with the material distributed present in the video-lesson. Each lesson lasts approximately 2 hours, with a break of 15 minutes between sessions. Lessons have the same structure and content as in *Vital Aging*-L and e-Learning versions (Table 1).

(iii) Vital Aging e-Learning. The program was supported by the UAM-Santander Inter-University Cooperation Program for Latin America (2010–2012), with the main goal of developing an e-learning methodology for senior citizens' university programs (PUM-e). In the first step, a pilot format of the program was implemented at UAM and the Catholic University of Chile, and subsequently assessed. Based on this pilot study, *Vital Aging* materials designed to be used on via Internet by Fernández-Ballesteros (http://www .vivirconvitalidad.com/) were adapted cross-culturally with the contribution from the three Latin American universities. Several changes were made to obtain an e-learning format that could be implemented through the Learning management System, LMS-Moodle Platform. Finally, the program was launched at the four participating universities: UAM, Catholic University of Chile, La Habana University (Cuba) and the National Autonomous University of Mexico. The *Vital Aging* e-Learning program requires around 65 hours of work, and was run over a period of three months. Students had a set of learning resources as follows. (1) Self-evaluation: in order to give the student a base-measure of his/her performance in each basic unit, a questionnaire is filled out, the responses being checked automatically. This self-evaluation is useful for making students aware of their status in relation

TABLE 1: Summary of *Vital Aging* versions: procedures for implementation and evaluation.

	Vital Ageing L	Vital Ageing M	Vital Ageing e-Learning
Date of implementation	1996–2003	2002–2012	2012
Duration each edition	3 months, 70 hours (3 hours/session; 2 sessions per week)	3 months, 48 hours (2–4 hours per session, 2 sessions per week)	3 months: 1 unit per 2 week
Trainers	Experts	Experts from Germany, Italy, and Spain Organized by a Tutor	Organized by a Virtual Tutor and an On-site tutor
Materials	Basic Text: Fernández-Ballesteros [11] Standard classes	Multimedia learning technology Video Lessons	Basic texts: http://www.vivirconvitalidad.com/ Learning management System, LMS-Moodle Platform
Financed	Institute of Older Adults and Social Services (IMSERSO)	European Commission (Vitalgell-C Project, 2002)	UAM-Santander Inter-University Cooperation Program for Latin America (PUM-e, 2010–2012)
Session procedure	(1) Introduction; (2) Pre-test; (3) Practice and exercises; (4) Post-test; (5) Conclusions and remarks	(1) Introduction; (2) Pre-test; (3) Practice and exercises; (4) Post-test; (5) Conclusions and remarks	(1) Introduction; (2) Pre-test; (3) Readings; (4) Practice and exercise; (5) Forums; (6) Tutorial; (7) Post-test in each unit
Recruitment	Announcements in newspapers, on radio and in UAM promotion systems	Announcements at selected Senior Citizens' Clubs and at UAM, to Students from University Programs for Older Adults	Students from University Programs for Older Adults at the four universities
Participants	240 volunteers attended the program (approximately 35 per course; Mean age = 72.3, range = 57–83, SD = 6.7; 70% women)	155 volunteers (around 10–22 per course; Mean age = 69.9, range = 60–94, SD = 6; 76% women)	88 volunteers: UAM ($N = 26$), La Habana University ($N = 20$), National University Autonomous of Mexico ($N = 23$) and Catholic University of Chile ($N = 19$) (Mean age = 64.2; SD: 7.57, range = 49–84; 84% women)

to each work module. (2) Readings: these provide useful, relevant, and proven information on the various topics addressed by the program. (3) Activities: two types of activity are involved, those used to verify self-knowledge related to the readings and those that serve for planning changes to be incorporated into daily life. (4) Forums: these are designed to promote discussion among students (including inter-country discussion) and the exchange of views about the various topics taught on the course. (5) Tutorial: the course offers the assistance of a Virtual tutor, who provides information about the execution of the task throughout the course and resolves any doubts that may arise regarding the materials and program content, and an On-site tutor, who deals with the technical difficulties that may arise on using the Moodle platform.

In order to allow comparisons of our materials and methods, Tables 1 and 2 show the procedures followed and the materials (domains, units, contents as well as the assessment and practice) for the three *Vital Aging* versions.

2.4. Vital Aging Program Hypothesis and Objectives. Our general hypothesis was that after *Vital Aging* programs, experimental individuals, in comparison to pre-test and controls, significantly, will attain the objectives of the program as measured by the instrument administered.

Objectives are the following: (a) to teach basic knowledge how to age well; (b) to promote healthy behavioral lifestyles;

(c) to train strategies for optimizing cognitive functioning and compensating potential decline; (d) to optimize positive affect and emotion, promoting control and coping styles; (e) to promote social relationships and participation throughout the life course using new technologies.

2.5. Teaching Materials. "*Vital Aging*-L," "*Vital Ageing*-M," and "*Vital Aging*-e" are multidimensional courses based on the same four-domain model of active aging. Therefore, materials (units, lesson content, assessment tests, and tasks for practical work) were developed on the basis of these four domains. The *Vital Aging* e-Learning version is less extensive than *Vital Aging* Life and Multimedia, but after a general introduction, the four domains are addressed. Table 2 shows a summary about Domains and Units, together with examples of Context and Assessment tests and Practice tasks for the three versions of *Vital Aging*.

3. Evaluation Studies on *Vital Aging* Programs

Four evaluation studies have been carried out on Active aging programs: following Scriven, formative evaluations were conducted at the beginning of both the *Multimedia* and *e-Learning* versions; [56] also, several summative or outcome evaluations were carried out for the *Life* and *Multimedia* programs; finally, since the *e-Learning* version is quite new,

TABLE 2: Domains, units, contents, and assessment and practice of vital aging versions.

Domains	Vital aging L and Vital aging M			Vital aging e-Learning		
	Units	Contents	Assessment and practice	Units	Contents	Assessment and practice
Aging well	Aging well	(i) General introduction to the Course (ii) Human development is lifelong (iii) Use it or lose it! (iv) What vital, successful, active, and productive ageing means: the four domains (v) Mechanisms for aging well: the SOC model (vi) Stereotypes and self-steretoypes of aging	(a) Your images about aging? (b) Which are aging well mechanism? (c) Level of your physical activity? (d) Your social relations? (e) Avoid state "I already cannot"	Aging well	(i) Active aging. Aging well (ii) Stereotypes and self-stereotypes of aging (Myths and realities about aging) (iii) Why "I cannot."	(a) What is aging well? (b) Active aging versus aging well task (c) How to identify my stereotypes and combat them? (d) How I am getting old? (e) Forum: Blessed versus damn old age
	Enjoy the Control of your life	(i) Importance of healthy lifestyles (ii) The concept of health (iii) How to learn new healthy habits (iv) Misconceptions about health (v) Health Crisis along life course (vi) Risk factors: how to control them (vii) Protective health factors (viii) How to improve self-esteem	(a) Assess what is going well/what can be improved (b) Target behaviours selection for change: (1) Short term (2) Long term			
Behavioral health and independence	Health and Nutrition: Good food, good life.	(i) Nutrition as one of the important aspects for health and aging (ii) Food as energy. Food guide Pyramid (iii) Nutrition fact (iv) How to build a healthy body (v) Changes in diet are required across lifespan (vi) How to cook healthy recipes	(a) Assess your food information (b) How calculate BMI (c) Assess your nutrition (d) Planning food for the next week/month	Take care of your body	(i) Physical activity: exercise and sport, its importance, and changes across life (ii) Good nutrition characteristics (iii) Take care of your teeth and your feet	(a) Identifying aging signs (b) How is your fitness? (c) How is your diet? (d) In what extent do you take care of your teeth and feet? (e) Plan your exercise (f) Plan your nutrition changes, and diet (g) Plan how your body caring (h) Forum: You will is you can
	Taking care of your body: Self-responsibility and self-management	(i) Body changes across the lifespan: a trip through the body across time (ii) Your 5 senses: where they are placed (iii) The importance of your teeth and your feet (iv) Self-responsibility to be independent in performing activities of daily living, choosing social contact, and personally meaningful interests (v) Older adults as social capital	(a) Take your mobility test (b) Take your balance test (c) Plan how to improve your body care (d) How to walk without risks (e) How to promote and maintain ADL			
	Regular exercise: the best formula for aging well	(i) Regular physical exercise and activity as one of the best means for ageing well physically and mentally (ii) Benefit of physical exercise at physiological, cognitive, emotional, and social levels (iii) Aerobic, strength, flexibility, and balance	(a) In what extent you exercise? (b) What do you do, what do you need? (c) Selecting physical activity and exercise to incorporate into your daily life (d) Make your plan (e) Assess you base line and following-up			

TABLE 2: Continued.

Domains	Vital aging L and Vital aging M			Vital aging e-Learning		
	Units	Contents	Assessment and practice	Units	Contents	Assessment and practice
Cognitive functioning	Train your mind: how to prevent brain ageing	(i) Change and Stability of cognitive functioning across life span (ii) Solving familiar and unfamiliar problems (iii) Managing everyday tasks (iv) Remember intended activities (v) Effects of cognitive training physical activities and psychological variables in brain functioning	(a) Test your cognitive functioning (b) Proposals of exercises and cognitive activities to train mental abilities and prevent brain ageing (c) Plan your brain training (d) Assess your base-line a continue following-up	Take care of your mind	(i) Cognitive functioning (ii) Change and Stability of cognitive functioning across life span (iii) Selection, optimization and compensation as mechanisms of adaptation to changes	(a) How do you take care of your mind? (b) Select your favourite cognitive activities. (c) Self-observation of your mental decline and stability (d) Check what you have learned (e) Plan your cognitive activity (f) Forum: Cognitive functioning among the very old
	Improve your memory	(i) Misconceptions about memory and ageing (ii) What is memory, how is it organized, and how does it work? (iii) Aging effects on memory. Memory problems (iv) How to improve memory through mnemonic	(a) Test your memory (b) Daily self-register of cognitive activity (c) Mnemonic skills training (d) Memory training			
	Wisdom: the expression of lifelong learning	(i) Wisdom: Lay (implicit), explicit, and expert theories (ii) Wisdom development across time (iii) Wisdom: in between intelligence and personality	(a) How you define "wisdom"? (b) Test your wisdom (c) How to train wisdom			
	The creative age	(i) What is creativity? (ii) Old people creativity (iii) Stereotypes about creative behaviour and ageing (iv) How to be creative	(a) Test your creativity (b) Choose preferred activities for expressing creativity			
Affect, control and coping styles	Self-efficacy Perception	(i) Primary and secondary control (ii) Self-efficacy as expression of control (iii) The belief of ageing successfully as predictor of aging well (iv) Self perception of aging	(a) You as a model of aging well (b) Others as modeling (c) Imageries of success (d) Solving life events across lifespan and solving life events in old age	Feel happy	(i) Emotion: pleasant activities and well-being (ii) Control and self-efficacy (iii) Coping with stress	(a) How do you feel? (b) Pleasant activities questionnaire (c) Weekly self-registration activities (d) Self-efficacy scale (e) How do you cope with stress? (f) Plan how to cope with stress
	Positive thinking	(i) We are what we think (ii) Attitudes and thought (iii) Thinking errors (iv) Positive thinking	(a) Test your positive thinking (b) Identify thinking errors (c) Turn negative experiences into positive ones			
	Coping with stress	(i) What is stress and anxiety? (ii) Coping with stress (iii) Active and passive coping (iv) Coping skills across life span	(a) Learn self-instructions, cognitive, emotional, and physiological coping strategies (b) How to apply them			

Table 2: Continued.

Domains	Vital aging L and Vital aging M			Vital aging e-Learning		
	Units	Contents	Assessment and practice	Units	Contents	Assessment and practice
	Death is also part of life	(i) Life and Death (ii) Bereavement (iii) Spiritual approach (iv) Transcendence (v) Meaning in life	(a) Test your fear to death (b) Think about you death (c) I think, I feel, I do.			
	Pleasant activities and well-being	(i) Activity as a source of life (ii) Feeling of depression (iii) Pleasant activities and well-being (iv) Use it or lose it	(a) Test your base line of activity (b) Plan pleasant activities: analysing resources and limitations (c) Plan and Self-monitoring your activity and well-being			
Social participation and engagement	How to improve relationships with family and friends	(i) Human relationships needs (ii) Family, friends and others: their benefits. (iii) Social relationships and independence (iv) Give and received (v) Social skills (vi) Emotional intelligence	(a) Test your social networks (b) How to improve social skills (c) Training empathy, assertiveness, say "no" say "yes" (d) Interpersonal conflict management	Get involved with others	(i) Family (ii) Friends (iii) The others: Social participation	(a) My relationships (b) Assess your social life (c) Friends' network (d) Forum: Spanish grandparents, looking after grandchildren
	The others need me too	(i) Importance of pro-social behaviour (ii) Stereotypes of personality changes (iii) Pro-social behaviours and well-being (iv) How to improve care relationships (v) Care and caring (vi) Volunteering	(a) Test your pro-social behaviour (b) Plan pro-social behaviours in common life (c) Train emotional self-control			
	Sexuality: beyond genitality	(i) What is sexuality? (ii) Stereotypes and social pressure in old people sexuality (iii) Sexuality beyond genitals: diverse modalities (iv) Aging and sex: physiological changes	(a) Sensitivity and sexuality (b) Train what you do not see (c) Pelvic floor muscles exercises			
	A new system of communication: Internet	(i) Healthy behaviours in computer used (ii) Stereotypes of old people using computers. (iii) Computers for hobbies, communication, navigation, and so forth	(a) How to use computers, Internet, and its different applications (b) All practice			

Fernández-Ballesteros, 2002 [12] (5 Volumes); http://www.vivirconvitalidad.com/.

a pilot outcome evaluation is reported. The formative evaluation focused on the materials used, on participants' views about the course and about changes that occurred, and finally on their satisfaction. Summative or outcome evaluations were performed on the basis of quasi-experimental/quasi-control designs (pre-post with control group), in order to test the objectives of the *Vital Aging* programs; that is, the extent to which they gave rise to expected changes [57].

3.1. Evaluation Studies. A first evaluation of *Vital Aging* M was carried out during 2002 and 2003. This study involved a comparison between *Vital Aging*-M participants living in residential facilities ($N = 13$, mean age = 79.3) and others living in the community (attending senior citizens' clubs; $N = 44$, mean age = 69.9). The control group was recruited in the same contexts, from those doing other activities ($N = 31$, mean age = 74.2). After 6 months, a follow-up of those participants living in the community was carried out. Participant characteristics, procedures, materials, and results are reported elsewhere [15].

In the second study, the *Vital-Aging*-M program ($N = 25$; Mean age = 69.5) was compared with *Vital aging* L ($N = 28$, mean age = 67.84). The two programs were also compared under similar quasi-experimental conditions to a control group ($N = 37$, mean age = 65.6). Control participants were recruited from among those attending other regular activities at the Community Centre. Participant characteristics, procedures, materials, and results are reported elsewhere [13, 14].

In our third study, participants were 115 people aged over 54. Of these, 73 had attended five different editions of the *Vital Aging-M* program (mean age = 62.56, 52.2% women) and 42 had not attended the program (though they were on the waiting list), though they filled out the same questionnaire at the same point; these latter participants made up the control group ($N = 42$, mean age = 62.29; 57.5% women) [17].

Finally, our fourth evaluation study refers to the *Vital Aging-e learning* program recently implemented (January–April 2012) and evaluated. Participants filled out the Formative and Summative protocol; only Formative results are going to be reported here, since summative evaluation is not yet finished; only some provisional data from the Spanish subsample will be reported. Sample characteristics of the four studies are summarized in Table 3.

In order to operationalize objectives two Protocols were set up with different assessment instruments administered during the program. Formative Evaluation Protocol covers the following variables: achievement tests (with the aim of checking whether there were effects on knowledge about the course units); appraisal of lessons (referring to aspects of the lesson itself); self-perceived changes (about expected changes in behavior and psychological characteristics), and satisfaction with the course. Based on the program objectives, Summative Evaluation Protocol contains a series of questions related to the following dependent variables: Views of aging (for testing changes in stereotypes and self-perceptions on aging), Activities performed (leisure, social, intellectual, cultural, etc.), Physical exercise and Nutrition (in order to assess lifestyles), Health problems, Social relationships (frequency, quality and satisfaction), and Life satisfaction. In

TABLE 3: Sample Characteristic of the four studies curried out.

Studies	Participants	N	Mean age
(1) *Vital Aging* M	Community	44	69.9
	Residential	13	79.3
	Control	31	74.2
(2) *Vital Aging* M versus *Vital aging* L	*Vital Aging* M	25	69.5
	Vital aging L	28	67.84
	Control	37	65.6
(3) *Vital Aging* M	*Vital Aging* M	73	62.56
	Control	42	62.29
(4) *Vital Aging* e-Learning	*Vital Aging* e-Learning	88	64.2
	Control	42	62.29

our third study the following variables were also included: subjective memory, mnemonic strategies, memory appraisal, self-efficacy for aging, and positive and negative affect.

For each study, statistical analyses were carried out separately for each group, since the interest reside in observing to what extent they showed similar patterns of results, means obtained before and after each version using a repeated-measures T test were performed. We also compared the pre- and post-test means of the experimental groups with that of the control group. Covariant analyses were performed in order to test potential effects of age and gender on results.

4. Summary of Results

4.1. Formative Evaluation

4.1.1. Achievement Test. First of all, based on the lesson's readings, trainers drew up ten questions for each lesson. Internal consistency and difficulty levels were assessed. In general, *Vital Aging-M* participants scored at least 50% correct answers in all achievement tests. Lessons yielding the highest scores were those on "Positive thinking," "Coping with stress," and "Sexual relationships: Beyond genitality." Those yielding the lowest scores (never lower than 50%) were "Creative aging," "Some basic facts about memory skills," and "Nutrition and health". These results were very helpful for improving lesson materials, since they allowed us to clear up some confusing aspects.

4.1.2. Appraisal of Lessons. The most positively rated lessons of *Vital Aging-M* were "Aging well" and "Taking care of your body" (both with all elements rated as equal to or above the mean score), while the lowest-rated were some of the lessons originally taught in a language other than Spanish and later translated and dubbed. All of these were rated below the mean score. Since there is a strong relationship between level of knowledge and rating of the different details of the lessons, several analyses were performed to identify which elements of the lessons are most closely related to the general level of achievement. The variable that best predicts the level of knowledge attained in a lesson is "Teacher's clarity of presentation" ($r = .607$), followed by "Interest of the exercises" ($r = .601$), "Usefulness of the exercises" ($r = .545$), and "Satisfaction with the lesson" ($r = .527$). In any case, it should be stressed that knowledge achievement correlates positively and significantly ($\alpha = 0.05$) with the opinions expressed.

Also, the appraisals of the lessons results were very helpful for improving materials.

4.1.3. Self-Perceived Changes.
At the end of the Course, participants reported the degree of change they perceived, with regard to each of the units involved. The results showed that "Enjoying life in general," "Thinking positively," "Improve memory," "Feeling self-efficacy," and "Pleasant events and well-being" were the domains in which participants perceived the most positive changes. On the other hand, "A new system of communication: Internet," "Sexual relationships," "Creative aging," and "Improving family and social relationships" were the areas in which they reported minor changes.

As regards *Vital Aging e-Learning* participants, 62% reported that they had made quite a few of or many of the changes suggested in the course. Seventy-six per cent (76%) of these changes referred to emotions (positive thinking, managing stress, enjoying life in general, feel effective, enjoyable activities); 73% were related to cognitive functioning (training the mind, memory, wisdom); 69% concerned social relationships (relations with family and friends); 51% referred to lifestyles (body care, nutrition, exercise); and finally, 48% concerned participation (volunteering and Internet use). Regarding the intention to introduce changes in the future, 59% reported that they are going to incorporate some changes proposed in the program, and 35% that they would plan to incorporate very many changes.

4.1.4. Satisfaction with the Course.
More than two-thirds of the *Vital Aging-M* course participants found the course very interesting, and no one reported low or none interest. The course met "fairly well" or "totally" the expectations of 98.8% of the participants, and 96.7% considered that the knowledge learnt had been useful or would be useful in the future. The difficulty of the course was considered low by 45.1%, while for 82.9% its content was already partially known, and 79.3% felt they had learned a great deal. General level of satisfaction was high (78.8%), and there were no participants with low satisfaction. The most negative aspect in relation to this evaluation concerns the fact that the participants scarcely consulted the reading materials available on the homepage, consulted the tutor by interview very little or not at all (78.5%), and made practically no use of the Internet at all (89.9%).

As far as *Vital Aging e-Learning* participants are concerned, 95.8% reported that the course was quite or very interesting; 80.6% considered that they performed all the program tasks proposed; 94% considered that their expectations about the course were sufficiently met; and 96% reported that the contents of the course were very helpful for improving daily living. Regarding the level of difficulty of the course, 59.7% considered the course was not easy or not very difficult, 33.3% reported that the difficulty of the program

was low, and only 6.9% perceived a high level of difficulty. Regarding satisfaction about the course, 77.5% reported that they were highly satisfied, and only 5.6% said that their level of satisfaction with the course was low. Finally, we asked participants to rate, on a scale of 1 (none) to 10 (maximum), to what extent the program would help them to grow-up as persons, the average score being 8.36 (SD = 1.93).

In summary, our formative evaluations served to improve our materials, but they also provided a subjectively positive view of the programs. Even so, our objective was not only to promote well-being, but also to produce changes in several target behaviors related to active aging, thus let introduce those outcomes.

4.2. Summative Evaluation.
First of all, it should be emphasized that our experimental and control groups did not significantly differ in the pretest with regard to the dependent variables and both sociodemographic variables, age, and gender do not have influences in any of the dependent variables. In comparisons between pre- and post-test measures in the experimental groups and between experimental and control post-test measures, significant differences were yielded in the following variables in the expected direction.

(1) Views of aging: Those participating in the *Vital Aging* programs were assessed (both *Vital Aging*-M and *Vital Aging*-L, and those living in residences and in the community) had a significantly better view of aging after the course, and also they considered themselves more efficient for facing the aging process. No significant pre-test/post-test differences were found in our third study for views of aging.

(2) Activity level: After the implementation of both *Vital Aging* programs assessed (Life and Multimedia), participants from both contexts (Community and Residence) reported higher frequency of cultural, intellectual and social activities while not changes were found among controls.

(3) All those participants living in the community attending *Vital Aging*-M or *Vital Aging*-L did significantly more *physical exercise* and significantly improved their *diet* after the course. These positive effects were not found in those participants living in residential settings.

(4) Regarding *Vital Aging*-M, no significant pre-test/post-test differences were found in our experimental groups in either context (residence or community) for the social relationships measures. Only participants in *Vital Aging*-L and those attending the program in the third study yielded positive results, reporting significant increases in the frequency of their social relationships.

(5) With respect to life satisfaction, participants in *Vital Aging*-M living in the community reported greater differences after the program in the first and the second studies. Nevertheless, no differences were found in those participants living in residences or in those

participating in the same *Vital Aging* program in our third study.

(6) In the follow-up carried out for our first study (after 6 months), all pre-post differences in the experimental group were maintained, but, as predicted, positive changes were found in health for the community group.

(7) All of these differences remained significant when the effect of age was controlled.

(8) In the third study, after attending *Vital Aging-M* participants reported better memory and more use of mnemonics, improved their hedonic balance, experienced fewer negative emotions, and increased the frequency of their social relationships.

(9) Regarding *Vital Aging e-Learning*, preliminary results obtained in the Spain subsample indicate that following the program, participants reported greater emotional balance, and higher leisure and productive activities. All of these results are consistent with the other *Vital Aging* versions.

5. Discussion

Although some findings are not totally consistent (mainly for life satisfaction and social relationships), *Vital Aging* programs yield quite encouraging results. Participants enrolled on *Vital Aging-Life* and *Multimedia* had a better view of aging, in accordance with what was presented in the program units. Likewise, they more frequently enjoy cultural, intellectual and social activities than they did before the course. With the exception of participants living in residences, all the experimental groups increase their physical exercise and significantly improve their diet. The results are in accordance with those from the literature on programs promoting physical exercise and healthy diet, and are similar to previous results about activity level [28, 58, 59].

Nevertheless, these positive results on physical activity and diet were not found in the Residence group. Therefore, it can be concluded that *Vital Aging-M* had much more impact in the community than in institutions. However, although these differences in favor of our participants living in the community could be attributed to the fact that they have much less control over their institutional context than those living in the community, it should also be attributed to age, since those living in residential settings participating in our study are older than those living in the community (a general pattern for residential settings in Spain). This pattern is in accordance with findings from the general literature in the field of programs implemented in institutions and in studies comparing implementations in the community and in residences, as reported by Dwyer et al., among others [60]; nevertheless, any conclusions would be premature, since the numbers of participants in our residence group was very small.

Satisfaction or well-being is one of the targets for most programs promoting active aging. Nevertheless, while the measure in our first Summative Evaluation Protocol was life

satisfaction, *Vital Aging-M* yielded a significant increase in life satisfaction only in the community group (not in residences) in the first and second studies, with no differences found in the third study. In sum, we failed to obtain changes in life satisfaction in two of our three studies. It should also be noted that when we introduced more specific variables of affect, in our third study, the *Vital Ageing-M* participants reported more positive emotional balance; that is positive affect is significantly higher than negative in the same direction as found in other studies [61, 62]. Although much more research is necessary, our results point to the stability of life satisfaction construct do not make it as a sensitive variable for evaluation purposes, as also reported by several other authors; [63] therefore, more specific measures of satisfaction and well-being must be used.

Participants in the *Vital Aging-M* program in the third study (the only study in which we used these variables) also reported better perceived health and significantly improved their appraisal of their memory, reporting the extensive use of mnemonics, improved their hedonic balance by experiencing fewer negative emotions, and increased the frequency of their social relationships. All of these results could be attributed to two circumstances. First, after our formative evaluation we made some changes in an attempt to improve our materials, and second, we introduced new measures in order to make more specific evaluations. Much more research needs to be carried out in order to disentangle these two hypotheses.

In addition, we should highlight our results regarding health (health-related problems). This variable referred to whether participants reported health-related problems (e.g., back problems). Our prediction was that health would not change in the post-test, with changes only reported in the follow-up. As predicted, in the first and second studies there were no differences between pre-test and post-test in this variable, but in the third study, both the experimental and control groups reported fewer health-related problems in the post-test. These results cannot easily be understood. However, bearing in mind that the Live and Multimedia programs had a duration of 3 months and did not include specific medical care, changes in health could not be expected, since they would only occur as a result of changes in lifestyles: on the other hand, as expected, positive changes in were indeed observed in our first study in the follow-up at 6 months.

It should also be stressed that the *Vital Aging* programs had only minor impact upon the hypothesized variables related to control (self-efficacy for aging) and social relationships (quality and satisfaction). New analyses have been carried out in order to learn more about these results. Since our participants improved their self-images of aging in both versions—Life and Multimedia (both in the community and in residences)— in our third study we added a new measure of self-efficacy for aging. However, in this study no changes at all were found after the program, though this measure showed a high level of reliability and construct validity [27].

Finally, we must add that we expect to have the summative results from the Vital Ageing e-Learning course available soon, since post-tests have already been administered in the four countries (Spain, Cuba, Mexico, and Chile) involved. From our preliminary results from the subsample in Spain it can be concluded that they are consistent with the other *Vital Aging* versions.

All of the studies reported here have some important limitations. First of all, our samples are small, and not representative. Our results can be generalized only to those older adults who are *willing* to age well and register in a program for promoting aging well. Second, changes produced refers mainly to immediate changes in behavioral life styles and not long term outcomes such as disability or survival and we carried out only one follow-up study, and the extent of the follow-up was quite limited. We are aware, this Program requires longer follow-up in order to test whether those changes in behaviors could produces effects on long term hard variables such as disability and healthy survival. In the near future, we are planning to follow up all our participants, since 1996, on the *Vital Aging* programs. Third, research on active aging is growing rapidly, so that active aging promotion programs cannot be "closed" in a particular set of units (or contents), since empirical evidence is increasing year on year, and new elements are continually being discovered, supported by empirical or experimental evidence, that can influence positive aging, so that they must be introduced in a flexible way. It is on the basis of this aspect that we have launched an Internet Site which can be updated for providing material to both users and professionals (http://www.vivirconvitalidad .com/). Fourth, as remarked by Fernandez-Ballesteros in a follow-up study on aging stereotypes, the media not only generate negative stereotypes in relation to the aging phenomenon, but can also produce positive changes in the mentality of new generations, embedding positive images about aging in line with the idea that individuals can be agents in their own aging process [64]. Therefore, we are aware that in the future it will be necessary to adjust the content and methodology of *Vital Aging* in accordance with a rapidly changing society—adapting them to generations of older adults who are increasingly demanding, better prepared, and better educated, so that we may need to introduce different levels of difficulty into our program. Finally, on the basis of our first study applied in Residences we have ceased the administration of *Vital Aging* in institutions, but we do believe that much more effort should be made to design a new version that could be implemented in institutions and in other settings.

Aging is an international phenomenon; it is an expression of the human being's capacity for adaptation, or plasticity—at both individual and population levels—and also a product of the level of development of our society and of its success. However, aging can also be considered a threat, as it is associated with illness and disability. National, regional and international institutions are calling for the implementation of initiatives, policies, and programs for extending health and well-being across the lifespan and into very old age, converting active aging into a kind of mantra. But active aging (or successful, optimal, productive, and *vital aging*) are also scientific concepts about which a substantial body of knowledge can be disseminated and applied at both the population and individual levels. It should not be overlooked that individuals themselves are the agents of their own

development and aging, and the most important resource for change. *Vital aging* represents only a modest step forward in this direction, and this paper is no more than a way station on the long, but fascinating, path in pursuit of better aging, as we try to convince people that, as well as adding years to life, they can always add life to years.

Acknowledgments

Vital Aging Programs were sponsored by the Institute for Older Adults and Social Services (IMSERSO-UAM Agreements 1997-00), the Socrates Minerva Program of the European Commission (AGE-LL-C, 2001-03), and the UAM-Santander Research Program for Latin America (PUM-e 2011-12).

References

[1] M. Roth, "Problems of an ageing population," *British Medical Journal*, vol. 1, no. 5181, pp. 1226–1230, 1960.

[2] J. F. Fries and L. M. Crapo, *Vitality and Aging*, Freeman, New York, NY, USA, 1981.

[3] J. F. Fries, "Aging, natural death, and the comprenssion of morbidity," *The New England Journal of Medicine*, vol. 303, pp. 130–135, 1980.

[4] J. F. Fries, *Aging Well*, Addison-Wesley, Reading, Mass, USA, 1989.

[5] K. Christensen, G. Doblhammer, R. Rau, and J. W. Vaupel, "Ageing populations: the challenges a head," *The Lancet*, vol. 374, no. 9696, pp. 1196–1208, 2009.

[6] J. W. Vaupel, "Biodemography of human ageing," *Nature*, vol. 464, no. 7288, pp. 536–542, 2010.

[7] P. B. Baltes and M. M. Baltes, "Psychological perspectives on successful aging: the model of selective optimization with compensation," in *Successful Aging: Perspectives from the Behavioural Sciences*, P. B. Baltes and M. M. Baltes, Eds., pp. 1–35, Cambridge University Press, Cambridge, UK, 1990.

[8] K. W. Schaie, "What can we learn from longitudinal studies of adult development?" *Research on Human Development*, vol. 2, pp. 133–158, 2005.

[9] WHO, *Active Ageing*, WHO, Geneva, Switzerland, 2002.

[10] R. Fernández-Ballesteros, *Active Aging. The Contribution of Psychology*, Hogrefe, Göttingen, Germany, 2008.

[11] R. Fernández-Ballesteros, "Hacia una vejez competente: Un reto para la ciencia y la sociedad. (Toward a competent aging. A challenge for science and society)," in *Psicología Evolutiva*, M. Carretero, Ed., vol. 3 of *Developmentalpsychology*, Alianza, Madrid, Spain, 1986.

[12] R. Fernández-Ballesteros, *Vivir con Vitalidad (Vital Aging)* , vol. 5 of *Vital Aging*, Pirámide, Madrid, Spain, 2002.

[13] R. Fernández-Ballesteros, "Evaluation of "Vital Aging-M": a psychosocial program for promoting optimal aging," *European Psychologist*, vol. 10, no. 2, pp. 146–156, 2005.

[14] M. G. Caprara, *Envejecimiento con éxito: valoración de un programa [Successfulaging: evaluation of a program] [Ph.D. thesis]*, Autonomous University of Madrid, 2005.

[15] R. Fernández-Ballesteros, M. G. Caprara, and L. F. García, "Vivir con Vitalidad-M: un Programa Europeo Multimedia," *Intervención Social*, vol. 13, pp. 65–85, 2004.

[16] R. Fernández-Ballesteros, M. G. Caprara, J. Iñiguez, and L. L. García, "Vivir con Vitalidad-M. A European multimedia programme," *Psychology in Spain*, vol. 9, pp. 1–12, 2005.

[17] M. G. Capara and R. Fernández-Ballesteros, *Promoting Active Aging: New Effects of Vital Aging Program*, UDIMA, Madrid, Spain, 2012.

[18] J. W. Rowe and R. L. Kahn, "Human aging: usual and successful," *Science*, vol. 237, no. 4811, pp. 143–149, 1987.

[19] A. Bandura, *Self-Efficacy: The Exercise of Control*, Freeman, New York, NY, USA, 1997.

[20] R. Fernández-Ballesteros, J. Botella, M. D. Zamarrón et al., "Cognitive plasticity in normal and pathological aging," *Clinical Intervention on Aging*, vol. 7, pp. 15–25, 2012.

[21] A. Pascual-Leone, C. Freitas, L. Oberman et al., "Characterizing brain cortical plasticity and network dynamics across the age-span in health and disease with TMS-EEG and TMS-fMRI," *Brain Topography*, vol. 24, pp. 302–315, 2011.

[22] R. Fernández-Ballesteros, "Envejecimiento satisfactorio, (Satisfactory aging)," in *Corazón Y Cerebro, Ecuación Crucial De Envejecimiento (Heart and Brain and Equation of Aging)*, M. Lage, Ed., Pfeizer, Madrid, Spain, 2002.

[23] R. Fernández-Ballesteros, R. Schettini, M. A. Molina, and M. Santacreu, *Testing a Four Domain Model of Aging Well*, Autonomous University of Madrid, Madrid, Spain, 2012.

[24] R. Fernández-Ballesteros, L. F. García, D. Abarca et al., "Lay concept of aging well: cross-cultural comparisons," *Journal of the American Geriatrics Society*, vol. 56, no. 5, pp. 950–952, 2008.

[25] R. Fernández-Ballesteros, L. F. García, D. Abarca et al., "The concept of "ageing well" in ten Latin American and European countries," *Ageing & Society*, vol. 30, pp. 41–56, 2010.

[26] R. Fernández-Ballesteros, M. A. Molina, R. Schettini, and M. Santacreu, "The semantic network of aging well," in *Healthy Longevity*, J. M. Robine, C. Jagger, and E. M. Crimmins, Eds., vol. 33, Annual Review of Gerontology and Geriatrics, 2013.

[27] R. Fernández-Ballesteros, M. D. Zamarrón, J. Diez-Nicolás et al., "Envejecer con éxito. Criterios y predictores," *Psicothema*, vol. 22, pp. 641–647, 2010.

[28] R. P. Bogers, M. R. Tijuis, B. M. Van Gelder, and D. Kromhout, Eds., *Final Report of the HALE (Healthy Aging: A Longitudinal Study in Europe Project)*, Centre for Prevention and Health Services Research, Bilthoven, The Netherlands, 2006.

[29] A. Haveman-Nies, L. C. P. G. M. de Groot, and W. A. van Staveren, "Dietary quality, lifestyle factors and healthy ageing in Europe: the SENECA study," *Age and Ageing*, vol. 32, no. 4, pp. 427–434, 2003.

[30] J. F. Fries, "Reducing disability in older age," *Journal of the American Medical Association*, vol. 288, no. 24, pp. 3164–3166, 2002.

[31] Y. Netz, M. J. Wu, B. J. Becker, and G. Tenenbaum, "Physical activity and psychological well-being in advanced age: a meta-analysis of intervention studies," *Psychology and Aging*, vol. 20, no. 2, pp. 272–284, 2005.

[32] F. Sofi, F. Cesari, R. Abbate, G. F. Gensini, and A. Casini, "Adherence to Mediterranean diet and health status: meta-analysis," *British Medical Journal*, vol. 11, pp. 337–344, 2008.

[33] A. Trichopoulou, P. Orfanos, T. Norat, B. Bueno-de-Mesquita et al., "Modified Mediterranean diet and survival: EPIC-elderly prospective cohort study," *British Medical Journal*, pp. 330–991, 2005.

[34] A. Trichopoulou and E. Vasilopoulou, "Mediterranean diet and longevity," *British Journal of Nutrition*, vol. 84, no. 2, pp. S205–S209, 2000.

[35] K. T. Knoops, L. C. de Groot, D. Kromhout, and M. S. Horng, "Healthy lifestyle and mediterranean diet decreases mortality in the elderly," *Journal of Clinical Outcomes Management*, vol. 11, no. 11, pp. 688–689, 2004.

[36] C. Bernis, "Gender, reproductive ageing, adiposity, fat distribution and cardiovascular risk factors in spanish women aged 45–65," *Anthropologist Special*, vol. 3, pp. 241–249, 2007.

[37] R. S. Wilson, L. L. Barnes, and D. A. Bennett, "Assessment of lifetime participation in cognitively stimulating activities," *Journal of Clinical and Experimental Neuropsychology*, vol. 25, no. 5, pp. 634–642, 2003.

[38] J. Verghese, R. B. Lipton, M. J. Katz et al., "Leisure activities and the risk of dementia in the elderly," *New England Journal of Medicine*, vol. 348, no. 25, pp. 2508–2516, 2003.

[39] K. Ball, D. B. Berch, K. F. Helmers et al., "Effects of cognitive training interventions with older adults: a randomized controlled trial," *Journal of the American Medical Association*, vol. 288, no. 18, pp. 2271–2281, 2002.

[40] P. Verhaeghen, *The Interplay of Growth and Decline: Theoretical and Empirical Aspects of Plasticity of Intellectual and Memory Performance in Normal Old Age*, Oxford University Press, NewYork, NY, USA, 2000.

[41] C. Hertzog, A. F. Kramer, R. S. Wilson, and U. Lindenberger, "Fit Body, Fit Mind?" *Scientific American Mind*, vol. 20, pp. 24–31, 2009.

[42] S. Colcombe and A. F. Kramer, "Fitness effects on the cognitive function of older adults: a meta-analytic study," *Psychological Science*, vol. 14, no. 2, pp. 125–130, 2003.

[43] S. D. Pressman and S. Cohen, "Does positive affect influence health?" *Psychological Bulletin*, vol. 131, no. 6, pp. 925–971, 2005.

[44] G. V. Ostir, K. J. Ottenbacher, and K. S. Markides, "Onset of frailty in older adults and the protective role of positive affect," *Psychology and Aging*, vol. 19, no. 3, pp. 402–408, 2004.

[45] U. M. Staudinger, A. M. Freund, M. Linden, and I. Maas, "Self, personality, and life regulation: facets of psychological resilience in old age," in *The Berlin Aging Study: Aging from 70 to 100*, P. B. Baltes and K. U. Mayer, Eds., pp. 302–328, Cambridge University Press, NewYork, NY, USA, 1999.

[46] G. Labouvie-Vief, "The psychology of emotions and ageing," in *The Cambridge Handbook of Age and Ageing*, M. L. Johnson, Ed., pp. 229–236, Cambridge University Press, Cambridge, UK, 2005.

[47] M. E. Lachman, "Perceived control over aging-related declines: adaptive beliefs and behaviors," *Current Directions in Psychological Science*, vol. 15, no. 6, pp. 282–286, 2006.

[48] M. E. Lachman and C. Andreoletti, "Strategy use mediates the relationship between control beliefs and memory performance for middle-aged and older adults," *Journals of Gerontology B*, vol. 61, no. 2, pp. P88–P94, 2006.

[49] M. E. Lachman and K. M. Firth, "The adaptive value of feeling in control during midlife," in *How Healthy Are We? A National Study of Well-Being at Midlife*, O. G. Brim, C. D. Ryff, and R. Kessler, Eds., pp. 320–349, University of Chicago Press, Chicago, Ill, USA, 2004.

[50] B. R. Levy, M. D. Slade, S. R. Kunkel, and S. V. Kasl, "Longevity increased by positive self-perceptions of aging," *Journal of Personality and Social Psychology*, vol. 83, no. 2, pp. 261–270, 2002.

[51] S. Wurm, C. Tesch-Römer, and M. J. Tomasik, "Longitudinal findings on aging-related cognitions, control beliefs, and health in later life," *Journals of Gerontology B*, vol. 62, no. 3, pp. 156–164, 2007.

[52] N. Morrow-Howell, J. Hinterlong, P. A. Rozario, and F. Tang, "Effects of volunteering on the well-being of older adults," *Journals of Gerontology B*, vol. 58, no. 3, pp. S137–S145, 2003.

[53] C. F. Mendes de Leon, T. A. Glass, and L. F. Berkman, "Social engagement and disability in a community population of older adults: the New Haven EPESE," *American Journal of Epidemiology*, vol. 157, no. 7, pp. 633–642, 2003.

[54] D. C. Park, A. H. Gutchess, M. L. Meade, and E. A. Stine-Morrow, "Improving cognitive function in older adults: nontraditional approaches," *The Journals of Gerontology B*, vol. 62, pp. 45–52, 2007.

[55] M. V. Zunzunegui, A. Rodriguez-Laso, A. Otero et al., "Disability and social ties: comparative findings of the CLESA study," *European Journal of Ageing*, vol. 2, no. 1, pp. 40–47, 2005.

[56] M. Scriven, *Evaluation Thesaurus Edition*, Sage, Newbury Park, Calif, USA, 4th edition, 1991.

[57] R. E. Millsap and A. Maydeu-Olivares, *The Sage Handbook of Quantitative Methods in Psychology*, Sage, Thousand Oaks, Calif, USA, 2009.

[58] ADA, "Position paper of the American Dietetic Association: nutrition across the spectrum of aging," *Journal of the American Dietetic Association*, vol. 105, no. 4, pp. 616–633, 2005.

[59] LIFE Study Investigators, "Effects of physical activity intervention on measures of Physical Performance: results of Life styles Interventions and Independence for Elders Pilot (LIFE-P) Study," *Journal of Gerontology*, vol. 61A, pp. 1157–1165, 2006.

[60] J. T. Dwyer, K. A. Coleman, E. Krall et al., "Changes in relative weight among institutionalized elderly adults," *Journals of Gerontology*, vol. 42, no. 3, pp. 246–251, 1987.

[61] R. Fernández-Ballesteros, G. Caprara, R. Schettini et al., "Effects of University Programs for Older Adults. Changes in cultural and group stereotypes, self-perception of aging, and emotional balance," *Educational Gerontology*. In press.

[62] R. Fernández-Ballesteros, M. A. Molina, R. Scgettini, and A. L. del Rey, "Promoting active aging through University Programs for Older Adults: an evaluation study," *Geropsychology*, vol. 25, no. 3, pp. 145–154, 2012.

[63] E. Diener, "Introduction to the special section on the structure of emotion," *Journal of Personality and Social Psychology*, vol. 76, no. 5, pp. 803–804, 1999.

[64] R. Fernández-Ballesteros, "GeroPsychology an applied field for the 21st century," *European Psychologist*, vol. 11, no. 4, pp. 312–323, 2006.

Subjective Memory Complaint and Depressive Symptoms among Older Adults in Portugal

Subjective Memory Complaint and Depressive Symptoms among Older Adults in Portugal

Mónica Sousa, Anabela Pereira, and Rui Costa

Aveiro University, Campus Universitário de Santiago, 3810-193 Aveiro, Portugal

Correspondence should be addressed to Mónica Sousa; m.sousa@ua.pt

Academic Editor: Gjumrakch Aliev

Background. Older adults report subjective memory complaints (SMCs) but whether these are related to depression remains controversial. In this study we investigated the relationship between the SMCs and depression and their predictors in a sample of old adults. *Methods.* This cross-sectional study enrolled 620 participants aged 55 to 96 years (74.04 ± 10.41). Outcome measures included a sociodemographic and clinical questionnaire, a SMC scale (QSM), a Geriatric Depression Scale (GDS), a Mini-Mental Status Examination (MMSE), and a Montreal Cognitive Assessment (MoCA). *Results.* The QSM mean total score for the main results suggests that SMCs are higher in old adults with depressed symptoms, comparatively to nondepressed old adults. The GDS scores were positively associated with QSM but negatively associated with education, MMSE, and MoCA. GDS scores predicted almost 63.4% of variance. Scores on QSM and MoCA are significantly predicted by depression symptomatology. *Conclusion.* Depression symptoms, lower education level, and older age may be crucial to the comprehension of SMCs. The present study suggested that depression might play a role in the SMCs of the older adults and its treatment should be considered.

1. Introduction

The aging process is complex and dynamic. For this reasons the cognitive performance over the lifespan is a heterogeneous process, associated with interindividual variability (diversity) and intraindividual variability (dispersion) [1, 2]. This complexity is also present in the controversial topic of the subjective memory complaint (SMC).

The SMCs are complains about memory problems of people in the absence, or not, of cognitive impairment [3]. Previous Portuguese studies have reported that 75.9% [4] and/or 80.4% [5] of older adults complain of memory problems.

Based on several meta-analyses, systematic reviews, and research studies, evidence that suggests that SMCs are associated with an increased risk of dementia is inconclusive [3]. Most postulate that SMCs increase with advancing of age, are a core cognitive criteria for the early diagnosis of MCI and prodromal Alzheimer disease (AD), and have value as a predictor of dementia [6, 7]. On the other hand, it is considered that SMC could not predict future conversion to dementia [8]. A Portuguese study shows that in a memory clinic setting the SMCs have no differences in the conversion to dementia [9]. Notably, a recent systematic review shows that approximately 2.3%–6.6% of older adults with SMCs will develop mild cognitive impairment (MCI) and dementia per year [10]. Therefore, it is believed that there is no treatment that can stop the progress of dementia, but with the early detection of signs the medical treatment can slow down this disease process [11].

The presence of preclinical AD in individuals with SMCs reinforces the importance of identifying modifiable risk factors associated with cognitive decline in middle-aged populations [12]. The recent study of the World Health Organization (WHO) [13] reveled that depression in the community is around 5%. In late life, depression is common [14]; however it is not a natural part of aging. There is still a dispute over whether SMCs reflect depressive disorder [14–17], rather than early memory impairment [7], or if depression can be an early marker of brain changes that characterize dementia [12].

Besides age, sex, and level of education, the most prominent factor strongly associated with SMC is depression [14–17]. Although SMC is not associated with greater risk of mortality, it was strongly associated with depression [14, 18]. According to Singh-Manoux [18], reporting to the doctor about memory complain was related to risk of mortality. However, this active seek for help can reflect more worries about memory [8].

There is a consistent evidence that untreated depression may lead to physical, cognitive, functional, and social impairment, as well as decreased quality of life. Appropriate treatment may allow the curing of depression; however the effect of this treatment on subsequent cognitive functioning is not well understood [12].

The present study explores how old adults with SMC and depressive or nondepressive symptoms rate their levels of memory complaint. In Portuguese older adults, there was a particular interest in whether SMCs are associated with poor performance in screening tests such as the Mini-Mental Status Examination (MMSE) [19] and the Montreal Cognitive Assessment (MoCA) [20] and whether SMCs are associated with measures of gender, age, education, and depression was also investigated in order to examine the factors that influence these SMCs. Moreover, to the best of our knowledge, most of the Portuguese research investigating the relationship between SMC and depression symptoms generally use homogenous or clinical patients samples [4] and excluded patients with major depression [5, 9]. For that reason, the central question of this study was to verify the difference in older adults with depressive symptomatology through the comparison with older adults without depressive symptomatology. It was further hypothesized that SMC is related to depression and we expected that older adults with depression are of older age and female, have a lower education level, and show lower scores in screenings tests.

2. Methods

2.1. Study Design and Participants.
This is a cross-sectional study with a convenience sample recruited at the local health center and nursing homes of different regions of Portugal (Coimbra and island of Madeira) where it was conducted.

The inclusion criteria included were old adults with age of 55 years and older willing to participate in the present study. The exclusion criteria were (i) age less than or equal to 54 years, (ii) presence of neurological or psychiatric disorder, (iii) chronic alcohol or drug abuse, (iv) inability to understand and cooperate, and (v) being nonnative Portuguese.

Informed consent was obtained from all participants and the study received ethical approval from the University of Aveiro and Institutional Ethics Committee.

2.2. Procedures.
A semi-structured interview was conducted by a trained psychologist to record sociodemographic and clinical information, psychiatric and neurological history, past habits, and medical history. A standard protocol comprising test and scales of neuropsychological assessment was carried out.

2.2.1. Memory Complaint.
The Portuguese version of SMC scale (QSM) [21] was used for the assessment of SMC. Scores ≥ 4 indicate clinically significant SMC.

2.2.2. Depressive Symptoms.
The presence of depressive mood was evaluated using Geriatric Depression Scale (GDS) [22]. A score < 10 in the GDS was used to consider the absence of depression symptoms.

2.2.3. Cognitive Domain.
The global cognitive status was assessed with the MMSE [19] and the MoCA [20], following the respective correspondence of the validation studies for Portuguese population participants scoring.

3. Statistical Analysis

Descriptive statistics are presented as means with standard deviations for continuous variables and as percentages for categorical variables. The analysis of differences between the two groups (nondepressed and depressed) was conducted by Chi-squared and independent t-tests. We examined the Pearson's correlation coefficients for the associations between demographic variables (age, gender, and education), MMSE, and MoCA, with the GDS and QSM total score. Linear regression models were used to predict SMC and depression performance scores adjusted by independent variables, namely, age, gender, education, MMSE, and MoCA, considering the Enter method.

All tests were two-tailed and a p value < 0.05 was assumed as statistically significant.

We performed the statistical analysis with the Statistical Package for the Social Sciences (SPSS) v22.0 package for Windows.

4. Results

Table 1 provides the sample characteristics and results of the neuropsychological assessment. The 620 participants included 449 women and 171 men with a mean age of 74.04 years (SD ± 10.41). The mean education level of the entire group was 3.61 ± 3.38 years. A total of 548 (88.4%) of participants only completed primary school or less, and 72 (11.6%) had secondary school education or higher. The mean total score of the SMC was 7.69 ± 4.28 and most of the participants had SMC (78.9%). Clinically significant depression symptoms were present in 46.3% ($n = 287$) of the participants.

There is no statistically significant association between gender and depression symptoms ($\chi^2(1) = 2.723$, $p = 0.09$). Depression symptoms were more frequent in SMC participants ($\chi^2(1) = 46.712$, $p = 0.00$) with lower education level ($\chi^2(5) = 44.370$, $p = 0.00$; $t(618) = 3.833$, $p = 0.00$) and older age ($t(610.82) = -3.965$, $p = 0.00$). The depressed participants showed significant improvement in QSM score ($t(618) = 17.981$, $p = 0.00$) but a significant decrease in MMSE score ($t(618) = -13.408$, $p = 0.00$) and MoCA $t(618) = 30.722$, $p = 0.00$ (Table 1).

Table 2 shows that there were no significant differences between both groups only in items (5) (*Do you often use notes to avoid forgetting things?*; $\chi^2(2) = 44.370$, $p = 0.18$) and (7) (*Did you ever lose your way in neighborhood?*; $\chi^2(1) = 0.009$, $p = 0.92$). The analysis of the other items suggests that

TABLE 1: Demographics and test scores of the study groups.

	Whole sample ($n = 620$)	GDS		p
		Not depressed (GDS < 10; $n = 333$)	Depressed (GDS ≥ 11; $n = 287$)	
Age (years) M ± SD	74.04 ± 10.41	72.52 ± 10.48	75.80 ± 10.06	0.00[b]
Female n (%)	449 (72.4)	232 (69.7)	217 (75.6)	0.09[a]
Education (years) M ± SD	3.61 ± 3.38	4.27 ± 3.55	2.85 ± 2.99	0.00[b]
No education completed n (%)	178 (28.7)	61 (18.3)	117 (40.8)	
Primary school n (%)	370 (59.7)	249 (74.8)	159 (55.4)	0.00[a]
Secondary school n (%)	56 (9)	9 (2.7)	9 (3.1)	
High school/university n (%)	16 (2.6)	14 (4.2)	2 (0.7)	
MMSE M ± SD (range)	24.85 ± 5.61 (6–30)	26.61 ± 4.38	22.80 ± 6.17	0.00[b]
MoCA M ± SD (range)	18.20 ± 7.93 (1–31)	20.97 ± 6.64	14.98 ± 8.08	0.00[b]
QSM M ± SD (range)	7.69 ± 4.28 (0–18)	5.80 ± 3.26	9.87 ± 4.29	0.00[b]
Clinically significant SMC n (%)	489 (78.9)	228 (68.5)	261 (90.9)	0.00[a]
GDS M ± SD (range)	9.28 ± 4.95 (0–20)			

MMSE: Mini-Mental State Examination; MoCA: Montreal Cognitive Assessment; QSM: Portuguese version of SMC scale; GDS: Geriatric Depression Scale.
[a]Chi-square test.
[b]Independent t-tests.

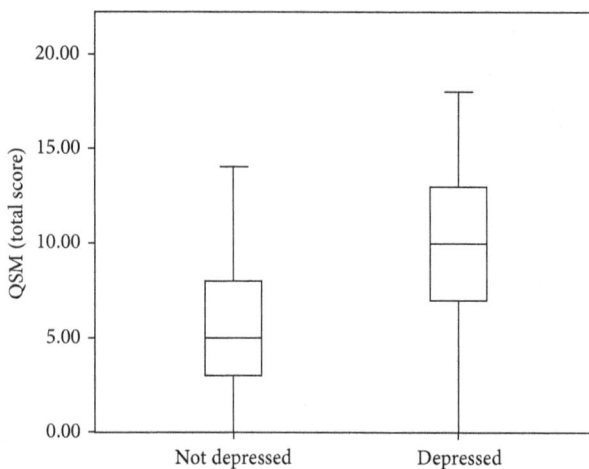

FIGURE 1: Total QSM score in the depressed and not depressed old adults.

depressed patients had generally answered the last option of the scoring.

As indicated in Figure 1, old adults with depression had higher scores on total SMC (9.87 ± 4.29; 0–14), comparatively to old adults without depression (5.80 ± 3.26; 0–18). Only one (0.3%) participant without depression symptoms and eight (2.8%) depression participants reported no memory complaint, in other words, had QSM equal to 0.

GDS score obtained significant weak negative correlation with education ($r = -0.29$, $p < 0.001$), MMSE ($r = -0.43$, $p < 0.001$), and MoCA ($r = -0.49$, $p < 0.001$) and only a significant weak positive correlation with age ($r = 0.24$, $p < 0.001$). QSM score showed a significant, weak, and positive correlation with age ($r = 0.14$, $p < 0.001$) and moderate

positive correlation with GDS ($r = 0.54$, $p < 0.001$). Education ($r = -0.13$, $p < 0.001$), MMSE, and MoCa ($r = -0.34$, $p < 0.001$) have significant weak negative correlation with QSM (Table 3).

Two multivariate logistic regressions were performed to identify the predictors of QSM and GDS scores. According to the results shown in Table 4, the QSM score was only influenced by education ($\beta = 0.14$, 95% confidence interval (CI) = -0.823–0.475), MMSE ($\beta = -0.11$, 95% CI = 0.034–0.241), and GDS scale scores ($\beta = 0.40$, 95% CI = -0.112–0.59). Age, gender, and MoCA were not influenced by QSM score (Table 3). The GDS performance were predicted by MoCA ($\beta = -0.402$, 95% CI = -0.341–-0.162) and QSM ($\beta = -0.419$, 95% CI = -0.408–0.561). These logistic regression models predicted 63.4% of total variations of GDS score and 31% of SMC score (Table 3).

5. Discussion

In the present study, we analyzed SMC and depression, and their relationship to sociodemographic and to the scores in MMSE and MoCA. The initial hypothesis that SMCs would be more reported by depressed old adults, as compared to nondepressed, was confirmed. However, in both groups, few participants had zero in the QSM total score. These findings are consistent with previous research on community samples, in which few participants also reported none memory difficulties measured by QSM [8].

On whole sample, the frequencies of SMC and depression are in line with those observed in other studies [14, 15, 18], highlighting the higher frequencies in the Portuguese old adults, independently of the characteristics of participants and settings where they are recruited [4, 5, 8, 9, 23].

TABLE 2: Results of the QSM.

Item	Subscore range	Participants score answers, %		χ^2	p
		Not depressed (GDS < 10; n = 333)	Depressed (GDS ≥ 11; n = 287)		
(1) Do you have any complaints concerning your memory?	0–3	0 = 6.9; 1 = 48.6; 2 = 26.4; 3 = 18	0 = 4.2; 1 = 19.5; 2 = 37.3; 3 = 39	69.541	0.00
(2) Do other people find you forgetful?	0–2	0 = 60.7; 1 = 27.3; 2 = 12	0 = 40.1; 1 = 31.7; 2 = 28.2	34.547	0.00
(3) Do you ever forget names of family members or friends?	0–3	0 = 69.4; 1 = 19.2; 2 = 9.6; 3 = 1.8	0 = 45.3; 1 = 19.5; 2 = 26.5; 3 = 8.7	55.253	0.00
(4) Do you often forget where things are left?	0–3	0 = 20.7; 1 = 51.7; 2 = 18.6; 3 = 9	0 = 25.1; 1 = 20.6; 2 = 28.9; 3 = 25.4	73.324	0.00
(5) Do you often use notes to avoid forgetting things?	0–2	0 = 84.4; 1 = 14.1; 2 = 1.5	0 = 82.9; 1 = 13.2; 2 = 3.8	3.371	0.18
(6) Do you ever have difficulties in finding particular words?	0-1	0 = 82; 1 = 18	0 = 59.9; 1 = 40.1	37.000	0.00
(7) Did you ever lose your way in neighborhood?	0-1	0 = 97; 1 = 3.0	0 = 96.9; 1 = 3.1	0.009	0.92
(8) Do you think more slowly than you used to?	0–2	0 = 28.2; 1 = 62.5; 2 = 9.3	0 = 11.8; 1 = 46.7; 2 = 41.5	92.862	0.00
(9) Do your thoughts ever become confused?	0–2	0 = 62.5; 1 = 29.7; 2 = 7.8	0 = 23.7; 1 = 31; 2 = 45.3	138.228	0.00
(10) Do you have concentration problems?	0–2	0 = 60.4; 1 = 30.6; 2 = 9	0 = 22; 1 = 36.6; 2 = 41.5	122.603	0.00

GDS: Geriatric Depression Scale; χ^2: Chi-square test.
Scoring of items (1), (3), and (4): 0: no; 1: yes, but no problem; 2: yes, problem; 3: yes, serious problem.
Scoring of items (2) and (5): 0: no; 1: yes, sometimes; 2: yes, often.
Scoring of items (6) and (7): 0: no; 1: yes.
Scoring of items (8)–(10): 0: no; 1: yes; 2: yes, serious problem.

TABLE 3: Correlation for the main variables and measures.

	GDS	QSM
Age	0.24**	0.14**
Education	−0.29**	−0.13**
MMSE	−0.43**	−0.34**
MoCA	−0.49**	−0.34**
GDS		0.54**

MMSE: Mini-Mental State Examination; MoCA: Montreal Cognitive Assessment; QSM: Portuguese version of SMC scale; GDS: Geriatric Depression Scale.
**p < 0.001.

Several studies have shown that older adults with depressive symptoms had significantly more SMCs, compared to older adults without these symptoms [15, 18, 24]. In this study, thus, depressive symptoms appear to be an important predictor of SMC and depression, age, education, and both screening instruments were significantly associated with QSM score. Despite the weak association, this result is analogous to the Portuguese studies [4, 23], observing positive correlations of depression with QSM score, and emphasizes that the lower cognitive performance influences the reports of memory dysfunction [14, 16].

The main findings were that participants without depression had more education, had higher scores on the MMSE and the MoCA, and had slightly minor QSM score than the participants with depression [14]. The poor cognitive function and inclination to SMC might be a reflection of a negative mental status and cognitive changes produced by anxiety and depression [14]. Therefore, overall, the Portuguese population of women over 64 years who completed primary education have a higher longevity [25, 26]. This research, based on self-reported measures of SMC and in a convenience sampling, illustrated this phenomenon. For this reason, these factors should be considered in the interpretation of the results.

Concerning the gender, no statistically significant differences were found for both SMC and depression symptoms. The influence of gender is not clear. Studies have demonstrated that there are no differences [8, 23], others that males have higher number of complaints [24], and others that women are at great risk for SMC [16].

Contrarily to previous research, in QSM items (5) (*Do you often use notes to avoid forgetting things?*) and (7) (*Did you ever lose your way in neighborhood?*), independently of whether depressed or nondepressed, few participants answered positively. Assessing the SMC with the same instrument [21], participants who were nonconverters to dementia had higher scores in item (5) [9] and participants from clinical and community sample also tend to score lower in item (7) [8]. A recent study performed in our population revealed the same higher option zero (0) in items (5) and (7) [5]. It also demonstrated that item (5) increased with

TABLE 4: Regression analysis of predictors of SMC and depression performance.

	QSM (n = 620)				GDS (n = 620)		
	β	(CI 95%)		p	β	(CI 95%)		p
Age	−0.008	3.790	10.632	0.649	−0.041	−0.056	0.017	0.296
Gender	−0.174	−0.042	0.026	0.599	−0.026	−0.980	0.413	0.425
Education	0.14	−0.823	0.475	0.009	−0.061	−0.200	0.023	0.118
MMSE	−0.11	0.034	0.241	0.035	0.074	−0.046	0.177	0.249
MoCA	−0.026	−0.215	−0.008	0.546	−0.402	−0.341	−0.162	0.000
GDS	0.40	−0.112	0.059	0.000				
QSM					0.419	0.408	0.561	0.000
R^2	31				63.4			
	$F(7.612) = 39.242.\ p < 0.001$				$F(6.613) = 68.659.\ p < 0.001$			

β: beta coefficient; 95% CI: 95% confidence interval; MMSE: Mini-Mental State Examination; MoCA: Montreal Cognitive Assessment; QSM: Portuguese version of SMC scale; GDS: Geriatric Depression Scale; R^2: Nagelkerke R Square.

the level of education and may be related to cognitive reserve and external strategies (listing dates or using schedules) [5].

In addition, the controversy between SMC and depression emphasizes that SMCs may have clinical usability to identify early cognitive changes self-described by old people [3, 6] but not so far detected in neuropsychological assessment. It also emphasizes that that depression can also increase the risk for dementia [12]. This study has significant implications for clinical practice, namely, the SMCs which should be considered clinically meaningful because they may have the potential to identify depressive symptoms.

Other possible limitations of the present investigation were the convenience sampling and the use of two cognitive screening tests. Future studies should include a larger sample that represents the Portuguese population, adopt random sampling, and should be evaluated with a comprehensive neuropsychological battery. However, the MMSE and MoCA were widely brief instruments that can provide important cognitive screening and are cost-effective for the clinical evaluation of adults' cognitive state [27]. This cross-sectional study might not provide causal information among variables and the majority of the sample was four years of education, opening the possibility to the presence of false positives. For this reason, we suggest that future studies should have a longitudinal design to deeply identify this causal relationship.

6. Conclusion

Our findings suggest that Portuguese old adults with age of 55 and older experience clinically significant depression symptoms and, as their age advances, lower education and lower cognitive function were significant predictors of the SMC. Approximately 78.9% of participants report significant SMC, with an increase form not depressed patients to depressed patients.

Based on these findings, we recommend that the clinicians, frequented by old adults with complaints of memory problems who seek help, should consider the different preventative measures and interventions that can be adopted to delay or reverse depression, and consequently the SMCs,

because this kind of complaints can be part of a scenario in which mood disorder is a symptom.

References

[1] L. Vaughan, I. Leng, D. Dagenbach et al., "Intraindividual variability in domain-specific cognition and risk of mild cognitive impairment and dementia," Current Gerontology and Geriatrics Research, vol. 2013, Article ID 495793, 10 pages, 2013.

[2] R. S. Siegler, "Inter- and intra-individual differences in problem solving across the lifespan," in Lifespan Cognition: Mechanisms of Change, pp. 285–296, University Press Scholarship Online, 2006.

[3] M. D. Mendonca, L. Alves, and P. Bugalho, "From subjective cognitive complaints to dementia: who is at risk?: a systematic review," American Journal of Alzheimer's Disease and Other Dementias, 2015.

[4] S. Ginó, T. Mendes, J. Maroco et al., "Memory complaints are frequent but qualitatively different in young and elderly healthy people," Gerontology, vol. 56, no. 3, pp. 272–277, 2010.

[5] A. A. João, J. Maroco, S. Ginó, T. Mendes, A. de Mendonça, and I. P. Martins, "Education modifies the type of subjective memory complaints in older people," International Journal of Geriatric Psychiatry, 2015.

[6] F. Jessen, B. Wiese, C. Bachmann et al., "Prediction of dementia by subjective memory impairment: effects of severity and temporal association with cognitive impairment," Archives of General Psychiatry, vol. 67, no. 4, pp. 414–422, 2010.

[7] M. Rönnlund, A. Sundström, R. Adolfsson, and L.-G. Nilsson, "Subjective memory impairment in older adults predicts future dementia independent of baseline memory performance: evidence from the Betula prospective cohort study," Alzheimer's & Dementia, vol. 11, no. 11, pp. 1385–1392, 2015.

[8] C. Pires, D. Silva, J. Maroco et al., "Memory complaints associated with seeking clinical care," International Journal of Alzheimer's Disease, vol. 2012, Article ID 725329, 5 pages, 2012.

[9] D. Silva, M. Guerreiro, C. Faria, J. Maroco, B. A. Schmand, and A. De Mendonça, "Significance of subjective memory complaints in the clinical setting," Journal of Geriatric Psychiatry and Neurology, vol. 27, no. 4, pp. 259–265, 2014.

[10] A. J. Mitchell, H. Beaumont, D. Ferguson, M. Yadegarfar, and B. Stubbs, "Risk of dementia and mild cognitive impairment in older people with subjective memory complaints: Meta-analysis," *Acta Psychiatrica Scandinavica*, vol. 130, no. 6, pp. 439–451, 2014.

[11] C. Jonker, M. I. Geerlings, and B. Schmand, "Are memory complaints predictive for dementia? A review of clinical and population-based studies," *International Journal of Geriatric Psychiatry*, vol. 15, no. 11, pp. 983–991, 2000.

[12] M. Baumgart, H. M. Snyder, M. C. Carrillo, S. Fazio, H. Kim, and H. Johns, "Summary of the evidence on modifiable risk factors for cognitive decline and dementia: a population-based perspective," *Alzheimer's & Dementia*, vol. 11, no. 6, pp. 718–726, 2015.

[13] WHO, "Depression is a common illness and people suffering from depression need support and treatment," WHO, http://www.who.int/mediacentre/news/notes/2012/mental_health_day_20121009/en/.

[14] Y. Balash, M. Mordechovich, H. Shabtai, N. Giladi, T. Gurevich, and A. D. Korczyn, "Subjective memory complaints in elders: depression, anxiety, or cognitive decline?" *Acta Neurologica Scandinavica*, vol. 127, no. 5, pp. 344–350, 2013.

[15] O. H. Del Brutto, R. M. Mera, V. J. Del Brutto et al., "Influence of depression, anxiety and stress on cognitive performance in community-dwelling older adults living in rural Ecuador: results of the Atahualpa Project," *Geriatrics & Gerontology International*, vol. 15, no. 4, pp. 508–514, 2015.

[16] L. D. S. V. e Silva, T. B. L. da Silva, D. V. D. S. Falcão et al., "Relations between memory complaints, depressive symptoms and cognitive performance among community dwelling elderly," *Revista de Psiquiatria Clinica*, vol. 41, no. 3, pp. 67–71, 2014.

[17] E. Holmes-Truscott, F. Pouwer, and J. Speight, "Further investigation of the psychometric properties of the insulin treatment appraisal scale among insulin-using and non-insulin-using adults with type 2 diabetes: results from diabetes MILES—Australia," *Health and Quality of Life Outcomes*, vol. 12, no. 1, article 87, 2014.

[18] A. Singh-Manoux, A. Dugravot, J. Ankri et al., "Subjective cognitive complaints and mortality: does the type of complaint matter?" *Journal of Psychiatric Research*, vol. 48, no. 1, pp. 73–78, 2014.

[19] J. Morgado, C. Rocha, C. Maruta, M. Guerreiro, I. Martins, and J. Morgado, "Novos valores normativos do mini-mental state examination," *Sinapse*, vol. 2, no. 9, pp. 10–16, 2009.

[20] S. Freitas, M. R. Simões, L. Alves, and I. Santana, "Montreal Cognitive Assessment (MoCA): normative study for the Portuguese population," *Journal of Clinical and Experimental Neuropsychology*, vol. 33, no. 9, pp. 989–996, 2011.

[21] S. Ginó, T. Mendes, F. Ribeiro, A. Mendonça, M. Guerreiro, and C. Garcia, "Escala de Queixas de Memória," in *Escalas e Testes na Demência*, A. Mendonça and M. Guerreiro, Eds., pp. 117–120, GEECD, Lisbon, Portugal, 2007.

[22] J. Barreto, A. Leuschner, F. Santos, and M. Sobral, "Escala de depressão geriátrica," in *Escalas e Testes na Demência*, A. Mendonça and M. Guerreiro, Eds., pp. 69–72, GEECD, Lisbon, Portugal, 2007.

[23] T. Mendes, S. Ginó, F. Ribeiro et al., "Memory complaints in healthy young and elderly adults: reliability of memory reporting," *Aging & Mental Health*, vol. 12, no. 2, pp. 177–182, 2008.

[24] J. Holmen, E. M. Langballe, K. Midthjell et al., "Gender differences in subjective memory impairment in a general population: the HUNT study, Norway," *BMC Psychology*, vol. 1, no. 1, article 19, 2013.

[25] Instituto Nacional de Estatística (INE), *Portuguese Official Statistics*, Instituto Nacional de Estatística, Lisbon, Portugal, 2011.

[26] A. Mota-Pinto, V. Rodrigues, A. Botelho et al., "A socio-demographic study of aging in the Portuguese population: the EPEPP study," *Archives of Gerontology and Geriatrics*, vol. 52, no. 3, pp. 304–308, 2011.

[27] M. Sousa, A. Pereira, R. Costa, and L. Rami, "Initial phase of adaptation of Memory alteration Test (M@T) in a Portuguese sample," *Archives of Gerontology and Geriatrics*, vol. 61, no. 1, pp. 103–108, 2015.

15

Geriatric Hip Fractures and Inpatient Services: Predicting Hospital Charges Using the ASA Score

Rachel V. Thakore, Young M. Lee, Vasanth Sathiyakumar, William T. Obremskey, and Manish K. Sethi

The Vanderbilt Orthopaedic Institute Center for Health Policy, Vanderbilt University, Suite 4200, South Tower, MCE, Nashville, TN 37221, USA

Correspondence should be addressed to Manish K. Sethi; manish.sethi@vanderbilt.edu

Academic Editor: Francesc Formiga

Purpose. To determine if the American Society of Anesthesiologist (ASA) score can be used to predict hospital charges for inpatient services. *Materials and Methods.* A retrospective chart review was conducted at a level I trauma center on 547 patients over the age of 60 who presented with a hip fracture and required operative fixation. Hospital charges associated with inpatient and postoperative services were organized within six categories of care. Analysis of variance and a linear regression model were performed to compare preoperative ASA scores with charges and inpatient services. *Results.* Inpatient and postoperative charges and services were significantly associated with patients' ASA scores. Patients with an ASA score of 4 had the highest average inpatient charges of services of \$15,555, compared to \$10,923 for patients with an ASA score of 2. Patients with an ASA score of 4 had an average of 45.3 hospital services compared to 24.1 for patients with a score of 2. *Conclusions.* A patient's ASA score is associated with total and specific hospital charges related to inpatient services. The findings of this study will allow payers to identify the major cost drivers for inpatient services based on a hip fracture patient's preoperative physical status.

1. Introduction

Hip fractures, the second leading cause of hospitalization in the elderly [1], cost over \$9.8 billion annually in treatment [2]. With the aging US population, it is estimated that over 458,000 to 1,037,000 hip fracture incidents will occur by the year 2050 [3]. As the rate of hip fracture cases increases, so will the costs associated with treating a primarily geriatric patient population that faces longer recovery periods [4], higher risks of opportunistic infections, and prolonged length of stay (LOS) [5–8]. As the Center of Medicare and Medicaid Services (CMS) moves toward a bundled payment model that will reimburse hospitals based on the expected costs of episodes of care, it has become important to understand potential risk factors that are associated with increased inpatient expenses for hip fracture patients. In this context, identifying patient factors that predict resource utilization during inpatient hospitalization can aid in the establishment of a risk-adjusted reimbursement system. One

potential risk-adjustment tool that has been considered by the government and other payers is the universally employed American Society of Anesthesiologist (ASA) classification system [9]. Utilized by anesthesiologists to assess a patient's preoperative health status, the ASA classification system assigns patients a score using a five-step scale ranging from normally healthy to moribund [10] (the appendix).

The ASA scoring system has been proven to be a reliable method for predicting LOS and costs associated with geriatric hip fracture patients [6, 11]. Garcia et al. recently demonstrated that a patient's ASA score was a stronger predictor of increased LOS and room and board charges than other well-known predictors of costs such as age, BMI, and comorbidities [6]. However, this study was limited in its scope, since service charges were not analyzed.

Based on the limitations of current literature, the distribution of costs and resources utilized within a patient's hospitalization remains extremely difficult to estimate. A few studies have demonstrated that comprehensive geriatric assessment (CGR)—a multidimensional series of screenings that evaluate a patient's medical, psychosocial, and functional status—may be predictive of surgical outcomes among elderly patients [12–14]. However, CGR is a complex, labor intensive evaluation that may not be feasible for use in all tertiary care centers [15]. A single, ubiquitous tool such as the ASA score that is used in all hospitals may be more widely adopted in predictive models of inpatient expenditure on patients with hip fractures. Therefore, the purpose of the present study was to investigate whether a patient's ASA score is significantly associated with the charges of inpatient services provided during hospitalization of patients with hip fractures.

2. Methods

Upon approval from our institutional review board, a retrospective chart review was conducted using our institution's electronic medical records system and the current procedural terminology (CPT) code system. CPT codes describe medical, surgical, and diagnostic services provided by physicians and other medical professionals. The amount of payment provided for services is based on Resource-Based Relative Value Scales (RBRVS), which are determined by calculating the resource costs needed to provide these services. Physician services are identified with the CPT code which is then submitted to insurance companies or Medicare for reimbursement [16].

Our institution is a level I trauma center that practices standard of care treatment where an orthopaedic surgeon is primarily responsible for the care of hip fracture patients. Gerontologists are consulted when needed. Patients were identified as study candidates using CPT code searches for those who had operative management of a hip fracture between January 1, 2000, and December 31, 2009 (CPT codes: 27125, 27236, 27236, 27238, 27244, and 27245). A total of 720 patients were identified using these inclusion criteria. Of these, 170 patients were excluded from analysis due to incomplete medical charts or age exclusion (<60 years). All patients were assigned ASA scores immediately before surgery. One patient with an ASA score of 1 and 2 patients with ASA scores of 5 were also excluded due to low sample sizes in those categories, leaving 547 patients for inclusion in this study.

The remaining 547 patients represented patients who underwent surgical management for an isolated low energy hip fracture who were also over 60 years of age and had complete medical records. The electronic medical charts of these patients were reviewed for information including age, gender, medical comorbidities, ASA score, date of admission, date of operation, date of hospital discharge, and type of operation via CPT code. The ASA score was assigned to each patient by the anesthesiologist before each operation. All inpatient services for these patients during their inpatient stays were obtained from the institution's financial services department. The tests and procedures for each patient were provided in line-item format via CPT code with associated charges for each item. These tests and procedures were subsequently organized into the six broad categories of CPT

codes defined by the American Medical Association (AMA): anesthesia, surgery, radiology, evaluation and management, pathology and laboratory, and medicine [17]. Anesthesia (00100–01999 and 99100–99150) included anesthesia administration by an anesthesiologist or nurse anesthetist in a general, regional, or local method. Surgery (10021–69990) included all surgical procedures within ten body systems, including surgical packages and separate procedures. Radiology (70010–79999) included diagnostic imaging and services provided by radiologists and radiology technicians. Evaluation and management (99201–99499) included consultations and services by physicians, nurse practitioners, clinical nurse specialists, certified nurse midwives, and physician assistants. Pathology and laboratory (80047–89398) included clinical laboratory tests related to the blood and lymph. Medicine (90281–99199, 99500–99607) included all medical services and procedures.

17 medical comorbidities were also collected from patient charts utilizing a data management database at our institution. These included a hypertension, myocardial infarction, cardiac dysrhythmia, atrial fibrillation, atrial flutter, congestive heart failure, heart block, cerebrovascular disease, bleeding disorder, chronic obstructive pulmonary disease, emphysema, current smoker, past smoker, renal insufficiency, dialysis dependency, cancer, and diabetes.

Prior to analysis, the normality of the variable distributions was assessed via histogram and Kolmogorov-Smirnov statistic. The charges by CPT code and total number of services provided were not normally distributed. Therefore, the relationship between the preoperative ASA and the total number of services provided during the inpatient stay was assessed using the Kruskal-Wallis nonparametric analysis of variance. Similarly, a Kruskal-Wallis analysis of variance was also performed to identify the relationship between ASA score and total charges of these tests and procedures during the inpatient stay. These analyses were repeated to exclude any inpatient days prior to the day of surgery in order to correlate ASA score to strictly postoperative tests and procedures. The significance of the difference for each of these analyses of variance was evaluated according to a Bonferroni correction at an alpha of $0.05/7 = 0.007$ to achieve a family-wise significance rate of 0.05 for each set of analyses. Linear regressions were performed using charges and number of services procedures performed as dependent variables with ASA score as an independent variable, controlled for age, gender, and the 17 comorbidities we collected during our chart review.

3. Results

720 patients who underwent hip fracture repair at our institution were found through our search. Patients who were under the age of 60 were excluded from analysis. Patients who had ASA scores of 1 ($n = 1$) or 5 ($n = 2$) were excluded from analysis due to the low sample size in these categories. After applying our exclusion criteria, 547 patients with complete medical records over the age of 60 were included in analysis. Table 2 provides demographic data

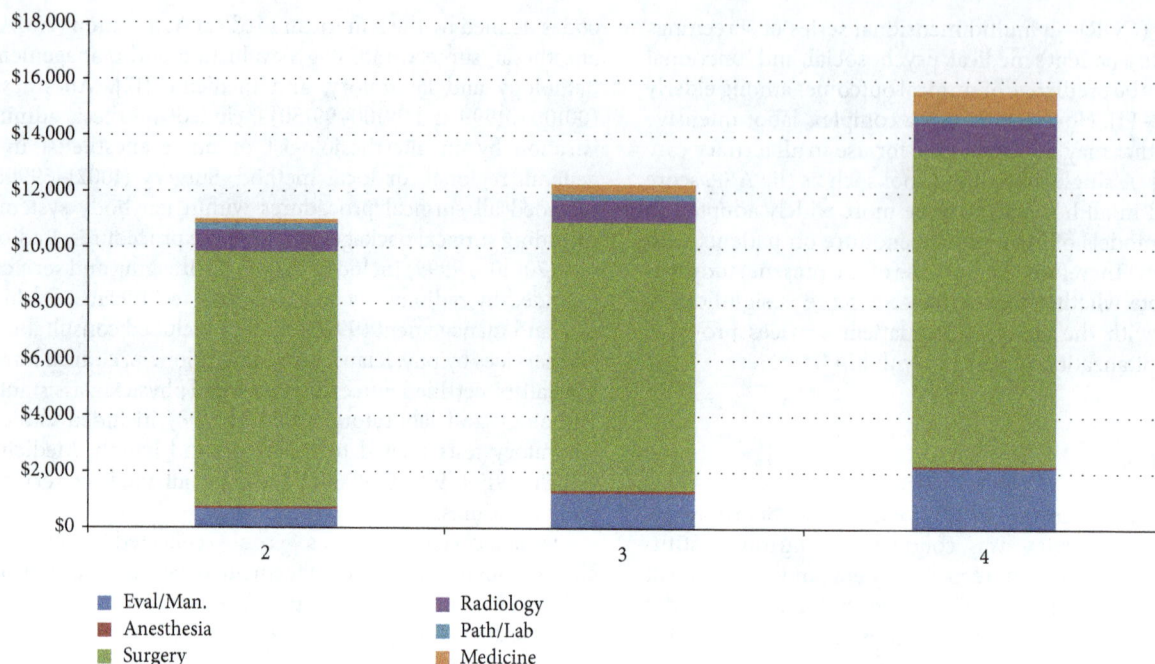

ASA class	Eval/Man. Mean (SD)	(%)	Anesthesia Mean (SD)	(%)	Surgery Mean (SD)	(%)	Radiology Mean (SD)	(%)	Path/Lab Mean (SD)	(%)	Medicine Mean (SD)	(%)	Total Mean (SD)
2	$685 (609)	6%	$78 (89)	1%	$9,103 (4,890)	83%	$771 (736)	7%	$236 (587)	2%	$127 (109)	1%	$10,923 (5,649)
3	$1,264 (1,429)	10%	$99 (122)	1%	$9,575 (5,922)	79%	$803 (842)	7%	$204 (391)	2%	$330 (545)	3%	$12,180 (7,559)
4	$2,199 (2,036)	14%	$86 (76.5)	1%	$11,214 (10,047)	72%	$1,069 (1153)	7%	$223 (423)	1%	$850 (1307)	5%	$15,555 (12,662)
P value	<0.001		0.647		0.010		0.003		0.829		<0.001		<0.001

*P value from linear regressions controlling for age, gender, and the 17 comorbidities

FIGURE 1: The average charge per patient within six categories of service based on patients' ASA scores. Total average charges are also presented.

for our patient population. The mean age of our patient population was 78 years. The majority of our patients were female (66.4%). Average BMI was within the normal range (24.7).

Figure 1 shows the average charge within six categories of service in relation to patients' assigned ASA scores. Average charges ranged from $10,923 to $15,555, with surgery comprising the highest proportion of charges for all three ASA classifications. Patients with an ASA score of 4 had the highest average inpatient charges ($15,555), followed by patients with a score of 3 ($12,180). Linear regression models controlled for age, gender, and 17 comorbidities showed that, for every increase in ASA score, there were statistically significant increases in charges for evaluation and management ($799.40, 95% CI $565.70–1033.10 $P < 0.001$), surgery ($1362.30, 95% CI $326.0–$2398.60, $P = 0.010$), radiology ($199.30, 95% CI $70.60–$331.04, $P = 0.003$), and medicine ($389.70, 95% CI $273.80–505.60, $P < 0.001$). There was also an increase in total charges by ASA score ($2751.30, 95% CI $1438.60–$4064.10, $P < 0.001$).

An ASA score of 4 was associated with the highest average number of services (45.3) while a score of 2 was associated with the lowest (24.1). Linear regression models controlled for age, gender, and comorbidities showed that, for every increase

in ASA score, there were statistically significant increases in number of services for evaluation and management (3.6, 95% CI 2.5–4.6, $P < 0.001$), surgery (1.0, 95% CI 0.5–1.4, $P < 0.001$), radiology (2.4, 95% CI 1.4–3.5, $P < 0.001$), and medicine (1.4, 95% CI 0.9–1.8, $P < 0.001$). There was also an increase in number of services by ASA score overall (11.2, 95% CI 8.3–14.1, $P < 0.001$) (Figure 2).

Figures 3 and 4 show the average frequency of postoperative services and associated charges, respectively, based on ASA scores. Patients with an ASA score of 4 had significantly higher average total charges and frequency of services provided for all postoperative tests compared to all other ASA scores. The lowest total charge was associated with an ASA score of 2 ($10,098), followed by scores of 3 ($10,996) and 4 ($13,364). Each increase in ASA score was significantly associated with increases in postoperative evaluation and management charges ($612.40, 95% CI $399.90–824.90, $P < 0.001$), surgical charges ($999.70, 95% CI 95.20–1904.20, $P = 0.30$), medicine charges ($210.60, 95% CI $123.40–297.80, $P < 0.001$), and total charges ($1876.10, 95% CI $763.60–2988.70, $P = 0.001$) (Figure 3). Similarly, an increase in ASA score was also significantly associated with the number of postoperative services provided. Specifically, ASA score was significantly associated with the number of evaluation

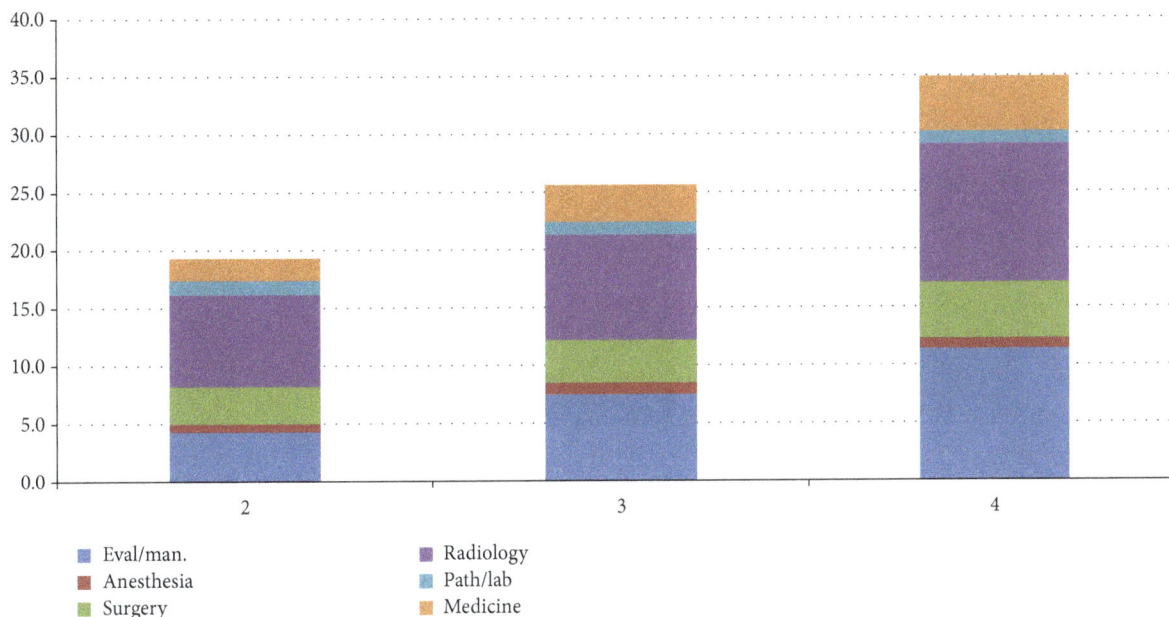

ASA class	Eval/man. Mean (SD)	(%)	Anesthesia Mean (SD)	(%)	Surgery Mean (SD)	(%)	Radiology Mean (SD)	(%)	Path/lab Mean (SD)	(%)	Medicine Mean (SD)	(%)	Total Mean (SD)
2	4.3 (3.9)	18%	0.7 (0.6)	3%	3.2 (2.1)	13%	8.0 (5.1)	33%	1.2 (1.6)	5%	1.9 (1.1)	8%	24.1 (10.1)
3	7.5 (6.4)	23%	1.0 (0.9)	3%	3.7 (2.7)	11%	9.1 (6.5)	28%	1.1 (1.6)	3%	3.2 (2.9)	10%	32.6 (18.7)
4	11.4 (8.0)	25%	0.9 (0.6)	2%	4.8 (4.2)	11%	12.0 (9.5)	26%	1.1 (1.6)	2%	4.7 (3.6)	10%	45.3 (23.1)
P value	**<0.001**		0.529		**<0.001**		**<0.001**		0.945		**<0.001**		**<0.001**

*P value from linear regressions controlling for age, gender, and the 17 comorbidities

FIGURE 2: The average frequency of services per patient based on patients' ASA scores. The total average frequency of services is also provided.

and management services (2.9, 95% CI 2.0–3.8, $P < 0.001$), number of surgical services (0.7, 95% CI 0.3–1.1, $P < 0.001$), number of radiological services (1.5, 95% CI 0.7–2.3, $P < 0.001$), number of medicine services (0.9, 95% CI 0.5–1.3, $P < 0.001$), and total number of services provided (7.1, 95% CI 4.6–9.6, $P < 0.001$) (Figure 4).

4. Discussion

Currently, more than 90% of hip fracture patients over the age of 65 have their hospitalization services covered by Medicare [4]. With the advent of the new bundled payment model, providers are reimbursed based on expected charges for episodes of care [18]. In this new system, reimbursement for treatment will be standardized for all patients, regardless of differences in patient factors that may increase the costs of care. While CGR may be a useful assessment of resource utilization in institutions where orthogeriatric specific management is utilized [19], several factors limit its feasibility in the hospitals where standard of care treatment is provided [15]. The ASA classification system, which is a simple and widely used method of ranking patients based on their preoperative physical status, may be a valuable measure to incorporate in the development of risk-adjusted reimbursement model instead of a global method of payment.

Our investigation demonstrated that ASA scores could be used to predict the number of times inpatient services are provided and the associated charges within six categories of service. Our findings are corroborated by previous studies that have studied the association between ASA scores and hospital charges for hip fracture patients. Garcia et al. recently reported that ASA score was associated with increased LOS which correlated to increased room and board charges at a charge of $4503 per day of hospitalization [6]. In our study, which investigated service charges instead of room and board, we found that the ASA score is a useful method for predicting the frequency and charges of services required for hip fracture patients in our institution and others were similar treatment models that are provided.

The ASA classification was originally developed for use by anesthesiologists to determine risk of operative morbidity [20] based on patients comorbidities. In our study, we have shown that the ASA score can also be used to predict surgical resource utilization. In fact, surgery was disproportionately the most expensive category of service, composing 72%–88% of all charges and only 11%–21% of services provided. Therefore, surgical services may be the best area to focus on quality improvement initiatives in order to most effectively lower costs among hip fracture patients with high ASA scores.

Several reasons explain why surgical charges may increase with ASA score, especially within the postoperative period.

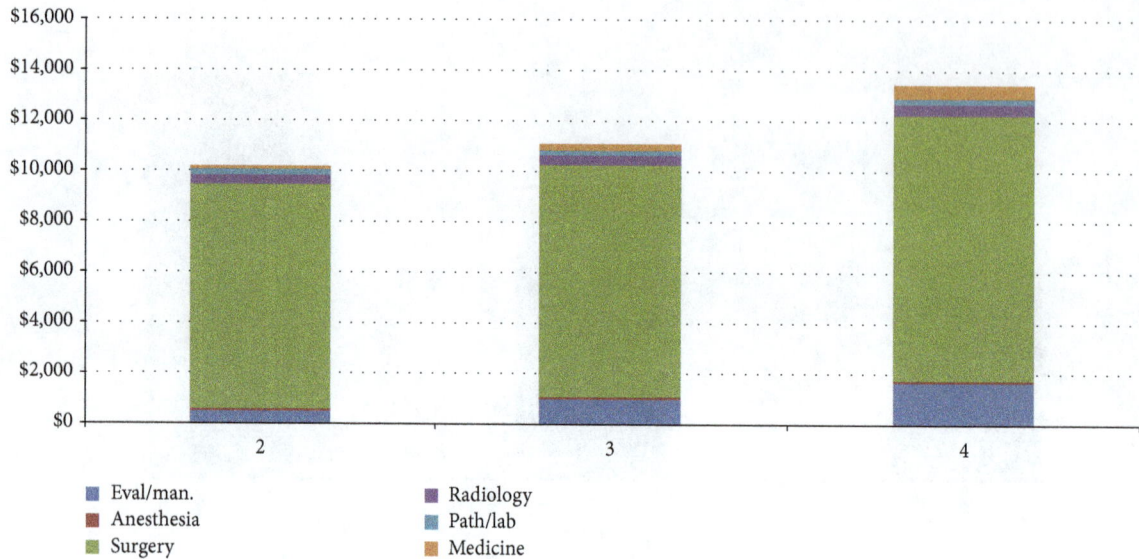

ASA class	Eval/man. Mean (SD)	(%)	Anesthesia Mean (SD)	(%)	Surgery Mean (SD)	(%)	Radiology Mean (SD)	(%)	Path/lab Mean (SD)	(%)	Medicine Mean (SD)	(%)	Total Mean (SD)
2	$501.8 (459)	5%	$78 (89)	1%	$8898 (4793)	88%	$359 (495)	4%	$236 (587)	2%	$103 (107)	1%	$10,098 (5460)
3	$985 (1342)	9%	$92 (104)	1%	$9188 (5306)	84%	$375 (571)	3%	$195 (385)	2%	$249 (459)	2%	$10,996 (6653)
4	$1682 (1765)	13%	$84 (75)	1%	$10493 (8166)	79%	$447 (526)	3%	$218 (417)	2%	$526 (919)	4%	$13,364 (9827)
P value	<0.001		0.612		0.030		0.140		0.762		<0.001		0.001

*P value from linear regressions controlling for age, gender, and the 17 comorbidities

FIGURE 3: The average charges per patient related to postoperative services based on patients' ASA scores. Total average charges are also presented.

The ASA classification system has been shown to be correlated with multiple factors that increase surgical resource utilization including infection [21], reoperations [22], intraoperative blood loss [23], and duration of surgery [24]. Similarly, hip fracture patients with a greater number of comorbidities have been shown to be more likely to suffer postoperative complications that would require diagnostics and imaging [25], which would explain the increase in radiology charges with ASA score.

The number of evaluation and management services and charges also increased significantly with ASA score. One major reason for this is that patients with higher ASA scores are more likely to develop complications. In fact, Donegan et al. recently showed that ASA classification is strongly associated with medical complications that require interventions by a medical specialist or internist after hip fracture surgery [11]. Furthermore, patients with higher ASA scores are likely to have even higher charges than those reported in our study due to repeated readmissions required for complications. In fact, Radcliff et al. reported that a higher ASA score was associated with worse outcomes thirty days after surgery for male hip fracture patients [26]. Therefore, when considering the future costs of readmissions, patients with higher ASA scores would become an even greater financial burden to hospitals and physicians in a global payment system than demonstrated in our study.

Alternatively, patients with higher ASA scores did not require significantly more anesthesia or pathology services during their hospitalization. This may be due to several reasons. Unlike other categories of service such as evaluation and management, services provided by anesthesiologists are not prolonged throughout a patient's duration of hospitalization. Pathology services are not commonly utilized for orthopaedic trauma patients who sustained fracture. In fact, most patients in our study required only one clinical laboratory service regardless of ASA scoring.

4.1. Study Limitations. Our study is limited as a retrospective chart review at a single level I trauma center. Although this study design minimized variability in hospital charges and patterns of practice, it also constrains the generalizability of our results to the general patient population and other medical centers. Because very few patients in our analysis were assigned an ASA score of 1 or 5, we could not include these patients in our analysis. We only controlled for 17 comorbidities in our linear regression model. Other medical comorbidities such as dementia and hepatic disease could also correlate to hospital resource utilization. We also did not consider whether medical conditions may have delayed surgical intervention for our patients. Moreover, the ASA classification system is limited by anesthesiologists' subjectivity in assigning scores, although moderate to substantial interrater

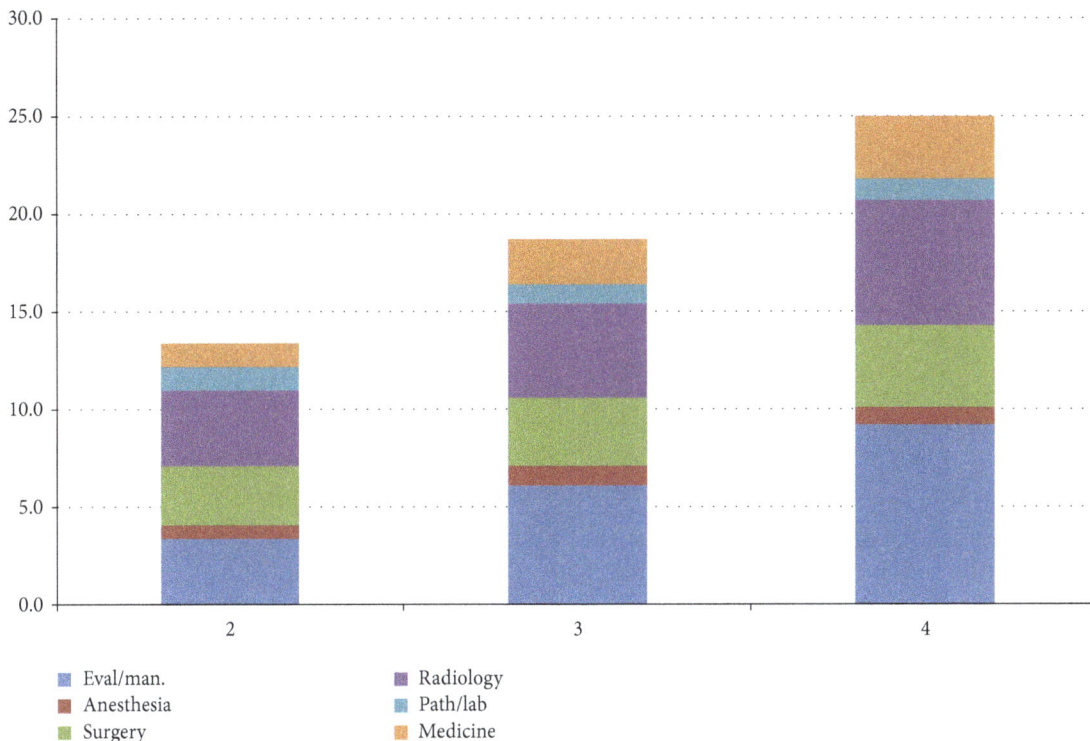

ASA class	Eval/man. Mean (SD)	(%)	Anesthesia Mean (SD)	(%)	Surgery Mean (SD)	(%)	Radiology Mean (SD)	(%)	Path/lab Mean (SD)	(%)	Medicine Mean (SD)	(%)	Total Mean (SD)
2	3.4 (3.1)	23%	0.7 (0.6)	5%	3.0 (1.7)	20%	3.9 (3.7)	26%	1.2 (1.6)	8%	1.2 (1.0)	8%	15.0 (8.7)
3	6.1 (5.8)	36%	1.0 (0.8)	6%	3.5 (2.3)	21%	4.8 (4.8)	28%	1.0 (1.5)	6%	2.3 (2.6)	14%	17.0 (16.3)
4	9.2 (7.3)	32%	0.9 (0.6)	3%	4.2 (3.0)	14%	6.4 (6.3)	22%	1.1 (1.6)	4%	3.2 (3.1)	11%	29.2 (18.2)
P value	**<0.001**		0.467		**<0.001**		**<0.001**		0.833		**<0.001**		**<0.001**

* P value from linear regressions controlling for age, gender, and the 17 comorbidities

FIGURE 4: The average frequency of postoperative services per patient based on patients' ASA scores. The total average frequency of services is also provided.

TABLE 1: American Society of Anesthesiology's physical status (ASA PS) class.

ASA score	Definition
1	A normal healthy patient
2	A patient with mild systemic disease
3	A patient with severe systemic disease
4	A patient with severe systemic disease that is a constant threat to life
5	A moribund patient who is not expected to survive without the operation
6	A declared brain-dead patient whose organs are being removed for donor purposes

reliability has been reported when limited to a single surgical specialty [27, 28]. A larger-scale, multi-institutional investigation would strengthen the argument of the use of the ASA

score as a tool for predicting inpatient charges and services among the hip fracture population.

5. Conclusion

In accordance with past investigations that have demonstrated the predictive power of the ASA classification system in the treatment of hip fracture patients, we have shown that a patient's ASA score is associated with services and charges provided during inpatient hospitalization. Further studies are needed to determine whether the charges associated with ASA score are due to potentially preventable outcomes, such as the development of complications and the need of reoperations, or are necessary expenditure related to severe presentation of injury. Additional studies to look at a day-by-day cost analysis would help identify the association between time and expenditure of resources on patients to help design future interventions to decrease cost. Although the new bundled payment model of reimbursement generalizes utilization

TABLE 2: Population demographic information.

	N	%
Age (yrs)		
60–74	202	13.3%
75+	345	63.1%
Mean	78.0 (9.9)	
Gender		
Male	184	33.6%
Female	363	66.4%
ASA score		
2	58	10.6%
3	371	67.8%
4	118	21.6%
Average BMI (kg/m^2)	24.7 (6.1)	

of hospital services by episode of care, individualized clinical characteristics of geriatric hip fracture patients, including severity of condition, can have a major influence on hospital expenditure. Because the ASA score is a universally applied method of classification, it should be considered in future reimbursement models in the care of hip fracture patients.

Appendix

See Table 1.

References

[1] K. Wilkins, "Health care consequences of falls for seniors," *Health Reports*, vol. 10, no. 4, pp. 47–55, 1999.

[2] News AAOS, "Academy Statement on Prevention of Hip Fractures," 2000, http://www2.aaos.org.proxy.library .vanderbilt.edu/aaos/archives/acadnews/2000news/c9-17.htm.

[3] C. A. Brown, A. Z. Starr, and J. A. Nunley, "Analysis of past secular trends of hip fractures and predicted number in the future 2010–2050," *Journal of Orthopaedic Trauma*, vol. 26, no. 2, pp. 117–122, 2012.

[4] US Congress OoTA, *Hip Fracture Outcomes in People Age 50 and Over—Background Paper*, US Government Printing Office, Washington, DC, USA, 1994.

[5] A. A. Fisher, M. W. Davis, S. E. Rubenach, S. Sivakumaran, P. N. Smith, and M. M. Budge, "Outcomes for older patients with hip fractures: the impact of orthopedic and geriatric medicine cocare," *Journal of Orthopaedic Trauma*, vol. 20, no. 3, pp. 172–178, 2006.

[6] A. E. Garcia, J. V. Bonnaig, Z. T. Yoneda RE et al., "Patient variables which may predict length of stay and hospital charges in elderly patients with hip fracture," *Journal of Orthopaedic Trauma*, vol. 26, no. 11, pp. 620–623, 2012.

[7] S. J. Long, K. F. Brown, D. Ames, and C. Vincent, "What is known about adverse events in older medical hospital inpatients? A systematic review of the literature," *International Journal for Quality in Health Care*, vol. 25, no. 5, pp. 542–554, 2013.

[8] L. Pousada, R. Leipzig, C. Smyth, S. Rosenfeld, P. Dooley, and R. D. Kennedy, "Effect of a geriatric consult team on length of acute-care hospital stay for hip fracture," *Einstein Quarterly*

Journal Of Biology & Medicine, vol. 9, no. 2, pp. 65–69, 1991.

[9] D. L. Davenport, E. A. Bowe, W. G. Henderson, S. F. Khuri, and R. M. Mentzer Jr., "National Surgical Quality Improvement Program (NSQIP) risk factors can be used to validate American Society of Anesthesiologists Physical Status Classification (ASA PS) levels," *Annals of Surgery*, vol. 243, no. 5, pp. 636–641, 2006.

[10] ASA Physical Classification System, American Society of Anesthesiologists, http://www.asahq.org/clinical/physicalstatus.

[11] D. J. Donegan, A. N. Gay, K. Baldwin, E. E. Morales, J. L. Esterhai Jr., and S. Mehta, "Use of medical comorbidities to predict complications after hip fracture surgery in the elderly," *The Journal of Bone & Joint Surgery*, vol. 92, no. 4, pp. 807–813, 2010.

[12] T. Fukuse, N. Satoda, K. Hijiya, and T. Fujinaga, "Importance of a comprehensive geriatric assessment in prediction of complications following thoracic surgery in elderly patients," *Chest*, vol. 127, no. 3, pp. 886–891, 2005.

[13] J. A. Overcash and J. Beckstead, "Predicting falls in older patients using components of a comprehensive geriatric assessment," *Clinical Journal of Oncology Nursing*, vol. 12, no. 6, pp. 941–949, 2008.

[14] N. Martinez-Velilla, B. Ibanez-eroiz, and J. Alonso-Renedo, "Is comprehensive geriatric assessment a better 1-year mortality predictor than comorbidity and prognostic indices in hospitalized older adults?" *Journal of the American Geriatrics Society*, vol. 61, no. 10, pp. 1821–1823, 2013.

[15] A. M. Horgan, N. B. Leighl, L. Coate et al., "Impact and feasibility of a comprehensive geriatric assessment in the oncology setting: a pilot study," *American Journal of Clinical Oncology*, vol. 35, no. 4, pp. 322–328, 2012.

[16] American Medical Association, "RBRVS: Resource-Based Relative Value Scale," http://www.ama-assn.org//ama/pub/ physician-resources/solutions-managing-your-practice/coding -billing-insurance/medicare/the-resource-based-relative-value -scale.page.

[17] M. Moisio, *Medical Terminology for Insurance and Coding*, Cengage Learning, 2009.

[18] Centers for Medicare & Medicaid Services, "Fact Sheets," 2013, http://www.cms.gov/apps/media/fact_sheets.asp.

[19] G. Pioli, M. L. Davoli, F. Pelliciotti, P. Pignedoli, and A. Ferrari, "Comprehensive care," *European Journal of Physical and Rehabilitation Medicine*, vol. 47, no. 2, pp. 265–279, 2011.

[20] M. Daabiss, "American Society of Anaesthesiologists physical status classification," *Indian Journal of Anaesthesia*, vol. 55, no. 2, pp. 111–115, 2011.

[21] S. Ridgeway, J. Wilson, A. Charlet, G. Katafos, A. Pearson, and R. Coello, "Infection of the surgical site after arthroplasty of the hip," *The Bone & Joint Journal*, vol. 87, no. 6, pp. 844–850, 2005.

[22] H. Palm, M. Krasheninnikoff, and K. Holck, "An algorithm for hip fracture surgery reduced the one-year reoperation rate from 18% to 12%," *The Bone & Joint Journal*, vol. 94, article 309, 2012.

[23] E. T. Newman, T. S. Watters, J. S. Lewis et al., "Impact of perioperative allogeneic and autologous blood transfusion on acute wound infection following total knee and total hip arthroplasty," *The Journal of Bone & Joint Surgery*, vol. 96, no. 4, pp. 279–284, 2014.

[24] U. Wolters, T. Wolf, H. Stützer, and T. Schröder, "ASA classification and perioperative variables as predictors of postoperative outcome," *British Journal of Anaesthesia*, vol. 77, no. 2, pp. 217–222, 1996.

[25] J. J. W. Roche, R. T. Wenn, O. Sahota, and C. G. Moran, "Effect of comorbidities and postoperative complications on mortality after hip fracture in elderly people: prospective observational cohort study," *British Medical Journal*, vol. 331, no. 7529, pp. 1374–1376, 2005.

[26] T. A. Radcliff, W. G. Henderson, T. J. Stoner, S. F. Khuri, M. Dohm, and E. Hutt, "Patient risk factors, operative care, and outcomes among older community-dwelling male veterans with hip fracture," *The Journal of Bone & Joint Surgery*, vol. 90, no. 1, pp. 34–42, 2008.

[27] R. Jacqueline, S. Malviya, C. Burke, and P. Reynolds, "An assessment of interrater reliability of the ASA physical status classification in pediatric surgical patients," *Paediatric Anaesthesia*, vol. 16, no. 9, pp. 928–931, 2006.

[28] K. G. Ringdal, N. O. Skaga, P. A. Steen et al., "Classification of comorbidity in trauma: the reliability of pre-injury ASA physical status classification," *Injury*, vol. 44, no. 1, pp. 29–35, 2013.

16

Prevalence and Determinants of Falls among Older Adults in Ecuador: An Analysis of the SABE I Survey

Carlos H. Orces

Department of Medicine, Laredo Medical Center, 1700 East Saunders, Laredo, TX 78041, USA

Correspondence should be addressed to Carlos H. Orces; corces07@yahoo.com

Academic Editor: Francesc Formiga

The present study based on a nationally representative sample of older adults living in the Andes mountains and coastal region of the country indicates that 34.7% of older adults had fallen in the previous year in Ecuador. Among fallers, 30.6% reported a fall-related injury. The prevalence of falls was higher in women and among older adults residing in the rural Andes mountains. In the multivariate model, women, subjects with cognitive impairment, those reporting urinary incontinence, and those being physically active during the previous year were variables found independently associated with increased risk of falling among older adults in Ecuador. Moreover, a gradual and linear increase in the prevalence of falls was seen as the number of risk factors increased. Falls represent a major public health problem among older adults in Ecuador. The present findings may assist public health authorities to implement programs of awareness and fall prevention among older adults at higher risk of falls.

1. Introduction

One-third of people over the age of 65 years who live in the community fall each year; this proportion increases to 50% by the age of 80 years. Although not all falls of older persons are injurious, about 5% of them result in a fracture, and other serious injuries occur in 5% to 10% of falls [1]. Approximately 30% of falls required medical treatment, often resulting in emergency department visits and subsequent hospitalizations, increasing the demand for healthcare services [2]. Previous studies have reported upward trends in fall-related injury hospitalizations and deaths in developed countries [3, 4]. Despite these facts, there is limited information about the epidemiology of falls among older adults in developing countries.

Reyes-Ortiz et al. (2005) reported that the prevalence of falls among adults aged 60 years or older across seven urban cities in Latin America ranged from 21.6% in Bridgetown, Barbados to 34% in Santiago, Chile [5]. In Brazil, the prevalence of falls found among older adults residing in urban areas was 27.6% [6]. Moreover, among studies in Latin America, the increased risk of falling has been associated with female gender, increased age, high depressive symptoms,

functional limitations, diabetes, arthritis, osteoporosis, and urinary incontinence [5–7].

In Ecuador, the proportion of persons aged 60 years or older was 6.2% in 1990 and it is expected to reach 11.9% by 2020 and 24.5% by 2050. These demographic changes may markedly increase the number of falls among older adults in the country [8]. Knowledge of the epidemiology of falls may assist public health authorities to implement prevention strategies among individuals at higher risk of falling. Thus, the aims of the present study were to estimate the prevalence of falls and to determine characteristics associated with fall risk among persons aged 60 years or older in Ecuador.

2. Subjects and Methods

The present study was based on cross-sectional data from older adults who participated in the first national survey of Health, Wellbeing, and Aging Study (SABE I), conducted between June and August of 2009. The SABE I survey is a probability sample of households with at least one person aged 60 years or older residing in the Andes mountains and coastal regions of Ecuador. In the primary sampling stage, a total of 317 sectors from the rural areas (<2,000 inhabitants) and 547 sectors from the urban areas of the Coastal and Andes Mountains regions of the country were selected from the 2001 population Census cartography. In the secondary sampling stage, 18 households within each sector were randomly selected based on the assumption that at least one person aged 60 years or older live in 24% and 23% of the households in the Coastal and Andes Mountains, regions, respectively. The objectives of the SABE I survey were to evaluate the health status, cognitive impairment, life style, access and utilization of health care, and functional limitations among older adults in Ecuador. Survey details, including operation manuals, are publicly available [9].

2.1. Falls Ascertainment. The prevalence of falls and recurrent falls were assessed by the following questions: "have you fallen in the past year" and "how many times have you fallen in the past year," respectively. Participants were characterized as recurrent fallers if they had reported two or more falls in the previous year. Participants who answered affirmatively to the question "did you need medical attention as a result of falls" were considered to sustain a fall-related injury.

2.2. Demographic and Health Characteristics. Age and sex were self-reported. Body height in centimeters and weight in kilograms were measured and the body mass index calculated (Kg/cm^2). Participants were asked about their living status (alone versus living with others) and area of residence (urban versus rural). The average use of alcohol per week during the previous three months was classified as none, one day, or two or more days per week.

Self-reported general health was defined as excellent, very good, good, fair, or poor. Medical conditions were assessed by asking the participants if they had been diagnosed by a physician with hypertension, diabetes mellitus, chronic obstructive pulmonary disease (COPD), arthritis, stroke, or cataracts. Urinary incontinence was defined as having involuntary incontinence of urine during the previous year.

Cognitive status was evaluated by the abbreviated Mini-Mental State Examination (AMMSE), which has been validated in the Chilean population. The AMMSE consists of 9 items and has a score from 0 to 19. A score of 12 or less was defined to identify participants with cognitive impairment [10]. The Geriatric Depression Scale was used to evaluate the presence of depressive symptoms. This 15-item scale has been validated in Spanish populations with a sensitivity of 81% and a specificity of 76%. Respondents with a score of 6 or more are considered to have symptoms of depression [11, 12]. The following activities of daily living (ADLs) were included in the present study: walking across a room, dressing, bathing, eating, getting in and out of bed, and using the toilet. Those participants who needed help or were unable to perform one or more of the six ADLs were considered functionally impaired. Physical activity was evaluated by the question "do you regularly exercise such as jogging, dance, or perform rigorous physical activity at least three times weekly for the past year." Those participants who responded affirmatively were defined as physically active. Lower extremity physical

limitation was present if the participants answered affirmatively to any of the following questions: "do you have any difficulty walking a few city blocks" or "do you have any difficulty walking a flight of stairs." The chair stand test was used to assess lower-limb muscle strength. This test is considered successfully completed if participants are able to stand-up five times from a chair with their arms folded within 60 seconds. Quartiles in seconds were created to analyze the association between lower-limb muscle strength and falls [13].

2.3. Statistical Analysis. The chi-square test for categorical variables and the t-test for continuous variables were used to compare the characteristics of participants who reported a fall in the previous year and those who did not. Subsequently, those variables statistically significant (P value < .05) in the univariate analyses were entered into a logistic regression model to evaluate the independent associations between falls and characteristics of the participants. Results of the regression model are presented as odds ratios (ORs) with their 95% confidence intervals (95% CI). The prevalence of falls was also examined according to the number of independent risk factors found in the multivariate model. Trend in fall prevalence according to the number of risk factors was examined with the chi-square test for trend. To adjust for the multistage sampling design of the SABE I survey, all analyses were weighted by using SPSS, Complex Sample Survey, version 17 software (SPSS Inc., Chicago, IL, USA) to generate national fall prevalence estimates.

3. Results

Of 5,227 participants with complete information on fall status, 37.4% (95% CI, 35.7–39.2) reported to have fallen in the previous year, representing an estimated 445,000 older adults in Ecuador. Recurrent falls (two or more) occurred in 23% (95% CI, 21.5–24.6) of the participants. Moreover, among those who had fallen 30.6% (95% CI, 27.9–33.5) sustained a fall-related injury.

The prevalence of falls increased gradually with advancing age and was higher among women (Figure 1). The prevalence of fall-related injuries also increased with age and was higher among women after age of 70 years. Figure 2 shows the prevalence of falls stratified by gender and area of residence. Overall, the prevalence of falls varies across regions of the country. However, the highest prevalence of falls in both genders was reported among those subjects residing in the rural Andes Mountains.

As displayed in Table 1, fallers were more likely to be older, women, residing in rural areas, having poor health status, comorbidities, being less physically active, having functional limitations on the lower extremities and personal ADLs, and having the lowest scores in the chair stand test as compared with non-fallers. In the final multivariate model, women (OR, 1.81; 95% CI, 1.32–2.48), subjects with cognitive impairment (OR, 1.71; 95% CI, 1.18–2.49), those reporting urinary incontinence (OR, 1.58; 95% CI, 1.13–2.22), and being those physically active during the previous year (OR, 1.68;

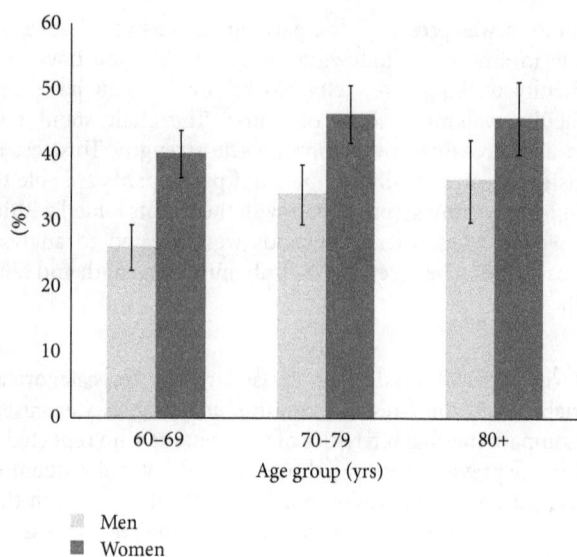

FIGURE 1: Prevalence of falls among older adults in Ecuador, SABE I.

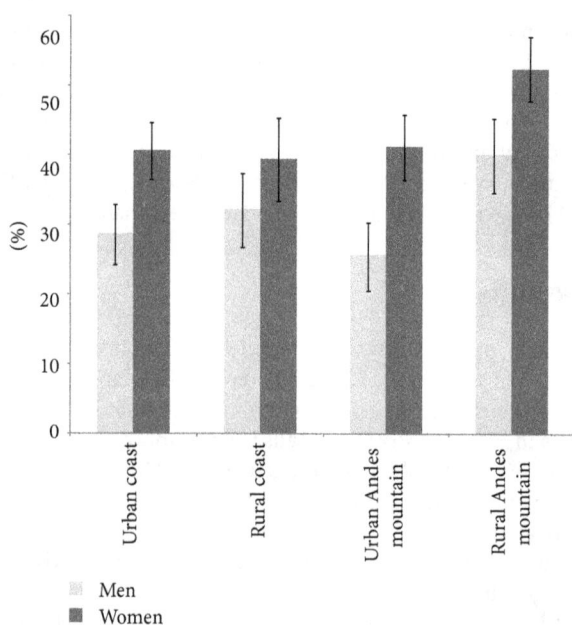

FIGURE 2: Prevalence of falls among older adults according to area of residence.

95% CI, 1.23–2.29) were variables found independently associated with increased risk of falling among older adults in Ecuador (Table 2). Although not statistically significant, a physician's diagnosis of stroke (OR, 0.86; 95% CI, 0.86–2.58) and drinking alcohol ≥ 2 days per week (OR, 1.47; 95% CI, 0.53–4.04) were also associated with increased risk of falling.

Figure 3 shows the prevalence of falls according to the number of risk factors. Overall, a gradual and linear increase in the prevalence of falls was seen as the number of risk factors increased from 19.6% among persons with no risk factors to

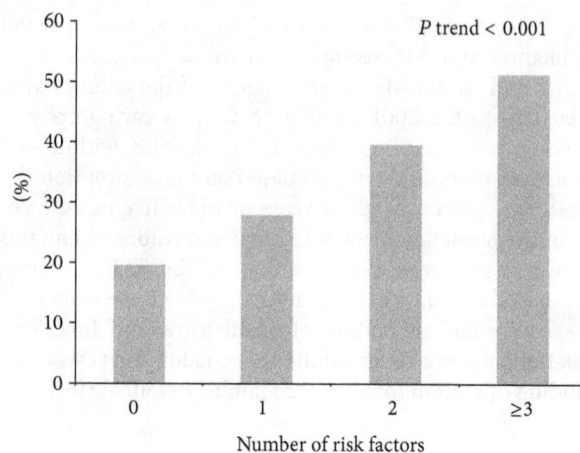

FIGURE 3: Number of risk factors and prevalence of falls among older adults in Ecuador.

51.3% among those with three or more risk factors (P trend < .0001).

4. Discussion

The present study estimates that 37.4% of community-dwelling older adults fall each year in Ecuador. These results indicate that the prevalence of falls in Ecuador is one the highest reported in the region compared to a previous study of fall prevalence among persons aged 60 years or older in Latin America [5]. Similarly, the prevalence of recurrent falls was higher than those reported in Santiago, Chile, Mexico City, and Sao Paulo, Brazil [5].

The proportion of fall-related injuries among older adults in Ecuador was similar to that reported among persons aged 65 years or older in the USA [14]. Moreover, the increased prevalence of falls and fall-related injuries with advancing age and among women is consistent with other published studies [5, 14–18]. Possible explanations for the higher incidence of fall-related injuries among women have been related to levels of physical activity, muscle weakness and loss of lower body strength, bone mass, circumstances surrounding the fall, and willingness to seek medical attention [17, 18].

Of interest, the highest prevalence of falls occurred among older men and women residing in the rural Andes Mountains. Consistent with this finding, a recent study reported a higher incidence of hip fractures among older adults residing in the Andes Mountains region of the country [19]. Similarly, a study in the USA demonstrated that rural residents have higher fall-related injury rates than urban and suburban residents [20]. Possible explanations for these disparities in fall-related injury may be associated with high-risk occupations such as farming, mining, forestry, and construction among adults residing in rural areas [20]. However, it is unknown whether the same occupational risk factors are present among older adults residing in rural areas of the country.

Table 1: Demographic and clinical characteristics of survey participants, SABE I.

	Fallers	Nonfallers	P value
Sex (n, %)			<.0001
Women	1,177 (62.3)	1,584 (49.2)	
Men	745 (37.7)	1,721 (50.8)	
Age, yrs	72.3 SD 8.8	70.8 SD 8.3	<.0001
BMI (Kg/m^2)	26.0 SD 4.8	26.0 SD 4.6	.837
Residing in rural areas (n, %)	942 (37.9)	1,408 (30.9)	<.0001
Alcohol use (n, %)			<.0001
None	1,572 (82.2)	2,591 (76.8)	<.0001
1 day	304 (15.0)	634 (21.0)	
≥2 days	45 (2.8)	78 (2.2)	
Self-reported health (n, %)			<.0001
Excellent	13 (0.8)	43 (1.6)	
Very good	22 (1.6)	105 (4.0)	
Good	282 (15.6)	730 (24.7)	
Fair	1,033 (53.5)	1,825 (52.9)	
Poor	569 (28.5)	597 (16.8)	
Comorbidities (n, %)			
Cognitive impairment	511 (29.0)	568 (17.0)	<.0001
Depression	533 (39.2)	618 (24.4)	<.0001
Hypertension	905 (49.8)	1,382 (43.9)	<.0001
Diabetes	266 (13.9)	396 (12.8)	<.0001
COPD[a]	192 (9.7)	221 (6.9)	<.0001
Arthritis	717 (40.0)	932 (28.0)	<.0001
Stroke	157 (8.9)	165 (4.8)	<.0001
Urinary incontinence	557 (31.8)	614 (19.6)	<.0001
Cataracts	548 (30.4)	803 (24.5)	<.0001
Physical activity (n, %)	577 (29.7)	1,078 (32.5)	<.0001
Lower extremity disability (n, %)	960 (70.1)	1,255 (62.3)	<.0001
ADLs limitation (n, %)[b]	685 (35.0)	713 (21.2)	<.0001
Chair stand test			<.0001
Q1 (4 to 9 sec)	346 (25.0)	842 (30.8)	
Q2 (10 to 11 sec)	313 (22.4)	727 (25.6)	
Q3 (12 to 14 sec)	367 (25.4)	704 (25.5)	
Q4 (unable and ≥15 sec)	385 (27.2)	531 (18.0)	

[a]Chronic obstructive pulmonary disease.
[b]Personal activities of daily living.

Table 2: Associations between characteristics of the participants and self-reported falls.

	Unadjusted OR (95% CI)	Adjusted OR (95% CI)
Sex		
Men	1.00 (Reference)	1.00 (Reference)
Women	1.70 (1.46–1.99)	**1.81 (1.32–2.48)**
Age groups, years		
60–69	1.00 (Reference)	1.00 (Reference)
70–79	1.34 (1.13–1.60)	1.13 (0.83–1.55)
≥80	1.40 (1.14–1.72)	0.95 (0.60–1.51)
Live in rural areas		
No	1.00 (Reference)	1.00 (Reference)
Yes	1.36 (1.17–1.58)	1.01 (0.76–1.34)
Alcohol use		
None	1.00 (Reference)	1.00 (Reference)
1 day per week	0.66 (0.54–0.81)	1.16 (0.77–1.73)
≥2 days per week	1.15 (0.70–1.91)	1.47 (0.53–4.04)
Self-reported health		
Excellent	1.00 (Reference)	1.00 (Reference)
Very good	0.81 (0.30–2.18)	0.22 (0.19–2.55)
Good	1.26 (0.57–2.78)	0.90 (0.13–6.20)
Fair	2.03 (0.93–4.40)	1.10 (0.16–7.38)
Poor	3.39 (1.55–7.41)	1.51 (0.22–10.4)
Comorbidities		
Cognitive impairment		
No	1.00 (Reference)	1.00 (Reference)
Yes	1.99 (1.65–2.40)	**1.71 (1.18–2.49)**
Depression		
No	1.00 (Reference)	1.00 (Reference)
Yes	1.99 (1.64–2.42)	1.14 (0.82–1.59)
Hypertension		
No	1.00 (Reference)	1.00 (Reference)
Yes	1.27 (1.09–1.48)	1.19 (0.90–1.58)
Diabetes		
No	1.00 (Reference)	1.00 (Reference)
Yes	1.10 (0.88–1.36)	1.07 (0.71–1.59)
COPD		
No	1.00 (Reference)	1.00 (Reference)
Yes	1.45 (1.10–1.89)	0.98 (0.60–1.59)
Arthritis		
No	1.00 (Reference)	1.00 (Reference)
Yes	1.72 (1.46–2.01)	1.03 (0.76–1.39)
Stroke		
No	1.00 (Reference)	1.00 (Reference)
Yes	1.91 (1.42–2.56)	1.49 (0.86–2.58)
Urinary incontinence		
No	1.00 (Reference)	1.00 (Reference)
Yes	1.91 (1.60–2.28)	**1.58 (1.13–2.22)**

An important finding of the present study was the strong and significant association between cognitive impairment and increased fall risk among older adults in Ecuador. This result is consistent with those from previous research [21–23]. In fact, a systematic review and meta-analysis of twenty-seven studies reported that impairment of global measures of cognition was associated with any fall, serious injuries, and distal radius fractures in community-dwelling older adults. Executive function was also associated with increased

TABLE 2: Continued.

	Unadjusted OR (95% CI)	Adjusted OR (95% CI)
Cataracts		
No	1.00 (Reference)	1.00 (Reference)
Yes	1.34 (1.13–1.59)	0.92 (0.66–1.29)
Physical activity		
No	1.00 (Reference)	1.00 (Reference)
Yes	1.14 (0.96–1.34)	**1.68 (1.23–2.29)**
Lower extremity disability		
No	1.00 (Reference)	1.00 (Reference)
Yes	1.41 (1.16–1.71)	1.20 (0.89–1.61)
Limitations in ADLs		
No	1.00 (Reference)	1.00 (Reference)
Yes	2.03 (1.73–2.39)	1.20 (0.86–1.67)
Chair stand test		
Q1 (4 to 9 sec)	1.00 (Reference)	1.00 (Reference)
Q2 (10 to 11 sec)	1.07 (0.84–1.38)	0.94 (0.63–1.39)
Q3 (12 to 14 sec)	1.23 (0.96–1.57)	0.87 (0.58–1.29)
Q4 (unable and ≥15 sec)	1.86 (1.45–2.38)	1.17 (0.78–1.77)

Bold numbers represent statistical significance in the final multivariate model.

risk for any fall and falls with serious injury in institution-dwelling older adults. A diagnosis of dementia of any type was associated with risk for any fall, but not serious injury [23]. Moreover, executive function has been associated to dual tasking and gait variability, supporting the idea that fall risk depends on this function [24]. More recently, results from a prospective cohort study demonstrate that, among community-dwelling older adults, the risk of future falls was predicted by performance on executive function and attention tests conducted five years earlier. In fact, individuals with the lowest score on executive function were more likely to fall sooner and more frequently during the follow-up period [25].

Urinary incontinence was also found an independent and significant risk factor for falls. The present finding is consistent with the results of a recent systematic review [26]. Falls related to incontinence are generally thought to result from loss of balance when rushing to the toilet. However, it is unclear whether incontinence is a primary cause of falls or it is simply a marker of generalized physical frailty [27].

Among the modifiable risk factors, regular alcohol use was associated with increased risk of falling among older adults. Although not statistically significant, there was a 1.4-fold higher risk of falling among older adults who drink on average two or more days per week compared to those who did not. These findings contrast with results from previous cohort studies that reported no significant association between alcohol use and fall risk among older adults [21, 22, 28, 29]. However, low alcohol concentrations among older adults, having considered to be safe for driving,

may affect the ability to successfully avoid sudden obstacles in the travel path. Moreover, it is suggested that many of alcohol-related falls are the results of the disruptive effects of alcohol on the online corrections of the ongoing gait pattern when walking under challenging conditions [30].

Several studies have shown that fall risk is closely related to ADLs capability and that difficulty in at least one activity of daily living double the risk of falling [5, 21, 22, 31, 32]. In Ecuador, the risk of falling was 1.2-fold higher among older adults with any impairment in ADLs. This finding confirms the results of a previous study showing that any ADLs limitation among older adults in Latin America and among Mexican-Americans increases significantly the risk of falling [5]. Limitations in ADLs often reflect poor mobility and lower-limb muscle strength, which are major risk factors for falling in older people [15, 33, 34]. In the present study, a significant association between lower-limb muscle strength and falls was found in the unadjusted regression model. However, after adjusting for covariates, a considerable attenuation of the association was observed suggesting that the increased risk of falls among participants with lower-limb muscle weakness was modified by demographic and health characteristics of the subjects. Of relevance, the risk of falling was significantly higher among participants who reported intense regular exercise during the previous year compared to those who did not. This finding may be partly explained by reported changes in postural control among older adults following moderate physical exercise, which may be related to fatigue levels [30]. However, environmental factors and terrain conditions should also be considered as determinants of moderate exercise-related falls among older adults in Ecuador.

As previously described by other researchers, a linear increase in the percentage falls is seen as the number of independent risk factors also increases [21, 22]. In Ecuador, the prevalence of falls among older adults with three or more risk factors was 51.3% compared to 19.6% among those with no risk factors. The principal clinical implication of this finding is that the risk of falling may be reduced significantly by modifying even a few risk factors [21].

The present study is the first to provide national estimates on the prevalence of falls among adults aged 60 years and older residing in the coastal and Andes mountains regions of Ecuador and identified demographic and health characteristics associated with increased risk of falling. However, several limitations must be mentioned in interpreting these results. First, the SABE I survey used a 12-month recall period, which is susceptible to recall bias. Second, these findings may also reflect nonresponse bias. Subjects who did not participate in the survey may have been older, frailer, and more likely to have fallen, which would result in underestimating falls. Third, older adults residing in the Amazon region of the country were not included in the SABE I survey. However, they represent only 3.3% of the population aged 60 years and older in Ecuador [35]. Fourth, other known factors associated with increased risk of falling such as gait disorder, orthostatic hypotension, dizziness, use of psychotropic drugs, or use of walking aid were not included in the analysis or collected in the survey.

In conclusion, falls represent a major public health problem among older adults in Ecuador. The present findings may assist public health authorities to implement programs of awareness and fall prevention among older adults at higher risk for falls.

References

[1] M. E. Tinetti and C. S. Williams, "Falls, injuries due to falls, and the risk of admission to a nursing home," *New England Journal of Medicine*, vol. 337, no. 18, pp. 1279–1284, 1997.

[2] K. A. Hartholt, J. A. Stevens, S. Polinder, T. J. van der Cammen, and P. Patka, "Increase in fall-related hospitalizations in the United States, 2001–2008," *Journal of Trauma*, vol. 71, no. 1, pp. 255–258, 2011.

[3] P. Kannus, J. Parkkari, S. Koskinen et al., "Fall-induced injuries and deaths among older adults," *Journal of the American Medical Association*, vol. 281, no. 20, pp. 1895–1899, 1999.

[4] C. H. Orces, "Trends in hospitalization for fall-related injury among older adults in the United States,1988–2005," *Ageing Research*, vol. 1, no. 1, pp. 1–4, 2010.

[5] C. A. Reyes-Ortiz, S. Al Snih, and K. S. Markides, "Falls among elderly persons in Latin America and the Caribbean and among elderly Mexican-Americans," *Revista Panamericana de Salud Publica*, vol. 17, no. 5-6, pp. 362–369, 2005.

[6] F. V. Siqueira, L. A. Facchini, and D. S. Silveira, "Prevalence of falls in elderly in Brazil: a countrywide analysis," *Cadernos de Saúde Pública*, vol. 27, no. 9, pp. 1819–1826, 2011.

[7] D. T. da Cruz, L. C. Ribeiro, T. Vieira Mde et al., "Prevalence of falls and associated factors in elderly individuals," *Revista de Saúde Pública*, vol. 46, no. 1, pp. 138–146, 2012.

[8] http://www.eclac.cl/celade/proyecciones/basedatos_BD.htm.

[9] http://anda.inec.gob.ec/anda/index.php/catalog/95.

[10] M. G. Icaza and C. Albala, "MInimental State Examinaitons (MMSE) del studio de la demencia en Chile: Análisis Estadístico—Serie Investigaciones en Salud Pública-Documentos Técnicos," Coordinación de Investigaciones, División de Salud y Desarrollo Humano, OPS, 1999, http://www.paho.org.

[11] J. A. Yesavage, T. L. Brink, T. L. Rose et al., "Development and validation of a geriatric depression screening scale: a preliminary report," *Journal of Psychiatric Research*, vol. 17, no. 1, pp. 37–49, 1982.

[12] J. Martínez De La Iglesia, M. C. Onís Vilches, R. Dueñas Herrero, C. Aguado Taberné, C. A. Colomer, and M. C. Arias Blanco, "Abbreviating the brief. Approach to ultra-short versions of the Yesavage questionnaire for the diagnosis of depression," *Atencion Primaria*, vol. 35, no. 1, pp. 14–21, 2005.

[13] A. R. Barbosa, J. M. Souza, M. L. Lebrão, R. Laurenti, and M. F. Marucci, "Functional limitations of Brazilian elderly by age and gender differences: data from SABE Survey," *Cadernos de Saúde Pública*, vol. 21, no. 4, pp. 1177–1185, 2005.

[14] J. A. Stevens, K. A. Mack, L. J. Paulozzi, and M. F. Ballesteros, "Self-reported falls and fall-related injuries among persons aged ≥65 years—United States, 2006," *Morbidity and Mortality Weekly Report*, vol. 57, no. 9, pp. 225–229, 2008.

[15] A. J. Campbell, G. F. Spears, and M. J. Borrie, "Examination by logistic regression modelling of the variables which increase the relative risk of elderly women falling compared to elderly men," *Journal of Clinical Epidemiology*, vol. 43, no. 12, pp. 1415–1420, 1990.

[16] M. E. Tinetti, J. Doucette, E. Claus, and R. Marottoli, "Risk factors for serious injury during falls by older persons in the community," *Journal of the American Geriatrics Society*, vol. 43, no. 11, pp. 1214–1221, 1995.

[17] J. A. Stevens and E. D. Sogolow, "Gender differences for non-fatal unintentional fall related injuries among older adults," *Injury Prevention*, vol. 11, no. 2, pp. 115–119, 2005.

[18] J. A. Stevens, M. F. Ballesteros, K. A. Mack, R. A. Rudd, E. Decaro, and G. Adler, "Gender differences in seeking care for falls in the aged medicare population," *American Journal of Preventive Medicine*, vol. 43, no. 1, pp. 59–62, 2012.

[19] C. H. Orces, "Trends in hip fracture rates in Ecuador and projections for the future," *Revista Panamericana de Salud Pública*, vol. 29, no. 1, pp. 27–31, 2011.

[20] H. Tiesman, C. Zwerling, C. Peek-Asa, N. Sprince, and J. E. Cavanaugh, "Non-fatal injuries among urban and rural residents: the National Health Interview Survey, 1997–2001," *Injury Prevention*, vol. 13, no. 2, pp. 115–119, 2007.

[21] M. E. Tinetti, M. Speechley, and S. F. Ginter, "Risk factors for falls among elderly persons living in the community," *New England Journal of Medicine*, vol. 319, no. 26, pp. 1701–1707, 1988.

[22] M. C. Nevitt, S. R. Cummings, S. Kidd, and D. Black, "Risk factors for recurrent nonsyncopal falls. A prospective study," *Journal of the American Medical Association*, vol. 261, no. 18, pp. 2663–2668, 1989.

[23] S. W. Muir, K. Gopaul, and M. Montero-Odasso, "The role of cognitive impairment in fall risk among older adults: a systematic review and meta-analysis," *Age and Ageing*, vol. 41, no. 3, pp. 299–308, 2012.

[24] T. Herman, A. Mirelman, N. Giladi, A. Schweiger, and J. M. Hausdorff, "Executive control deficits as a prodrome to falls in healthy older adults: a prospective study linking thinking, walking, and falling," *Journals of Gerontology A*, vol. 65, no. 10, pp. 1086–1092, 2010.

[25] A. Mirelman, T. Herman, M. Brozgol et al., "Executive function and falls in older adults: new findings from a five-year prospective study link fall risk to cognition," *PLoS One*, vol. 7, no. 6, Article ID e40297, 2012.

[26] P. E. Chiarelli, L. A. Mackenzie, and P. G. Osmotherly, "Urinary incontinence is associated with an increase in falls: a systematic review," *Australian Journal of Physiotherapy*, vol. 55, no. 2, pp. 89–95, 2009.

[27] S. Lord, C. Sherrington, H. Menz, and J. Close, *Falls in Older People*, Cambridge, UK, 2011.

[28] D. E. Nelson, R. W. Sattin, J. A. Langlois, C. A. DeVito, and J. A. Stevens, "Alcohol as a risk factor for fall injury events among elderly persons living in the community," *Journal of the American Geriatrics Society*, vol. 40, no. 7, pp. 658–661, 1992.

[29] A. C. Grundstrom, C. E. Guse, and P. M. Layde, "Risk factors for falls and fall-related injuries in adults 85 years of age and older," *Archives of Gerontology and Geriatrics*, vol. 54, no. 3, pp. 421–428, 2012.

[30] J. Hegeman, V. Weerdesteyn, B. J. F. Van Den Bemt, B. Nienhuis, J. Van Limbeek, and J. Duysens, "Even low alcohol concentrations affect obstacle avoidance reactions in healthy senior individuals," *BMC Research Notes*, vol. 3, article 243, 2010.

[31] F. Bloch, M. Thibaud, B. Dugué, C. Brèque, A. S. Rigaud, and G. Kemoun, "Episodes of falling among elderly people: a systematic review and meta-analysis of social and demographic pre-disposing characteristics," *Clinics*, vol. 65, no. 9, pp. 895–903, 2010.

[32] R. W. Sattin, J. G. Rodriguez, C. A. Devito, and P. A. Wingo, "Home environmental hazards and the risk of fall injury events among community-dwelling older persons," *Journal of the American Geriatrics Society*, vol. 46, no. 6, pp. 669–676, 1998.

[33] S. R. Lord, J. A. Ward, P. Williams, and K. J. Anstey, "Physiological factors associated with falls in older community-dwelling women," *Journal of the American Geriatrics Society*, vol. 42, no. 10, pp. 1110–1117, 1994.

[34] M. E. den Ouden, M. J. Schuurmans, I. E. Arts, and Y. T. van der Schouw, "Association between physical performance characteristics and independence in activities of daily living in middle-aged and elderly men," *Geriatrics & Gerontology International*, 2012.

[35] http://www.inec.gob.ec/inec/index.php?option=com_remository&Itemid=420&func=select&id=74&lang=ki.

17

Menopausal Symptoms and Its Correlates: A Study on Tribe and Caste Population of East India

Doyel Dasgupta, Priyanka Karar, Subha Ray, and Nandini Ganguly

Department of Anthropology, University of Calcutta, 35 Ballygunge Circular Road, Kolkata, West Bengal 700019, India

Correspondence should be addressed to Doyel Dasgupta; doel.dasgupta83@gmail.com

Academic Editor: Fulvio Lauretani

Present study aimed to compare the incidence of menopausal problems and concomitants between tribe and caste population. This cross section study was conducted in five villages of West Bengal, a state in the eastern part of India. This study was conducted between two different ethnic groups—one of the "Particularly Vulnerable Tribal Groups (PTG)" of India named as "Lodha" and the other was a Bengali speaking caste population. A total number of 313 participants were finally recruited for this study. Study participants were married, had at least one child, had no major gynaecological problems, and had stopped menstrual bleeding spontaneously for at least 1 year. Additionally, data on sociodemographic status and menstrual and reproductive history were collected using a pretested questionnaire/schedule. Bivariate analyses (chi square test) revealed that significantly more number of caste participants suffered from urinary problems than their tribe counterpart. The reverse trend has been noticed for the frequency of vaginal problems. Multivariate analyses (binary logistic regression) show that sociodemographic variables and menstrual and reproductive history of the present study participants seem to be the concomitants of menopausal symptoms. Tribe and caste study population significantly differed with respect to the estrogen deficient menopausal problems and the concomitants to these problems.

1. Introduction

Menopause is associated with reduction in the normal estrogen levels and subsequent incidence of menopausal symptoms [1]. Studies stated that, during the early postmenopausal period, the prevalence of vasomotor symptoms ranges from 30 to 80 percent and, during later period, vaginal dryness from 25 to 47 percent [2]. The prevalence of urogenital complaints has been reported to increase at menopause and is more common in women than men, implicating menopause [3–5].

For most women, natural menopause takes place between the ages of 45 and 55 years [6, 7]. In most developed countries, this event occurs around the age of 50 years [8]. But in developing countries like India there has been a trend in advancement of age at menopause [9]. Thus, along with increase in life expectancy growing number of these women can expect to live for several decades after menopause. Furthermore, several studies have shown that the frequency of reporting of menopausal symptoms of Indian women varies with culture and also with sociodemographic status [10, 11].

In Indian subcontinent, one may find an appreciable quantum of literature on menopause. To the best of the understanding of the authors, few studies addressed the menopausal issues of any indigenous ethnic group (tribe). Although in this globalised world we observe some radical change to have occurred in different societies, the indigenous ethnic group maintains homogeneity in the form of practicing endogamy and in maintaining traditional cultural beliefs. They differ from the other ethnic groups in terms of their biological and cultural identity such as mating structure and social tradition. This inequality in social and cultural characteristics is likely to affect the reproductive characteristics, including reproductive aging or menopause of the indigenous groups differentially.

Under this circumstance, the present study aims to find out the prevalence of menopausal problems between tribe and caste population of West Bengal, a state of east India.

2. Material and Methods

2.1. Study Area. The present study has been conducted in one of the indigenous ethnic groups known as "Lodha" of West Bengal, a state located in eastern India. Lodha population have been declared as one of the "Particularly Vulnerable Tribal Groups" of this country on the basis of certain characteristics like low level of literacy, preagricultural level of technology, and declining or stagnant population. In West Bengal they mainly lived in the district of West Medinipur. We selected them from 5 villages of West Medinipur district. Caste population have been recruited from the same villages. Study areas have been selected using multistage random sampling techniques, considering one local administrative unit (*gram panchayat*) from the district and five villages from *gram panchayat*. Each of the administrative units was randomly selected.

2.2. Study Population. We identified 404 postmenopausal (221 Lodha and 183 caste participants) participants on the basis of the criteria fixed for the study: the participants were between the ages of 40 and 55 years, had attained natural menopause, were married, had at least one child, and had no history of hysterectomy or other major gynaecological problems. We have excluded childless participants from the study to ensure that all participants have been exposed to certain reproductive events/behaviour in life (like pregnancy, lactation, and parity) that modify the reproductive hormonal levels of participants. Finally 313 of these participants (172 Lodha and 141 caste participants) were available or volunteered to participate. Thus the total participation rate was 77.5.9% (lodha 77.8% and schedule caste 77.0%). The menopausal state was ascertained following the classification of the World Health Organization [8].

Prior to collection of data, the nature of research was explained and consent was taken from all the participants.

2.3. Data Types and Data Collection Techniques. A pretested and structured questionnaire was used to collect the data on sociodemographic status that include age of the participants at the time of interview, years of education, working status, per capita monthly household expenditure in Indian rupees, use of tobacco, and consumption of black tea or alcohol. Data on menstrual history includes ages at menarche, history of menstrual regularity, and history of heavy and scanty menstrual discharge; reproductive history includes age at marriage, use of oral contraceptive pills, number of live births, duration of breastfeeding (months), and history of sterilization. Barring the variable "age at menarche," information on other menstrual and reproductive factors pertains to the stage after the last child birth. Data collection techniques have been discussed elsewhere [12]. Menopausal problems of the participants were collected (last 30 days' recall) with the help of a "menopausal problem list" used in study on the Bengali speaking Hindu women of West Bengal [13]. The procedural details of using this questionnaire have been discussed elsewhere [13].

The present study is conducted during the period of March 2009 to July 2012. The study protocol has been approved by the "Research Ethics Committee" of the University of Calcutta, India (reference number: BEHR/1095/2304).

2.4. Methods of Analyses. We applied descriptive statistics (frequency and mean calculation) to compare the trend in the sociodemographic variables and menstrual and reproductive history and menopausal problems between tribe and caste postmenopausal participants. We also used t-test and χ^2 test in bivariate comparisons.

Binary multivariate logistic regression (using enter method) analyses were done to find out the concomitants that significantly associated with menopausal problems. In these analyses, the presence or absence of menopausal problems were considered dependent variables. All the sociodemographic, menstrual, and reproductive variables were entered together in the analysis as independent variables. The following were the reference categories (in parenthesis) for each of the categorical variables: working status (nonworking), history of heavy or scanty menstrual discharge (absent), oral contraceptive pill (ever used), history of reproductive wastage (absent), sterilisation (absent), use of tobacco (no), and consumption of black tea (no). The rest of the variables, such as age of the participants at the time of interview, per capita monthly household expenditure, years of education, duration of breast feeding, and number of live births, were treated as continuous variables. The colinearity of the independent variables is checked and the values are found to be within the acceptable limit (SE = 0.001 to 5.0). In the text, values of odds ratio and 95% CI are presented only for those variables that showed significant association ($P \leq 0.05$) with a particular menopausal problem. We excluded the variables like alcohol consumption from the multivariate analyses as none of the caste population and few sections of tribal women consume it.

3. Results

Table 1 shows that an overwhelming section of tribal participants had no formal education whereas more than half of the caste women got it. Larger section of caste participants belonged to nonworking category, but higher number of tribal participants were mostly engaged in day labour, small scale business, and agricultural activities. Per capita monthly household expenditure was significantly more in caste than in tribal participants. Significantly higher number of tribal participants were tobacco chewers and majority of participants consumed black tea. A few sections of tribal participants consume alcohol, but none of the caste ones consumes it. No significant differences have been observed between tribe and caste participants regarding mean age at menarche. An overwhelming section of participants had the history of menstrual regularity, whereas significantly higher number of tribal participants had the history of heavy and scanty menstrual discharge. Mean ages at marriage, first pregnancy, and last pregnancy and duration of breastfeeding were significantly earlier in tribal than caste participants. Mean number of live births was similar among both groups. Use of oral contraceptive and history of reproductive wastage

TABLE 1: Socio demographic variables, menstrual and reproductive history.

	Tribe ($n = 172$)	Caste ($n = 141$)	P value
Mean age of participants at the time of interview (years)	49.09 ± 4.7	48.85 ± 4.2	0.052
Years of education			NA
0	163 (94.6)	66 (46.8)	
1–4	5 (3.0)	13 (9.2)	
5–8	3 (1.8)	37 (26.2)	
9-10	1 (0.6)	18 (12.8)	
≥11	0 (0.0)	7 (5.0)	
Working status			0.097
Nonworking	50 (29.1)	110 (78.0)	
Working	122 (70.9)	31 (22.0)	
Mean per capita monthly household expenditure (in Indian rupees)	998.35 ± 22.2	1080.96 ± 27.8	0.001
Use of tobacco (at least once in a week)	122 (70.9)	28 (19.9)	0.001
Consumption of black tea (at least once in a week)	145 (84.3)	120 (85.1)	0.844
Consumption of alcohol (at least once in a week)	13 (7.6)	0 (0.0)	NA
Mean age at menarche (years)	13.94 ± 1.4	14.10 ± 1.6	0.443
History of menstrual regularity	169 (98.3)	335 (98.2)	0.990
Had periods with heavy discharge	69 (40.1)	63 (18.5)	0.001
Had periods with scanty discharge	47 (27.3)	30 (8.8)	0.001
Mean age at marriage (years)	15.07 ± 2.5	17.29 ± 3.4	0.001
Mean age at first pregnancy (years)	18.23 ± 2.4	20.05 ± 3.1	0.001
Mean age at last pregnancy (years)	25.96 ± 5.4	27.21 ± 4.8	0.009
Mean number of live births	3.70 ± 1.77	3.75 ± 1.5	0.738
Mean duration of breastfeeding of the last child (months)	51.16 ± 20.8	37.81 ± 32.2	0.001
Ever use of oral contraceptive pills	1 (0.6)	15 (10.6)	0.001
History of reproductive wastage	12 (7.0)	29 (20.5)	0.004
History of sterilisation	121 (70.3)	85 (60.3)	0.040
Mean age at menopause (years)	41.69 ± 5.6	40.65 ± 5.0	

Figures in the parentheses indicate percentage.

was significantly higher in caste than tribe participants, whereas significantly higher number of tribal participants have the history of sterilization. Tribal participants attained menopause at an earlier age than caste women.

Table 2 shows the frequency of menopausal symptoms of tribe and caste participants. Vasomotor problems like hot flush and night sweats did not differ significantly between tribe and caste participants. Urinary problems like inability to hold urine and urine leakage were significantly higher in caste participants than intribal ones. On the other hand, vaginal problems such as vaginal dryness, discharge, and bad smell were significantly higher among tribal than caste participants.

Table 3 shows that the chance of hot flush in tribal and caste participants increased with early age at menarche and early age at last pregnancy, respectively. The history of reproductive wastage increased the chance of night sweat among tribal participants. On the other hand the chance of this problem significantly increased in caste women with early onset of menarche, with history of scanty menstrual bleeding, and never use of oral contraceptive pills. Among the tribe, history of heavy menstrual discharge significantly increased the likelihood of the problem like painful urination but, among caste, late onset of menarche and age at marriage

TABLE 2: Prevalence of menopausal symptom types.

	Tribe	Caste	P value
Vasomotor domain			
Hot flush	66 (38.4)	57 (40.4)	0.400
Night sweats	94 (54.7)	76 (53.9)	0.492
Urinary domain			
Painful urination	44 (25.6)	25 (17.7)	0.062
Inability to hold urine	81 (47.1)	91 (64.5)	0.001
Frequent urination	50 (29.1)	54 (38.3)	0.054
Urine leakage	41 (23.8)	72 (51.1)	0.001
Vaginal domain			
Vaginal dryness	79 (45.9)	10 (7.1)	0.001
Burning sensation	16 (9.3)	7 (5.0)	0.105
Vaginal discharge	56 (32.6)	19 (13.5)	0.001
Vaginal itching	24 (14.0)	17 (12.1)	0.374
Bad smell	20 (11.6)	3 (2.1)	0.001

Figures in the parentheses indicate percentage.

seemed to be the factors associated with this problem. Tribal participants who consume black tea and caste ones who use

TABLE 3: Correlates of menopausal symptoms.

	Tribe	Exp(B), 95% C.I., P value	Caste	Exp(B), 95% C.I., P value
Hot flush	Age at menarche (in years)	0.139 (0.027–0.719) 0.019	Age at last pregnancy (in years)	0.251 (0.091–0.692) 0.008
Night sweat	History of reproductive wastage (absent)	1.001 (1.000–1.003) 0.046	Age at menarche (in years)	0.916 (0.854–0.983) 0.015
			Scanty menstrual discharge (absent)	0.694 (0.511–0.944) 0.020
			Use of OCP (ever used)	1.678 (1.081–2.603) 0.021
Painful urination	Heavy menstrual discharge (absent)	1.894 (0.816–0.978) 0.015	Age at menarche (in years)	1.547 (1.058–2.264) 0.024
			Age at marriage (in years)	1.431 (1.019–2.009) 0.039
Inability to hold urine	Consumption of black tea (no)	3.029 (1.140–8.049) 0.026	Use of OCP (ever used)	0.738 (0.548–0.994) 0.046
Frequent urination	Consumption of black tea (no)	1.606 (1.041–2.477) 0.032	Use of OCP (ever used)	0.716 (0.526–0.974) 0.033
Urine leakage during laughing & coughing	Present age (years)	1.906 (0.829–0.989) 0.028	Use of OCP (ever used)	0.670 (0.499–0.900) 0.008
Vaginal dryness	Heavy menstrual discharge (absent)	0.326 (0.141–0.754) 0.009	History of sterilisation (absent)	1.288 (1.000–1.659) 0.050
	Present age (years)	1.894 (0.816–0.978) 0.015	Scanty menstrual discharge (absent)	0.112 (1.161–3.840) 0.014
Vaginal discharge	Heavy menstrual discharge (absent)	0.369 (0.146–0.934) 0.035	Present age (years)	1.029 (1.006–1.054) 0.015
	Duration of breastfeeding last child	0.130 (0.071–0.060) 0.013		
Burning sensation at vagina	Duration of breastfeeding last child	0.6977 (0.5283–0.9212) 0.014	Years of education	0.932 (0.881–0.987) 0.016
			Scanty menstrual discharge (absent)	2.391 (1.203–4.749) 0.013
Vaginal itching	Per capita monthly household expenditure (in Indian rupees)	0.396 (0.189–0.832) 0.014	Scanty menstrual discharge (absent)	0.827 (1.081–3.087) 0.024
Bad smell at vagina	Duration of breastfeeding last child	0.364 (0.207–0.639) 0.001	Number of live births	0.07 (0.11–0.25) 0.012

Only significant concomitants have been presented here.

the oral contraceptive pills were more likely to be affected by inability to hold urine and frequent urination. Present age was a concomitant for urine leakage in tribal participants, whereas use of oral contraceptive pills and sterilization were found to be the concomitants for this problem for caste women. Presence of heavy and scanty type of menstrual discharge increased the chance of vaginal dryness in tribe and caste participants, respectively. In tribal participants present age, history of heavy menstrual discharge, and short duration of breastfeeding significantly increased the chance of vaginal discharge whereas present age was the only factor for caste participants. Concomitants like short duration of breastfeeding increased the chance of burning sensation of tribe; on the other hand fewer years of education and presence of scanty menstrual discharge significantly increased the likelihood of this problem in caste participants. Decrease in per capita monthly household expenditure and history of scanty menstrual discharge increased the chance of vaginal itching in tribe and caste participants, respectively, whereas decreased duration of breastfeeding and decreased number of live births significantly increased the likelihood of bad smell in vagina in tribe and caste participants, respectively.

4. Discussion

Menopause may have profound implications for subsequent morbidity and mortality [14]. Studies show that women who attain menopause at an early age are at a greater risk of being affected by cardiovascular disease [15], osteoporosis [16], and rheumatoid arthritis [17], while late menopause carries a higher risk of breast [18] and endometrial [19] cancer. The estrogen deficient menopausal problems lead to an increase in the progression of cytokines such as GM-CSF, IL-1, and IL-6, and that could potentially induce autoimmune responses in systemic autoimmune diseases such as SLE and rheumatoid arthritis [17, 20]. Aging is also associated with progressive decline in T cell functions, including decreased response to various antigens, and production of IL-2, and defect in signalling pathway resulting in the increase in frequency of cancer [21, 22].

Studies stated the relationship between hot flashes and certain reproductive history variables, such as age at menarche, age at first and last pregnancy, and parity; however it revealed the inconsistent result [13, 23, 24]. However, the present study showed that the likelihood of hot flush was more in the participants who attained menarche at an early age and had last pregnancy at their early age. Early onset of menarche might be associated with early exhaustion of ova [25] and early age at last pregnancy might be related with faster rate of atresia [26]. The ovarian shortage of oocytes for both reproductive events could formulate the fluctuation of oestrogen level during menopausal transition and occurrence of hot flush [27].

Consumption of black tea seemed to be the factor of urinary incontinences (inability to hold urine and frequent urination) of tribe participants whereas, along with the use of oral contraceptive pills, lower incidence of sterilization seemed to be the factor of urinary incontinences of caste ones.

In this context, it has been stated that the development of UI symptoms can also be affected by caffeine intake in the form of black tea. A study on women from USA reported that the incidence of UI was positively associated with caffeine ingestion, and a high level of intake increased the risk of urge but not stress or mixed incontinence [28]. Present study was corroborated with that finding. It has been found that caffeine has diuretic effect; thus intake of such substance can lead to rise in the pressure that is exerted inwards by the detrusor urinae muscles of the bladder wall, and this detrusor instability may produce urinary incontinence [29, 30]. Furthermore, earlier study stated that both the current and the former use of oral hormone therapy increased the risks of urinary incontinence (UI) among postmenopausal participants [31, 32]. Use of the hormone changed the collagen composition of the bladder and makes it contractile. Increased bladder contractility has been proposed as some potential explanations of the occurrence of UI [31, 32]. As OCP use was significantly more in caste study participants of this study compared to tribe ones, that might be a reason of more prevalence of urinary symptoms in caste participants.

Oestrogen is a dominant regulator of vaginal physiology. It has been found that oestrogen-receptor density is highest in the vagina [33–35]. Several features of the vaginal microenvironment change have been noticed with increasing age, mostly in response to alterations of oestrogen levels [35]. Present study was consistent with this finding. During menopause, the vaginal mucosa becomes weakened, loses its rugae, and appears pale and almost transparent because of decreased vascularity [36]. Present study showed that tribal study participants who had the history of heavy menstrual discharge and breastfeed their child for short time are more likely to be affected with the estrogen deficient symptoms like vaginal problems during her menopausal life. Whereas for a caste study participants, who had the history of scanty menstrual discharge and less number of live births, the chance of these types of problems increased. In this regard it has been said that short duration of breastfeeding and lower number of live births lead to the fast depletion of ovarian follicles [37]. As follicular decline results in lowered levels of oestrogen, faster exhaustion of ovarian follicle might be a reason of fluctuation of oestrogen that might be associated with occurrence of vaginal problems. Moreover, oestrogen deficiency was one of the reasons for heavy or scanty menstrual discharge [38]. So women who had the history of scanty menstrual discharge were more likely to suffer from vaginal symptoms during menopause [13].

Menopausal health of women is determined by their menstrual and reproductive histories, sociodemographic variable, and types of diet. They are susceptible to health problems by reason of either their genetics or their lifestyles and, finally, their access to adequate health care [13, 39, 40]. Thus, inclusion of the data on dietary practices and genetics would give a better understanding of menopausal symptoms of the two different populations of the present study. Moreover, the findings of the present study suggest that variation exists in the menopausal experience and its socio demographic and reproductive concomitants between two ethnic groups living in the same geographical area. However, they are limited in generalizability due to the small sample size. Our volunteer sample may not be representative of the broader population of postmenopausal women from each of the ethnic groups.

Acknowledgments

The authors wish to thank the study participants for their valuable efforts and time and the University Grant Commission, India, for providing financial support.

References

[1] M. L. Traub and N. Santoro, "Reproductive aging and its consequences for general health," *Annals of the New York Academy of Sciences*, vol. 1204, pp. 179–187, 2010.

[2] L. Dennerstein, E. C. Dudley, J. L. Hopper, J. R. Guthrie, and H. G. Burger, "A prospective population-based study of menopausal symptoms," *Obstetrics & Gynecology*, vol. 96, no. 3, pp. 351–358, 2000.

[3] D. E. Irwin, I. Milsom, S. Hunskaar et al., "Population-based survey of urinary incontinence, overactive bladder, and other lower urinary tract symptoms in five countries: results of the EPIC study," *European Urology*, vol. 50, no. 6, pp. 1306–1315, 2006.

[4] S. Correia, P. Dinis, F. Rolo, and N. Lunet, "Prevalence, treatment and known risk factors of urinary incontinence and overactive bladder in the non-institutionalized Portuguese population," *International Urogynecology Journal*, vol. 20, no. 12, pp. 1481–1489, 2009.

[5] A. Tinelli, A. Malvasi, S. Rahimi et al., "Age-related pelvic floor modifications and prolapse risk factors in postmenopausal women," *Menopause*, vol. 17, no. 1, pp. 204–212, 2010.

[6] M. Meschia, F. Pansini, A. B. Modena et al., "Determinants of age at menopause in Italy: results from a large cross-sectional study," *Maturitas*, vol. 34, no. 2, pp. 119–125, 2000.

[7] A. Biri, C. Bakar, I. Maral, O. Karabacak, and M. A. Bumin, "Women with and without menopause over age of 40 in Turkey: consequences and treatment options," *Maturitas*, vol. 50, no. 3, pp. 167–176, 2005.

[8] World Health Organization, "Research on the menopause in the 1990s. Report of a WHO scientific group," WHO Technical Report Series 866, World Health Organization, Geneva, Switzerland, 1996.

[9] Indian Institute of Population Sciences (IIPS) and ORC Macro, *National Family and Health Survey-3, 2005-2006*, IIPS, Mumbai, India, 2007.

[10] T. S. Syamala and M. Sivakami, "Menopause: an emerging issue in India," *Economic and Political Weekly*, vol. 40, pp. 4923–4930, 2005.

[11] V. Kakkar, D. Kaur, K. Chopra, A. Kaur, and I. P. Kaur, "Assessment of the variation in menopausal symptoms with age, education and working/non-working status in north-Indian sub population using menopause rating scale (MRS)," *Maturitas*, vol. 57, no. 3, pp. 306–314, 2007.

[12] D. Dasgupta, B. Pal, and S. Ray, "Factors that discriminate age at menopause: a study of Bengali Hindu women of West Bengal," *American Journal of Human Biology*, 2015.

[13] D. Dasgupta and S. Ray, "Vasomotor and urogenital problems at midlife: a study on rural and urban women in India," *Annals of Human Biology*, vol. 42, no. 3, pp. 268–275, 2015.

[14] B. K. Jacobsen, I. Heuch, and G. Kvåle, "Age at natural menopause and all-cause mortality: a 37-year follow-up of 19,731 Norwegian women," *American Journal of Epidemiology*, vol. 157, no. 10, pp. 923–929, 2003.

[15] Y. T. Schouw, Y. Graaf, E. W. Steyerberg, M. J. C. Eijkemans, and J. D. Banga, "Age at menopause as a risk factor for cardiovascular mortality," *The Lancet*, vol. 347, no. 9003, pp. 714–718, 1996.

[16] D. Kritz-Silverstein and E. Barrett-Connor, "Early menopause, number of reproductive years, and bone mineral density in postmenopausal women," *American Journal of Public Health*, vol. 83, no. 7, pp. 983–988, 1993.

[17] D. Deon, S. Ahmed, K. Tai et al., "Cross-talk between IL-1 and IL-6 signaling pathways in rheumatoid arthritis synovial fibroblasts," *The Journal of Immunology*, vol. 167, no. 9, pp. 5395–5403, 2001.

[18] D. Trichopoulos, B. MacMahon, and P. Cole, "Menopause and breast cancer risk," *The Journal of the National Cancer Institute*, vol. 48, no. 3, pp. 605–613, 1972.

[19] A. Kalandidi, A. Tzonou, L. Lipworth, I. Gamatsi, D. Filippa, and D. Trichopoulos, "A case-control study of endometrial cancer in relation to reproductive, somatometric, and life-style variables," *Oncology*, vol. 53, no. 5, pp. 354–359, 1996.

[20] M. Feldmann, F. M. Brennan, and R. N. Maini, "Role of cytokines in rheumatoid arthritis," *Annual Review of Immunology*, vol. 14, pp. 397–440, 1996.

[21] S. Gupta, R. Bi, K. Su, L. Yel, S. Chiplunkar, and S. Gollapudi, "Characterization of naïve, memory and effector CD8+ T cells: effect of age," *Experimental Gerontology*, vol. 39, no. 4, pp. 545–550, 2004.

[22] J.-N. Cao, S. Gollapudi, E. H. Sharman, Z. Jia, and S. Gupta, "Age-related alterations of gene expression patterns in human CD8$^+$ T cells," *Aging Cell*, vol. 9, no. 1, pp. 19–31, 2010.

[23] K. Ford, M. Sowers, M. Crutchfield, A. Wilson, and M. Jannausch, "A longitudinal study of the predictors of prevalence and severity of symptoms commonly associated with menopause," *Menopause*, vol. 12, no. 3, pp. 308–317, 2005.

[24] S. Sabia, A. Fournier, S. Mesrine, M.-C. Boutron-Ruault, and F. Clavel-Chapelon, "Risk factors for onset of menopausal symptoms: results from a large cohort study," *Maturitas*, vol. 60, no. 2, pp. 108–121, 2008.

[25] F. Parazzini, "Determinants of age at menopause in women attending menopause clinics in Italy," *Maturitas*, vol. 56, no. 3, pp. 280–287, 2007.

[26] D. W. Cramer, H. Xu, and B. L. Harlow, "Does 'incessant' ovulation increase risk for early menopause?" *American Journal of Obstetrics & Gynecology*, vol. 172, no. 2, pp. 568–573, 1995.

[27] D. C. Deecher and K. Dorries, "Understanding the pathophysiology of vasomotor symptoms (hot flushes and night sweats) that occur in perimenopause, menopause, and postmenopause life stages," *Archives of Women's Mental Health*, vol. 10, no. 6, pp. 247–257, 2007.

[28] Y. H. Jura, M. K. Townsend, G. C. Curhan, N. M. Resnick, and F. Grodstein, "Caffeine intake, and the risk of stress, urgency and mixed urinary incontinence," *The Journal of Urology*, vol. 185, no. 5, pp. 1775–1780, 2011.

[29] S. M. Creighton and S. L. Stanton, "Caffeine: does it affect your bladder?" *British Journal of Urology*, vol. 66, no. 6, pp. 613–614, 1990.

[30] R. J. Maughan and J. Griffin, "Caffeine ingestion and fluid balance: a review," *Journal of Human Nutrition and Dietetics*, vol. 16, no. 6, pp. 411–420, 2003.

[31] F. Grodstein, K. Lifford, N. M. Resnick, and G. C. Curhan, "Postmenopausal hormone therapy and risk of developing urinary incontinence," *Obstetrics & Gynecology*, vol. 103, no. 2, pp. 254–260, 2004.

[32] S. L. Hendrix, B. B. Cochrane, I. E. Nygaard et al., "Effects of estrogen with and without progestin on urinary incontinence," *Journal of the American Medical Association*, vol. 293, no. 8, pp. 935–948, 2005.

[33] M. B. Hodgins, R. C. Spike, R. M. Mackie, and A. B. MacLean, "An immunohistochemical study of androgen, oestrogen and progesterone receptors in the vulva and vagina," *British Journal of Obstetrics and Gynaecology*, vol. 105, no. 2, pp. 216–222, 1998.

[34] G. D. Chen, R. H. Oliver, B. S. Leung, L.-Y. Lin, and J. Yeh, "Estrogen receptor alpha and beta expression in the vaginal walls and uterosacral ligaments of premenopausal and postmenopausal women," *Fertility and Sterility*, vol. 71, no. 6, pp. 1099–1102, 1999.

[35] J. B. Gebhart, D. J. Rickard, T. J. Barrett et al., "Expression of estrogen receptor isoforms alpha and beta messenger RNA in vaginal tissue of premenopausal and postmenopausal women," *American Journal of Obstetrics and Gynecology*, vol. 185, no. 6, pp. 1325–1331, 2001.

[36] S. L. Hofland and J. Powers, "Sexual dysfunction in the menopausal woman: hormonal causes and management issues," *Geriatric Nursing*, vol. 17, no. 4, pp. 161–165, 1996.

[37] J. Ginsburg, "What determines the age at the menopause? The number of ovarian follicles seems the most important factor," *British Medical Journal*, vol. 302, no. 6788, pp. 1288–1289, 1991.

[38] B. L. Sweeney, K. Dennis, and A. Desai, "Gynecologic and obstetric disorders: contraception, hormone replacement therapy and endometriosis," in *Gibaldi's Drug Delivery Systems in Pharmaceutical Care*, M. Lee and A. Desai, Eds., pp. 321–344, American Society of Health-System Pharmacists, Bethesda, Md, USA, 2007.

[39] Pan American Health Organization (PAHO), *Midlife and Older Women in Latin America and the Caribbean*, Pan American Health Organization, Washington, DC, USA, 1989.

[40] C. Bernis and D. S. Reher, "Environmental contexts of menopause in Spain: comparative results from recent research," *Menopause*, vol. 14, no. 4, pp. 777–787, 2007.

18

Anthropometric Measures and Frailty Prediction in the Elderly: An Easy-to-Use Tool

Vera Elizabeth Closs,[1] Patricia Klarmann Ziegelmann,[2,3] João Henrique Ferreira Flores,[3] Irenio Gomes,[1] and Carla Helena Augustin Schwanke[1]

[1]*Graduate Program in Biomedical Gerontology, Institute of Geriatrics and Gerontology (IGG), Pontifical Catholic University of Rio Grande do Sul (PUCRS), Av. Ipiranga 6681, Prédio 81, 7 Andar, Sala 703, 90619-900 Porto Alegre, RS, Brazil*
[2]*Postgraduate Program in Epidemiology and Postgraduate Program in Cardiovascular Sciences, Federal University of Rio Grande do Sul (UFRGS), Av. Bento Gonçalves 9500, Prédio 43-111, Agronomia, 91509-900 Porto Alegre, RS, Brazil*
[3]*Department of Statistics, Federal University of Rio Grande do Sul (UFRGS), Av. Bento Gonçalves 9500, Prédio 43-111, Agronomia, 91509-900 Porto Alegre, RS, Brazil*

Correspondence should be addressed to Carla Helena Augustin Schwanke; schwanke@pucrs.br

Academic Editor: Fulvio Lauretani

Purpose. Anthropometry is a useful tool for assessing some risk factors for frailty. Thus, the aim of this study was to verify the discriminatory performance of anthropometric measures in identifying frailty in the elderly and to create an easy-to-use tool. *Methods.* Cross-sectional study: a subset from the Multidimensional Study of the Elderly in the Family Health Strategy (EMI-SUS) evaluating 538 older adults. Individuals were classified using the Fried Phenotype criteria, and 26 anthropometric measures were obtained. The predictive ability of anthropometric measures in identifying frailty was identified through logistic regression and an artificial neural network. The accuracy of the final models was assessed with an ROC curve. *Results.* The final model comprised the following predictors: weight, waist circumference, bicipital skinfold, sagittal abdominal diameter, and age. The final neural network models presented a higher ROC curve of 0.78 (CI 95% 0.74–0.82) ($P < 0.001$) than the logistic regression model, with an ROC curve of 0.71 (CI 95% 0.66–0.77) ($P < 0.001$). *Conclusion.* The neural network model provides a reliable tool for identifying prefrailty/frailty in the elderly, with the advantage of being easy to apply in the primary health care. It may help to provide timely interventions to ameliorate the risk of adverse events.

1. Introduction

Frailty is common among the elderly, and several pathophysiological processes are related to its development. It was also observed that there is a close relationship between frailty and weight loss, sarcopenia, obesity, body composition, and nutritional aspects. Frail older people are more likely to become dependent and vulnerable to adverse health outcomes, such as disability, falling, the need for long-term care, and mortality [1]. However, thus far, health care systems do not fully consider this to be an important issue [2].

Although several tools to diagnose frailty have been developed [3], most of them, including the widely accepted Fried Phenotype, can be difficult to apply in clinical practice, especially in primary health care (PHC) settings [4].

In this context, anthropometry is a useful and easy-to-apply tool to assess nutritional status, functional decline, and chronic health conditions, which are important risk factors for frailty [5]. However, in specific scientific literature related to the area of geriatrics and gerontology, there is a lack of studies that provide in-depth information about the anthropometric parameters of frailty in the elderly [6], and the World Health Organization [7] emphasizes the need for values pertaining to specific populations, such as the elderly.

Faced with the difficulty of applying the Fried Phenotype in older adults who were assisted at PHC centers, the purpose of this study was to verify the discriminatory performance of anthropometric measures in identifying frailty in the elderly assisted at the Family Health Strategy [8] and to create an easy-to-use tool for this population.

2. Materials and Methods

2.1. Study Design and Population. This is a cross-sectional study that is part of the Multidimensional Study of the Elderly in the Family Health Strategy (EMI-SUS), whose methodology is described in Gomes et al. [9]. The Family Health Strategy is part of the Brazilian Unified Health System (Sistema Único de Saúde) [8]. The sample comprised 583 older adults aged 60 years or older (sample size calculated between 418 and 799). More details about health characteristics of individuals assessed are described in Closs et al. [10].

2.2. Data Collection Procedures. Sociodemographic data were obtained through a general questionnaire administered at the subjects' homes. A multidisciplinary team collected data for the determination of the Fried Phenotype [11] according to the following procedures: (A) self-reported unintentional weight loss in the past 12 months (weight loss); (B) grip strength (weakness); (C) self-reported exhaustion (exhaustion); (D) walking speed (slowness); (E) weekly energy expenditure (low physical activity). Frailty (outcome) was dichotomized as frailty (frailty + prefrailty ≥ 1 component) and robustness (0 components). Nutritionists, trained by the International Society for the Advancement of Kinanthropometry [12], collected 26 anthropometric measures: weight; height; knee height; circumferences of the arm, calf, forearm, hip, neck, thigh, and waist (at the umbilical level, at the smaller point, and at the midpoint between the iliac crest and the costal edge); abdominal, bicipital, calf, pectoral, suprailiac, subscapular, thigh, and triceps skinfolds; sagittal abdominal diameter at six points (at the umbilical level, at the smaller waist, at the midpoint between the iliac crest and the costal edge, at the iliac crest level, at the largest waist, and in the orthostatic position). The anthropometric measures used were chosen according to the International Standards for Anthropometric Assessment and considered all the basic measurements items, skinfolds, and circumferences most frequently used in the evaluation of adults and elderly [12].

2.3. Statistical Analysis. Data were presented as mean (standard deviation) or frequency (percentage). To build a predictive rule to detect frailty, we used both logistic regression (LR) and artificial neural network (NN). NN can generate models with better results since it can include interactions among predictors [13–15]. Predictive models should be tested in order to evaluate their prognostic ability. Therefore, the original sample (N = 583) was divided into a learning sample (n = 439) and a testing sample (n = 144). The common rule of four participants in the learning group to one participant in the test group was used and the samples were selected, divided by the frailty subgroups. That is, approximately 80% of the individuals classified as frail and 80% of those classified as robust were randomly selected from the original sample to form the learning sample. The learning sample was used to develop the tool to identify frailty and the test sample was used to compare the prognostic ability of the tool. LR models (unadjusted and adjusted for age and gender) were constructed for each anthropometric predictor

(considered to be continuous) to evaluate their predictive ability with regard to frailty. The LR linear assumption was checked by incorporating a quadratic effect in the model and testing its significance ($P < 0.05$). In addition, the accuracy of each univariate model in correctly identifying older adults with frailty was assessed by estimating the area under the Receiver Operating Characteristic ($_{au}$ROC) curve. ROC curves were generated using the predicted probabilities estimated by the LR models. Potential predictors to build a multivariable model were selected based on the significance level and clinical practice. First, predictors with $P > 0.20$ in the univariable model were discarded. Second, for the measurements that were taken at more than one distinct anatomical point, just the one most cited in the literature (including international guidelines) was selected.

The multivariable model was built using a backward strategy and keeping age and gender as potential confounders. Neural networks are generally formed by a three-layer neuron structure, and a similar network structure was used in this study. The Multilayer Perceptron (MLP) NN is formed of neurons in the input, hidden, and output layers. A feedforward NN with the backpropagation learning algorithm was used [13]. The final model was selected after a series of tests with different configurations over the hidden layer. The accuracy of the final models was assessed by $_{au}$ROC curve, sensitivity (Se), specificity (Sp), and predictive values (positive and negative) [16]. $_{au}$ROC > 0.7 was considered to indicate sufficient predictive accuracy [16]. Predictive rules were constructed based on the multivariable LR model and the NN model using three criteria: higher Youden Index (YiC), Se of at least 0.80 (SeC), and Sp of at least 0.60 (SpC) [17]. All data analysis was performed using SPSS for Windows 17.0 [18] and R 3.1.1 [19].

2.4. Ethical Considerations. The study was approved by the Research Ethics Committee of PUCRS (protocol number CEP-10/04967) and by the Municipal Health Secretary of Porto Alegre (protocol number 001.021434.10.7). Informed consent was obtained from all participants.

3. Results

A total of 439 older adults (learning sample) (63.8% female) with a mean age of 68.7 ± 7.2 years (ranging from ages 60 to 103) were included in the study. The estimated prevalence of frailty (frailty + prefrailty) among the elderly was 70.8% (95% CI: 66.3–75.1). Table 1 presents the characteristics of the participants according to the frailty diagnosis.

Table 2 presents the results for both unadjusted and age-adjusted LR univariable models and the $_{au}$ROC. The sample size varied for each predictor due to missing values. Those results show the ability of each anthropometric variable as predictor of prefrailty + frailty.

All anthropometric measures individually lacked adequate predictive accuracy ($_{au}$ROC > 0.7). Therefore, a multivariable model was adjusted. Three predictors (neck circumference, suprailiac skinfold, and abdominal skinfold) were discarded because they present $P > 0.20$. The three waist circumference measurements generated $P < 0.20$. For the final

TABLE 1: Sociodemographic characteristics of older adults who were assisted at primary health care centers.

Characteristics*	Total N (%)	Frail + prefrail N = 311 N (%)	Robust N = 128 N (%)
Gender (female)	280 (63.8)	216 (69.5)	64 (50.0)
Age in years (mean ± SD)	68.7 ± 7.2	69.4 ± 7.7	66.7 ± 5.3
Age group (years)			
60–64.9	158 (36.0)	105 (33.8)	53 (41.4)
65–69.9	109 (24.8)	70 (22.5)	39 (30.5)
70–74.9	82 (18.7)	59 (19.0)	23 (18.0)
75–79.9	52 (11.8)	42 (13.5)	10 (7.8)
≥80	38 (8.7)	35 (11.2)	3 (2.3)
Race/ethnicity			
White	290 (67.3)	191 (62.6)	99 (78.6)
Black	76 (17.6)	44 (14.4)	10 (7.9)
"Mulatto"/brown-skinned	54 (12.5)	60 (19.7)	16 (12.7)
Native Indian	11 (2.6)	10 (3.3)	1 (0.8)
Education			
Illiterate	72 (16.7)	65 (21.3)	7 (5.5)
Incomplete elementary	117 (27.1)	88 (28.9)	29 (22.8)
Complete elementary	180 (41.7)	114 (37.4)	66 (52.0)
Complete middle school	38 (8.8)	23 (7.5)	15 (11.8)
Complete high school	21 (4.9)	13 (4.3)	8 (6.3)
Higher education	4 (0.9)	2 (0.7)	2 (1.6)
Marital status			
Married	162 (37.3)	107 (34.7)	55 (43.7)
Separated/divorced	71 (16.4)	45 (14.6)	26 (20.6)
Single	71 (16.4)	52 (16.9)	19 (15.1)
Widowed	130 (30.0)	104 (33.8)	26 (20.6)
Monthly income (MS†)			
Up to 2	382 (93.4)	273 (93.5)	109 (93.2)
>2 MS to 4	20 (4.9)	15 (5.1)	5 (4.3)
>4 MS to 6	7 (1.7)	4 (1.4)	3 (2.6)

Notes. *The number of subjects with missing values was eight for race/ethnicity, seven for education, five for marital status, and 30 for monthly income. †MS: minimum salary = R$ 540 (=US$270).

model the midpoint between the iliac crest and the costal edge was chosen, due to its scientific relevance (most commonly cited in the literature). Likewise, the six sagittal abdominal diameter measurements had $P < 0.20$, and the selected one was at the umbilical level. Therefore, 16 predictors (weight, height, and knee height; arm, forearm, waist midpoint, hip, thigh, and calf circumferences; subscapular, pectoral, triceps, bicipital, thigh, and calf skinfolds; sagittal abdominal diameter at umbilical level and age) were included in the multivariable model (Table 2).

The multivariable model started with two components (linear and quadratic) for those predictors with the quadratic element in the univariable model and one component (linear) for the others. In the backward procedure, both the linear and the quadratic components could be removed from the model independently. The final model comprised weight (WE) and waist circumference at the midpoint between the iliac

crest and the costal edge (WC), bicipital skinfold (BS), sagittal abdominal diameter at the umbilical level (SAD), and age.

Table 3 individually presents the prognostic predictive ability for these five predictors and that of the final RL multivariable model (learning and test sample). The results are presented by each of the three criteria, namely, SeC, SpC, and YiC. It can be seen that the predictors alone did not achieve simultaneously satisfactory values of Se and Sp.

The estimated frailty probability produced by the final multivariable LR model can be obtained by the equation: predicted probability = $\exp(g)/(1 + \exp(g))$, where g = $15.639022 + 0.073423 * BS + 0.003939 * SAD^2 + 0.001822 * WC^2 - 0.350425 * WC - 0.0621702 * WE + 0.044818 * Age$ (years).

In the univariate models, the frailty predictive ability of the predictors achieved values that did not exceed 80.2% of Se, and Sp ranged from 31.3% to 75.0%. The final multivariable

TABLE 2: Logistic regression univariable models and $_{au}$ROC results for the learning sample.

Anthropometric measures	N	Unadjusted		Adjusted for age	
		$\beta\ (P)^{*}$	$_{au}$ROC (95% CI)	$\beta\ (P)^{*}$	$_{au}$ROC (95% CI)
Weight^2	436	0.001 (0.003)	0.58 (0.52–0.63)‡	0.001 (0.005)	0.63 (0.58–0.69)†
Height	436	−5.313 (<0.001)	0.64 (0.58–0.69)†	−4.731 (<0.001)	0.66 (0.61–0.72)†
Knee height	436	−0.098 (0.004)	0.60 (0.54–0.65)‡	−0.091 (0.008)	0.64 (0.58–0.69)†
Circumference					
Neck	429	−0.050 (0.128)	0.54 (0.48–0.60)	−0.032 (0.331)	0.60 (0.54–0.65)‡
Arm^2	438	0.021 (<0.001)	0.61 (0.55–0.67)†	0.020 (0.001)	0.66 (0.60–0.71)†
Forearm	432	−0.097 (0.014)	0.58 (0.52–0.64)‡	−0.068 (0.100)	0.61 (0.55–0.66)†
Umbilical level^2	417	0.002 (0.003)	0.58 (0.52–0.64)‡	0.002 (0.003)	0.65 (0.59–0.70)†
Smaller waist^2	415	0.002 (0.011)	0.57 (0.52–0.63)‡	0.002 (0.009)	0.64 (0.58–0.69)†
Waist midpoint^2	413	0.002 (0.007)	0.58 (0.53–0.64)‡	0.002 (0.005)	0.64 (0.58–0.70)†
Hip^2	412	0.002 (0.009)	0.56 (0.50–0.62)	0.002 (0.010)	0.63 (0.58–0.69)†
Thigh^2	416	0.006 (0.018)	0.57 (0.51–0.62)‡	0.005 (0.034)	0.62 (0.56–0.67)†
Calf^2	434	0.015 (0.016)	0.55 (0.49–0.60)	0.014 (0.033)	0.61 (0.56–0.67)†
Skinfold					
Subscapular^2	438	0.003 (0.031)	0.53 (0.48–0.59)	0.003 (0.045)	0.62 (0.56–0.67)†
Pectoral^2	430	0.004 (0.085)	0.56 (0.50–0.61)	0.004 (0.091)	0.62 (0.57–0.68)†
Triceps	435	0.039 (0.005)	0.58 (0.53–0.64)‡	0.043 (0.003)	0.64 (0.59–0.70)†
Bicipital	432	0.059 (0.005)	0.58 (0.52–0.63)‡	0.067 (0.002)	0.65 (0.59–0.70)†
Suprailiac	417	0.008 (0.515)	0.53 (0.47–0.59)	0.014 (0.270)	0.60 (0.54–0.66)‡
Abdominal	418	0.001 (0.941)	0.52 (0.46–0.58)	0.008 (0.542)	0.59 (0.53–0.65)‡
Thigh	417	0.022 (0.033)	0.57 (0.51–0.62)‡	0.021 (0.042)	0.61 (0.56–0.67)†
Calf	428	0.048 (0.001)	0.60 (0.54–0.66)‡	0.045 (0.002)	0.64 (0.59–0.70)†
Sagittal abdominal diameter					
Umbilical level^2	397	0.021 (0.012)	0.57 (0.51–0.63)‡	0.022 (0.010)	0.63 (0.57–0.69)†
Smaller waist^2	397	0.026 (0.008)	0.56 (0.50–0.61)	0.027 (0.007)	0.62 (0.57–0.58)†
Midpoint^2	397	0.021 (0.014)	0.57 (0.51–0.63)‡	0.022 (0.011)	0.63 (0.57–0.69)†
Iliac crest level^2	397	0.022 (0.009)	0.58 (0.52–0.64)‡	0.023 (0.007)	0.63 (0.57–0.69)†
Orthostatic position^2	400	0.013 (0.019)	0.58 (0.52–0.64)‡	0.014 (0.018)	0.63 (0.57–0.69)†
Larger waist^2	397	0.023 (0.008)	0.59 (0.53–0.65)‡	0.023 (0.007)	0.64 (0.58–0.69)†

Notes. Exponent 2 means that the quadratic term of the predictor was included in the model, along with the linear term. *Logistic regression; $^{\dagger}P\ (_{au}$ROC) < 0.001; $^{\ddagger}P\ (_{au}$ROC) < 0.005.

LR model (predictors grouped) is translated into an improved capability to predict frailty: approximately the same Se (80%) but with higher Sp (range 48–79.2%).

As shown at the bottom of Table 3, the test sample results for SeC were slightly higher in both Se and Sp (81.7% versus 48.5%) than those obtained in the learning sample (80.1% versus 48.0%), suggesting that these values could be used for classification. The final multivariable LR model presented an $_{au}$ROC of 0.71 (95% CI 0.66–0.77).

In order to further explore the predictive ability of the anthropometric predictors the five predictors left at the final multivariable LR model were used as the input layer of NN models that were built using an input layer, a hidden layer, and a single, continuous, output layer. We ran MLP models using three to six hidden layers. These limits were selected

based on the amount of data available. Figure 1 presents the architecture of the models.

The result from the final NN (output neuron) model is a continuous value ranging from zero (robust) to one (frail) depending on the predictors values. Although those values are not estimated as probabilities they have similar interpretation as the probabilities estimated by the LR model. The resulting equation from the NN final model is implemented in an Excel spreadsheet (Supplementary Appendix S1 in Supplementary Material available online at https://doi.org/10.1155/2017/8703503). The prognostic ability to predict frailty using the NN final model results is shown in Table 4 for the learning and the test samples. It can be seen that, in general, the results bare superiority to those found by the LR final model. In the learning sample, when the SpC cut-off point is

TABLE 3: Prognostic ability of anthropometric measures as predictors of prefrailty + frailty in older adults who were assisted at primary health care centers.

Predicted probability of anthropometric measures	Frailty			Se	Sp	PPV	NPV
	Total prevalence N (%)	Yes N (%)	No N (%)				
Weight							
>0.6253[SeC]	335 (76.8)	247 (80.2)	88 (68.8)	0.802	0.313	0.737	0.396
>0.6777[SpC]	233 (53.6)	183 (59.4)	50 (39.4)	0.594	0.602	0.785	0.381
>0.7102[YiC]	188 (43.1)	156 (50.6)	32 (25.0)	0.506	0.750	0.829	0.387
Waist circumference at midpoint[2]							
>0.6161[SeC]	303 (73.4)	229 (80.1)	74 (58.3)	0.801	0.417	0.755	0.481
>0.6508[YiC]	254 (61.5)	197 (68.9)	57 (44.9)	0.689	0.551	0.775	0.440
>0.6680[SpC]	223 (54.0)	172 (60.1)	51 (40.2)	0.601	0.600	0.771	0.400
Bicipital skinfold							
>0.6211[SeC]	274 (71.5)	210 (77.5)	64 (57.1)	0.800	0.375	0.766	0.440
>0.6888[SpC]	239 (55.3)	188 (61.8)	51 (39.8)	0.618	0.602	0.786	0.399
>0.7138[YiC]	199 (46.1)	162 (53.3)	37 (28.9)	0.533	0.711	0.814	0.390
Sagittal abdominal diameter at umbilical level[2]							
>0.6095[SeC]	294 (74.2)	216 (73.5)	78 (61.9)	0.801	0.381	0.734	0.470
>0.6161[YiC]	284 (71.5)	213 (78.6)	71 (56.3)	0.786	0.437	0.750	0.486
>0.6637[SpC]	207 (52.1)	157 (57.9)	50 (39.7)	0.579	0.603	0.758	0.400
Logistic regression model (learning sample)							
>0.6158[SeC]	282 (71.2)	217 (80.1)	65 (52.0)	0.801	0.480	0.769	0.526
>0.6486[SpC]	245 (61.9)	195 (72.0)	50 (40.0)	0.720	0.600	0.795	0.496
>0.7137[YiC]	182 (46.0)	156 (57.6)	26 (20.8)	0.576	0.792	0.857	0.462
Logistic regression model (testing sample)							
>0.6158[SeC]	75 (72.1)	58 (81.7)	17 (51.5)	0.817	0.485	0.773	0.551
>0.6486[SpC]	66 (63.5)	51 (71.8)	15 (45.5)	0.718	0.546	0.772	0.473
>0.717[YiC]	49 (47.1)	38 (53.5)	11 (33.3)	0.535	0.667	0.775	0.400

Notes. Se: sensitivity; Sp: specificity; PPV: positive predictive value; NPV: negative predictive value; SeC: sensitivity ≈ 80%; SpC: specificity ≈ 60%; YiC: Youden Index. Exponent 2 means that the quadratic term of the predictor was included in the model, along with the linear term.

TABLE 4: Prognostic ability of anthropometric measures as predictors of frailty in older adults who were assisted at primary health care centers via artificial neural models.

Predicted probability of anthropometric measures	Frailty			Se	Sp	PPV	NPV
	Total prevalence N (%)	Yes N (%)	No N (%)				
Neural network (learning sample)							
>0.5648[SpC]	268 (67.2)	220 (79.7)	48 (17.9)	0.797	0.610	0.820	0.572
>0.7176[YiC]	217 (54.4)	188 (68.1)	29 (23.6)	0.681	0.764	0.866	0.516
>0.5621[SeC]	271 (68.3)	221 (80.1)	50 (41.3)	0.801	0.587	0.815	0.563
Neural network (testing sample)							
>0.5648[SpC]	69 (68.3)	54 (81.8)	15 (42.9)	0.818	0.571	0.782	0.625
>0.7176[YiC]	53 (53.0)	46 (69.7)	7 (20.6)	0.697	0.794	0.867	0.574
>0.5621[SeC]	72 (71.3)	54 (81.8)	18 (51.4)	0.818	0.486	0.750	0.586

Notes. Se: sensitivity; Sp: specificity; PPV: positive predictive value; NPV: negative predictive value; SeC: sensitivity ≈ 80%; SpC: specificity ≈ 60%. YiC: Youden Index.

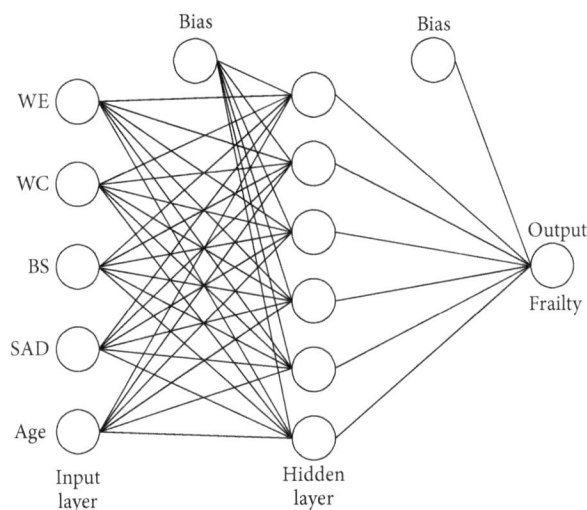

FIGURE 1: Neural network configuration of anthropometric measures and frailty in older adults who were assisted at primary health care centers. WE: weight; WC: waist circumference; BS: bicipital skinfold; SAD: sagittal abdominal diameter.

used, the Se is higher for the NN model (Se = 0.797) when compared to the LR model (Se = 0.720). Also, for the SeC cutoff the NN model has Sp = 0.486 while the LR model has Sp = 0.480. In the sample test, all cut-off points resulted in better Se and Sp. The NN final model presented an $_{au}$ROC of 0.78 (95% CI 0.74–0.82), indicating greater predictive accuracy ($P < 0.001$) than the LR model.

4. Discussion

The purpose of this study was to investigate the ability of anthropometric measures to predict prefrailty/frailty in older adults assisted at PHC centers. The main finding was that, among the 26 anthropometric measures analyzed, those that together predicted frailty were WE, WC, BS, and SAD for both the LR and the NN model. With regard to the method used to determine the predictive value of frailty, the NN proved to be more efficient than the LR model in predicting frailty in the older adults assessed.

To the best of our knowledge, this is the first investigation carried out in a sample of older adults who were assisted at PHC centers to verify the performance of several anthropometric measures in identifying frailty from the NN model. In addition, the resulting algorithm can be applied in the evaluation of older adults from the Family Health Strategy with satisfactory results.

Surveys often investigate the relationship of frailty with measures commonly used to evaluate nutritional status, such as the body mass index or body composition [20–22]. In our study, we used pure and simple measures, not combined into equations, with the objective of obtaining an algorithm that was as simple as possible, using easily obtained measurements in the PHC. The importance of identifying prefrailty or frailty in older adults is associated with the fact that interventions can help to prevent, delay, reverse, or reduce the severity of frailty as well as preventing or reducing adverse health outcomes in those whose frailty is not reversible. Effective

interventions can promote benefits for elderly individuals, their families, and the whole society [23–25].

Anthropometric measures have been studied due to their ability to identify certain health parameters, such as nutritional status, due to their relationship with diseases and with physical function status [5, 26] and all conditions involved in the course of frailty [1]. However, the molecular, physiological, and clinical course of frailty, in turn, presents nonuniform features of pathways for an individual to become frail: people with the same level of frailty may have reached this stage in a variety of ways and present decline in their physiological reserve, whether in the neuromuscular, metabolic, or immune system [1]. Concerning the relationship between frailty and anthropometric measures, we observed that frailty stems from a set of observations and that the relationship between one such observation with certain anthropometric parameters is sometimes already known, while for others it is completely unknown [1]. This set of predictors that are connected to various shapes and weights motivated the use of NN, a model capable of handling nonlinear relationships [27].

Even considering that the strength or the predictive value is established by the set of predictors, it may be interesting to analyze the individual characteristics of the measures included in the final model (WE, WC, BS, and SAD).

It is known that WE on average tends to decrease after the age of 60 years, and the contribution of fat mass to this weight loss is relatively small, but the fat tends to be redistributed toward the abdomen, that is, increasing visceral fat deposits [5]. SAD and WC are measures that are positively related to abdominal adiposity [28], and some evidence has pointed to a possible connection between abdominal adiposity, cardiovascular diseases, and frailty in older people [22, 29, 30]. However, in aging, lean body mass is lost, while fat mass may be preserved or even increased. This state is named sarcopenic obesity [31] and it is known that sarcopenia is involved in the pathogenesis of frailty [1]. Previous study, evaluating the association of anthropometric measurements with frailty, in the same population, demonstrated that frailty was associated with muscle mass loss. The frail elderly had lower measures of size and complexion [32]. This pattern of increase of intramuscular and visceral fat with aging is accompanied by changes in subcutaneous fat, which can be evaluated through the measurement of BS [33]. Many frail elderly are thin, weak, and undernourished; however, there is also strong evidence that excessive adiposity contributes to frailty [21].

When grouped, it was possible to observe that the prognostic predictive ability of the predictors achieved better performance. The result of the LR was translated into improved predictive capability for prefrailty/frailty, with similar Se but higher Sp. However, it was noted that in relation to the LR model NN showed an improved predictive capability for prefrailty/frailty. For the three cut-off points assessed, both Se and Sp were considered superior and satisfactory to avoid false negative and positive screenings [17]. The accuracy of the final NN models, as assessed by $_{au}$ROC, was higher than that of the LR model, overcoming the value considered to have sufficient predictive accuracy [16].

The main results of this paper were the demonstration of the following: (a) the performance capabilities of anthropometric measures to identify prefrailty/frailty; (b) the superior performance of the NN for prefrailty/frailty prediction with heterogeneous data—NN explores other relationships that can generate models with better results [15]; (c) early stages of frailty that are more commonly seen in the older adults of the community—therefore, identification and screening tools must be applied in this population [23].

This study has some positive aspects that must be noted. First, it includes the evaluation of a large set of anthropometric measurements. Second, the method used to investigate the ability of various anthropometric measures to identify prefrailty/frailty in the older adults is particularly innovative, specifically, the analytical methodology chosen to investigate this ability. Third, the model is capable of providing a noninvasive tool for the large-scale screening of prefrailty/frailty.

The limitations of the study include the following: (a) the cross-sectional design prevented the establishment of a cause-and-effect relationship; (b) the available data (small sample) restricted the configurations of the NN models. To overcome the second issue, we used the same variables of the LR model in the input layer and the backpropagation learning algorithm, method recommended for those cases [15]; however, further research should be carried out to resolve these limitations.

In conclusion, our data suggest that grouped anthropometric measures can be recommended as good predictors of prefrailty/frailty in older adults who were assisted at PHC centers. The possibility of having a simple tool in PHC to identify prefrailty/frailty allows for the implementation of an individual treatment plan that can prevent, reverse, or treat the complications that can lead to frailty while preserving the autonomy of the elderly.

In addition to promoting health benefits and quality of life in the elderly through the identification, prevention, and treatment of frailty, these measures can reduce health care costs. Further research is needed to establish the clinical utility of the instrument developed.

Authors' Contributions

Closs, Gomes, and Schwanke were responsible for study concept and design. Closs and Gomes were responsible for data collection. Closs, Ziegelmann, and Flores were responsible for analysis and interpretation of data. Closs was responsible for initial draft of manuscript. Closs, Ziegelmann, and Schwanke were responsible for critical revision of manuscript.

Acknowledgments

This work was supported by the Foundation for the Support of Research in the State of Rio Grande do Sul (Fundação de Amparo à Pesquisa do Estado do Rio Grande do Sul, FAPERGS), Proclamation 02/2009 PPSUS (09/0075-7, 09/0055-0), and scholarship from Coordination for the Improvement of Higher Education Personnel Foundation (Coordenação de Aperfeiçoamento de Pessoal de Nível Superior, CAPES) (Vera Elizabeth Closs).

References

[1] J. Walston, E. C. Hadley, L. Ferrucci et al., "Research agenda for frailty in older adults: toward a better understanding of physiology and etiology: summary from the American geriatrics society/national institute on aging research conference on frailty in older adults," *Journal of the American Geriatrics Society*, vol. 54, no. 6, pp. 991–1001, 2006.

[2] B. Vellas, P. Cestac, and J. E. Morley, "Editorial implementing frailty into clinical practice: we cannot wait," *The Journal of Nutrition, Health & Aging*, vol. 16, no. 7, pp. 599-600, 2012.

[3] M. Kuzuya, "Process of physical disability among older adults-contribution of frailty in the super-aged society," *Nagoya Journal of Medical Science*, vol. 74, no. 1-2, pp. 31–37, 2012.

[4] G. Abellan Van Kan, Y. Rolland, H. Bergman, J. E. Morley, S. B. Kritchevsky, and B. Vellas, "The I.A.N.A. task force on frailty assessment of older people in clinical practice," *The Journal of Nutrition, Health & Aging*, vol. 12, no. 1, pp. 29–37, 2008.

[5] J. C. Seidell and T. L. S. Visscher, "Body weight and weight change and their health implications for the elderly," *European Journal of Clinical Nutrition*, vol. 54, no. 3, pp. S33–S39, 2000.

[6] A. R. Barbosa, J. M. P. Souza, M. L. Lebrão, R. Laurenti, and M. D. F. N. Marucci, "Anthropometry of elderly residents in the city of São Paulo, Brazil," *Cadernos de saúde público*, vol. 21, no. 6, pp. 1929–1938, 2005.

[7] World Health Organization, "Physical status: the use and interpretation of anthropometry," Report of a WHO Expert Committee, Worl Health Organization, Geneva, Switzerland, 1995.

[8] J. Macinko and M. J. Harris, "Brazil's family health strategy - Delivering community-based primary care in a universal health system," *The New England Journal of Medicine*, vol. 372, no. 23, pp. 2177–2181, 2015.

[9] I. Gomes, E. L. Nogueira, P. Engroff, and et al., "The multidimensional study of the elderly in the family health strategy in Porto Alegre (EMI-SUS)," *Pan American Journal of Aging Research*, vol. 1, no. 1, pp. 20–24, 2013.

[10] V. E. Closs, P. K. Ziegelmann, I. Gomes, and C. H. A. Schwanke, "Frailty and geriatric syndromes in elderly assisted in primary health care," *Acta Scientiarum - Health Sciences*, vol. 38, no. 1, pp. 9–18, 2016.

[11] L. P. Fried, C. M. Tangen, J. Walston et al., "Frailty in older adults: evidence for a phenotype," *The Journals of Gerontology: Medical Sciences*, vol. 56, no. 3, pp. M146–M156, 2001.

[12] M. Marfell-Jones, T. Olds, A. Stewart, and J. E. Lindsay Carter, *International Standards for Anthropometric Assessment*, International Society for the Advancement of Kinanthropometry, School of Biokinetics, Recreation and Sport, 2006.

[13] P. E. Puddu and A. Menotti, "Artificial neural network versus multiple logistic function to predict 25-year coronary heart disease mortality in the Seven countries study," *European Journal of Cardiovascular Prevention and Rehabilitation*, vol. 16, no. 5, pp. 583–591, 2009.

[14] A. Kupusinac, E. Stokić, and R. Doroslovački, "Predicting body fat percentage based on gender, age and BMI by using artificial neural networks," *Computer Methods and Programs in Biomedicine*, vol. 113, no. 2, pp. 610–619, 2014.

[15] S. Haykin, *Redes Neurais: Princípios e Prática*, Bookman, Porto Alegre, Brazil, 2nd edition, 2001.

[16] F. H. Wians Jr., "Clinical laboratory tests: which, why, and what do the results mean?" *LabMedicine*, vol. 40, no. 2, pp. 105–113, 2009.

[17] H. Blake, M. McKinney, K. Treece, E. Lee, and N. B. Lincoln, "An evaluation of screening measures for cognitive impairment after stroke," *Age and Ageing*, vol. 31, no. 6, pp. 451–456, 2002.

[18] "SPSS Inc. *SPSS Statistics for Windows*, Version 17.0, Chicago, Illinois, USA, 2008".

[19] R Development Core Team, *R: A Language and Environment for Statistical Computing*, R Foundation for Statistical Computing, Vienna, Austria, 2011.

[20] X. Song, A. Mitnitski, C. MacKnight, and K. Rockwood, "Assessment of individual risk of death using self-report data: an artificial neural network compared with a frailty index," *Journal of the American Geriatrics Society*, vol. 52, no. 7, pp. 1180–1184, 2004.

[21] S. Izawa, H. Enoki, Y. Hirakawa et al., "The longitudinal change in anthropometric measurements and the association with physical function decline in Japanese community-dwelling frail elderly," *British Journal of Nutrition*, vol. 103, no. 2, pp. 289–294, 2010.

[22] K. N. Porter Starr, S. R. McDonald, and C. W. Bales, "Obesity and physical frailty in older adults: a scoping review of lifestyle intervention trials," *Journal of the American Medical Directors Association*, vol. 15, no. 4, pp. 240–250, 2014.

[23] R. E. Hubbard, I. A. Lang, D. J. Llewellyn, and K. Rockwood, "Frailty, body mass index, and abdominal obesity in older people," *The Journals of Gerontology. Series A, Biological Sciences and Medical Sciences*, vol. 65, no. 4, pp. 377–381, 2010.

[24] T. M. Gill, E. A. Gahbauer, H. G. Allore, and L. Han, "Transitions between frailty states among community-living older persons," *JAMA Internal Medicine*, vol. 166, no. 4, pp. 418–423, 2006.

[25] X. Chen, G. Mao, and S. X. Leng, "Frailty syndrome: an overview," *Clinical Interventions in Aging*, vol. 9, pp. 433–441, 2014.

[26] R. Daniels, S. Metzelthin, E. van Rossum, L. de Witte, and W. van den Heuvel, "Interventions to prevent disability in frail community-dwelling older persons: an overview," *European Journal of Ageing*, vol. 7, no. 1, pp. 37–55, 2010.

[27] F. Landi, G. Onder, A. Russo et al., "Calf circumference, frailty and physical performance among older adults living in the community," *Clinical Nutrition*, vol. 33, no. 3, pp. 539–544, 2014.

[28] E. D. B. Goulet, A. Hassaine, I. J. Dionne et al., "Frailty in the elderly is associated with insulin resistance of glucose metabolism in the postabsorptive state only in the presence of increased abdominal fat," *Experimental Gerontology*, vol. 44, no. 11, pp. 740–744, 2009.

[29] P. C. Anunciação, R. C. L. Ribeiro, M. Q. Pereira, and M. Comunian, "Different measurements of waist circumference and sagittal abdominal diameter and their relationship with cardiometabolic risk factors in elderly men," *Journal of Human Nutrition and Dietetics*, vol. 27, no. 2, pp. 162–167, 2014.

[30] N. A. Ricci, G. S. Pessoa, E. Ferriolli, R. C. Dias, and M. R. Perracini, "Frailty and cardiovascular risk in community-dwelling elderly: a population-based study," *Clinical Interventions in Aging*, vol. 9, pp. 1677–1685, 2014.

[31] M. C. Moretto, R. M. A. Alves RMA, A. L. Neri, and M. H. Guariento, "Relação entre estado nutricional e fragilidade em idosos brasileiros," *Revista da Sociedade Brasileira de Clínica Médica*, vol. 10, no. 4, pp. 1–5, 2012.

[32] V. E. Closs, L. S. Rosemberg, B. G. Ettrich, I. Gomes, and C. H. Schwanke, "Medidas antropométricas em idosos assistidos na atenção básica e sua associação com gênero, idade e síndrome da fragilidade: dados do EMI-SUS," *Scientia Medica*, vol. 25, no. 3, pp. 1–7, 2015.

[33] R. M. Collard, H. Boter, R. A. Schoevers, and R. C. Oude Voshaar, "Prevalence of frailty in community-dwelling older persons: a systematic review," *Journal of the American Geriatrics Society*, vol. 60, no. 8, pp. 1487–1492, 2012.

Age-Friendliness and Life Satisfaction of Young-Old and Old-Old in Hong Kong

Alma M. L. Au, Stephen C. Y. Chan, H. M. Yip, Jackie Y. C. Kwok, K. Y. Lai, K. M. Leung, Anita L. F. Lee, Daniel W. L. Lai, Teresa Tsien, and Simon M. K. Lai

Department of Applied Social Sciences, The Hong Kong Polytechnic University, Hung Hom, Hong Kong

Correspondence should be addressed to Stephen C. Y. Chan; sccy.chan@connect.polyu.hk

Academic Editor: Fulvio Lauretani

Age-friendliness, promoted by the World Health Organization (WHO), aims to enable and support individuals in different aspects of life for fostering life satisfaction and personal well-being as they age. We identified specific aspect(s) of age-friendliness associated with life satisfaction and examined similarities and differences in age-friendliness and life satisfaction in young-old and old-old adults. Six hundred and eighty-two ageing adults were asked to complete a survey questionnaire consisting of the Age-friendly City Scale, Satisfaction with Life Scale, and sociodemographic variables. Multiple linear regression analysis was used to examine the effects of various domains of age-friendliness on life satisfaction among the young-old adults (aged 65 to 74, $n = 351$) and the old-old adults (aged 75 to 97, $n = 331$). Common domains associated with life satisfaction in both young-old and old-old groups were transportation and social participation. Community and health services were associated with life satisfaction for the young-old group only. On the other hand, civic participation and employment was significantly associated with the old-old group only. Social participation is important for the young-old and the old-old. Ageing older adults can be a resource to the society. Implications for promoting and implementing age-friendliness were discussed in the context of successful and productive ageing and the need for a more refined taxonomy of social activities.

1. Introduction

As in other Asian countries, Hong Kong is encountering increasing population ageing. According to the Hong Kong Population Projections Report, the population of adults 65 and over will increase from 15% in 2014 to 31% in 2044 [1]. Hong Kong has the longest life expectancy in the world, and the average lifespan for both genders is around 84 years [2]. With the aged population boom and longer life expectancy, the Hong Kong Government has provided targeted services and subsidies. The age of 65 is the typical benchmark to define eligibility for most of the relevant welfare supports, including the Old Age Living Allowance [3]. Building an age-friendly environment is one of the major targets highlighted in the 2016 Policy Address of the Hong Kong Government [4]. In addition to addressing the financial burden of the ageing population in terms of retirement protection, medical care, and elderly services, the Policy Address underscored

that the new generation of aged adults will be healthier, better educated, and fully capable of making further contributions to the community. Initiatives include enhancing barrier-free access, outdoor facilities, and providing a safe and comfortable home environment and digital inclusion for age individuals.

The age-friendly city concept is based on the framework for active ageing defined by the World Health Organization (WHO), rooted in the belief that a supportive and inclusive environment will enable residents to optimize health, participation, and well-being as they age successfully in the place in which they are living without the need to move [5–7]. The eight domains or features of age-friendly city encompass aspects ranging from physical infrastructure to social environment and include (i) outdoor spaces and buildings, (ii) transportation, (iii) housing, (iv) social participation, (v) respect and social inclusion, (vi) civic participation and employment, (vii) communication and information, and (viii) community and health services [8]. This framework has been applied in various countries to gauge the age-friendliness of retirement communities [9] and of transport and health services [10, 11]. According to a study conducted in two districts in Hong Kong, many age-friendly features exist but there is still substantial room for improvement in developing more comprehensive and specific long-term action and evaluation plans. The authors recommended that mechanisms be established to involve all aged adults, government officials, politicians, and service providers in conducting a baseline assessment and developing a three-year age-friendly action plan [12]. This study described in this paper is a part of this follow-up initiative [13].

The purpose of this study was to identify specific aspect(s) of age-friendliness associated with life satisfaction and examine similarities and differences in age-friendliness and life satisfaction in young-old and old-old adults. The concept of age-friendly city has based its formulation on active ageing [5–7]. Various definitions of active and successful ageing have been proposed. These concepts and models can be helpful in furthering our understanding of how age-friendly models can contribute to the well-being of aged adults. Active and successful ageing includes having a positive sense of oneself and relations with others, acceptance of the past and the present, autonomy and control over one's environment, participation in activities, and having a purpose in life [14]. More recent criteria have highlighted the need for testable components, including healthy lifestyle, maintaining high functioning levels, and active social engagement [5, 15]. Process-orientated models such as the selective optimization with compensation model depict the flexible adjustment of goals in relation to age-related losses [16]. The socioemotional selectivity theory underscores that the sense of limited future time motivates aged people to prioritize goals intended to derive emotional meaning from life [17]. The differentiation of process from outcomes enables the inclusion of age-graded expectations and the subjective criteria of psychological experience such as life satisfaction or psychological well-being [18].

Neugarten and colleagues considered age norms in regulating the life course [19]. These norms are culturally affected and act as a "social clock" to inform individuals of the appropriate time for a certain life event. Neugarten has also suggested that there might be differences in age norms even among aged adults [20, 21]. She identifies two major groups of aged adults: the "young-old," aged 55 to 75, and the "old-old," aged 75 or above. Different aged individuals are able to judge and set their corresponding social clocks. Satisfaction or distress may result based on the subjective evaluation of personal life.

With reference to successful or active ageing, there is a close association between subjective well-being and life satisfaction [22]. Life satisfaction, the cognitive component of well-being, refers to an individual's evaluation of their life [23]. A great number of aged adults have reported higher well-being linked to participation in social and leisure activities [24].

According to a study by Jeste et al. [25], despite physical and cognitive declines, older age was found to be associated with higher levels of resilience and lower levels of depression. Explanations put forward include contentedness with accomplishments in life and a more realistic appraisal of one's own strengths and limitations include after surviving various hardships. Resilience is often understood as response to acute stress. At the same time, adaptive self-appraisal may be an important aspect of maintaining well-being in the context of losses in functioning with ageing.

With the emergence of Neugarten's view of young-old and old-old, more researchers have focused on these categories. However, existing studies have focused more on the young-old, since they shared some common characteristics. For instance, they are entering their first retirement and are relatively healthy, better educated, and active in social and political participation. One study has shown higher levels of well-being associated with volunteering among young-old adults [26]. With respect to group differences, the young-old have been found to possess higher positive well-being and self-perceived successful ageing than the old-old [27, 28]. Concerning mental or physical health issues, the prevalence of depressive symptoms has been found to be highest in oldest-old adults compared to other aged groups [29]. Another study identified significant associations between depression and malnutrition in the young-old but not the old-old [30]. In a previous study of 254 aged adults, Au and her colleagues found that while life satisfaction was significantly related to the fulfilment of achievement and affiliation for the young-old, life satisfaction was significantly associated with the fulfilment of altruistic goals for the old-old [31].

While previous studies have examined differences in ageing experiences between age groups of aged adults, to our knowledge, no studies have examined the specific relationship between age-friendliness and life satisfaction with reference to the young-old and old-old. Neugarten's model can have important implications for the understanding of how age-friendly concepts can contribute to the life satisfaction of aged adults. Therefore, the aims of the present study include (1) to examine the relationship between specific sociodemographic variables and life satisfaction among young-old and old-old adults, (2) to assess the relationship between specific domains of age-friendliness and life satisfaction with controlled sociodemographic variables, and (3) to identify similarities and differences in specific domains of age-friendliness associated with life satisfaction between young-old and old-old adults.

2. Materials and Methods

2.1. Participants. Study participants were recruited mainly from community centres and nongovernmental organizations (NGOs) in Kowloon East Region including Kowloon City and Kwun Tong, using a convenience sampling approach. Inclusion criteria for participants included being Cantonese speakers, having comprehensive understanding without wearing a hearing aid, and being mentally sound. The original study aimed at exploring the age-friendliness of Hong Kong as perceived by individuals aged 18 or older. For the purpose of this study, we only select adults aged 65 and above for data analysis.

2.2. Measures.

All participants were asked to complete a structured questionnaire, which consisted of three main parts: the Age-friendly City Scale, the Satisfaction with Life Scale, and basic demographic variables.

2.2.1. The Age-Friendly City Scale (AFCS).

Based on the WHO age-friendly city guidelines, it was adopted and translated into Chinese [32]. Eight domains were assessed using 53 items. Participants were asked to rate their views on each item using a 6-point Likert-type scale ranging from 1 ("strongly disagree") to 6 ("strongly agree"). Responses for each domain were averaged as a mean score. The reliability (Cronbach's alpha) estimate for each domain ranged from .66 to .81. Example items for each domain are included in Appendix.

2.2.2. The Satisfaction with Life Scale (SWLS).

It was used to measure the cognitive component of subjective well-being [33]. It consisted of five items, such as "I am satisfied with my life." Participants rated each item on a 7-point Likert-type scale ranging from 1 ("strongly disagree") to 7 ("strongly agree"). The average score of this scale was used for analysis. The reliability of SWLS was .87 and over .90 in this study and our previous study, respectively [31].

2.2.3. Sociodemographic Variables.

Sociodemographic variables including age, gender, education level, health status, marital status, income, and expenditure were used in the analysis as factors to be controlled statistically. These variables have been consistent in predicting life satisfaction in previous research [34]. Gender was coded as 1 ("male") or 2 ("female"). Participants aged 65 to 74 were categorized as "young-old" and those aged 75 or as "old-old." Education level was measured in eight categories referring to the local education system, ranging from 1 ("never") to 8 ("degree level or above"). Health condition and expenditure were measured using 5-point Likert-type scales, ranging from 1 ("bad") to 5 ("excellent") and from 1 ("very insufficient") to 5 ("very sufficient"), respectively. Income was categorized into 14 options ranging from 1 ("less than $2000") to 14 ("more than 100,000"). Although educational level and income were grouped as presented in Table 1, original values were used for data analyses.

2.3. Procedures.

Participants were introduced the background of our study by research helpers, who were trained master students and research assistants in the field of Psychology as well as members from the Institute of Active Ageing. After signing the informed consent form, a set of questionnaires would be given. A few aged participants had difficulties in reading or writing, and research helpers assisted these participants to complete the questionnaire by reading out the questions and asking them to denote their response to each item. Participants were given a supermarket coupon after completing the questionnaire.

2.4. Statistical Analyses.

Multiple linear regression analyses were performed using IBM SPSS Statistics 23. It tested the direction and strength of the association between predictor(s) and dependent variable(s). The predictors of SWLS were formed into two blocks and analysed hierarchically using the ENTER method. The first block of predictors includes sociodemographic variables and were evaluated as statistically controlled factors of SWLS. The second block of predictors included dimensions of AFCS and their predictive effects on SWLS were evaluated with the sociodemographic variables adjusted.

3. Results

3.1. Descriptive Statistics.

Differences in sociodemographic variables between young-old and old-old participants are shown in Table 1. The respective mean age of young-old and old-old participants was 68.91 (SD = 2.82) years and 80.29 (SD = 4.27), and most participants were women. Young-old participants reported a higher overall education level, with nearly 80% reporting primary or secondary education, while around 70% of old-old participants reported no education or primary education. In general, both young-old and old-old participants reported an adequate living standard, with around 15% reporting "bad" health status and around 15% reporting "insufficient" expenditure.

The mean AFSC domain scores of young-old and old-old participants are presented in Table 2. The scores for SWLS and six out of eight AFSC domains (outdoor spaces and buildings, transportation, housing, social participation, respect and social inclusion, and community, and health services) reported by old-old participants were significant higher than the scores reported by young-old participants ($p < .05$). There was no difference in scores for domains of civic participation and employment ($p = .071$) and communication and information ($p = .091$) between young-old and old-old participants. Both groups rated the social participation domain the highest and the community and health services domain lowest among the eight AFSC domains.

3.2. Association between Sociodemographic Variables and Life Satisfaction.

The results of analyses for the first research question, the association between sociodemographic variables and life satisfaction, are presented in Tables 3 and 4. In both young-old and old-old groups, SWLS scores were significantly correlated ($p < .05$) with sociodemographic variables of expenditure ($r = .36$ and $r = .34$), income ($r = .17$ and $r = .11$), and health status ($r = .24$ and $r = .39$). Gender was significantly correlated with SWLS score only in the young-old group ($r = -.12$). The results of the regression analysis show that gender, marital status, educational level, income, and expenditure explained a significant amount of variance in SWLS score in both young-old ($R^2 = .18$, $F(6, 344) = 12.17$, $p < .01$) and old-old ($R^2 = .23$, $F(6, 324) = 16.04$, $p < .01$) groups. In both groups, expenditure ($\beta = .31$ and $\beta = .25$, $p < .05$) and health ($\beta = .16$ and $\beta = .33$, $p < .05$) had significant positive regression weights on SWLS

TABLE 1: Descriptive statistics of sociodemographic variables (mean and SD in age) by age group.

Variables		Young-old (n = 365)	Old-old (n = 354)
Age	Mean ± SD	68.91 (2.82)	80.29 (4.27)
	Levels	Percentage	
Gender	Female	72.1%	65.8%
	Male	27.9%	34.2%
Marital status	Single	6.8%	2.3%
	Married	60.8%	44.9%
	Widowed	24.7%	47.7%
	Divorced	6.6%	4.3%
	Others	1.1%	0.8%
Education level	Never	12.6%	32.2%
	Primary school	39.6%	41.5%
	Secondary	39.8%	23.2%
	Diploma or higher diploma	2.8%	2%
	Degree or above	5.2%	1.1%
Health	Bad	15.1%	15.8%
	General	52.1%	50.0%
	Good	19.7%	22.1%
	Very good	10.4%	9%
	Excellent	2.7%	3.1%
Expenditure	Very insufficient	1.4%	1.7%
	Insufficient	14.5%	13.6%
	Just enough	64.1%	66.1%
	Sufficient	17.5%	16.9%
	Very sufficient	2.5%	1.7%
Income	<6000	54.8%	76.3%
	6001–10000	20%	11.8%
	10001–20000	11.5%	5.4%
	20001 or above	4.7%	2.5%
	N/A	9%	4%

score, indicating that those who perceived they had more than enough to spend and better health status would show better life satisfaction.

3.3. Association between Age-Friendly City Domains and Life Satisfaction. The results of analyses addressing the second research question, the association between AFCS and life satisfaction, are presented in Tables 5 and 6. SWLS scores were positively associated with scores on all AFCS domains. After controlling the effect of demographic variables, results of the regression analyses showed the association of AFCS scores with SWLS scores, with a statistically significant model for young-old ($\Delta R^2 = .14$, $F(14, 336) = 11.1$, $p < .01$) and old-old ($\Delta R^2 = .15$, $F(14, 316) = 8.95$, $p < .01$) groups. Similarities and differences in domains of age-friendliness associated with life satisfaction between young-old and old-old groups were then addressed within the models. The domain scores for transportation ($\beta = .14$ and $\beta = .14$, $p < .05$) and social participation ($\beta = .21$ and $\beta = .15$,

$p < .05$) were significantly associated with SWLS scores in both young-old and old-old, respectively. In addition, the domain score for community and health services was significantly correlated with SWLS scores only in the young-old group ($\beta = .19$, $p < .05$), while the domain score for civic participation and employment was significantly associated with SWLS only in the old-old group ($\beta = .12$, $p < .05$). In other words, young-old adults tended to be more satisfied in an environment with good transportation, social participation, and community and health services, while old-old adults were more satisfied with an environment with good transportation, social participation, and civic participation and employment.

4. Discussion

In this study, old-old participants reported significantly higher scores in most of the age-friendly city domains as well as the Satisfaction with Life Scale, compared to young-old

TABLE 2: Mean scores of age-friendly city domains and satisfaction with Life Scale of young-old and old-old participants.

Domain	Young-old		Old-old		p value
	Mean	SD	Mean	SD	
Outdoor spaces and buildings	4.10	0.72	4.21	0.68	.049
Transportation	4.39	0.63	4.56	0.53	<.01
Housing	3.97	0.93	4.15	0.97	.013
Social participation	4.56	0.68	4.68	0.67	.024
Respect and social inclusion	4.22	0.78	4.34	0.78	.028
Civic participation and employment	4.01	0.88	4.13	0.95	.071
Communication and information	4.16	0.77	4.26	0.74	.091
Community and health services	3.85	0.78	4.10	0.69	<.01
SWLS	4.59	0.95	4.88	1.00	<.01

participants. These findings support the idea of "paradox of well-being," in which older adults maintain high subjective well-being even when facing different challenges [35]. Old-old adults have been reported to be more capable of shifting motivation from pursuing information to achieving emotional satisfaction under time-constraints, as postulated by the socioemotional selectivity theory [36]. This motivational shift allows for changes in attitude, including a better evaluation and acceptance of individual strengths and limitations [37]. As aged adults have been reported to perceive their stressors as less severe when compared to younger generations [38], it would be a plausible interpretation for the higher rating of life satisfaction among old-old participants than young-old participants.

Variables such as economic status and perceived health situation were positively correlated with life satisfaction in both young-old and old-old groups. These results support the findings of previous studies [34, 39–41]. The standardized Beta weight for health among old-old participants was greater than among young-old participants, indicating that perceived good health may be a more vital determinant of life satisfaction in later life. Marital status and educational level did not show any correlation with life satisfaction in the study sample, and, with women reporting lower levels of life satisfaction, gender was found to correlate with life satisfaction in the young-old but not the old-old group. These findings are largely consistent with the findings of previous studies [42–44]. However, the specific reasons are not identified in the present study. Possible reasons include adoption of multiple caregiving roles [43].

The main purpose of this study was to investigate the association between age-friendliness and life satisfaction after controlling for sociodemographic variables. In both

young-old and old-old groups, all age-friendly domains were correlated with life satisfaction, and most of the domains were correlated moderately. With respect to the regression model, both transportation and social participation were significant correlates of life satisfaction for both young-old and old-old groups, indicating that aged adults are more satisfied if these two domains are fulfilled. Mobility (the ability to move oneself, including walking or using transportation) [45] and social participation are essential components of successful ageing and have been associated with proximity to resources and recreational facilities, social support, and having a driving license [15, 46]. The Hong Kong Government has launched the Public Transport Fare Concession Scheme, intended to enable elderly people to travel on designated public transport modes and services at a concessionary fare of two dollars per trip [47]. Greater availability of choices and cheaper fees for transportation might allow elderly people to engage more actively in society. On the other hand, the domains of civic participation and employment were significantly associated with life satisfaction for the old-old group.

Social and civic participation also emerged as major themes from the data generated from the eight focus groups involving eight-five older adults in Kwun Tong and Kowloon City [48, 49]. Participants remarked that there were a variety of affordable activities that they could participate in community settings. However, more quota and more convenient locations were suggested. Apart from leisure activities, participants also highlighted a need for more productive activities like volunteering and even employment. Moreover, there was a need for more regular channels for older adults to express their opinions. Finally, more relief provisions were underscored to facilitate the participation of caregivers.

Making communities more age-friendly involves both physical and social infrastructure to enable older adults to participate in life-long activities in meaningful ways. Through personal and social engagement in the community, social inclusion is promoted and social capital is enhanced [50, 51]. This engagement could be achieved through contributions to paid and unpaid work, such as voluntary work [6]. Arguing that there can be more than one pathway through which social engagement can promote well-being, the ascribed value as well as purpose/goal or the meaning of the activities can be crucial [24]. Critical reviews of successful ageing have challenged the notion of promoting normative ideals for ageing in the context of social and civic engagement [52]. By implying the measurement of the value of a person based doing rather than being, we may fail to take into account the notion that there are structural inequalities in access to prescribed contributory roles for some marginalized groups due to differences in education, income, gender, social connections, health problems, and job opportunities [28, 53]. Thus, various crucial barriers are needed to be addressed before promoting social engagement for aged adults: profound involvement in caregiving, compulsory altruism, personal resources, and objective perceived and subjectively available engagement opportunities [54]. As such, an alternative model of ageing should be based on equal regard for all persons, taking

TABLE 3: Correlations and results from regression analyses of demographic variables in association with SWLS score in young-old participants.

| Variables | Pearson correlation (r) | | | | | | [B]β |
	[A]SWLS	Gender	Marriage	Education level	Expenditure	Income	
Gender	−.12*						−.122*
Marriage	−.06	.14*					.011
Education level	.04	−.22*	−.21*				−.076
Expenditure	.36*	.01	−.14*	.16*			.312*
Income	.17*	.04	−.09	.16*	.30*		.079
Health	.24*	−.17*	−.10*	.17*	.21*	.11*	.161*

*Statistically significant at $p < .05$ level.
Note. [A]SWLS referred to the Satisfaction with Life Scale.
[B]Standardized coefficients beta of predictors of SWLS score are presented.

TABLE 4: Correlations and results from regression analyses of demographic variables in association with SWLS score in old-old participants.

| Variables | Pearson correlation (r) | | | | | | [B]β |
	[A]SWLS	Gender	Marriage	Education level	Expenditure	Income	
Gender	.07						.096
Marriage	.01	.26*					.018
Education level	−.08	−.31*	−.14*				−.101
Expenditure	.34*	−.06	−.08	.16*			.253*
Income	.11*	.00	−.13*	.13*	.28*		.009
Health	.39*	−.13*	−.08	.05	.32*	.13*	.328*

*Statistically significant at $p < .05$ level.
Note. [A]SWLS referred to the Satisfaction with Life Scale.
[B]Standardized coefficients beta of predictors of SWLS score are presented.

TABLE 5: Correlations and results from regression analyses of AFC scores in association with SWLS score in young-old participants.

| | Pearson Correlation (r) | | | | | | | | [B]β |
	[A]SWLS	Outdoor spaces and buildings	Transportation	Housing	Social participation	Respect and social inclusion	Civic participation and employment	Communication and information	
Outdoor spaces and buildings	.23*								−.030
Transportation	.29*	.70*							.141*
Housing	.25*	.42*	.39*						.088
Social participation	.30*	.41*	.45*	.41*					.207*
Respect and social inclusion	.21*	.53*	.55*	.37*	.59*				−.136
Civic participation and employment	.09*	.34*	.35*	.27*	.39*	.49*			−.090
Communication and information	.19*	.46*	.38*	.38*	.41*	.56*	.41*		.050
Community and health services	.31*	.51*	.53*	.42*	.43*	.57*	.34*	.49*	.194*

*Statistically significant at $p < .05$ level.
Note. [A]SWLS referred to the Satisfaction with Life Scale.
[B]Standardized coefficients beta of predictors of SWLS score are presented.

TABLE 6: Correlations and results from regression analyses of AFC score in association with SWLS score in old-old participants.

	[A]SWLS	Outdoor spaces and buildings	Transportation	Housing	Social participation	Respect and social inclusion	Civic participation and employment	Communication and information	[B]β
				Pearson correlation (r)					
Outdoor spaces and buildings	.29*								−.021
Transportation	.36*	.63*							.136*
Housing	.33*	.42*	.41*						.049
Social participation	.35*	.43*	.44*	.47*					.147*
Respect and social inclusion	.30*	.51*	.48*	.43*	.51*				.002
Civic participation and employment	.35*	.38*	.37*	.31*	.38*	.47*			.117*
Communication and information	.27*	.37*	.34*	.34*	.44*	.46*	.38*		.065
Community and health services	.34*	.42*	.50*	.35*	.40*	.44*	.42*	.41*	.060

*Statistically significant at $p < .05$ level.

Note. [A]SWLS referred to the Satisfaction with Life Scale.

[B]Standardized coefficients beta of predictors of SWLS score are presented.

into account of the diversity of aged adults and ageing processes as well as the oldest-old who are suffering from functional deterioration. These present findings have highlighted the importance of providing both young-old and old-old with an opportunity to contribute in the society leading to a sense of accomplishment and satisfaction [55, 56].

Community and health services were significantly associated with life satisfaction for the young-old group but not the old-old. These findings also echo previous findings in Hong Kong Chinese population. Cheng [57] measured aspiration–achievement discrepancies in three specific areas—material resources, social relationships, and health—in groups of older, middle-aged, and younger adults. Older adults had significantly smaller discrepancies in material resources and social relationships than the younger age groups but larger health discrepancies. However, though aspiration–achievement discrepancies in health increased with age, it had smaller effects on subjective well-being as compared to discrepancies in relationships. While some explanation may be provided in the context of the socioemotional selectivity theory [36], further investigations will be needed for ageing in the very old who may have adjusted to the health system.

The present study has also indicated suggestions for improvement in future research. Since the concept of age-friendly city was adopted from the WHO guidelines, some questions may not be pertinent in local context. For instance, cycle paths are not common facilities in all areas of Hong Kong. Moreover, volunteering may involve both social and civic participation [58]. Levasseur and her colleagues conducted a systematic review on how to define social participation in gerontology. They have suggested a common definition and a taxonomy of social activities linked with the ecological model [59]. This alternative conceptualization may suggest flexibility to integrate items in the domain of social participation and civic participation and employment for further investigation. Nevertheless, social and psychological functioning may change over time until very old age. For example, the association between social networks and social participation for middle-aged and elderly adults is confirmed in their longitudinal study [60]. A longitudinal design is advised to investigate the effect and changes at different time points so that clearer relationships between variables could be revealed. This is vital as the importance of social participation persists in the old-old.

5. Conclusion

Age-friendliness is significantly related to the life satisfaction of the ageing population. Social participation is important for the young-old and the old-old. Ageing older adults can be a resource to the society. The findings of this study have delineated some of the similarities and differences of needs between young-old and old-old adults. Future directions will need to work on a more specific taxonomy of possible social activities and social participation and how they can take place in the living environment of aged adults to enhance their well-being and their contribution to the younger generations.

Appendix

See Table 7.

TABLE 7

Domain	Sample item
Outdoor spaces and buildings	Public areas are clean and pleasant
Transportation	Public transportation costs are consistent, clearly displayed and affordable
Housing	Sufficient and affordable home maintenance and support services are available
Social participation	Activities and events can be attended alone or with a companion
Respect and social inclusion	Older people are regularly consulted by public, voluntary and commercial services on how to serve them better
Civic participation and employment	A range of flexible options for older volunteers is available, with training, recognition, guidance and compensation for personal costs
Communication and information	Regular information and broadcasts of interest to older people are offered
Community and health services	Home care services include health and personal care and housekeeping

Competing Interests

The authors declare that they have no competing interests.

Acknowledgments

The authors acknowledge the support of The Hong Kong Jockey Club Charities Trust for The Jockey Club Age-friendly City Project. For subject recruitment, the authors are also very grateful for the help of the staff of the District Elderly Community Centres and Neighbourhood Elderly Centres in Kwun Tong and Kowloon City. Finally, the authors wish to thank the senior members and administrative staff of The Institute of Active Ageing at The Hong Kong Polytechnic University for their generous support of the project.

References

[1] Census and Statistics Department, 2015, http://www.statistics.gov.hk/.

[2] "Life expectancy at birth, total (years)," 2014 http://data.worldbank.org/indicator/SP.DYN.LE00.IN?year_high_desc=true.

[3] Social Welfare Department, http://www.swd.gov.hk/en/index/site_pubsvc/page_elderly/.

[4] 2016 Policy Address, 2016, http://www.policyaddress.gov.hk/2016/eng/.

[5] World Health Organization, *Active Ageing: A Policy Framework*, World Health Organization, Non-communicable Disease Prevention and Health Promotion Department, Geneva, Switzerland, 2002.

[6] World Health Organization, *Global Age-Friendly Cities: A guide*, World Health Organization, Geneva, Switzerland, 2007.

[7] World Health Organization, *Measuring the Age-Friendliness of Cities: A Guide to Using Core Indicators*, World Health Organization, Geneva, Switzerland, 2015.

[8] C.-W. Lui, J.-A. Everingham, J. Warburton, M. Cuthill, and H. Bartlett, "What makes a community age-friendly: a review of international literature," *Australasian Journal on Ageing*, vol. 28, no. 3, pp. 116–121, 2009.

[9] J. Liddle, T. Scharf, B. Bartlam, M. Bernard, and J. Sim, "Exploring the age-friendliness of purpose-built retirement communities: evidence from England," *Ageing and Society*, vol. 34, no. 9, pp. 1601–1629, 2014.

[10] K. Broome, L. Worrall, K. McKenna, and D. Boldy, "Priorities for an age-friendly bus system," *Canadian Journal on Aging*, vol. 29, no. 3, pp. 435–444, 2010.

[11] S. Chiou and L. Chen, "Towards age-friendly hospitals and health services," *Archives of Gerontology and Geriatrics*, vol. 49, supplement 2, pp. S3–S6, 2009.

[12] M. Wong, P. H. Chau, F. Cheung, D. R. Phillips, and J. Woo, "Comparing the age-friendliness of different neighbourhoods using district surveys: an example from Hong Kong," *PLoS ONE*, vol. 10, no. 7, Article ID e0131526, 2015.

[13] Building Hong Kong into an Age-Friendly City—Elderly Services—Community & Charities—The Hong Kong Jockey Club, http://charities.hkjc.com/charities/english/community-contributions/hkjc-130-story-elderly-building.aspx.

[14] C. D. Ryff, "Beyond Ponce de Leon and life satisfaction: new directions in quest of successful ageing," *International Journal of Behavioral Development*, vol. 12, no. 1, pp. 35–55, 1989.

[15] J. W. Rowe and R. L. Kahn, "Successful aging," *Gerontologist*, vol. 37, no. 4, pp. 433–440, 1997.

[16] P. B. Baltes and M. M. Baltes, "Psychological Perspectives on Successful Ageing: The Model of Selective Optimization with Compensation," in *Successful Ageing*, pp. 1–34, Cambridge University Press, New York, NY, USA, 1990.

[17] L. L. Carstensen, "Social and emotional patterns in adulthood: support for socioemotional selectivity theory," *Psychology and aging*, vol. 7, no. 3, pp. 331–338, 1992.

[18] S.-T. Cheng, "Defining successful aging: the need to distinguish pathways from outcomes," *International Psychogeriatrics*, vol. 26, no. 4, pp. 527–531, 2014.

[19] B. L. Neugarten, J. W. Moore, and J. C. Lowe, "Age norms, age constraints, and adult socialization," *AJS; American journal of sociology*, vol. 70, no. 6, pp. 710–717, 1965.

[20] B. L. Neugarten, "Age groups in American Society and the rise of the young-old," *The Annals of the American Academy of Political and Social Science*, vol. 415, no. 1, pp. 187–198, 1974.

[21] B. L. Neugarten, "The future and the young-old," *Gerontologist*, vol. 15, no. 1, pp. 4–9, 1975.

[22] A. Au, T. Tsien, A. Tsui et al., "A study on evaluating the effectiveness of elderly centre services of Tung Wah Group of hospitals to fulfil the needs of young old: a report jointly prepared by the Hong Kong Polytechnic University and Tung Wah Group of Hospitals Community Services Division (Elderly Services) for the Social Welfare Department," 2013.

[23] W. Pavot, E. Diener, and J. N. Butcher, "Review of the satisfaction with life scale," *Psychological Assessment*, vol. 5, no. 2, pp. 164–172, 1993.

[24] K. B. Adams, S. Leibbrandt, and H. Moon, "A critical review of the literature on social and leisure activity and wellbeing in later life," *Ageing & Society*, vol. 31, no. 4, pp. 683–712, 2010.

[25] D. V. Jeste, G. N. Savla, W. K. Thompson et al., "Association between older age and more successful aging: critical role of resilience and depression," *American Journal of Psychiatry*, vol. 170, no. 2, pp. 188–196, 2013.

[26] T. D. Windsor, K. J. Anstey, and B. Rodgers, "Volunteering and psychological well-being among young-old adults: how much is too much?" *Gerontologist*, vol. 48, no. 1, pp. 59–70, 2008.

[27] J. Smith, M. Borchelt, H. Maier, and D. Jopp, "Health and well-being in the young old and oldest old," *Journal of Social Issues*, vol. 58, no. 4, pp. 715–732, 2002.

[28] A. S. Martin, B. W. Palmer, D. Rock, C. V. Gelston, and D. V. Jeste, "Associations of self-perceived successful aging in young-old versus old-old adults," *International Psychogeriatrics*, vol. 27, no. 4, pp. 601–609, 2015.

[29] J. Yu, J. Li, P. Cuijpers, S. Wu, and Z. Wu, "Prevalence and correlates of depressive symptoms in Chinese older adults: A Population-based Study," *International Journal of Geriatric Psychiatry*, vol. 27, no. 3, pp. 305–312, 2012.

[30] K. Yoshimura, M. Yamada, Y. Kajiwara, S. Nishiguchi, and T. Aoyama, "Relationship between depression and risk of malnutrition among community-dwelling young-old and old-old elderly people," *Aging and Mental Health*, vol. 17, no. 4, pp. 456–460, 2013.

[31] A. Au, E. Ng, S. Lai et al., "Goals and Life satisfaction of Hong Kong Chinese older adults," *Clinical Gerontologist*, vol. 38, no. 3, pp. 224–234, 2015.

[32] World Health Organization, *Checklist of Essential Features of Age-Friendly Cities*, World Health Organization, 2007, http://www.who.int/ageing/publications/Age_friendly_cities_checklist.pdf.

[33] E. Diener, R. A. Emmons, R. J. Larsem, and S. Griffin, "The satisfaction with life scale," *Journal of Personality Assessment*, vol. 49, no. 1, pp. 71–75, 1985.

[34] E. Macia, P. Duboz, J. M. Montepare, and L. Gueye, "Exploring life satisfaction among older adults in dakar," *Journal of Cross-Cultural Gerontology*, vol. 30, no. 4, pp. 377–391, 2015.

[35] D. K. Mroczek and C. M. Kolarz, "The effect of age on positive and negative affect: a developmental perspective on happiness," *Journal of Personality and Social Psychology*, vol. 75, no. 5, pp. 1333–1349, 1998.

[36] L. L. Carstensen, J. A. Mikels, and M. Mather, "Aging and the intersection of cognition, motivation, and emotion," *Handbook of the Psychology of Aging*, pp. 343–362, 2006.

[37] D. V. Jeste and A. J. Oswald, "Individual and societal wisdom: explaining the paradox of human ageing and high well-being," *Psychiatry: Interpersonal and Biological Processes*, vol. 77, no. 4, pp. 317–330, 2014.

[38] D. M. Almeida, "Resilience and vulnerability to daily stressors assessed via diary methods," *Current Directions in Psychological Science*, vol. 14, no. 2, pp. 64–68, 2005.

[39] S. Kim, K. A. Sargent-Cox, D. J. French, H. Kendig, and K. J. Anstey, "Cross-national insights into the relationship between wealth and wellbeing: a comparison between Australia, the United States of America and South Korea," *Ageing and Society*, vol. 32, no. 1, pp. 41–59, 2012.

[40] C. G. Dumitrache, L. Rubio, and R. Rubio-Herrera, "Perceived health status and life satisfaction in old age, and the moderating role of social support," *Aging & Mental Health*, pp. 1–7, 2016.

[41] T. R. Adams, L. A. Rabin, V. G. Da Silva, M. J. Katz, J. Fogel, and R. B. Lipton, "Social support buffers the impact of depressive symptoms on life satisfaction in old age," *Clinical Gerontologist*, vol. 39, no. 2, pp. 139–157, 2016.

[42] P. J. Rentfrow, C. Mellander, and R. Florida, "Happy States of America: a state-level analysis of psychological, economic, and social well-being," *Journal of Research in Personality*, vol. 43, no. 6, pp. 1073–1082, 2009.

[43] M. Pinquart and S. Sörensen, "Gender differences in self-concept and psychological well-being in old age: a meta-analysis," *Journals of Gerontology—Series B Psychological Sciences and Social Sciences*, vol. 56, no. 4, pp. P195–P213, 2001.

[44] E. L. Waddell and J. M. Jacobs-Lawson, "Predicting positive well-being in older men and women," *The International Journal of Aging and Human Development*, vol. 70, no. 3, pp. 181–197, 2010.

[45] S. C. Webber, M. M. Porter, and V. H. Menec, "Mobility in older adults: a comprehensive framework," *The Gerontologist*, vol. 50, no. 4, pp. 443–450, 2010.

[46] M. Levasseur, M. Généreux, J.-F. Bruneau et al., "Importance of proximity to resources, social support, transportation and neighborhood security for mobility and social participation in older adults: Results from A Scoping Study," *BMC Public Health*, vol. 15, Article ID 503, 2015.

[47] Labour and Welfare Bureau, 2016 http://www.lwb.gov.hk/fare_concession/index_e.html#s2.

[48] A. Au and H. M. Yip, *Age-Friendly City: Baseline Assessment Report of Kowlooon City*, The Hong Kong Jockey Club Charities Trust, 2016.

[49] A. Au and H. M. Yip, *Age-Friendly City: Baseline Assessment Report of Kwun Tong*, The Hong Kong Jockey Club Charities Trust, Hong Kong, 2016.

[50] O. Huxhold, K. L. Fiori, and T. D. Windsor, "The dynamic interplay of social network characteristics, subjective well-being, and health: the costs and benefits of socio-emotional selectivity," *Psychology and Aging*, vol. 28, no. 1, pp. 3–16, 2013.

[51] A. E. Scharlach and A. E. Lehning, *Creating Aging-Friendly Communities*, Oxford University Press, New York, NY, USA, 2016.

[52] M. Martinson and J. Halpern, "Ethical implications of the promotion of elder volunteerism: a critical perspective," *Journal of Aging Studies*, vol. 25, no. 4, pp. 427–435, 2011.

[53] D. V. Jeste and B. W. Palmer, "A call for a new positive psychiatry of ageing," *British Journal of Psychiatry*, vol. 202, no. 2, pp. 81–83, 2013.

[54] J. Rozanova, N. Keating, and J. Eales, "Unequal social engagement for older adults: constraints on choice," *Canadian Journal on Aging*, vol. 31, no. 1, pp. 25–36, 2012.

[55] E. H. Erikson, J. M. Erikson, and H. Q. Kivnick, *Vital Involvement in Old Age*, Norton, New York, NY, USA, 1986.

[56] N. Morrow-Howell, J. Hinterlong, P. A. Rozario, and F. Tang, "Effects of volunteering on the well-being of older adults," *Journals of Gerontology—Series B Psychological Sciences and Social Sciences*, vol. 58, no. 3, pp. S137–S145, 2003.

[57] S.-T. Cheng, "Age and subjective well-being revisited: a discrepancy perspective," *Psychology and Aging*, vol. 19, no. 3, pp. 409–415, 2004.

SABE Colombia: Survey on Health, Well-Being, and Aging in Colombia—Study Design and Protocol

Fernando Gomez,[1] **Jairo Corchuelo,**[2] **Carmen-Lucia Curcio,**[1]
Maria-Teresa Calzada,[2] **and Fabian Mendez**[2]

[1]*Research Group on Geriatrics and Gerontology, International Association of Gerontology and Geriatrics Collaborative Center,*
 University of Caldas, Manizales, Colombia
[2]*Escuela de Salud Pública, Universidad del Valle, Research Group of Epidemiology and Population Health (GEPH),*
 Cali, Colombia

Correspondence should be addressed to Fernando Gomez; gomez.montes@ucaldas.edu.co

Academic Editor: Marco Malavolta

Objective. To describe the design of the SABE Colombia study. The major health study of the old people in Latin America and the Caribbean (LAC) is the Survey on Health, Well-Being, and Aging in LAC, SABE (from initials in Spanish: SAlud, Bienestar & Envejecimiento). *Methods.* The SABE Colombia is a population-based cross-sectional study on health, aging, and well-being of elderly individuals aged at least 60 years focusing attention on social determinants of health inequities. Methods and design were similar to original LAC SABE. The total sample size of the study at the urban and rural research sites (244 municipalities) was 23.694 elderly Colombians representative of the total population. The study had three components: (1) a questionnaire covering active aging determinants including anthropometry, blood pressure measurement, physical function, and biochemical and hematological measures; (2) a subsample survey among family caregivers; (3) a qualitative study with gender and cultural perspectives of quality of life to understand different dimensions of people meanings. *Conclusions.* The SABE Colombia is a comprehensive, multidisciplinary study of the elderly with respect to active aging determinants. The results of this study are intended to inform public policies aimed at tackling health inequalities for the aging society in Colombia.

1. Introduction

The major health study of the old people in Latin America and the Caribbean (LAC) is the SABE study Survey on Health, Well-Being, and Aging in Latin America and the Caribbean; SABE (from initials in Spanish: SAlud, Bienestar & Envejecimiento) is a multicenter project originally conducted by the Pan-American Health Organization (PAHO) [1–4]. The study included 10,891 individuals, 60+ years of age, living in seven big cities of the region (Bridgetown, Buenos Aires, Havana, Mexico City, Montevideo, Santiago, and Sao Paulo) and was based on a probabilistic, stratified, multistage, cluster-sampling design of noninstitutionalized elderly population of the seven participating cities. The study represented a milestone in the field of population aging in the

region and could provide enough information to study the phenomenon of aging in detail. Results of SABE increased our understanding of the aging processes and the formulation of public policy toward the well-being of the LAC populations and provided a solid base for a second generation of studies in the region [2]. For example, on the basis of this research second panel data was analyzed in Chile and Brazil [5, 6].

After the SABE study was conducted in Latin America, several cross-sectional studies have been carried out in the region. Between 2009 and 2010 in Ecuador, a similar study with emphasis on aborigine population (10.4% of total population) was conducted: SABE Ecuador [7, 8]. As expected, ethnicity is a critical factor in poverty, inequity, and social exclusion among aborigines in the region [9]. Recently, with a similar methodology of the SABE study, a cross-sectional survey was conducted in the urban zone of Bogotá (Colombia) including 2000 people of 60+ years [10]. In Peru a SABE study is ongoing by 2016.

More than 40 papers from SABE study have been published during the last decade including different topics like gender, chronic conditions, hypertension, diabetes mellitus, obesity, anemia, cancer, anthropometric measures, oral health, mobility, frailty and sarcopenia, disability, falls, depression, cognitive function, and caregivers [11, 12].

Colombia is a country of approximately 48 million inhabitants, with some 5.2 million being aged 60 years and above. Currently, life expectancy in Colombia is 72.3 years and by 2025 it will be 77.6 years for women and 69.8 years for men. Colombia is experiencing demographic changes including population aging, decreasing fertility, rapid urbanization, and changes in the epidemiological profile with the persistence of communicable diseases and a concomitant increase in noncommunicable chronic diseases [13]. Despite long-term adverse social conditions related to inequities and violence, elderly population has characteristics in their aging process similar to other areas around the world [13]. However, many aspects included in SABE Latin America have not been explored in Colombian older people. The aim of this paper is to describe the design of the SABE Colombia study.

2. Materials and Methods

This is a cross-sectional study of community-dwelling elderly individuals living in urban and rural areas of Colombia. The target population for SABE Colombia includes all adults aged 60 years and above who reside in households. Following conventional practice for population surveys, institutionalized persons (of prisons, jails, nursing homes, and long-term or dependent care facilities) were excluded. The methods and procedures were based on those used in the SABE international study to reach comparability [4] but included an analytical approach based on active aging as recommended by WHO to understand factors, processes, or "determinants" that influence individuals, families, and nations over the life course [14].

Individuals for the SABE Colombia were selected following a multistage area probability sampling design. In particular, sampling was developed using a multistage cluster-sampling technique with stratification of the units at the highest levels of aggregation. The sample included four distinct selection stages. The primary stage of sampling was carried out with a probability proportionate to size (PPS) selection of municipalities as primary sampling units (PSUs). The secondary sampling units (SSU) were area segments (i.e., blocks) randomly selected within PSUs. The third stage of sample selection was preceded by a complete listing (enumeration) of all housing units (HUs) that were physically located within the bounds of the selected SSU. The third sampling stage was a systematic selection of housing units from the HU listings for the sampled SSU. The fourth and final stage in the multistage design was the selection of the household unit within a sample HU. The SABE Colombia is integrated within the general framework of the Colombian National Surveys System, which has a common sampling

design inside the national master sample ("muestra maestra") for country population surveys in Colombia. This is the first study of aging in Colombia that is conducted nationwide with a sample framework included in the national survey system. Given the political situation, relevant aspects of violence, displacement, housing, and income networks integrated into a conceptual model from the social determinants of health and active aging were included in the survey.

The estimated sample size was 24553 individuals, and assuming an 80% response the target sample was 30691 individuals. However, at fieldwork after implementing several strategies to achieve the overall sample and prevent nonparticipation, response proportion was about 70% and varied by region and urban/rural distributions. Specifically, data collection took place between April and September 2015, and response proportion ranged from about 62% in urban areas to 77% in rural sites. It should be kept in mind that all interviews were face to face, and the fieldwork included large metropolitan areas, where traditionally there is more reluctance to provide a survey interview than in more rural areas. Also, a very few areas in our country were considered unsafe for fieldwork and were excluded from the sample. In consequence, we are confident that the nonresponse was not related to main issues analyzed in the survey and that the sample obtained represents well all groups and regions of the target population. The final sample size achieved, including 244 municipalities across all departments (i.e., states) of the country, was 23.694 elderly Colombians.

Participants were included if they were 60+ years of age, were capable of communicating with the research team, and provided written informed consent. Individuals were excluded at the beginning of the interview if they had a total score of less than 13 in the revised version of the Folstein Mini-Mental State Examination, known as MMSE [15]. Low scores in the MMSE were considered indicative of inability to complete the study procedures, and therefore a proxy interview was developed. The percentage of interviews applied to proxies was 17,5%.

Active aging is defined as the dynamic, lifelong interplay of risk and protection within the person and within the environment [16]. Active aging has proven to be influential in guiding policies and research agendas throughout the world. In agreement with the original active aging policy framework, we adopted an analytical approach to assess determinants as recommended by the WHO [14]. The approach not only helped us to define operative categories of analysis but also added comparability to our data with research on determinants of active aging produced in North America and Europe.

In particular, for data analysis we grouped variables based on categories of active aging determinants as follows: economic, social environment, physical environment, personal factors, behavioral, and health and social services systems. In addition, given that active aging includes the role of culture and gender as cross-cutting factors influencing all other determinants in the SABE study, we included key analysis variables related with demographic indicators, socioeconomic status, geographical regions, and race/ethnicity.

All data were collected and managed using a database program specifically designed for the SABE Colombia

(Synkron, folder synchronization). Quality control and quality assurance procedures were implemented in the field and using telephone verification of registered data to control for erroneous or missing values. Only trained and authorized personnel were able to access the database system. All participants were interviewed and their responses registered on mobile capture devices (tablets), while in some circumstances (insecurity and no internet access to upload questionnaires) printed versions of the questionnaire were applied and later were digitalized. All information was stored using a security protocol to assure safety and confidentiality of collected data. All collected source data are maintained and stored at the Epidemiological Office in National Health Ministry, Bogotá Colombia. Contact information can be found at the following website: https://www.minsalud.gov.co/. The SABE Colombia data set includes a range of sensitive personal information about individuals. It is essential that privacy is protected and that confidentiality is maintained; we use a series of measures to ensure this. Maintenance and use of the data set are overseen by a Steering Committee and every project is considered by this committee. Researchers interested in collaborative work are invited to contact delegate from the Ministry of Health: Herney Rengifo. All information related with results of SABE Colombia is available at https://www.minsalud.gov.co/sites/rid/Lists/BibliotecaDigital/RIDE/VS/ED/GCFI/Socializacion-Resultados-SABE-2016.zip.

Trained health investigators performed physical examination and medical laboratory technicians collected blood samples and laboratory tests. They all were instructed to follow the standardized clinical and laboratory protocols.

Data analyses were carried out using statistical methods appropriated for multistage sampling techniques. Descriptive and inferential statistics were developed taking into account the probability of selection of individuals in the sample to calculate the expansion factors. A focus on social determinants of health is a core component of the data analysis, in order to identify and characterize health inequities among elderly individuals. In particular, the prevalence of various geriatric and chronic conditions and related factors was estimated according to age, gender, ethnicity, place of living, employment, and other key socioeconomic variables to illustrate health disparities among individuals. Statistical analyses were conducted using STATA version 13 (Stata Corp LP, College Station, Texas, USA) and SPSS version 22.0 statistical package (SPSS Inc., Chicago, Ill., USA).

Ethics committees of both University of Caldas and University of Valle reviewed and approved the study protocol. Participants provided written informed consent (including permission to use secondary data and blood samples) before enrolling in the study and completing the first examination. Participants were informed that they could choose to withdraw from the study at any time. Interviews were conducted in a separate room to protect the participants' privacy. The procedures were in accordance with institutional guidelines and were approved by an institutional review committee. Institutional review boards at both universities involved in developing the SABE Colombia approved the study protocol, and a written informed consent was obtained from every individual before inclusion.

3. Results

Before starting fieldwork, a pilot study with 84 individuals was conducted to evaluate questionnaire application among different ethnic groups and cultures participating in the study. Standard Operating Procedures (SOPs) were written for all procedures in the protocol and a study manual was set to guide fieldwork. In addition, research and field staff was trained in all aspects of data collection, questionnaire administration, and development of physical measurements. Interviewers received the same standard training based on protocol instructions and data entry forms. In particular, the core research staff coordinated the development of training of all interviewers focusing on the study manual of procedures and using role-playing.

In addition to the questionnaire covering active aging determinants the survey included anthropometric measurements, taking blood pressure, assessment of physical function, and taking blood samples for biochemical and hematological measures. Furthermore, the SABE study was composed also of two additional components (Table 1): (1) a subsample survey among family caregivers and (2) a qualitative study with gender and cultural perspectives of quality of life to understand different dimensions of people meanings.

Table 2 shows the sociodemographic indicators of participants at recruitment in 2015 by residence and by sex.

Data collection and analysis were guided with the following categories of determinants.

3.1. Economic Determinants. Socioeconomic factors were assessed with regard to work history: current occupation, most long-term occupation, and reasons for no work at the moment of interview; income: detailed data on subjective and objective financial status, household income, and expenditures; and social protection: pensions and social transfers. Furthermore, marital status and ethnicity were obtained [17].

3.2. Social Environment Determinants. Information in this section included educational attainment and degree of literacy; assessment of frequency, size, and closeness of social support and social networks to provide information about the social environment of Colombian older people; living arrangements, social environments, and perception to neighborhood safety. Also, under a life-course perspective, early-life circumstances (first 15 years) and childhood adversity, abuse, mistreatment, and perceived discrimination were assessed to identify disparities across socioeconomic status originated in childhood [18]. Participants were also asked about their social participation in 18 most common activities reported in previous studies, including hobbies and traveling [19]. Because of specific characteristics of violence in Colombian urban and rural regions, emphasis on characteristics of abuse, mistreatment, and social exclusion (perceived discrimination) and reasons of migration and displacement in the last 5 years were also assessed.

3.3. Physical Environment Determinants. Enabling and supportive environments for older people were one of the central goals at the Second World Assembly on Ageing, Madrid,

TABLE 1: Operative categories of analysis based on active aging determinants in the SABE Colombia study.

Classification	Measures and instruments
Economic determinants	Work history: occupation, employment, current occupation, and reasons for no work. Income: subjective and objective financial status, household income, and expenditures. Social protection: pensions and social transfers. Marital status, ethnicity.
Social environment determinants	Educational attainment and degree of literacy. Assessment of frequency, size, and closeness of social support and social networks. Living arrangements and perception in respect to neighborhood safety. Early-life circumstances (first 15 years) and childhood adversity, abuse, mistreatment, and perceived discrimination. Social participation. Migration and displacement.
Physical environment determinants	Housing characteristics, housing safety, and environmental risks. Use of technology. Transportation services, built environment, and public services.
Personal determinants	Spirituality, sexuality, subjective health status, life space assessment, and functioning: physical and instrumental ADL limitations; mobility disability (Nagi questionnaire), grip strength, short physical performance battery (SPPB): balance, gait speed, and chair stands.
Behavioral determinants	Habits: smoking and alcohol. Physical activity: Advanced Activities of Daily Living scale. Mini-Nutritional Assessment. Anthropometry: height; weight; body mass index; circumference of waist, calf, and arm. Oral health.
Health and social services systems	Multimorbidity, chronic conditions (hypertension, osteoarthritis, diabetes, cardiovascular disease, osteoporosis, chronic obstructive pulmonary disease, cancer, and stroke), sensory impairments (vision and hearing loss), diseases linked to the aging processes (depression, dementia, falls and fear of falling, urinary incontinence, and frailty), mental well-being, and medications use (polypharmacy, hypnotics, homeopathic products, and adherence). Access and utilization of healthcare services.
Blood assays	Hemoglobin and hematocrit, total cholesterol, LDL, HDL cholesterol, and triglycerides.
Family caregiving	Caregiver characteristics, perceived burden, caregiver health, and training.
Qualitative data	Interactions and participation, physical and psychological well-being, experiences, relationships, social contacts and support, and living environment.

ADL: activities of daily living.

2002. Housing conditions were assessed in a similar way of original SABE study [3]. Items included housing characteristics, housing safety, and environmental risks. Use of technology was explored in relation to access to information and communication technologies and daily use of technological tools such as microwave oven, automatic cashier, or cell phone. Transportation services, built environment, and public services were also assessed.

3.4. Personal Determinants. In original active aging determinants, cognitive capacity is included among personal determinants; however, SABE survey included cognitive impairment; as a consequence, it is included in health determinants section. Other determinants as spirituality, sexuality, subjective health status, life space assessment, and functioning were assessed. Functioning was assessed with activities of daily living (ADL) evaluation using two types of questionnaires: a Spanish-adapted version of physical level ADL (Barthel Index) [20] and an adapted instrumental level ADL scale recommended for epidemiological studies in the elderly people [21]. Mobility disability was defined as having difficulty in walking 400 m or climbing a flight of stairs without resting [22]. Grip strength was assessed by using the average of two Takey hydraulic dynamometer (the Smedley Hand

Dynamometer III) attempts, and the reported stronger hand category measure was included for analyses. Physical performance was assessed by the validated Spanish version of short physical performance battery (SPPB) [23]. The SPPB includes three timed tests of lower body function: a hierarchical test of standing balance, a 4 m walk, and five repeated chair stands.

3.5. Behavioral Determinants. Habits as cigarette smoking and alcohol consumption (current and past behavior) were assessed; current physical activity was assessed by an adaptation of Reuben's Advanced Activities of Daily Living scale [24]. The participants were classified into four categories according to their answers: frequent vigorous exercisers, frequent long walkers, frequent short walkers, and persons who did not exercise frequently (sedentary group).

Nutritional status was assessed by using the longer, original version of the Mini-Nutritional Assessment (MNA) [25]. Anthropometry measurements include height and body weight; a portable stadiometer (SECA 213) and an electronic scale (Kendall platform scale graduated) were used. Body mass index (kg/m^2) was calculated. Blood pressure and pulse rate were measured using an electronic manometer (HEM-7113, Omron Healthcare Co., Ltd., Kyoto, Japan). Values were recorded after 5 min of rest in the sitting position and three

TABLE 2: Sociodemographic characteristics of participants at recruitment, 2015 (SABE Colombia).

| | Residence | | | | Sex | | | | | | |
| | Urban | | Rural | | Men | | Women | | Total | |
	%	95% CI	%	95% CI	%	95% CI	%	95% CI	%	95% CI
Age group										
60–64	77	61,5–87,6	23	12,4–38,5	47,1	44,4–49,7	52,9	50,3–55,6	30,6	28,8–32,5
65–69	79,3	63,9–89,3	20,7	10,7–36,1	46,6	43,4–49,8	53,4	50,2–56,6	26,6	24,6–28,7
70–74	76,3	60,9–86,9	23,7	13,1–39,1	45,5	43,1–47,9	54,5	52,1–56,9	16,8	16,0–17,7
75–79	80,6	66,9–89,5	19,4	10,5–33,1	43,5	38,9–48,1	56,5	51,9–61,1	13,4	12,7–14,2
80 and above	78,5	63,7–88,4	21,5	11,6–36,3	41,2	38,8–43,6	58,8	56,4–61,2	12,6	11,8–13,4
Skin color										
Light	84,5	70,0–92,7	15,5	7,3–30,0	41	39,1–42,8	59	57,2–60,9	54,2	46,2–61,9
Medium	72,3	55,7–84,4	27,7	15,6–44,3	49,8	46,1–53,4	50,2	46,6–53,9	34,7	30,3–39,5
Dark	65	47,2–79,5	35	20,5–52,8	54,2	50,2–58,2	45,8	41,8–49,8	11,1	7,6–15,9
Socioeconomic status										
1	55,6	41,4–68,9	44,4	31,1–58,6	46,8	44,5–49,3	53,2	50,7–55,5	28,4	19,5–39,4
2	78,8	61,6–89,5	21,2	10,5–38,4	45,1	43,2–47,0	54,9	53,0–56,8	39,6	36,5–42,8
3-4	97,2	89,8–99,3	2,8	0,7–10,2	45,7	43,7–47,8	54,3	52,2–56,3	30	22,1–39,4
5-6	99,7	97,7–100,0	0,3	0,0–2,3	28,7	16,7–44,8	71,3	55,2–83,3	2	1,3–3,1
Region										
Atlántico	75,4	47,6–91,2	24,6	8,8–52,4	46,1	42,4–49,9	53,9	50,1–57,6	19	8,0–38,9
Oriental	66,9	29,2–90,8	33,1	9,2–70,8	46	43,2–48,8	54	51,2–56,8	17,9	6,9–39,1
Central	77,5	34,9–95,7	22,5	4,3–65,1	45,3	42,4–48,1	54,7	51,9–57,6	27,1	9,4–57,4
Pacific	71	27,2–94,1	29	5,9–72,8	45,2	43,8–46,5	54,8	53,5–56,2	17,5	5,2–45,4
Orinoquia and Amazonia	96,3	83,3–99,3	3,7	0,7–16,7	47,8	43,7–51,8	52,2	48,2–56,3	1,4	0,4–4,4
Bogotá	99,8	96,7–100,0	0,2	0,0–3,3	44,5	44,5–44,5	55,5	55,5–55,5	17	2,5–62,1
Main cities										
Medellín	100		0		41,5	41,5–41,5	58,5	58,5–58,5	9,4	1,4–42,7
Cali	99,2	88,3–99,9	0,8	0,1–11,7	45,5	45,4–45,7	54,5	54,3–54,6	6,9	1,0–35,5
Barranquilla	100		0		36,6	36,6–36,6	63,4	63,4–63,4	3,6	0,5–22,7
Total	78,1	63,2–88,1	21,9	11,9–36,8	45,5	44,2–46,7	54,5	53,3–55,8	80,1	55,2–93,0

consecutive measures were obtained, waiting for at least 30 s between readings. Waist circumference was measured over the midpoint between the lower border of the ribs and iliac crest in the midaxillary plane. Calf and mid-arm circumferences were measured at the largest point of the calf and arm, respectively. Oral health determinant was assessed by several items including self-reporting of presence or missing of teeth and access to dental care. In the SABE, the Geriatric Oral Health Assessment Index (GOHAI) scale was used to quantify the "unmet needs for oral health services" of older adults [26]. Preventive breast and cervical cancer screening among women and prostate cancer screening among men in the last two years were assessed.

3.6. Health and Social Services Systems. Medical information includes multimorbidity, chronic conditions adapted from the original SABE study (hypertension, osteoarthritis, diabetes, cardiovascular disease, osteoporosis, chronic obstructive pulmonary disease, cancer, and stroke), sensory impairments (vision and hearing loss), diseases linked to the aging processes (depression, dementia, falls and fear of falling, urinary incontinence, and frailty), mental well-being,

and medications use (polypharmacy, hypnotics, homeopathic products, and adherence). Medication use and access and utilization of healthcare services (hospitalization, out-patients services, and preventive programs use) were evaluated using questions of the Economic Commission for Latin America and the Caribbean (ECLAC) questions set recommended for epidemiological studies in the elderly people [21].

3.7. Blood Analysis. After an overnight fast, blood and urine samples were collected in the morning. Blood samples were centrifuged for 10 min at 3000 rpm 30 min after sampling. All samples were delivered to a single central laboratory (Dinamica Laboratories, Bogotá, Colombia) for analysis within 24 h. Biochemical tests include hemoglobin and hematocrit, total, LDL, and HDL cholesterol, and triglycerides. Residual samples were stored at −80°C for future analysis.

3.8. Family Caregiving. A family caregiver was defined as a member, relative, or friend at the age of 18 years and above who provides unpaid assistance to an elderly care recipient in at least one ADL or IADL. The caregiver could be staying in the same household or another household (e.g., married daughter). The effects of being a family caregiver, though sometimes positive, are generally negative, with high rates of burden and psychological morbidity as well as social isolation, physical ill-health, and financial hardship. We assessed characteristics of care, perceived burden, caregiver health, and formal or informal training to care for the elderly [27].

3.9. Qualitative Data. WHO defines quality of life as individuals' perception of their position in life in the context of the culture and value systems in which they live and in relation to their personal goals, expectations, standards, and concerns [28]. As part of the SABE Colombia, a qualitative study from gender and culture perspectives was developed to understand the quality of life meanings and to evaluate their particular dimensions (interactions and participation, physical and psychological well-being, experiences, relationships, social contacts and support, and living environment). A pilot study was carried out to adapt the procedures and to build a guide for individual interviews and focus groups. Using a symbolic interactionism approach, a total of 123 interviews and 11 focus groups, including men and women, were done in urban and rural areas of Colombia. Data analyses were conducted using ATLAS Ti (for Windows).

4. Discussion

This study protocol describes the design and methods used in the SABE Colombia study. The SABE Colombia study is designed to assess socioeconomic variables, health status, nutrition, cognition, depression, anthropometric and biological measures, and social support and networks in community-dwelling elderly persons in Colombia. This broad investigative scope has allowed the sample to be well characterized, collecting an extensive array of factors (biomedical, physical, lifestyle, behavioral, and sociodemographic) that contribute to the health and well-being status of participants. Furthermore, in this study, we focus on not only quantitative approach of epidemiological studies, but also a qualitative approach to identify participant's meanings of quality of life. In addition, blood-sampling approach provided a nationally representative sample and will allow inferences about metabolic and hematological status of Colombian older population. Moreover, samples from participants have also been stored for future analysis.

There are several strengths in this study. First, this study has a large sample size, with enough statistical power to detect mild to moderate associations. Second, this study was well designed with stratified randomized sampling methods, taking place in all geographical areas of Colombia. Third, the use of variables included in active aging determinants permits us to change from "needs-based" approach to a "rights-based" approach of older people; we need a better understanding of the pathways that explain how these broad determinants actually affect health and well-being in developing world. Fourth, the face-to-face interview method may be useful in obtaining accurate information, especially among the elderly who may not immediately understand or respond to the questionnaire. Fifth, this study recruited the elderly from both urban and rural areas, and it will be useful to investigate geriatric health under different geographic and socioeconomic environments and lifestyles. However, this study also has certain limitations. No institutionalized elderly participants were included in this study; therefore some conclusions might not be directly applied to individuals living in long-term institutions. Furthermore, given that this is a cross-sectional study without follow-up, this may not assist in determining causal associations between predicted determinants of health and outcomes and may not be used to obtain trajectories of geriatric health over time.

The SABE will provide epidemiological information about determinants of active aging in Colombian elderly people. We expect our data to help find substantial body of evidence on how these determinants (and the interplay between them) have an influence during all life autonomy and independence. At the same time we expect identifying good predictors of health, for both individuals and populations, that permit the maintenance of autonomy and independence in aging. We insist on operationalizing active aging for epidemiological studies that in a near future could be compared among different cultures.

Two more features make SABE Colombia a highly valuable source for genuine cross-cultural comparisons. First, SABE Colombia is closely modeled and harmonized with its parent studies SABE in Latin America and Health Retirement Study in USA. This model has sparked and informed new research on aging over the world. Thus SABE Colombia is into a truly global perspective that permits comparisons with other epidemiological studies as SHARE (Europe), ELSA (England), or LASA (Amsterdam). Second, SABE Colombia is a nationwide survey including a large rural and urban sample. Thus cross-national comparisons will be made with other epidemiological studies in Colombia as SABE Bogotá and International Mobility in Aging Study (IMIAS).

The national survey system including SABE Colombia has projected system update thematic surveys every 10 years, so during that period this study will be the baseline for policy adjustment to aging. Through the Ministry of Health, the database will be released in the course of the first term of 2017 to be consulted not only by decision makers at the local, regional, and national level, but also by research groups interested in the elderly.

Comprehensive health data obtained from SABE Colombia based on active aging determinants is expected to contribute to policy formulation and planning of healthcare services, welfare management, and other social services for elderly persons in Colombia.

Competing Interests

The authors declare that they have no competing interests.

Acknowledgments

This study is supported by a fund (2013, no. 764) from Colciencias y Ministerio de Salud y la Protección Social de Colombia.

References

[1] A. Palloni, M. Peláez, and R. Wong, "Introduction: aging among Latin American and Caribbean populations," *Journal of Aging and Health*, vol. 18, no. 2, pp. 149–156, 2006.

[2] R. Wong, M. Peláez, A. Palloni, and K. Markides, "Survey data for the study of aging in Latin America and the Caribbean: selected studies," *Journal of Aging and Health*, vol. 18, no. 2, pp. 157–179, 2006.

[3] A. Palloni, M. McEniry, R. Wong, and M. Peláez, "The tide to come: elderly health in Latin America and the Caribbean," *Journal of Aging and Health*, vol. 18, no. 2, pp. 180–206, 2006.

[4] C. Albala, M. L. Lebrao, E. M. Léon Díaz et al., "The health, well-being, and aging (SABE) survey: methodology applied and profile of the study population," *Revista Panamericana de Salud Publica*, vol. 17, no. 5-6, pp. 307–322, 2005.

[5] C. Albala, C. García, and L. Lera, "Condiciones de salud de los ancianos en América Latina y el Caribe. Encuesta sobre salud, bienestar y envejecimiento en Santiago, Chile. Estudio SABE Chile," *Santiago de Chile, Instituto de Nutrición y Tecnología de los Alimentos, Universidad de Chile, Organización Panamericana de la Salud*, 2007.

[6] M. L. Lebrao and Y. A. O. Duarte, "Desafios de um estudo longitudinal: o projeto SABE," *Saúde Coletiva*, vol. 5, no. 24, pp. 166–167, 2008.

[7] C. H. Orces, "Prevalence and determinants of falls among older adults in ecuador: an analysis of the SABE i survey," *Current Gerontology and Geriatrics Research*, vol. 2013, Article ID 495468, 7 pages, 2013.

[8] W. B. Freire and W. F. Waters, "Condiciones de salud en los adultos mayores en el Ecuador: Desafíos presentes y futuros. Encuesta nacional de salud, bienestar y envejecimiento SABE I Ecuador 2009-2010," http://www.alapop.org/Congreso2012/DOCSFINAIS_PDF/ALAP_2012_FINAL212.pdf.

[9] W. F. Waters and C. A. Gallegos, Salud y Bienestar del adulto mayor indígena (Health and Wellbeing of Aborigen Older Adult), April 2016, https://www.usfq.edu.ec/programas_academicos/colegios/cocsa/institutos/ISYN/Documents/salud_bienestar_del_adulto_mayor_indigena.pdf.

[10] C. Gómez-Restrepo, M. N. Rodríguez, N. Díaz, C. Cano, and N. Tamayo, "Depresión y satisfacción con la vida en personas mayores de 60 años en Bogotá: Encuesta de Salud, Bienestar y Envejecimiento (SABE)," *Revista Colombiana de Psiquiatría*, vol. 43, pp. 65–70, 2013.

[11] A. Palloni and M. McEniry, "Aging and health status of elderly in Latin America and the Caribbean: preliminary findings," *Journal of Cross-Cultural Gerontology*, vol. 22, no. 3, pp. 263–285, 2007.

[12] F. Gomez and C. L. Curcio, "Geriatrics in Latin America," in *Textbook of Geriatric Medicine and Gerontology*, chapter 121, 8th edition.

[13] F. Gómez, C.-L. Curcio, and G. Duque, "Health care for older persons in Colombia: a country profile," *Journal of the American Geriatrics Society*, vol. 57, no. 9, pp. 1692–1696, 2009.

[14] World Health Organization, Active Ageing: A Policy Framework, World Health Organization, Geneva, Switzerland, 2002, http://apps.who.int/iris/bitstream/10665/67215/1/WHO_NMH_NPH_02.8.pdf.

[15] M. G. Icaza and C. Albala, *Minimental State Examination (MMSE) del Estudio de Demencia en Chile: Análisis Estadístico. Proyecto SABE 7. Investigaciones en Salud Publica. Documentos Técnicos*, Organización Panamericana de la Salud, Washington, DC, USA, 1999.

[16] International Longevity Centre Brazil (Centro Internacional de Longevidade Brasil), *Active Ageing: A Policy Framework in Response to the Longevity Revolution*, International Longevity Centre Brazil (Centro Internacional de Longevidade Brasil), Rio de Janeiro, Brazil, 1st edition, 2015, http://envejecimiento.csic.es/documentos/documentos/ActiveAgeingPolicyFramework_2015.pdf.

[17] E. Telles, R. D. Flores, and F. Urrea-Giraldo, "Pigmentocracies: educational inequality, skin color and census ethnoracial identification in eight Latin American countries," *Research in Social Stratification and Mobility*, vol. 40, pp. 39–58, 2015.

[18] P. Braveman and C. Barclay, "Health disparities beginning in childhood: a life-course perspective," *Pediatrics*, vol. 124, supplement 3, pp. S163–S175, 2009.

[19] Instituto de Mayores y Servicios Sociales (IMSERSO), Participación Social de las Personas Mayores. Colección Estudios Serie Personas Mayores No. 11005, Madrid, Spain, 2008.

[20] J. J. Baztán-Baztán, J. Perez de Molino, and T. Alarcón, "Indice de Barthel: Instrumento válido para la valoración funcional de pacientes con enfermedad cerebrovascular," *Revista Española de Geriatría y Gerontología*, vol. 28, pp. 32–40, 1993.

[21] ECLAC, Directrices para la elaboración de módulos sobre envejecimiento en las encuestas de hogares, CELADE—División de Población de la CEPAL, Serie manuales 60, Santiago de Chile, noviembre de 2008, http://www.cepal.org/es/publicaciones/5499-directrices-para-la-elaboracion-de-modulos-sobre-envejecimiento-en-las-encuestas.

[22] S. Z. Nagi, "An epidemiology of disability among adults in the United States," *Milbank Memorial Fund Quarterly, Health and Society*, vol. 54, no. 4, pp. 439–467, 1976.

[23] J. F. Gómez Montes, C.-L. Curcio, B. Alvarado, M. V. Zunzunegui, and J. Guralnik, "Validity and reliability of the Short Physical Performance Battery (SPPB): A Pilot Study on Mobility in the Colombian Andes," *Colombia Medica*, vol. 44, no. 3, pp. 165–171, 2013.

[24] D. B. Reuben, L. Laliberte, J. Hiris, and V. Mor, "A hierarchical exercise scale to measure function at the advanced activities of daily living (AADL) level," *Journal of the American Geriatrics Society*, vol. 38, no. 8, pp. 855–861, 1990.

[25] Y. Guigoz, "The Mini-Nutritional Assessment (MNA®) review of the literature—what does it tell us?" *Journal of Nutrition, Health and Aging*, vol. 10, no. 6, pp. 466–487, 2006.

[26] H. Singh, R. G. Maharaj, and R. Naidu, "Oral health among the elderly in 7 Latin American and Caribbean cities, 1999-2000: A Cross-Sectional Study," *BMC Oral Health*, vol. 15, no. 1, article 46, 2015.

[27] J. R. García, Los tiempos del cuidado, El impacto de la dependencia de los mayores en la vidacotidiana de suscuidadores, Premio IMSERSO 'Infanta Cristina' 2009 *Premioa Estudios e Investigaciones Sociales*, Ministerio de Sanidad y Política Social Secretaría General de Política Social y Consumo Instituto de Mayores y Servicios Sociales (IMSERSO), *Colección Estudios Serie Dependencia* no. 12011, 2010.

[28] WHOQOL Group, "The World Health Organization quality of life assessment (WHOQOL): position paper from the World Health Organization," *Social Science & Medicine*, vol. 41, no. 10, pp. 1403–1409, 1995.

Physical Activity Scale for the Elderly: Translation, Cultural Adaptation, and Validation of the Italian Version

Antonio Covotta,[1] Marco Gagliardi,[1] Anna Berardi,[1] Giuseppe Maggi,[2] Francesco Pierelli (iD),[3,4] Roberta Mollica,[5] Julita Sansoni,[6] and Giovanni Galeoto (iD)[6]

[1]Sapienza, University of Rome, Italy
[2]Policlinico" Umberto I, Sapienza University of Rome, Italy
[3]IRCCS Neuromed, Pozzilli, Italy
[4]Department of Medical Surgical Sciences and Biotechnologies, Sapienza University of Rome, Italy
[5]Department of Anatomical, Histological, Forensic and Orthopaedic Sciences, "Sapienza" University of Rome, Italy
[6]Department of Public Health, Sapienza University of Rome, Italy

Correspondence should be addressed to Giovanni Galeoto; giovanni.galeoto@uniroma1.it

Academic Editor: Charles P. Mouton

Objective. The aim of the study was to translate and culturally adapt the Physical Activity Scale for the Elderly into Italian (PASE-I) and to evaluate its psychometric properties in the Italian older adults healthy population. *Methods.* For translation and cultural adaptation, the "Translation and Cultural Adaptation of Patient-Reported Outcomes Measures" guidelines have been followed. Participants included healthy individuals between 55 and 75 years old. The reliability and validity were assessed following the "Consensus-Based Standards for the Selection of Health Status Measurement Instruments" checklist. To evaluate internal consistency and test-retest reliability, Cronbach's α and Intraclass Correlation Coefficient (ICC) were, respectively, calculated. The Berg Balance Score (BBS) and the PASE-I were administered together, and Pearson's correlation coefficient was calculated for validity. *Results.* All the PASE-I items were identical or similar to the original version. The scale was administered twice within a week to 94 Italian healthy older people. The mean PASE-I score in this study was 159 ± 77.88. Cronbach's α was 0.815 ($p < 0.01$) and ICC was 0.977 ($p < 0.01$). The correlation with the BBS was 0.817 ($p < 0.01$). *Conclusions.* The PASE-I showed positive results for reliability and validity. This scale will be of great use to clinicians and researchers in evaluating and managing physical activities in the Italian older adults population.

1. Introduction

Over the last 30 years, several studies have shown that physical activity can prevent age-related diseases, such as cardiovascular disease [1–3], diabetes mellitus [3–7], certain types of cancer [8], osteoporosis [9–11], respiratory disease [12, 13], and dementia [14, 15]. It has also been established that physical activity can improve body mass index (BMI) [16] and mental health [17] and conserve energy balance, reduce the risk of falling [18], and help a person to extend their life expectancy and maintain their independence [19].

As in other developed countries, the age ratio in present-day Italy is strongly imbalanced. In 2015, people aged 65 and older accounted for 22% of the population, and this figure is estimated to increase to 33% by 2065 [20]. The percentage of Italian older people who follow the World Health Organization's (WHO) [21] recommended levels of physical activity for adults aged 65 and older is still very low [22]. In Italy, the number of people between the ages of 65 and 74 years who claimed to take part in physical activities reached 11% in 2015, which was 60% higher than in 2005. Sports participation tends to decrease with age. From the age of 65, almost half of the population declares themselves to be sedentary (45%), and the most sedentary people are 75 years old or older (70%). However, there has been a strong increase in the older adults population's participation in sports over the last 10 years, which has almost doubled from 6% to 11% in that time [22].

As the older adults population in Italy has increased, the concepts of healthy aging and chronic disease protection have become more important. Knowledge of older adults' physical activity levels is vital to determining their health statuses and protective and preventive approaches to chronic disease. In other words, it is both necessary and important to record and measure the current physical activity levels of Italian older adults. The cross-cultural adaptation of a health status measurement tool for use in multiple countries is also essential. It is now recognized that if measurements are to be used across cultures, the items must not only be well translated but also culturally adapted so that the content validity of the instrument is maintained at a conceptual level from culture to culture.

To assess physical activity, this study used objective tools, such as accelerometers, and subjective tools that featured self-report measurements. In 2012, Williams et al. [23] conducted a systematic review and analysis of 104 self-reportable physical activity measurements, which included 35 items that had been designed to assess an older adults population. Of these, the Physical Activity Questionnaire [24], which was composed of 55 questions, and the Physical Activity Scale for the Elderly (PASE), which was composed of only 10 items, were the only scales of measurement that could be self-administered. Compared to other measurement scales, the advantages of the PASE include its brevity (five minutes), easy scoring process, and application by way of letter or phone. Furthermore, the PASE evaluates activities other than exercise. The inclusion of activities common to most older adults, such as household and caregiving activities, helps to ensure that the instrument provides a comprehensive assessment of overall physical activity.

The PASE was developed in 1993 by Washburn et al. [25], specifically to assess physical activity in epidemiologic studies of the older people. In 1999, Washburn et al. [26] evaluated the PASE to quantify the level, duration, and frequency of the physical activity that older adults engaged in. The PASE consists of 10 items that focus on the following 3 domains of activity over a period of 7 days: leisure (5 components), household (4 components), and work-related (1 component) activities. Participation in leisurely activities is recorded by frequency (e.g., never, seldom, sometimes, and often) and duration (e.g., less than an hour, 2–4 hours, or more than 4 hours); paid or unpaid work is recorded by total hours of work per week; and housework, lawn work, home repair, outdoor gardening, and care for others are recorded with yes or no answers. The total PASE score is calculated by multiplying activity participation (yes/no) or the amount of time spent on each activity (hours/week) by the weights of the items that were obtained in the original study.

The PASE was originally developed for use in Britain and North America [25, 26] and has since seen use in the Netherlands [27], Japan [28], Canada [29], China [30], Malaysia [31], and Turkey [32]. The validity and reliability of PASE were also examined in the U.S. in 1999 for patients with knee pain and physical disability [33], in 1998 for patients with moderate to severe chronic obstructive pulmonary disease [34], and in 2001 for patients with end-stage renal disease [35]. Beyond the aforementioned countries, its validity and

reliability were tested in Norway in 2012 for patients with hip osteoarthritis [36], in Taiwan in 2013 for cancer survivors [37], in Switzerland in 2014 for patients who had undergone total knee arthroplasties [38] and total hip arthroplasties [39], and in Australia in 2015 for lung cancer survivors [40].

Over the past three years, several studies have used the PASE to assess the Italian population [41–48]. In spite of this, the lack of an Italian version of the scale that has been adapted to account for the country's culture has prevented its regular use in studies that assess Italy's older adults population. Thus, this study aims to translate the current PASE scale into Italian, to culturally adapt the tool, and to assess its validity and reliability.

2. Methods

This study was conducted by a research group composed of medical doctors and rehabilitation professionals from the "Sapienza" University of Rome and from "Rehabilitation and Outcome Measure Assessment" (ROMA) association. ROMA association in the last few years has dealt with the validation of many outcome measures in Italy [49–57].

Once the consent of the developers of the PASE is received, following the "Translation and Cultural Adaptation of Patient-Reported Outcomes Measures—Principles of Good Practice" guidelines [58] the original tool was translated from English to Italian.

Translation and Cultural Adaptation. The original English version of the PASE [25] was translated into three independent Italian literal translations by one Italian physiotherapist familiar with English and two native English speakers. The results were synthesized by an independent native speaker of the target language who had not been involved in the forward translations. Without having seen the original version, three Italian translators then translated the questionnaire back into English. The original version and the back-translated version of the tool were then compared. Finally to adapt the translated version to the Italian culture, a focus group composed of two physiotherapists and a proofreader familiar with both English and Italian checked the final translation and corrected any remaining spelling, diacritical, grammatical, or other errors and then reworded and reformulated some items to minimize any differences from the original English version.

Participants. According to preceding validations of the PASE [25–32] to be included in the study participants had to be aged 55 to 75; have their personal physician's clearance; have adequate mental status; and have no evidence of clinical depression.

Individuals with emotional or psychiatric problems (as determined by clinical screening) were excluded from the study. All participants were informed about the study, and their interest in taking part in it was recorded; those who entered the study gave their consent before inclusion [59]. Recruited participants who met the study inclusion criteria were scheduled for two testing sessions. Following the "Consensus-Based Standards for the Selection of Health Status Measurement Instruments" (COSMIN) checklist [60], the reliability and validity of the culturally adapted scale were assessed.

Reliability. The PASE-I was given to the population by two physiotherapists. The internal consistency of the PASE-I was examined by Cronbach's alpha (α) that should be at least 0.7 as an indicator of the satisfactory homogeneity of the items within the total scale [61]. The PASE-I was administered twice within a week to a representative, randomized subgroup of the population by the same professionals. To measure test-retest reliability, the Intraclass Correlation Coefficient (ICC) was calculated and the scale was considered stable with an ICC of > 0.70.

Validity. According to the original validation [26], concurrent validity was assessed using Pearson's correlation analyses to determine the association between the PASE-I and the Italian version of the Berg Balance Scale (BBS) [62, 63]. The BBS is a 12-item questionnaire designed to assess the subject's ability to successfully complete tasks such as standing from a sitting position, turning to look behind them, standing with their eyes closed, and standing on one foot. Each item is scored on a 0–4 metric with possible total scores ranging from 0 to 48 [62]. The Italian version of the BBS and the PASE-I were administered together by the same rater.

All statistical analyses were done using IBM-SPSS version 23.00.

3. Results

Translation and Cultural Adaptation. Following guidelines for translation and cultural adaptation,[40] after forward and backward translation, and after a consensus meeting, the translated scale was formed and all item results were identical or similar to the original version. However, the experts agreed that some of the examples used to describe leisure time activities needed an adaptation to the Italian culture to improve comprehensibility and applicability. Activities such as shuffleboard, baseball, and softball were likely to be unknown or not very common to individuals living in Italy and may not have been reflective of values related to the Italian population. Therefore, we deleted or modified examples in items 3, 4, 5, and 6 (e.g., hunting has been changed with dancing or shuffleboard has been changed with boules).

Participants. Participants were community-dwelling older adults recruited from September 2017 through a primary care doctor in Rome. Of the 100 recruited participants, 94 met the inclusion criteria; all agreed to participate and were enrolled in the study (mean age ± standard deviation (SD) = 62.88±7.16). The Italian version of the PASE (PASE-I) was administered from September 29, 2017. The demographic characteristics of the participants are summarized in Table 1, and the mean ± SD of the PASE-I is summarized in Table 2.

Reliability. The PASE-I was found to have a good degree of internal consistency, with a Cronbach's α of 0.815 (p < 0.01). A randomized subgroup of the population (n = 48) was

involved in the test-rest reliability procedures. The PASE-I was reliable with respect to test-retest reliability with an ICC of 0.977 (p < 0.01) and > 0.967 (p < 0.01) in each domain, as reported in Table 3.

Validity. The Italian version of the BBS [63] was also administered to the population. The Pearson's correlation coefficient of the total score of the PASE-I with the Italian version of the BBS [63] was 0.817 (p < 0.01), indicating that the PASE-I has good concurrent validity. The Pearson's correlation coefficient of each item is reported in Table 4.

4. Discussion

We translated the PASE to Italian (PASE-I) and adapted it to Italian culture. The PASE is brief (five minutes) and easily scored [25]. Its brevity makes its use in large-scale epidemiologic studies, where there is limited time to assess physical activity, feasible [25]. This instrument, which has not previously been made available in Italian, is well-suited to studies on the health and physical activity of older adults populations.

Comparison with Other Studies. In this study, we assessed the validity and reliability of the PASE-I while working with 94 healthy and Italian older adults. The results of the study suggest that the Italian version of the tool has strong measurement properties and that it is valid and reliable for research and practice fields.

While the mean PASE scores in previous studies have varied between 94.96 [31] and 131.3 [29], the mean PASE score in this study was 159 ± 77.88. As with other studies [25–32], the current study identified a significant decline of physical activity with age. For example, adults who were 75-years old or older exhibited lower levels of physical activity than those who were 65 years old or younger. The higher total score in this study may have been linked to the participants' younger mean age (62.88 ± 7.16). The greatest contributor to the total physical activity score was household activity (52.8%), which is in line with the results from previous studies [25, 28, 31]. As in other studies [25–32], the PASE-I scores also did not significantly differ between men and women.

Lolan et al.'s [64] and Ayvat et al.'s [32] studies are the only previous studies to have calculated Cronbach's alpha (0.73 and 0.71, respectively). Regardless, the value for Cronbach's alpha in the current study was higher (0.815), which could be attributed to the rigorous cultural adaptation process that was involved in the translation of the examples that were used to describe leisurely activities.

As in other studies, we included the BBS to determine the association between balance and PASE scores. The correlation between static balance and PASE scores was discussed in the original PASE article [26] and subsequent papers. In the current study, work-related activities correlated with higher BBS scores, which is consistent with the findings from previous studies. According to existing research, individuals who more confidently perform activities that challenge their balance have also been proven to be more physically active [26, 28, 29].

TABLE 1: Demographic characteristics for the 194 participants in the reliability study (PASE-I).

	Sample = 96
Age Mean (SD)	62.88 (7.16)
Gender men %	50.5
Education (%)	
Elementary school 4%	4
Middle school 12%	12
High school 36.4%	36.5
University 47.5%	47.5
Marital Status (%)	
Married/Cohabitant	88.9
Single/Widow/Divorced	11.1
Cardio circulatory Disease (%)	
Yes	18.2
No	81.8
Hypertension (%)	
Yes	36.7
No	63.3
Neoplasms	
Yes	4
No	96
Recent Recovery (last 3 years) (%)	
Yes	20.2
No	79.8
Arthritis (%)	
Yes	5.1
No	94.9
Weekly Working Hours (%)	
0	40.4
1-39	32.3
More than 40	27.3
Smoker (%)	
Yes	16.2
No	83.8

TABLE 2: Mean±SD PASE-I scores and BBS scores.

	Test Mean±Standard Deviation
PASE LEISURE TIME ACTIVITIES	29.94±29.63
PASE HOUSE HOLD ACTIVITIES	84.55±45.41
PASE WORK-RELATED ACTIVITIES	44.51±58.86
PASE TOTAL SCORE	159±77.88
BERG BALANCE SCALE	46.63±1.72

Limitations of the Study. As in previous studies, limitations include our exclusion of individuals with mobility issues and cognitive impairment [29]. Expanding the study to include all older people with various health statuses and living conditions could help to form a database that considers a wider older adults population [32].

We agree with the authors of previous validation studies [27–32] in that the PASE itself also contains potential limitations. For example, one limitation is that leisurely activities can be influenced by climate. Furthermore, while the last item on the scale has four possible answers that gauge difficulty, this information excludes those who have worked while sitting (e.g., in an office) and is only assessed if a participant has or has not worked in the past seven days. Assessments of physical activity in the older adults could be improved if they were to differentiate between those

TABLE 3: Test-retest reliability, range of ICC parameters of each item on 48 participants (PASE-I).

	Test mean±SD	Re-Test mean±SD	ICC	IC 95%
PASE LEISURE TIME ACTIVITIES	23.18±22.22	27.71±21.7	0.993	0.988-0.996
PASE HOUSE HOLD ACTIVITIES	76.67±45	78.56±46.83	0.989	0.981-0.994
PASE WORK-RELATED ACTIVITIES	45.87±59.74	49.12±61.1	0.967	0.941-0.981
PASE TOTAL SCORE	145.72±75	150.4±76.17	0.977	0.959-0.987

TABLE 4: Gold standard analysis, Pearson's correlation between PASE-I and the Italian version of BBS.*p < 0.01.

	Berg Balance Scale
PASE LEISURE TIME ACTIVITIES	0.459*
PASE HOUSE HOLD ACTIVITIES	0.495*
PASE WORK-RELATED ACTIVITIES	0.713*
PASE TOTAL SCORE	0.817*

who work standing up (answer 2) and those whose work involves carrying loads that exceed 22 kg (answer 4). The current study only compared the Italian version of the PASE with studies that evaluated balance. As such, other objective measurements should be considered to provide more precise and accurate estimates of physical activity and to reduce measurement errors that are related to these issues.

5. Conclusions

As the older adults population has increased, the concepts of healthy aging and chronic disease protection have become more important. To determine the health status of older adults and protective and preventive strategies against chronic disease, it is important to identify the levels of physical activity that older adults practice. As such, the present study can guide Italian physiotherapists and other health and rehabilitation professionals who work in this area [32]. To inform health policy recommendations, the use of a culturally appropriate instrument is also critical to obtaining valid population-based physical activity data. In conclusion, the Italian version of the PASE is a valid and reliable tool for the evaluation and measurement of physical activity levels in Italian older adults. Thus, this scale can prove useful to clinicians and researchers who have been charged with evaluating and managing the physical activities of the Italian older adults population.

Ethical Approval

All procedures followed were in accordance with the ethical standards of the responsible committee on human experimentation (institutional and national) and with the Helsinki Declaration of 1975, as revised in 2008.

References

[1] J. A. Berlin and G. A. Colditz, "A meta-analysis of physical activity in the prevention of coronary heart disease," *American Journal of Epidemiology*, vol. 132, no. 4, pp. 612–628, 1990.

[2] A. S. Leon, J. Connett, D. R. Jacobs Jr., and R. Rauramaa, "Leisuretime physical activity levels and risk of coronary heart disease and death," *The Journal of the American Medical Association*, vol. 258, no. 17, pp. 2388–2395, 1987.

[3] N. Haapanen, S. Miilunpalo, I. Vuori, P. Oja, and M. Pasanen, "Association of leisure time physical activity with the risk of coronary heart disease, hypertension and diabetes in middle-aged men and women," *International Journal of Epidemiology*, vol. 26, no. 4, pp. 739–747, 1997.

[4] S. P. Helmrich, D. R. Ragland, R. W. Leung, and R. S. Paffenbarger, "Physical activity and reduced occurrence of non-insulindependent diabetes mellitus," *The New England Journal of Medicine*, vol. 325, no. 3, pp. 147–152, 1991.

[5] J. E. Manson, E. B. Rimm, M. J. Stampfer et al., "Physical activity and incidence of non-insulindependent diabetes mellitus in

women," *The Lancet*, vol. 338, no. 8770, pp. 774–778, 1991.

[6] J. E. Manson, D. M. Nathan, A. S. Krolewski, M. J. Stampfer, W. C. Willett, and C. H. Hennekens, "A prospective study of exercise and incidence of diabetes among US male physicians," *Journal of the American Medical Association*, vol. 268, no. 1, pp. 63–67, 1992.

[7] F. B. Hu, R. J. Sigal, J. W. Rich-Edwards et al., "Walking compared with vigorous physical activity and risk of type 2 diabetes in women: A prospective study," *Journal of the American Medical Association*, vol. 282, no. 15, pp. 1433–1439, 1999.

[8] R. J. Shephard and R. Futcher, "Physical activity and cancer: how may protection be maximized?" *Critical Reviews in Oncogenesis*, vol. 8, no. 2-3, pp. 219–272, 1997.

[9] S. R. Cummings, J. L. Kelsey, M. C. Nevitt, and K. J. O'Dowd, "Epidemiology of osteoporosis and osteoporotic fractures," *Epidemiologic Reviews*, vol. 7, pp. 178–208, 1985.

[10] M. E. Farmer, J. H. Madans, R. B. Wallace, J. Cornoni-Huntley, and L. R. White, "Anthropometric indicators and hip fracture. The NHANES I epidemiologic follow-up study," *Journal of the American Geriatrics Society*, vol. 37, no. 1, pp. 9–16, 1989.

[11] E. Gregg, J. Cauley, and D. Seeley, "Physical activity and osteoporotic fracture risk in older women. Study of Osteoporotic Fractures Research Group," *Annals of Internal Medicine*, vol. 91, no. 12, pp. 81–88, 1998.

[12] Y. Lacasse, E. Wong, G. H. Guyatt, D. King, D. J. Cook, and R. S. Goldstein, "Meta-analysis of respiratory rehabilitation in chronic obstructive pulmonary disease," *The Lancet*, vol. 348, no. 9035, pp. 1115–1119, 1996.

[13] J. Garcia-Aymerich, P. Lange, M. Benet, P. Schnohr, and J. M. Antó, "Regular physical activity modifies smoking-related lung function decline and reduces risk of chronic obstructive pulmonary disease: a populationbased cohort study," *American Journal of Respiratory and Critical Care Medicine*, vol. 175, no. 5, pp. 458–463, 2007.

[14] US Department of Health & Human Services, *Physical Activity and Health: A Report of The Surgeon General*, Department of Health & Human Services, GA, USA, 1996.

[15] M. Reiner, C. Niermann, D. Jekauc, and A. Woll, "Long-term health benefits of physical activity: a systematic review of longitudinal studies," *BMC Public Health*, vol. 13, no. 1, article 813, pp. 1–9, 2013.

[16] J.-M. Kvamme, T. Wilsgaard, J. Florholmen, and B. K. Jacobsen, "Body mass index and disease burden in elderly men and women: The Tromsø Study," *European Journal of Epidemiology*, vol. 25, no. 3, pp. 183–193, 2010.

[17] S. J. Parker, S. J. Strath, and A. M. Swartz, "Physical activity measurement in older adults: Relationships with mental health," *Journal of Aging and Physical Activity*, vol. 16, no. 4, pp. 369–380, 2008.

[18] D. A. Ganz, G. E. Alkema, and S. Wu, "It takes a village to prevent falls: Reconceptualizing fall prevention and management for older adults," *Injury Prevention*, vol. 14, no. 4, pp. 266–271, 2008.

[19] K. E. Chad, B. A. Reeder, E. L. Harrison et al., "Profile of physical activity levels in community-dwelling older adults," *Medicine & Science in Sports & Exercise*, vol. 37, no. 10, pp. 1774–1784, 2005.

[20] https://www.istat.it/it/anziani/popolazione-e-famiglie.

[21] http://www.who.int/dietphysicalactivity/factsheet_olderadults/en/.

[22] https://www.istat.it/it/files/2017/10/Pratica-sportiva2015.pdf?title= La+pratica+sportiva+in+Italia++-+19%2Fott%2F2017+-+Testo+ integrale++e+nota+metodologica.pdf.

[23] K. Williams, A. Frei, A. Vetsch, F. Dobbels, M. A. Puhan, and K. Rüdell, "Patient-reported physical activity questionnaires: A systematic review of content and format," *Health and Quality of Life Outcomes*, vol. 10, article no. 28, 2012.

[24] B. Liu, J. Woo, N. Tang, K. Ng, R. Ip, and A. Yu, "Assessment of total energy expenditure in a Chinese population by a physical activity questionnaire: Examination of validity," *International Journal of Food Sciences and Nutrition*, vol. 52, no. 3, pp. 269–282, 2001.

[25] R. A. Washburn, K. W. Smith, A. M. Jette, and C. A. Janney, "The physical activity scale for the elderly (PASE): Development and evaluation," *Journal of Clinical Epidemiology*, vol. 46, no. 2, pp. 153–162, 1993.

[26] R. A. Washburn, E. McAuley, J. Katula, S. L. Mihalko, and R. A. Boileau, "The Physical Activity Scale for the Elderly (PASE): Evidence for validity," *Journal of Clinical Epidemiology*, vol. 52, no. 7, pp. 643–651, 1999.

[27] A. J. Schult, E. G. Schonten, K. R. Westerterp, and W. H. M. Saris, "Validity of the Physical Activity Scale for the Elderly (PASE): According to energy expenditure assessed by the doubly labeled water method," *Journal of Clinical Epidemiology*, vol. 50, no. 5, pp. 541–546, 1997.

[28] A. Hagiwara, N. Ito, K. Sawai, and K. Kazuma, "Validity and reliability of the Physical Activity Scale for the Elderly (PASE) in Japanese elderly people," *Geriatrics & Gerontology International*, vol. 8, no. 3, pp. 143–151, 2008.

[29] K. Vaughan and W. C. Miller, "Validity and reliability of the Chinese translation of the Physical Activity Scale for the Elderly (PASE)," *Send to Disabil Rehabil*, vol. 35, no. 3, pp. 191–197, 2012.

[30] S. Ngai, R. Cheung, P. Lam, J. Chiu, and E. Fung, "Validation and reliability of the Physical Activity Scale for the Elderly in Chinese population," *Journal of Rehabilitation Medicine*, vol. 44, no. 5, pp. 462–465, 2012.

[31] N. Ismail, F. Hairi, W. Y. Choo, N. N. Hairi, D. Peramalah, and A. Bulgiba, "The Physical Activity Scale for the Elderly (PASE): Validity and reliability among community-dwelling older adults in Malaysia," *Asia-Pacific Journal of Public Health*, vol. 27, pp. 62–72, 2015.

[32] E. Ayvat, M. Kilinç, and N. Kirdi, "The Turkish version of the physical activity scale for the elderly (PASE): Its cultural adaptation, validation, and reliability," *Turkish Journal of Medical Sciences*, vol. 47, no. 3, pp. 908–915, 2017.

[33] K. A. Martin, W. J. Rejeski, M. E. Miller, M. K. James, W. H. Ettinger Jr., and S. P. Messier, "Validation of the PASE in older adults with knee pain and physical disability," *Medicine & Science in Sports & Exercise*, vol. 31, no. 5, pp. 627–633, 1999.

[34] J. L. Larson, M. C. Kapella, S. Wirtz, M. K. Covey, and J. Berry, "Reliability and Validity of the Functional Performance Inventory in Patients with Moderate to Severe Chronic Obstructive Pulmonary Disease," *Journal of Nursing Measurement*, vol. 6, no. 1, pp. 55–73, 1998.

[35] K. L. Johansen, P. Painter, J. A. Kent-Braun et al., "Validation of questionnaires to estimate physical activity and functioning in end-stage renal disease," *Kidney International*, vol. 59, no. 3, pp. 1121–1127, 2001.

[36] I. Svege, E. Kolle, and M. Risberg, "Reliability and validity of the Physical Activity Scale for the Elderly (PASE) in patients with hip osteoarthritis," *BMC Musculoskeletal Disorders*, vol. 13, article no. 26, 2012.

[37] C.-C. Su, K.-D. Lee, C.-H. Yeh, C.-C. Kao, and C.-C. Lin, "Measurement of physical activity in cancer survivors: A validity study," *Journal of Cancer Survivorship*, vol. 8, no. 2, pp. 205–212, 2014.

[38] S. Bolszak, N. C. Casartelli, F. M. Impellizzeri, and N. A. Maffiuletti, "Validity and reproducibility of the Physical Activity Scale for the Elderly (PASE) questionnaire for the measurement of the physical activity level in patients after total knee arthroplasty," *BMC Musculoskeletal Disorders*, vol. 15, no. 1, article no. 46, 2014.

[39] N. C. Casartelli, S. Bolszak, F. M. Impellizzeri, and N. A. Maffiuletti, "Reproducibility and validity of the physical activity scale for the elderly (PASE) questionnaire in patients after total hip arthroplasty," *Physical Therapy in Sport*, vol. 95, no. 1, pp. 86–94, 2015.

[40] C. L. Granger, S. M. Parry, and L. Denehy, "The self-reported Physical Activity Scale for the Elderly (PASE) is a valid and clinically applicable measure in lung cancer," *Supportive Care in Cancer*, vol. 23, no. 11, pp. 3211–3218, 2015.

[41] F. Curcio, I. Liguori, M. Cellulare et al., "PASE (Physical Activity Scale for the Elderly) Score Is Related to Sarcopenia in Noninstitutionalized Older Adults," *Journal of Geriatric Physical Therapy*, p. 1, 2018.

[42] C. Gagliardi, R. Papa, D. Postacchini, and C. Giuli, "Association between cognitive status and physical activity: Study profile on baseline survey of the my mind project," *International Journal of Environmental Research and Public Health*, vol. 13, no. 6, article no. 585, 2016.

[43] A. Muscari, G. Bianchi, C. Conte et al., "No Direct Survival Effect of Light to Moderate Alcohol Drinking in Community-Dwelling Older Adults," *Journal of the American Geriatrics Society*, vol. 63, no. 12, pp. 2526–2533, 2015.

[44] C. De Nunzio, F. Presicce, R. Lombardo et al., "Physical activity as a risk factor for prostate cancer diagnosis: A prospective biopsy cohort analysis," *BJU International*, vol. 117, no. 6, pp. E29–E35, 2016.

[45] E. Bacchi, C. Bonin, M. E. Zanolin et al., "Physical activity patterns in normal-weight and overweight/obese pregnant women," *PLoS ONE*, vol. 11, no. 11, Article ID e0166254, 2016.

[46] U. Tarantino, J. Baldi, M. Scimeca et al., "The role of sarcopenia with and without fracture," *Injury*, vol. 47, pp. S3–S10, 2016.

[47] M. Noale, S. Maggi, W. Artibani et al., "Pros-IT CNR: an Italian prostate cancer monitoring project," *Aging Clinical and Experimental Research*, vol. 29, no. 2, pp. 165–172, 2017.

[48] C. Giuli, R. Papa, R. Bevilacqua et al., "Correlates of perceived health related quality of life in obese, overweight and normal weight older adults: An observational study," *BMC Public Health*, vol. 14, no. 1, 2014.

[49] G. Galeoto, A. Lauta, A. Palumbo, S. F. Castiglia, R. Mollica, and V. Santilli, "The Barthel Index: Italian translation, adaptation and validation," *International Journal of Neurology and Neurotherapy*, vol. 2, no. 2, pp. 1–7, 2015.

[50] G. Galeoto, A. Berardi, R. De Santis et al., "Validation and cross-cultural adaptation of the Van Lieshout test in an Italian population with cervical spinal cord injury: a psychometric study," *Spinal Cord Series and Cases*, vol. 4, no. 1, 2018.

[51] G. Culicchia, M. Nobilia, M. Asturi et al., "Cross-Cultural Adaptation and Validation of the Jebsen-Taylor Hand Function Test in an Italian Population," *Rehabilitation Research and Practice*, Article ID 8970917, 2016.

[52] S. Castiglia, "The culturally adapted Italian version of the Barthel Index (IcaBI): assessment of structural validity, inter-rater reliability and responsiveness to clinically relevant improvements in patients admitted to inpatient rehabilitation centers," *Functional Neurology*, vol. 32, no. 4, p. 221, 2017.

[53] M. A. Marquez, R. De Santis, V. Ammendola et al., "Cross-cultural adaptation and validation of the "Spinal Cord Injury-Falls Concern Scale" in the Italian population," *Spinal Cord*, vol. 56, no. 7, pp. 712–718, 2018.

[54] G. Galeoto, J. Sansoni, M. Scuccimarri et al., "A Psychometric Properties Evaluation of the Italian Version of the Geriatric Depression Scale," *Depression research and treatment*, Article ID 1797536, 2018.

[55] M. Murgia, A. Bernetti, M. Delicata, C. Massetti, E. M. Achilli, and M. Mangone, "Inter-and intra-interviewer reliability of Italian version of Pediatric Evaluation of Disability Inventory," *Annali di Igiene*, vol. 30, pp. 153–161, 2018.

[56] A. Berardi, R. De Santis, M. Tofani et al., "The Wheelchair Use Confidence Scale: Italian translation, adaptation, and validation of the short form," *Disability and Rehabilitation: Assistive Technology*, pp. 1–6, 2017.

[57] M. Tofani, C. Candeloro, M. Sabbadini et al., "The psychosocial impact of assistive device scale: Italian validation in a cohort of nonambulant people with neuromotor disorders," *Assistive Technology*, pp. 1–6, 2018.

[58] D. Wild, A. Grove, M. Martin et al., "Principles of good practice for the translation and cultural adaptation process for patient-reported outcomes (PRO) measures: report of the ISPOR Task Force for Translation and Cultural Adaptation," *Value in Health*, vol. 8, no. 2, pp. 94–104, 2005.

[59] G. Galeoto, R. Mollica, O. Astorino, and R. Cecchi, "Informed consent in physiotherapy: proposal of a form," *Giornale Italiano di Medicina del Lavoro ed Ergonomia*, vol. 37, no. 4, pp. 245–254, 2015.

[60] L. B. Mokkink, C. B. Terwee, D. L. Patrick et al., "The COSMIN checklist for assessing the methodological quality of studies on measurement properties of health status measurement instruments: an international Delphi study," *Quality of Life Research*, vol. 19, no. 4, pp. 539–549, 2010.

[61] J. C. Nunnally, *Psychometric Theory*, McGraw-Hill, NY, USA, 1978.

[62] K. O. Berg, S. L. Wood-Dauphinee, J. I. Williams, and B. Maki, "Measuring balance in the elderly: Validation of an instrument," *Canadian Journal of Public Health*, vol. 83, pp. S7–S11, 1992.

[63] M. Ottonello, G. Ferriero, E. Benevolo, P. Sessarego, and D. Dughi, "Psychometric evaluation of the Italian version of the Berg Balance Scale in rehabilitation inpatients," *European Journal of Physical and Rehabilitation Medicine*, vol. 39, no. 4, pp. 181–189, 2003.

[64] N. W. Loland, "Reliability of the Physical Activity Scale for Elderly (PASE)," *European Journal of Sport Science*, vol. 2, no. 5, pp. 1–12, 2002.

Assessment of Osteoporosis in Injured Older Women Admitted to a Safety-Net Level One Trauma Center: A Unique Opportunity to Fulfill an Unmet Need

Elisabeth S. Young,[1,2] May J. Reed,[2] Tam N. Pham,[3] Joel A. Gross,[4] Lisa A. Taitsman,[5] and Stephen J. Kaplan[2,6]

[1]*University of Hawaii College of Medicine, Honolulu, HI, USA*
[2]*Division of Geriatrics and Gerontology, Department of Medicine, Harborview Medical Center, University of Washington, Seattle, WA, USA*
[3]*Department of Surgery, Harborview Medical Center, University of Washington, Seattle, WA, USA*
[4]*Department of Radiology, Harborview Medical Center, University of Washington, Seattle, WA, USA*
[5]*Department of Orthopedics and Sports Medicine, Harborview Medical Center, University of Washington, Seattle, WA, USA*
[6]*Section of General, Thoracic, and Vascular Surgery, Department of Surgery, Virginia Mason Medical Center, Seattle, WA, USA*

Correspondence should be addressed to Stephen J. Kaplan; stephen.kaplan@virginiamason.org

Academic Editor: Francesc Formiga

Background. Older trauma patients often undergo computed tomography (CT) as part of the initial work-up. CT imaging can also be used opportunistically to measure bone density and assess osteoporosis. *Methods.* In this retrospective cohort study, osteoporosis was ascertained from admission CT scans in women aged ≥65 admitted to the ICU for traumatic injury during a 3-year period at a single, safety-net, level 1 trauma center. Osteoporosis was defined by established CT-based criteria of average L1 vertebral body Hounsfield units <110. Evidence of diagnosis and/or treatment of osteoporosis was the primary outcome. *Results.* The study cohort consisted of 215 women over a 3-year study period, of which 101 (47%) had evidence of osteoporosis by CT scan criteria. There were no differences in injury severity score, hospital length of stay, cost, or discharge disposition between groups with and without evidence of osteoporosis. Only 55 (59%) of the 94 patients with osteoporosis who survived to discharge had a documented osteoporosis diagnosis and/or corresponding evaluation/treatment plan. *Conclusion.* Nearly half of older women admitted with traumatic injuries had underlying osteoporosis, but 41% had neither clinical recognition of this finding nor a treatment plan for osteoporosis. Admission for traumatic injury is an opportunity to assess osteoporosis, initiate appropriate intervention, and coordinate follow-up care. Trauma and acute care teams should consider assessment of osteoporosis in women who undergo CT imaging and provide a bridge to outpatient services.

1. Introduction

Adults aged 65 and older constitute over 25% of trauma related admissions and are the fastest growing trauma patient population, with a significant proportion sustaining fractures [1]. Osteoporotic fractures, particularly hip fracture, are a significant cause of morbidity and mortality in these patients [2]. Older women are particularly vulnerable to osteoporosis as declining estrogen contributes to an increased rate of bone loss and thus reduced bone mineral density (BMD) that contributes to fracture risk. As the population ages, osteoporosis is a growing individual and public health concern with more than 40 million Americans at risk for this diagnosis [2–4]. The lifetime risk of developing a fracture in patients with underlying osteoporosis is estimated to be up to 50% in women and 20% in men [2].

Over 80 million CT scans are performed annually in the United States and many of these scans are performed on older patients who have undiagnosed chronic conditions. In the routine evaluation of patients with traumatic injury, thorough imaging via computed tomography (CT) is often obtained [5]. Nevertheless, the implications of routine opportunistic utilization of CT scans for the assessment of osteoporosis in acute care settings have not been previously evaluated. Aside from the immediate needs of addressing traumatic injury, harnessing the diagnostic power of routine evaluations in acute care settings may provide significant health and cost benefits.

This repurposing of diagnostic imaging is not a new idea. CT-derived BMD is an established method to identify chronic bone loss, diagnose vertebral fractures, and improve reliability of BMD estimates in patients with aortic calcification [6]. Others have reported diagnosing osteopenia and osteoporosis with CT scans ordered for other reasons and noted substantial opportunities for savings with respect to obviating the expense of additional imaging and the cost of preventable fractures [7, 8].

The use of computed tomography to evaluate bone mineral density has been broadly described, although it has not been widely accepted as a gold standard for routine outpatient screening. Specifically, Pickhardt et al. compared CT-derived BMD to Dual Energy X-ray Absorptiometry (DXA) measures in over 2000 paired comparisons and found highly predictive values for osteoporosis diagnosis (area under the curve [AUC] = 0.83, 95% CI 0.81–0.85) [8]. Subsequent authors have independently demonstrated significant predictive values and correlations between DXA and CT [7, 9–11].

The US Preventive Service Task Force (USPSTF) recommends that all women over 65 years of age should be screened for osteoporosis and that women below 65 years of age should be tested in the presence of additional risk fractures, such as a fragility fracture [2, 3]. Despite these guidelines, many older women do not undergo formal BMD evaluation, even in the context of falls or known fall risk [1, 2].

The purpose of this study was to assess the prevalence of osteoporosis by opportunistic CT imaging in older adult women admitted for trauma, a high-risk population, and measure recognition of this chronic disease by acute care providers in a safety-net hospital.

2. Methods

2.1. Study Design and Participants. This retrospective cohort study included all women of age ≥ 65 who were in-state residents, sustained traumatic injury without serious head injury (maximum head abbreviated injury severity [AIS] score < 3), had CT imaging of L1 within 7 days of admission, and were admitted to the intensive care unit (ICU) at a safety-net, level one trauma center from January 2011 to February 2014. Our target population was chosen because women are a traditionally at-risk population, with female to male 4 : 1 prevalence of osteoporosis in the US [2]. We also restricted our analysis to patients admitted to the ICU because severely injured patients were more likely to undergo truncal CT evaluation on admission. Inclusion of only in-state residents allowed for readmissions and mortality linkage using state registries as described below. Women who died within 24

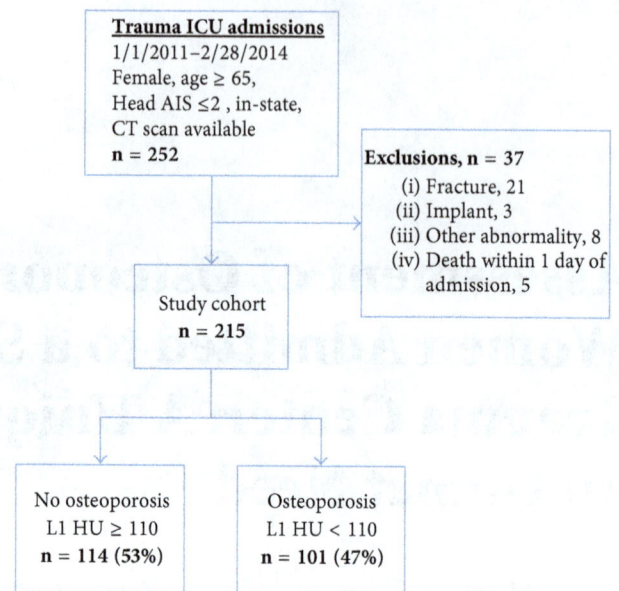

FIGURE 1: Flow diagram of study patients, showing inclusion and exclusion criteria, grouping of study cohort.

hours of admission or whose L1 imaging was inadequate for analysis were excluded (Figure 1).

2.2. Study Setting. This study was conducted at a level one trauma center, which serves the surrounding metropolitan area, state, and surrounding four-state region. In addition to being the only level one adult trauma, pediatric trauma, and burn center in the state, the facility also serves as the state's main safety-net hospital. Fifteen percent of the state population is ≥65 years old; 12% of the population is living in poverty (income below 100% of the federal poverty line). Sixty-two percent of patients visiting this hospital qualify for Medicaid or premium subsidies under the state Health Insurance Marketplace. Nearly 50% of the service population are members of racial and/or ethnic minorities; more than 8% are non-English speaking; and more than 2% are indigents without third-party coverage.

2.3. Definition of Osteoporosis by CT. Patients were divided into groups by presence or absence of osteoporosis, which was defined as average vertebral body Hounsfield units (HU) < 110 (90% specificity) as described by Pickard et al., 2013 [7, 8, 10, 11].

2.4. Covariates. Patient data, injury details, and clinical measures were queried through the state trauma registry. Ground-level falls were determined according to ICD-9 E codes (E880.1, E884.2, E884.3, E884.4, E884.6, E885.9, E888.1, and E888.8). To determine outcomes after trauma, the registry was linked to the Comprehensive Hospital Abstract Reporting System (CHARS), a statewide database that contains hospital admission information. Only the first nonelective readmission after the index trauma hospitalization was included (identified by categorization in CHARS).

Trauma Registry and CHARS datasets were further linked to the Washington State Death Registry to assess 30-day and 1-year mortality.

2.5. Evidence of Osteoporosis Recognition and Treatment by Inpatient Providers. Recognition of osteoporosis was ascertained from problem list; patient education materials; discharge summary; or treatment of osteoporosis (calcium, vitamin D, bisphosphonate, teriparatide, or denosumab) that was abstracted from the discharge medication list.

2.6. Image Analysis Protocol. In the sagittal midline plane, the L1 vertebral body was identified by locating the superior aspect of the sacrum and labeling the immediately superior vertebral body as L5. Identification of L1 was confirmed by absence of ribs at that level. T12 was utilized if L1 was excluded due to Genant Grade II or III compression fracture, neoplastic lesion, hemangioma, or any compromising abnormality that resulted in nonhomogenous bone. L2 was utilized if T12 required exclusion. The most superior axial plane of the chosen vertebral body, which minimized presence of cortical bone and excluded comprising abnormalities, was chosen. Vertebral BMD was assessed by placing a single elliptical region of interest (ROI) 100–120 mm^2 on the central part of the vertebral body excluding cortical bone, sclerotic bone, or fracture lines. Average HU measurement and SD from the selected vertebra was recorded. Intra- and Interrater reliability of HU measurements was confirmed using intraclass correlation coefficients utilizing the first 32 patients included in the study. The images were analyzed separately by a trauma radiologist (J. A. G.), a research scholar and surgical resident (S. J. K.), and a medical student (E. S. Y.). Intraclass correlation coefficients were 0.98 [95% Cl 0.96–0.99] for HU calculation and 0.99 [95% Cl 0.993–0.999] for axial image selection. All three evaluators excluded the same three patients due to a compromising abnormality.

2.7. Statistical Analysis. Data normality was evaluated with the Shapiro-Wilk test and histogram visualization. Continuous, normally distributed data are reported as mean ± standard deviation (SD) and compared between groups using the *t*-test. Discrete and skewed continuous data are reported as median (interquartile range [IQR]) and compared using the Mann–Whitney U test. Categorical data are reported as count (proportion) and compared using Pearson's χ^2 or Fisher's exact test, as appropriate. Confidence intervals for relative proportions of CT-identified osteoporosis and the subset of patients who did not have a diagnosis or medication listed in discharge data were calculated using the thresholds described by Pickhardt et al. [8]. All statistical calculations were performed with Stata/SE 14.1 (StataCorp LP, College Station, TX) using an a priori two-sided significance level of 0.05.

3. Results

Of the 252 women ≥ 65 years old who met inclusion criteria, 37 patients were excluded for death within 24 hours of admission (n = 5) or inadequate imaging/unusable vertebral bodies at or adjacent to the L1 level (n = 32). The remaining 215 comprised the study cohort. Using the threshold described above, 101 women (47%) retrospectively had evidence of osteoporosis by CT scan, leaving 114 (53%) without osteoporosis.

Women with osteoporosis were older (81.4 ± 8.2 versus 77.3 ± 8.3, p < 0.001) and more likely to have sustained a ground-level fall (41 [40.6%] versus 29 [25.4%], relative risk [RR] 1.59 [95% CI 1.08–2.36], p = 0.02). Demographics and clinical characteristics between osteoporotic and nonosteoporotic groups were otherwise relatively similar (Table 1). Twenty patients died in hospital. There were no differences between groups with regard to any of the following outcomes: hospital length of stay, discharge disposition, inpatient cost, 30-day readmission, 30-day mortality, and 1-year mortality.

Among survivors to discharge, 63 (67.0%) of osteoporotic patients were discharged to a skilled nursing facility (SNF) compared to 55 (54.5%) of nonosteoporotic patients. This difference approached significance on multivariate analysis (RR 1.23 [95% CI 0.98–1.55], p = 0.07).

Only 55 (59%) of the 94 patients with CT-identified osteoporosis who survived to discharge had a listed osteoporosis diagnosis and/or corresponding evaluation/treatment plan: 24 had a medication prescribed before their traumatic injury; the other 31 of 55 had a new medication prescribed at time of discharge. The remaining thirty-nine (41%) patients with retrospectively identified osteoporosis did not have a marker for the recognition of osteoporosis by the acute care team. Undiagnosed and untreated osteoporosis proportions did not differ markedly using more sensitive, less specific criteria (Table 2) [8]. Among women with retrospectively identified osteoporosis, the proportion of osteoporosis recognition did not differ between women who sustained a ground-level fall and those with other injury mechanisms (17 [45%] versus 22 [39%], p = 0.60).

4. Discussion

In this retrospective study, we utilized routine admission CT in an opportunistic fashion to evaluate older women for low L1 BMD. We found that nearly half of those admitted for traumatic injuries had underlying osteoporosis using the most specific of criteria of <110 HU. However, 41% of those women did not have documentation conveying this finding, either in the discharge summary or problem list, or the documentation of medications used to treat osteoporosis. Of the women with evidence of osteoporosis by CT, we found that just 12% were deemed osteoporotic in the problem list or discharge summary.

DXA remains the objective gold standard in BMD assessment (osteoporosis defined as a T-score of <−2.5) during routine outpatient care. Despite increased fracture risk and increased mortality in the population with falls, screening for chronic bone loss remains underutilized even in this patient population [1, 12]. It is worth noting that DXA is not reimbursed in the inpatient setting and is largely delegated to outpatient providers. As a result, appropriate follow-up for this chronic disease is susceptible to the communication

TABLE 1: Patient demographics and clinical characteristics.

	No osteoporosis (L1 HU ≥ 110) N = 114	Osteoporosis (L1 HU < 110) N = 101	p value
Age, years	77.3 ± 8.3	81.4 ± 8.2	<0.001
CCI, score	0 (0–2)	1 (0–2)	0.08
Type of injury			
Fall	62 (54.4)	61 (60.4)	
Blunt	49 (43.0)	38 (37.6)	0.76
Penetrating	1 (0.9)	0	
Other	2 (1.8)	2 (2.0)	
Ground-level fall	29 (25.4)	41 (40.6)	0.02
ISS	14 (10–21)	14 (10–18)	0.67
Head AIS			
0	86 (75.4)	82 (81.2)	0.51
1	4 (3.5)	4 (4.0)	
2	24 (21.1)	15 (14.9)	
Received mechanical ventilation	33 (29.0)	23 (22.8)	0.30
ICU LOS, days	2.3 (1.3–4.7)	2.2 (1.5–4.7)	0.75
Hospital LOS, days	6 (4–10)	7 (5–11)	0.20
Disposition			
Home with assist	3 (2.6)	4 (4.0)	
Home	37 (32.5)	25 (24.8)	
Outpatient acute care	1 (0.9)	1 (1.0)	0.21
Rehab	5 (4.4)	1 (1.0)	
SNF	55 (48.3)	63 (62.4)	
In-hospital death	13 (11.4)	7 (6.9)	
Inpatient Cost, $1k	29.3 (17.1–47.7)	29.8 (17.3–51.7)	0.79
Discharged with either osteoporosis diagnosis or medication[a]	42 (41.6)	55 (58.5)	0.02
Preadmission diagnosis/medication	22 (46.8)	26 (45.6)	0.90
New diagnosis/medication	25 (53.2)	31 (54.4)	
Readmission within 30 days[b]	19 (19.8)	18 (19.4)	0.94
30-day mortality[b]	1 (1.0)	3 (3.2)	0.36
1-year mortality[b]	5 (5.2)	8 (8.6)	0.36

Data displayed as n (%) for categorical data; mean ± standard deviation for continuous, normally distributed data; and median (interquartile range) for discrete or nonnormally distributed continuous data; HU, Hounsfield unit; CCI, updated Charlson Comorbidity Index; ISS, injury severity score; AIS, abbreviated injury score; ICU, intensive care unit; LOS, length of stay; SNF, skilled nursing facility. [a]Among the 195 patients who survived to discharge; [b]among the 189 patients who survived to discharge and have readmission/mortality data available.

TABLE 2: Frequencies and proportion estimates of osteoporosis diagnosis via retrospective CT stratified by diagnostic threshold.

Osteoporosis diagnostic threshold	Patients with osteoporosis by retrospective CT diagnosis		Patients with osteoporosis but without diagnosis or medication in discharge data[a]	
Average HU	N	% (95% CI)	N	% (95% CI)
<110	94	48 (41–55)	39	41 (32–52)
<135	142	73 (66–79)	66	46 (38–55)
<160	169	87 (81–91)	79	47 (39–54)

CT, computed tomography; HU, Hounsfield unit; CI, confidence interval. [a]Among the 195 patients who survived to discharge.

breakdowns that are common when transitioning from inpatient to outpatient settings [13].

Of the 94 women with evidence of osteoporosis by CT who survived to discharge, only 31 (31%) were prescribed new medications during admission and only 26 (25%) were on previously prescribed medications that could benefit osteoporosis. It is possible that some acute care providers deferred initiation of bone modifying medications, such as bisphosphonates, because of the theoretical concern that these medications impair fracture healing [14, 15]. In order to improve sensitivity, we also included vitamin D and/or calcium as additional surrogates for initiation of osteoporosis treatment. Still, a substantial number of older women with osteoporosis did not receive any medications to promote bone health.

Of note, there were also a number of patients who did not meet the CT-based threshold for osteoporosis but yet had evidence of osteoporosis recognition based on their medication list or diagnosis list (42 [41%] among survivors to discharge). This is likely an effect of the highly specific, but poorly sensitive HU-based threshold of 110. When more sensitive thresholds are considered, more patients are considered osteoporotic (Table 2). However, regardless of threshold used, the estimated proportion of patients with osteoporosis by CT criteria who are discharged without medications or formal diagnoses remains between 41 and 47% in this study cohort.

Osteoporosis evaluation and treatment is largely considered within the purview of primary care: a perspective that may explain the limited evaluation and treatment initiation in an at-risk population during an admission for trauma. Multiple investigations have focused on improving the transition to outpatient care and referral for evaluation of osteoporosis after discharge [16, 17]. These studies have demonstrated improved treatment and evaluation with such methods as a dedicated osteoporosis health professional, fracture liaison nurse, or a letter to the patient's primary care provider. However, diagnosis by CT-derived BMD could streamline initiation of interventions, reduce risk of missed communication, and provide considerable cost savings.

Fragility fractures are a significant public health issue and treatment of osteoporosis has been found to be effective in reducing morbidities, such as secondary fracture prevention [18, 19]. Many of the organizations and countries that have financial responsibility for covered lives have instituted formal protocols for identifying and treating fragility fractures and osteoporosis, ultimately to the benefit of the patient [20, 21]. The ability to utilize existing CT scans to assess osteoporosis could be beneficial for patients and the health care system. Simply providing patients with information regarding their diagnosis of osteoporosis improves the likelihood that a patient will have their osteoporosis addressed by their primary care provider [22].

Opportunistic diagnosis of osteoporosis using CT scans could also serve an unmet need in hospitals that serve as a safety-net, such as ours [23]. By definition, safety-net hospitals serve low income, medically, and socially vulnerable patients regardless of their ability to pay. Economically disadvantaged individuals with chronic conditions have high rates of readmission and emergency department usage following initial hospitalization. Additionally, this population faces greater challenges in receiving pre- and postinjury care [24]. Point-of-care diagnosis could be valuable in the acute care setting, as hospitalization is an opportunity for the patient to be assessed for osteoporosis by CT BMD in a cost- and time-effective manner. Recognition of low BMD as part of trauma care may improve care transitions and lead to efficient arrangement of subsequent interventions and appointments. In a safety-net hospital, CT could also provide an early diagnosis of bone loss in the late-middle age population (55–64 years of age), who do not typically qualify for insurance coverage of outpatient DXA [2, 25].

The present study has several limitations. It is retrospective and excludes patients without imaging, which contributed to a smaller sample size. Participants are exclusively from an ICU population, so severity of injuries is greater than that of a typical population of older adults admitted with trauma. We note that patients admitted to general orthopedic services, especially those with medicine comanagement, are more likely to receive a diagnosis and subsequent plan of care for osteoporosis.

5. Conclusion

Trauma patients often undergo routine CT imaging, which provides a unique opportunity to diagnose older women with osteoporosis. Osteoporosis poses a significant risk factor for fractures, future falls, and death. Trauma and other acute care teams should consider using opportunistic imaging to assess older women for osteoporosis, especially those in safety-net settings, and provide a bridge to outpatient services.

Disclosure

The content is solely the responsibility of the authors and does not necessarily represent the official views of the sponsoring institutions or supporting agencies.

Acknowledgments

The authors wish to acknowledge Mamatha Damodarasamy for assistance with the manuscript and Zeyno Shorter, Ph.D., MPH, for data acquisition. Additionally, they thank Itay Bentov, MD, Ph.D., Steven H. Mitchell, MD, and Saman Arbabi, MD, MPH, and the Geriatric Injury Workgroup at Harborview Medical Center, for their assistance on this project. This work was supported in part by the John A. Hartford Foundation Center of Excellence in Geriatric Medicine and Training at the University of Washington, the Medical Student Training in Aging Research Program at the University of California, Los Angeles, and the Patterson Surgery Research Endowment at Benaroya Research Institute/Virginia Mason.

References

[1] P. Ayoung-Chee, L. McIntyre, B. E. Ebel, C. D. MacK, W. McCormick, and R. V. Maier, "Long-term outcomes of ground-level falls in the elderly," *Journal of Trauma and Acute Care Surgery*, vol. 76, no. 2, pp. 498–503, 2014.

[2] K. E. Ensrud and C. J. Crandall, "Osteoporosis," *Annals of Internal Medicine*, vol. 167, no. 3, pp. ITC17–ITC32, 2017.

[3] U.S. Preventive Services Task Force, "Screening for osteoporosis: U.S. Preventive Services Task Force recommendation statement," *Annals of Internal Medicine*, vol. 154, no. 5, pp. 356–364, 2011.

[4] N. C. Wright, A. C. Looker, K. G. Saag et al., "The recent prevalence of osteoporosis and low bone mass in the United States based on bone mineral density at the femoral neck or lumbar," *Journal of Bone and Mineral Research*, vol. 29, no. 11, pp. 2520–2526, 2014.

[5] S. J. Kaplan, T. N. Pham, S. Arbabi et al., "Association of radiologic indicators of frailty with 1-year mortality in older trauma patients: Opportunistic screening for sarcopenia and osteopenia," *JAMA Surgery*, vol. 152, no. 2, article e164604, 2017.

[6] S. Kinsella, K. Murphy, M. Breen et al., "Comparison of single CT scan assessment of bone mineral density, vascular calcification and fat mass with standard clinical measurements in renal transplant subjects: The ABC HeART study," *BMC Nephrology*, vol. 16, no. 1, article 188, 2015.

[7] C. F. Buckens, G. Dijkhuis, B. de Keizer, H. J. Verhaar, and P. A. de Jong, "Opportunistic screening for osteoporosis on routine computed tomography? An external validation study," *European Radiology*, vol. 25, no. 7, pp. 2074–2079, 2015.

[8] P. J. Pickhardt, B. D. Pooler, T. Lauder, A. M. del Rio, R. J. Bruce, and N. Binkley, "Opportunistic screening for osteoporosis using abdominal computed tomography scans obtained for other indications," *Annals of Internal Medicine*, vol. 158, no. 8, pp. 588–595, 2013.

[9] O. Emohare, M. Wiggin, P. Hemmati, and J. Switzer, "Assessing bone mineral density following acute hip fractures: the role of computed tomography attenuation," *Geriatric Orthopaedic Surgery & Rehabilitation*, vol. 6, no. 1, pp. 16–21, 2015.

[10] M. K. Choi, S. M. Kim, and J. K. Lim, "Diagnostic efficacy of Hounsfield units in spine CT for the assessment of real bone mineral density of degenerative spine: correlation study between T-scores determined by DEXA scan and Hounsfield units from CT," *Acta Neurochirurgica*, vol. 158, no. 7, pp. 1421–1427, 2016.

[11] S. Y. Lee, S.-S. Kwon, H. S. Kim et al., "Reliability and validity of lower extremity computed tomography as a screening tool for osteoporosis," *Osteoporosis International*, vol. 26, no. 4, pp. 1387–1394, 2015.

[12] D. Bliuc, D. Alarkawi, T. V. Nguyen, J. A. Eisman, and J. R. Center, "Risk of subsequent fractures and mortality in elderly women and men with fragility fractures with and without osteoporotic bone density: The dubbo osteoporosis epidemiology study," *Journal of Bone and Mineral Research*, vol. 30, no. 4, pp. 637–646, 2015.

[13] C. J. Yates, M.-A. Chauchard, D. Liew, A. Bucknill, and J. D. Wark, "Bridging the osteoporosis treatment gap: Performance and cost-effectiveness of a fracture liaison service," *Journal of Clinical Densitometry*, vol. 18, no. 2, pp. 150–156, 2015.

[14] S. Larsson and N. L. Fazzalari, "Anti-osteoporosis therapy and fracture healing," *Archives of Orthopaedic and Trauma Surgery*, vol. 134, no. 2, pp. 291–297, 2014.

[15] V. Hegde, J. E. Jo, P. Andreopoulou, and J. M. Lane, "Effect of osteoporosis medications on fracture healing," *Osteoporosis International*, vol. 27, no. 3, pp. 861–871, 2016.

[16] K. Bell, H. Strand, and W. J. Inder, "Effect of a dedicated osteoporosis health professional on screening and treatment in outpatients presenting with acute low trauma non-hip fracture: a systematic review," *Archives of Osteoporosis*, vol. 9, article 167, 2014.

[17] W. W. Hung, K. A. Egol, J. D. Zuckerman, and A. L. Siu, "Hip fracture management: Tailoring care for the older patient," *Journal of the American Medical Association*, vol. 307, no. 20, pp. 2185–2194, 2012.

[18] H. S. Bawa, J. Weick, and D. R. Dirschl, "Anti-osteoporotic therapy after fragility fracture lowers rate of subsequent fracture: Analysis of a large population sample: Analysis of a large population sample," *Journal of Bone and Joint Surgery - American Volume*, vol. 97, no. 19, pp. 1555–1562, 2014.

[19] E. F. Ekman, "The role of the orthopaedic surgeon in minimizing mortality and morbidity associated with fragility fractures," *American Academy of Orthopaedic Surgeon*, vol. 18, no. 5, pp. 278–285, 2010.

[20] S. Drew, S. Sheard, J. Chana, C. Cooper, M. K. Javaid, and A. Judge, "Describing variation in the delivery of secondary fracture prevention after hip fracture: an overview of 11 hospitals within one regional area in England," *Osteoporosis International*, vol. 25, no. 10, pp. 2427–2433, 2014.

[21] K. Ganda, M. Puech, J. S. Chen et al., "Models of care for the secondary prevention of osteoporotic fractures: a systematic review and meta-analysis," *Osteoporosis International*, vol. 24, no. 2, pp. 393–406, 2013.

[22] M. J. Gardner, R. H. Brophy, D. Demetrakopoulos et al., "Interventions to improve osteoporosis treatment following hip fracture: a prospective, randomized trial," *The Journal of Bone & Joint Surgery—American Volume*, vol. 87, no. 1, pp. 3–7, 2005.

[23] R. V. Maier, "Seattle's Harborview Medical Center, 1877–2003," *Archives of Surgery*, vol. 139, no. 1, pp. 14-15, 2004.

[24] S. Hewner, S. Casucci, and J. Castner, "The roles of chronic disease complexity, health system integration, and care management in post-discharge healthcare utilization in a low-income population," *Research in Nursing & Health*, vol. 39, no. 4, pp. 215–228, 2016.

[25] S. Nayak, M. S. Roberts, and S. L. Greenspan, "Cost-effectiveness of different screening strategies for osteoporosis in postmenopausal women," *Annals of Internal Medicine*, vol. 155, no. 11, pp. 751–761, 2011.

23

Investigation of Geriatric Patients with Abdominal Pain Admitted to Emergency Department

Pınar Henden Çam ⓘ,[1] Ahmet Baydin ⓘ,[1] Savaş Yürüker,[2] Ali Kemal Erenler ⓘ,[3] and Erdinç Şengüldür[1]

[1]*Ondokuz Mayıs University, Department of Emergency Medicine, Samsun, Turkey*
[2]*Ondokuz Mayıs University, Department of General Surgery, Samsun, Turkey*
[3]*Hitit University, Department of Emergency Medicine, Çorum, Turkey*

Correspondence should be addressed to Pınar Henden Çam; drhenden@yahoo.com

Academic Editor: Jacek Witkowski

Introduction. The aim of this study is to detect the possible reasons of abdominal pain in the patients aged 65 and older admitted to emergency department (ED) with complaint of abdominal pain which is not related to trauma, to determine the length of hospitalization of old (65–75 age) and elderly (aged 75 and older) patients, and to define the hospitalization and mortality rates. *Material and Methods.* In the study, 336 patients were included. Groups were compared in respect to gender, internal or surgical prediagnoses, complaints accompanying abdominal pain, vital findings, comorbidities, requested consultations, hospitalizing service, waiting time in the ED and in the hospital, and treatment methods. *Results.* Of the patients, 48.2% were male, and 51.8% were female. While 52.4% of the patients were in 65–74 age group, 47.6% of them were aged 75 years and above. An internal disease was detected in 76.8% of the patients as an origin of abdominal pain. Most common prediagnoses were biliary diseases and diseases related to biliary tract followed by nonspecific abdominal pain, abdominal pain secondary to malignity, ileus, and acute gastroenteritis, respectively. The most frequent finding accompanying abdominal pain was vomiting. The most frequent chronic disease accompanying abdominal pain was hypertension in both age groups. We observed that 75.9% of the patients required consultation. We detected that 48.8% of the patients with abdominal pain were hospitalized and they were hospitalized mostly by gastroenterology ward (24.8%). Surgical treatments were applied to the 17.6% of the patients with abdominal pain. *Conclusion.* Clinical findings become indistinct by age, and differential diagnosis of abdominal pain gets more difficult in geriatric patients. Therefore, physicians should consider age related physiological changes in order to distinguish geriatric patients admitted to emergency service with abdominal pain from pathological cases requiring immediate surgical operation.

1. Introduction

The number of elderly people (≥65 years old) is increasing both in Turkey and internationally due to improved living conditions and decreased mortality rates. Knowing the characteristics of elderly patients admitted to emergency departments can provide guidance for diagnosis and treatment approaches [1]. As the number of elderly patients increases, the number of elderly patients admitted to the EDs increases. Various studies have shown that percentage of geriatric patients admitted to EDs vary between 9 and 19% and these patients are known to present with more severe clinical situation when compared to younger patients [2–5]. While abdominal pain is about 10% of all complaints presenting to EDs, 20% of these patients are known to be geriatric patients. More than half of these patients are being hospitalized and surgical intervention is performed to 1/3 of the patients. Fagbohun et al. reported that biliary system diseases are the most common source of abdominal pain and the primary reason for surgery [6]. Mortality rate for patients older than 65 years has been reported to vary between 11 and 14%. Mc Namara et al. reported that reasons for high mortality rate in geriatric patients were related to comorbidities, former surgical procedures, multiple drug use, impotent immune system, and delayed recognition of serious conditions in the ED [7]. Despite improvements in management of geriatric patients in the ED, geriatric patients remain to be a clinical challenge for ED physicians. In this study, our aim was to investigate reasons, prevalence, hospitalization rates, demographic features, and morbidity and mortality rates of patients older than 65 years admitted to our ED due to abdominal pain and guide physicians and hospital managers in geriatric patient care.

2. Material and Methods

After ethical approval, medical records of patients older than 65 years admitted to our ED with abdominal pain in the last year were investigated retrospectively. Inclusion criteria were patients with abdominal pain older than 65 years. Medical records of the patients were detected for age, gender, vital signs, complaints accompanying abdominal pain (nausea-vomiting, loss of appetite, constipation, intestinal gas extraction inability, diarrhea, dysuria, jaundice), comorbidities, duration of abdominal pain, length of ED stay (0–6, 6–12, 12–24 and over 24 hours), prediagnosis in the ED, consultations required (internal medicine, general surgery, urology, gynecology, etc.), wards that the patients were admitted to (ED, internal medicine, general surgery, intensive care, etc.), length of stay (LOS) of the patients in the hospital (1 day, 1–4 days, 4–10 days, more than 10 days), choice of treatment (medical, surgical), and outcomes (recovery, vegetative stage, exitus). The patients were divided into subgroups according to age (65–74 years and above 75 years) and diagnoses (medical and surgical). Patients under 65 years and with traumatic abdominal pain were excluded from the study.

Data were analyzed using Statistical Package for Social Sciences (SPSS) for Windows® 21.0 programme. Frequency (n) and percentage (%) were given for categorical variables. Median, minimum, and maximum values were given for continuous variables. In comparison of categorical variables, Pearson's chi-square test and Student T-test were used. For comparison of body temperature between patient groups, Mann–Whitney U test was used. $p < 0.05$ was considered as statistically significant.

3. Results

Into the study, 336 patients over 65 years with abdominal pain were included between the study periods. Of the patients, 162 were male (48.2%) and 174 female (51.8%). While 176 patients were involved in 65–74 years group (52.4%), 160 were involved in 75 years and above group (47.6%).

Mean age of the patients was 74.8 ± 6.5 years (min: 65 years, max: 96 years). While mean age of female patients was 75.3 ± 6.0, mean age of male patients was 74.2 ± 6.0. Mean age of the patients according to gender was not statistically significant ($p > 0.05$). Comparison of patient characteristics according to age groups is summarized in Table 1.

When source of abdominal pain was investigated, 258 patients had a medical source (76.8%) and 78 had a surgical source (23.2%). Of the patients with medical diagnoses, 53.5%

were in 65–74 years group and 46.5% were in 75 years and above group. Of the patients with surgical diagnoses, 48.7% were in 65–74 years group and 51.3% were in 75 years and above group. No statistical significance could be determined when patients were investigated according to age, gender, and source of abdominal pain ($p > 0.05$). When complaints accompanying abdominal pain were compared between age groups, no statistical significance could be determined.

When complaints accompanying abdominal pain were compared, nausea/vomiting and gas extraction inability were found to be statistically significant in males ($p < 0.05$).

Additionally, when complaints were compared as medical and surgical sources, diarrhea, jaundice in medical sources, and gas extraction inability in surgical sources were found significantly higher ($p > 0.05$). Table 2 summarizes the findings of the patients in respect to sources of the diseases.

In 77.4% of the patients, a chronic illness was determined. Cerebrovascular diseases (CVD) were statistically significant in patient group above 75 years ($p = 0.027$).

When chronic diseases were compared according to gender, hypertension (HT) in males and Diabetes Mellitus (DM) and congestive heart failure (CHF) in females were found to be statistically significant ($p < 0.05$).

When accompanying diseases were compared between medical and surgical sources of abdominal pain, HT and liver cirrhosis were significant in medical sources ($p < 0.05$).

Mean values of vital signs of the patients on admission to ED were as follows: systolic blood pressure: 120.0 ± 20.4 mmHg, heart beat: 84.0 ± 13.4 beats/minute, and temperature: 36.6 ± 0.6°C. Blood pressure was found to be significantly higher in females than males ($p = 0.008$).

When medical histories of the patients were investigated, it was determined that 29.8% of the patients have undergone surgery in the past. Malignity was the leading cause for surgery (8%), followed by cholecystectomy (7.1%) and appendectomy (2.9%).

When patients were classified according to duration of abdominal pain (less than 24 hours, more than 24 hours), no statistical significance could be determined between gender, age, and prediagnoses.

For 265 patients (75.9%), a consultation was required. Of the patients admitted, 133 (50.2%) were in 65–74 age group and 132 (49.8%) were in 75 age and above group. When consultations were investigated, 118 (44.5%) patients consulted with internal medicine specialists, 72 (27.2%) with general surgery specialists, 50 (18.9%) with both internal medicine and general surgery specialists, and 25 (9.4%) with other specialists.

The most common diagnosis was biliary and biliary tract diseases (19.6%) followed by nonspecific abdominal pain (11.9%) and abdominal pain related to malignity (9.8%). Subgroups of biliary and biliary tract diseases were choledocholithiasis (11.3%), cholangitis (5.1%), cholecystitis (2.1%), and cholelithiasis (1.2%).

Of the patients, 164 (48.8%) were hospitalized, 131 (39.0%) were discharged from ED, and 41 (12.2%) have died. Of those who were discharged, 107 (81.7%) were discharged with full recovery and 24 (18.3%) rejected treatment and left the ED with written consent.

TABLE 1: Comparison of patient characteristics according to age groups.

Characteristics	Group I: 65–74 years (n, %)		Group II: above 75 years (n, %)	
Total patient number	176	52.4	160	47.6
Gender				
Male	94	58	68	42
Female	82	47.1	92	52.9
Vital signs				
Blood pressure (mmHg)	110 ± 19.09		120 ± 21.9	
Heart rate (beats/min)	80 ± 13.8		86 ± 12.8	
Fever	36.6 ± 0.7		36.6 ± 0.5	
Complaints accompanying abdominal pain				
Nausea	88	50,3	78	48.8
Vomiting	72	41,1	62	38.8
Loss of appetite	22	12.6	13	8.1
Constipation	28	16	17	10,6
Intestinal gas extraction inability	25	14,3	13	8,1
Diarrhea	19	10,9	18	11.3
Dysuria	19	10,9	16	9.4
Jaundice	19	10,9	19	11.9
Length of ED stay				
0–6 hours	74	42	68	42.5
6–12 hours	49	27.9	61	38.1
12–24 hours	24	13.7	11	6.9
Over 24 hours	29	16.4	20	12.5
Duration of abdominal pain				
0–24 hours	35	20	140	80
Over 24 hours	33	20.6	127	79.4
Length of stay in the hospital				
1 day	76	43.2	64	40
1–4 days	20	11.4	25	15.6
4–10 days	38	21.6	33	20.6
More than 10 days	42	23.8	38	23.8
Choice of treatment				
Medical	151	85.8	126	78.8
Surgical	25	14.2	34	21.2
Consultation				
Internal medicine	60	45.1	58	43.5
General surgery	35	26.3	37	28.2
Internal medicine and general surgery	22	16.5	28	21.4
Other consultations	16	12	9	6.9
Outcomes				
Recovery	73	41,5	58	36,3
Vegetative stage	88	50	76	47.5
Exitus	15	8.5	26	16.2

While majority of the geriatric patients (41.8%) were followed in the observation room of the ED, 24.7% were followed in gastroenterology and 17.6% were followed in general surgery wards.

When LOS of patients were investigated, majority of the patients were determined to stay 0–6 hours. Patients with abdominal pain of medical source had significantly longer LOS ($p < 0.05$).

TABLE 2: Comparison of groups according to diagnoses.

Characteristics	Internal prediagnoses (n, %)		Surgical prediagnoses (n, %)		p value
Total patient number	258	76.8	78	23.2	
Gender					
Male	121	46,9	41	52,6	
Female	137	53,1	37	47,4	
Vital signs					
Blood pressure (mmHg)		120 ± 19.1		$120 \pm 24,1$	
Heart rate (beats/min)		84 ± 12.7		84 ± 15.7	
Fever		36.6 ± 0.6		36.7 ± 0.5	
Complaints accompanying abdominal pain					
Nausea	123	47.7	43	55.1	
Vomiting	96	37.7	38	48.7	
Loss of appetite	31	12	4	5.1	
Constipation	31	12	14	17.9	
Inability to intestinal gas extraction	14	5,4	24	30.4	0,001
Diarrhea	34	13.2	3	3.8	0,021
Dysuria	28	10.9	7	9	
Jaundice	36	14	2	2.6	0,005
Length of ED stay					
0–6 hours	117	45,3	24	30,8	
6–12 hours	73	28,3	38	48,7	0,002
12–24 hours	25	9,7	10	12,8	
Over 24 hours	43	16.7	6	7,7	
Duration of abdominal pain					
0–24 hours	55	21,3	13	16,7	
Over 24 hours	203	78,7	65	83,3	
Length of stay in the hospital					
1 day	126	48.8	13	16,7	
1–4 days	30	11.6	15	19,2	0,001
4–10 days	48	18.6	23	29,5	
More than 10 days	54	21	27	34,6	
Choice of treatment					
Medical	251	97,3	26	33,3	0,001
Surgical	7	2,7	52	66,7	
Consultation					
Internal medicine	114	59,7	4	5,4	
General surgery	22	11,5	50	67,6	0,001
Internal medicine and general surgery	33	17,3	3	4,1	
Other consultations	22	11,5	17	23	
Outcomes					
Recovery	120	46,5	11	14,1	
Vegetative stage	113	43,8	51	65,4	0,001
Exitus	25	9,7	16	20,5	

Of the patients with a prediagnosis of medical source, 2.7% have undergone surgical treatment; of patients with a prediagnosis of surgical source, 26% have undergone medical treatment. We also determined that medical treatment was more likely to be performed when compared to surgical treatment in geriatric patients with abdominal pain.

4. Discussion

As the life expectancy of the community increases, number of geriatric patients admitted to EDs increases. Studies on geriatric patients have shown that rate of admission of geriatric patients to EDs varies between 9 and 15% [2, 5, 7, 8]. In our study, percentage of geriatric patients was found to be 21.2%. The reason of the high percentage in our study may be related to characteristics of our hospital as a district hospital that serves as a last step hospital to the city and surroundings.

When complaints of geriatric patients on admission to ED were investigated, Kılıçarslan et al. reported that the most common complaints were chest pain, abdominal pain, shortness of breath, and headache, respectively. Of the patients, 5.7% were admitted due to abdominal pain [9]. Gallenger et al. reported that 5–8% of complaints on admission to EDs were abdominal pain [10]. Additionally, in a study by Fagbohun et al. this rate was reported to be 10% [6]. In concordance with the literature, results of our study revealed that 4.4% of the geriatric patients were admitted due to abdominal pain to our ED.

In the literature, it was well-defined that majority of the patients presented to EDs are females [11–14]. Gardner et al. reported in a study that 60% of the patients were females [15]. Our studies also revealed that majority of the patients were females. Our study also revealed that mean age of women was higher than that of men. Longer life expectancy in women may be the reason for this finding.

The reason for abdominal pain in geriatric patients may originate from both biliary tract infection and pancreatitis. As age progresses, contraction ability of the gallbladder, in response to cholecystokinin enzyme, decreases. Additionally, increased cholesterol and phospholipid content of the bile causes gallbladder stones and increased biliary tract diameter results in biliary diseases [16–18]. In our study, we determined biliary tract diseases in 19.6% and pancreatitis in 4.8% of the patients. Another reason for high rate of biliary tract diseases is related to high transfer rate of the patients for Endoscopic Retrograde Cholangiopancreatography from surrounding cities.

In various studies, the most common complaint accompanying abdominal pain was reported to be nausea/vomiting [4, 11]. In our study, 20.8% of the patients were admitted due to isolated abdominal pain, and nausea and vomiting were the most common accompanying complaints. In surgical source group, gas and stool extraction inability was the most common complaint and this finding was compatible with the results of Staniland et al. [12]. This result is also compatible with the fact that biliary tract diseases are the most common diseases among elderly patients. Its typical clinical presentations are known to be fever, right upper quadrant pain, nausea, and vomiting [19].

In the literature, it was reported that 75–90% of the geriatric patients have a chronical illness [2, 20–22]. Loloğlu et al. reported that the most common chronical illnesses in geriatric patients were as follows: HT (40.8%), coronary artery disease (CAD) (26.6%), and DM (22.4%). In our study, 77.4% of the patients had a chronical illness. The most common illnesses in our study were HT (47.2%), DM (25.7%), and malignity (24%). We also determined that, in 75 years and above group, neurological diseases (Alzheimer's Disease, Parkinson, CVD, etc.) were more common than in 65–74 years group. This finding is reasonable because advanced age is known to be related to higher neurological disease incidence. It is well-described in the literature that HT is a common problem in geriatric patients with a prevalence as high as 60 to 80% [23]. In a study by Salvi et al., it was reported that the most common diagnoses in elderly patients were atrial fibrillation, congestive heart failure, pneumonia, and stroke [24]. In another study, mental status alterations were reported to be present in 1/4 of the elder patients [25]. Additionally, among these diagnoses, neoplasms were determined to have the highest risk for mortality [26].

It is known that the elderly tend to be exposed to infectious diseases, and high body temperature may be a late finding in this patient group [27]. Age is a risk factor for alterations in vital signs [1]. In our study, compatible with the literature, mean body temperature was found to be 36.6 ± 0.6°C. However, we could not find any significance in vital signs when patients were compared according to age groups.

The most common surgical source for abdominal pain in elderly was reported to be biliary and biliary tract diseases [7, 27]. Kauvar et al. reported that acute appendicitis was the third cause of abdominal pain in elderly requiring surgery [28]. In the literature, it is reported that ileus is determined in 10% of the patients with abdominal pain of surgical origin [29–31]. It was also reported that ileus was three times frequent in elderly when compared to younger patients [32]. In our study, the most common reasons for surgery history were malignity, cholecystectomy, and appendectomy. This finding may be related to advanced facilities on malignity surgery in our hospital.

Chronical analgesic use may obscure severity of abdominal pain in elderly [27]. Durukan et al. reported that delayed admittance to hospital in geriatric patients was common (after 97.1 ± 160.8 hours after the onset of the pain). They also reported that signs, symptoms, and findings in these patients might be insignificant, and defense and rigidity might be absent [4]. In our study, tenderness was determined in 79.4%, defense was determined in 20.9%, and rebound was determined in 10.4% of the patients. In concordance with the findings of Pappas et al. [33], abdominal pain in our patients was determined to occur within 24 hours.

The leading lethal condition in patients with abdominal pain is known to be abdominal aortic aneurysm (AAA) rupture [27]. Bengtsson et al. reported that AAA rupture has a prevalence of 2–4% in patients under 50 years. However, prevalence rises up to 10% in patients over 50 years [34]. Another lethal condition in elderly is known to be mesentery ischemia [35]. Despite improvement in diagnostic tests, mortality in mesentery ischemia remains as 60–90% [36, 37].

In our study, 0.3% of our patients had AAA and 3 of our patients had mesentery ischemia. Those with a diagnosis of mesentery ischemia have died after surgery.

It is fact that threshold for consultation in geriatric patients is recommended to be low [7]. Mert et al. reported that 45.4% of the patients with abdominal pain consulted with internal medicine and/or general surgery specialists. It was also reported that the number of consultations was higher in patients above 65 years [1]. In our study a consultation was required for 75.9% of the patients. The higher rate in our study is related to our study design. We only included geriatric patients into our study and consultation rates appeared to be high.

Nonspecific abdominal pain—abdominal pain without a specific origin—is common among young patients. Bavunoğlu et al. reported that nonspecific abdominal pain is seen in less than 15% of geriatric patients [38]. Gün et al. reported in a study that the cause of abdominal pain in 30.6% of the geriatric patients could not be determined and these patients were diagnosed with nonspecific abdominal pain [39]. In our study, incidence of nonspecific abdominal pain was found to be 11.9%. When all ages are considered, nonspecific abdominal pain is the most common complaint in ED; however, in the elderly, biliary tract diseases are known to be more common [40]. Our findings are compatible with the literature.

As age advances, infectious diseases are seen more frequently in elderly patients due to immune system weakening [4]. Our study revealed that the most frequent infectious disease was gastroenteritis followed by urinary tract infections. However, in a study, Saçar et al. reported that urinary tract infection was the most common infection followed by gastroenteritis in geriatric patients [41].

It is well-known that acute appendicitis is more common in young patients when compared to geriatric patients. Numerous studies revealed that the frequency of acute appendicitis in geriatric patients is 5–10% [5, 42, 43]. Durukan et al. reported this rate as 4.5% in their study [4]. In our study, 1.8% of the patients had appendicitis and majority of the patients were involved in 65–74 age group. This finding is compatible with previous findings that incidence of appendicitis decreases by age.

In a study, Türker et al. reported that 33% of the patients with abdominal pain have been discharged with full recovery following medical treatment. Of these patients, 18.4% were discharged for outpatient follow-up, 18.7% were hospitalized in general surgery ward, 9.4% were hospitalized in internal medicine ward, 4.5% were discharged following ED observation, 1.9% left the ED voluntarily, and 0.4% have died [44]. In another study, in 45–64 age group, discharge rate from the ED was reported as 78.6% and hospitalization rate was reported to be 19.6%, while in 65 years and above group, discharge rate from the ED was reported to be 51.7% and hospitalization rate was reported to be 44.5% [1]. In our study, 41.7% of the patients were discharged from the ED, 48.8% were hospitalized, and 12.2% have died. Higher rates of hospitalization and mortality in our study may be related to higher incidence of concomitant chronical illnesses and admittance of patients with bad general condition.

In the literature, it is reported that mortality rates in geriatric patients related to emergency surgery vary between 11% and 37% [45–47]. In our study, mortality rate related to abdominal pain of medical origin was 9.7% and of surgical origin was 20.5%. In the literature there is an ongoing controversy about relationship between gender and mortality. Ağalar et al. reported that mortality rate in males is high when compared to females [48]. However, Reis et al. reported that gender did not have any influence on mortality rates [49]. In our study, mortality rate was found to be higher in both 75 years and above group and female gender.

In our study, the most common ward where the patients were hospitalized was found to be internal medicine, particularly gastroenterology ward. It was previously reported that hospitalization rates of patients with abdominal pain vary between 18.9% and 63.2% [4, 5, 43]. Pappas et al. reported that patients above 65 years were more likely to be hospitalized in internal medicine wards [42]. Mert et al. reported that general surgery was the most commonly preferred ward for patients with abdominal pain [1].

In a report by Chan et al., it was stated that 1.4–2.9% of the patients admitted to EDs leave the ED without being seen by a physician due to prolonged LOS in the ED [50]. This rate was reported to be 1% by Serinken et al. [51]. In our study, 68% of the patients had to wait more than 6 hours in the ED. Of the patients, 7.1% refused treatment and left the ED. While refusal rate in patients with abdominal pain of medical origin was found to be 8.5%, it was 2.6% in surgical origin group. This may be a result of prolonged LOS and delay in diagnosis of patients with abdominal pain of medical origin.

In the literature, medical treatment is the most common treatment method in geriatric patients with abdominal pain [42, 52, 53]. On the contrary, Pappas et al. could not find any difference between medical and surgical procedures in patients under 65 and above 65 years [33]. In our study, we determined that surgical treatment was performed to 17.6% of our patients. In 65–74 years group, surgery rate was 14.2%, and in 75 years and above group, surgery rate was 21.2%.

5. Conclusion

Results of our study revealed that the most common cause for abdominal pain in geriatric patients is biliary tract disorders. We also determined that majority of the patients with abdominal pain have a concomitant chronical illness. The most common complaints accompanying abdominal pain are nausea/vomiting and gas extraction inability. Mortality rate in geriatric patients with abdominal pain is 12.2% and higher in males. As the age advances, both rates of surgical procedures and mortality rate increase.

References

[1] D. K. Mert, "Acil servise karın ağrısı şikayeti ile başvuran 45–64 yaş ile 65 yaş ve üzerihastaların karşılaştırılması ve tanılarının fizyolojik değişikliklerle ilişkisinin değerlendirilmesi," *Uludağ Üniversitesi Tıp Fakültesi Acil Tıp Anabilim Dalı, Bursa, Uzmanlık Tezi*, pp. 1–35, 2014.

[2] A. Loloğlu, L. Ayrik, C. Köse et al., "Acil servise başvuran travma dışı geriatrik olguların demografik özelliklerinin incelenmesi," *Turkish Journal of Emergency Medicine*, pp. 13–171, 2013.

[3] G. R. Strange, E. H. Chen, and A. B. Sanders, "Use of emergency departments by elderly patients: Projections from a multicenter data base," *Annals of Emergency Medicine*, vol. 21, no. 7, pp. 819–824, 1992.

[4] P. Durukan, M. Yildiz, and Y. Çevik, "Acil servise karın ağrısıyla başvuran yaşlı hastaların değerlendirilmesi," *Türk Geriatri Dergisi*, vol. 8, pp. 111–114, 2005.

[5] A. Ünsal, A. A. Çevik, S. Metintaş et al., "Yaşlı hastaların acil servis başvuruları," *Türk Geriatri Dergisi*, vol. 6, pp. 83–88, 2003.

[6] C. F. Fagbohun, E. C. Toy, and B. Baker III, "The evaluation of acute abdominal pain in the elderly patient," *Primary Care Update for OB/GYNS*, vol. 6, no. 6, pp. 181–185, 1999.

[7] R. McNamara, "Abdominal pain in the elderly," in *Emergency Medicine; A Comprehensive Study Guide*, J. E. Tintinalli, G. D. Kelen, and J. S. Stapczynski, Eds., pp. 515–519, McGraw-Hill, New York, NY, USA, 5th edition, 2000.

[8] E. Mert, "Geriatrik hastaların acil servis kullanımı," *Turk Geriatri Dergisi*, vol. 9, pp. 70–74, 2006.

[9] I. Kilicaslan, H. Bozan, C. Oktay, and E. Goksu, "Demographic properties of patients presenting to the emergency department in Turkey," *Turkish Journal of Emergency Medicine*, vol. 5, pp. 5–13, 2005.

[10] E. J. Gallenger, "Gastrointestinal emergency: Acute abdominal pain," in *Emergency Medicine; A Comprehensive Study Guide*, J. E. Tintinalli, G. D. Kelen, and J. S. Stapczynski, Eds., pp. 356–366, McGraw-Hill, New York, NY, USA, 5th edition, 2000.

[11] A. B. MacKersie, M. J. Lane, R. T. Gerhardt et al., "Nontraumatic acute abdominal pain: Unenhanced helical CT compared with three-view acute abdominal series," *Radiology*, vol. 237, no. 1, pp. 114–122, 2005.

[12] J. R. Staniland, J. Ditchburn, and F. T. De Dombal, "Clinical presentation of the acute abdomen: Study of 600 patients," *British Medical Journal*, vol. 3, no. 5823, pp. 393–398, 1972.

[13] L. Agreus, K. Svardsudd, O. Nyren et al., "The epidemiology of abdominal symptoms: prevalance and demographic characteristics in a Swedish adult population: a report from the abdominal symptom study," *Scandinavian Journal of Gastroenterology*, vol. 29, no. 2, pp. 102–109, 2009.

[14] S. M. Abbas, T. Smithers, and E. Truter, "What clinical and laboratory parameters determine significant intra abdominal pathology for patients assessed in hospital with acute abdominal pain?" *World Journal of Emergency Surgery*, vol. 2, no. 1, article no. 26, 2007.

[15] R. L. Gardner, R. Almeida, J. H. Maselli, and A. Auerbach, "Does Gender Influence Emergency Department Management and Outcomes in Geriatric Abdominal Pain?" *The Journal of Emergency Medicine*, vol. 39, no. 3, pp. 275–281, 2010.

[16] B. Rossetti, A. Spizzirri, C. Migliaccio et al., "Acute pancreatitis in the elderly: Our experience," *BMC Geriatrics*, vol. 9, no. 1, article no. A47, 2009.

[17] M.-J. Xin, H. Chen, B. Luo, and J.-B. Sun, "Severe acute pancreatitis in the elderly: Etiology and clinical characteristics," *World Journal of Gastroenterology*, vol. 14, no. 16, pp. 2517–2521, 2008.

[18] J. Affronti, "Billiary disease in the elderly patient," *Clinics in Geriatric Medicine*, vol. 15, pp. 571–578, 1999.

[19] R. Spangler, T. Van Pham, D. Khoujah, and J. P. Martinez, "Abdominal emergencies in the geriatric patient," *International Journal of Emergency Medicine*, vol. 7, no. 1, 2014.

[20] L. Ragsdale and L. Southerland, "Acute Abdominal Pain in the Older Adult," *Emergency Medicine Clinics of North America*, vol. 29, no. 2, pp. 429–448, 2011.

[21] C. Fadıloğlu and Y. Tokem, "Geriatrik rehabilitasyonda hemşirenin rolü," *Turk Geriatri Dergisi*, vol. 7, pp. 241–246, 2004.

[22] L. Ozdemir, G. Kocoğlu, H. Sumer, N. Nur, and H. Polat, "Sivas il merkezinde yaşlı nufusta bazı kronik hastalıkların prevalansı ve risk faktorleri," *Cumhuriyet Universitesi Tıp Fakultesi Dergisi*, vol. 27, pp. 89–94, 2005.

[23] F. O. Çakan, "Hypertension in the Elderly," *Archives of the Turkish Society of Cardiology*, vol. 45, Suppl 5, pp. 29–31, 2017.

[24] F. Salvi, A. Mattioli, E. Giannini et al., "Pattern of use and presenting complaints of older patients visiting an Emergency Department in Italy," *Aging Clinical and Experimental Research*, vol. 25, no. 5, pp. 583–590, 2013.

[25] N. Samaras, T. Chevalley, D. Samaras, and G. Gold, "Older patients in the emergency department: a review," *Annals of Emergency Medicine*, vol. 56, no. 3, pp. 261–269, 2010.

[26] Y. Shen, Y. C. Tay, E. W. K. Teo, N. Liu, S. W. Lam, and M. E. H. Ong, "Association between the elderly frequent attender to the emergency department and 30-day mortality: A retrospective study over 10 years," *World Journal of Emergency Medicine*, vol. 9, no. 1, pp. 20–25, 2018.

[27] M. Ersel, "Acute abdominal pain in geriatric patient," *Ege Journal of Medicine*, vol. 53, 2637 pages, 2014.

[28] D. R. Kauvar, "The geriatric acute abdomen," *Clinics in Geriatric Medicine*, vol. 9, pp. 547–558, 1993.

[29] K. W. Kizer and M. J. Vassar, "Emergency department diagnosis of abdominal disorders in the elderly," *The American Journal of Emergency Medicine*, vol. 16, no. 4, pp. 357–362, 1998.

[30] T. F. Bugliosi, T. D. Meloy, and L. F. Vukov, "Acute abdominal pain in the elderly," *Annals of Emergency Medicine*, vol. 19, no. 12, pp. 1383–1386, 1990.

[31] A. Sonnenberg, "Demographic characteristics of hospitalized IBD patients," *Digestive Diseases and Sciences*, vol. 54, no. 11, pp. 2449–2455, 2009.

[32] S. Telfer, G. Fenyo, P. R. Holt, and F. T. de Dombal, "Acute abdominal pain in patients over 50 years of age," *Scandinavian Journal of Gastroenterology Supplement*, vol. 144, pp. 47–50, 1998.

[33] A. Pappas, H. Toutouni, S. Gourgiotis et al., "Comparative approach to non-traumatic acute abdominal pain between elderly and non elderly in the emergency department: a study in rural Greece," *Journal of Clinical Medicine Research*, vol. 4, pp. 300–304, 2013.

[34] H. Bengtsson, D. Bergqvist, and N. H. Sternby, "Increasing prevalence of abdominal aorticaneurysms: A necropsy study," *The European Journal of Surgery*, pp. 19–23, 1992.

[35] R. A. Ruotolo and S. R. Evans, "Mesenteric ischemia in the elderly," *Clinics in Geriatric Medicine*, vol. 15, pp. 527–557, 1999.

[36] W. T. Kassahun, T. Schulz, O. Richter, and J. Hauss, "Unchanged high mortality rates from acute occlusive intestinal ischemia: six

year review," *Langenbeck's Archives of Surgery*, vol. 393, no. 2, pp. 163–171, 2008.

[37] W. M. Park, P. Gloviczki, K. J. Cherry Jr. et al., "Contemporary management of acute mesenteric ischemia: Factors associated with survival," *Journal of Vascular Surgery*, vol. 35, no. 3, pp. 445–452, 2002.

[38] I. Bavunoğlu and F. Sirin, "Akut cerrahi karını taklit eden cerrahi dışı nedenler," *Türkiye Klinikleri Cerrahi Tıp Bilimleri*, vol. 10, pp. 30–35, 2005.

[39] B. Gün, S. Yolcu, V. Değerli et al., "Multi-detector angio-CT and the use of D-dimer for the diagnosis of acute mesenteric ischemia in geriatric patients," *Ulusal Travma ve Acil Cerrahi Dergisi*, vol. 20, no. 5, pp. 376–381, 2014.

[40] G. Cervellin, R. Mora, A. Ticinesi et al., "Epidemiology and outcomes of acute abdominal pain in a large urban Emergency Department: Retrospective analysis of 5,340 cases," *Annals of Translational Medicine*, vol. 4, no. 19, article 362, 2016.

[41] S. Saçar, D. H. Cenger, A. Asan et al., "Geriatrik infeksiyonların 50 olguda değerlendirilmesi," *Pamukkale Tıp Dergisi*, vol. 1, pp. 84–86, 2008.

[42] A. Ciccone, J. R. Allegra, D. G. Cochrane, R. P. Cody, and L. M. Roche, "Age-related differences in diagnoses within the elderly population," *The American Journal of Emergency Medicine*, vol. 16, no. 1, pp. 43–48, 1998.

[43] G. Gurleyik and E. Gurleyik, "Age-related clinical features in older patients with acute appendicitis," *European Journal of Emergency Medicine*, vol. 10, no. 3, pp. 200–297, 2003.

[44] S. K. Türker, N. G. Beceren, Ş. Yolcu et al., "Acil servisimize bir yıl süreyle başvuran travma dışı erişkin karın ağrılı hastaların incelemesi," *Genel Tıp Derg*, vol. 25, pp. 1–7, 2015.

[45] G. Fenyö, "Acute abdominal disease in the elderly. Experience from two series in Stockholm," *The American Journal of Surgery*, vol. 143, no. 6, pp. 751–754, 1982.

[46] R. Reiss and A. A. Deutsch, "Emergency abdominal procedures in patients above 70," *The Journal of Gerontology. Series A, Biological Sciences and Medical Sciences*, vol. 40, no. 2, pp. 154–158, 1985.

[47] F. Ağalar, M. Özdoğan, Ç. E. Daphan et al., "Akut karınla başvuran geriatrik hastalarda cerrahi tedavi ve sonuçları," *Geriatri*, vol. 1, pp. 1–4, 1999.

[48] Z. Kekeç, F. Koç, and S. Büyük, "Acil serviste yaşlı hasta yatışlarının gözden geçirilmesi," *The Journal of Academic Emergency Medicine*, vol. 8, pp. 21–24, 2009.

[49] T. C. Chan, J. P. Killeen, D. Kelly, and D. A. Guss, "Impact of rapid entry and accelerated care at triage on reducing emergency department patient wait times, lengths of stay, and rate of left without being seen," *Annals of Emergency Medicine*, vol. 46, no. 6, pp. 491–497, 2005.

[50] H. J. Hoekstra, "Cancer surgery in the elderly," *European Journal of Cancer*, vol. 37, pp. 235–244, 2001.

[51] Ş. K. Türker, N. G. Beceren, S. Yolcu et al., "Acil servisimize bir yıl süreyle başvuran travma dışı erişkin karın ağrılı hastaların incelemesi," *Genel Tıp Derg*, vol. 25, pp. 1–7, 2015.

[52] M. Serinken, I. Turkcuer, M. Ozen, E. Uyanik, H. Elicabuk, and E. Karsli, "A Retrospective analysis of patients who visited the emergency department and left by their own choice in a university hospital," *Journal of Academic Emergency Medicine*, vol. 12, no. 3, pp. 126–129, 2013.

[53] M. Calışkan, A. Coşkun, A. Acar et al., "Multivariate prospective evaluation of patients admitted with acute abdominal pain in emergency surgery clinics," *The Journal of Academic Emergency Medicine*, vol. 9, pp. 75–82, 2010.

24

Pancreatic Surgery in the Older Population: A Single Institution's Experience over Two Decades

Bhaumik Brahmbhatt,[1] Abhishek Bhurwal,[1] Frank J. Lukens,[1] Mauricia A. Buchanan,[2] John A. Stauffer,[3] and Horacio J. Asbun[3]

[1]*Division of Gastroenterology and Hepatology, Mayo Clinic, 4500 San Pablo Road, Jacksonville, FL 32224, USA*
[2]*Clinical Studies Unit, Mayo Clinic, 4500 San Pablo Road, Jacksonville, FL 32224, USA*
[3]*Division of General Surgery, Mayo Clinic, 4500 San Pablo Road, Jacksonville, FL 32224, USA*

Correspondence should be addressed to Bhaumik Brahmbhatt; brahmbhatt.bhaumik@mayo.edu

Academic Editor: Francesc Formiga

Objectives. Surgery is the most effective treatment for pancreatic cancer. However, present literature varies on outcomes of curative pancreatic resection in the elderly. The objective of the study was to evaluate age as an independent risk factor for 90-day mortality and complications after pancreatic resection. *Methods*. Nine hundred twenty-nine consecutive patients underwent 934 pancreatic resections between March 1995 and July 2014 in a tertiary care center. Primary analyses focused on outcomes in terms of 90-day mortality and postoperative complications after pancreatic resection in these two age groups. *Results*. Even though patients aged 75 years or older had significantly more postoperative morbidities compared with the younger patient group, the age group was not associated with increased risk of 90-day mortality after pancreatic resection. *Discussion*. The study suggests that age alone should not preclude patients from undergoing curative pancreatic resection.

1. Introduction

The older population, defined as older than 65 years of age, is an important section of the United States (US) population [1]. The US 2010 census reported that the older population increased at a faster rate (15.7%) than the entire US population (9.7%) in the last decade [1]. This expanding older population has also been reported to have a higher incidence of pancreatic cancer. From 2008–2012, 39.6% of pancreatic cancers were diagnosed in patients older than 75 years of age [2]. The Surveillance, Epidemiology, and End Results program estimated that, in 2015, there were 48,960 new cases of pancreatic cancer and 40,560 people died of this disease [2]. Pancreatic cancer is the third leading cause of cancer death in the United States [2]. The 5-year survival rate for pancreatic cancer is 7.2% [2]. To date, surgery has proven to be the most effective treatment for pancreatic cancer. Despite the recent advances that have reduced the overall operative risks [3–6], there is still conflicting evidence regarding the outcomes of surgery in older patients.

The majority of the studies published on the topic have been retrospective, with small sample sizes, conducted at highly specialized, high-volume centers [4, 7–12]. Some studies have reported age to be a risk factor in postoperative morbidity after pancreatic resection [6, 11, 13–16], while others reported that increased age alone does not prohibit pancreatic surgery [7, 10, 12, 17]. Recently, Lee et al. reported that increased age is not a risk factor for postoperative mortality based on information from the American College of Surgeons National Surgical Quality Improvement Program (NSQIP) database [3]. However, NSQIP is a voluntary program, and it does not represent all hospitals in the US. Furthermore, the NSQIP database is built on a sample from a particular patient population, so it does not include the total number of patients treated at each participating institution. It is, therefore, difficult to correctly make a conclusion based on the current available findings.

The aim of this study was to compare the outcomes of pancreatic surgery, including 90-day morbidity and mortality, for patients aged 75 years or older to those younger than 75 years in a high-volume tertiary center.

2. Methods

A retrospective review of a prospectively maintained pancreas database was performed. All patients who had undergone pancreatic resection at our tertiary care center from March 1995 to July 2014 were included in the study. Institutional Review Board approval was obtained. All pancreatectomies were performed by the surgical group at our institution within the time period. This resulted in a sample of 934 pancreatic resections in 929 different patients. To optimize clinical outcome after pancreatic resection, preoperative decisions were preceded by individualized evaluations for the entire cohort. Every patient's cardiologist and/or pulmonologist for those with a medical history of cardiac or pulmonary disease, respectively, were consulted prior to the procedure for optimization of medical conditions including hypertension and diabetes. Ultimately, the decision to offer surgery was made by the attending surgeon after reviewing subspecialist evaluations and preoperative testing results and by assessing each patient's functional status via evaluation of an individual's capacity to perform activities of daily living independently. Our primary analysis focused on comparing morbidity and 90-day mortality of older patients undergoing pancreatic surgery to those younger than 75 years of age.

2.1. Data Collection and Outcomes. For baseline characteristics, age, gender, race, American Society of Anesthesiologists class, comorbidities, preoperative symptoms, and preoperative laboratory values were compared. For surgical details, type of resection, operative time, technique of pancreaticojejunostomy, gastrojejunostomy, and/or duodenojejunostomy, and pathology of the resected lesion were compared. For outcomes data, postoperative stay, including Intensive Care Unit (ICU) days, perioperative packed red blood cell transfusion, postoperative complications, and lab values; follow-up information; and postoperative mortality were compared. The primary outcome measures were to compare morbidities and 90-day mortality in the postoperative period between patients aged 75 years or older and those younger than 75 years.

2.2. Statistical Analysis. Continuous variables were summarized using the sample median with range and numbers with percentage. Comparison was done using t-test for continuous variables and chi-square test for categorical variables. Additionally, multivariate stepwise logistic regression was performed to estimate odds ratios for factors associated with 90-day mortality and the occurrence of major complications. p values less than 0.05 were considered significant. All statistical analyses were performed using SPSS for Windows version 17 (SPSS, Inc., Chicago, IL). This was not a funded study.

3. Results and Discussion

3.1. Results. The study sample included 934 pancreas resections: 737 aged younger than 75 years (range 18 years to 75

years) and 197 aged 75 years or older (range 75 years to 90 years of age). Patient demographics and comorbidities are shown in Table 1. Patients aged 75 years or older at the time of surgery were more likely to have a history of cardiovascular and pulmonary comorbidities and higher Eastern Cooperative Oncology Group (ECOG) status (Table 1). Active tobacco use was significantly lower in patients aged 75 years or older when compared to patients younger than 75 years (6% versus 19%). Patients younger than 75 years, as expected, were likely to have better health status as indicated by higher levels of hemoglobin (13.04 versus 12.51, $p < 0.001$), lower elevations of aspartate aminotransferase (50.61 versus 70.61, $p = 0.003$) and alkaline phosphatase (203 versus 283, $p < 0.001$), higher levels of albumin (4.04 versus 3.88, $p < 0.001$), and better renal functions (glomerular filtration rate 65.71 versus 61.18, $p = 0.007$). Overall, patients aged 75 years or older had higher morbidities than the patients younger than 75 years at the time of surgery.

Pathology of the resected lesions is shown in Table 1. Patients aged 75 years or older had a significantly higher incidence of pancreatic ductal adenocarcinoma (42.6% versus 31%) as compared to patients younger than 75 years. Surgical details of the resected specimen are shown in Table 2. Over the period of 20 years, there was a statistically significant trend towards pylorus preserving pancreaticoduodenectomy as compared to standard PD (p value <0.001). Patients aged 75 years or older were more likely to have pylorus preserving pancreaticoduodenectomy (PD) (32.9% versus 29.5%) and standard PD (22.3% versus 19.8%). There was no significant difference between the two groups in terms of operating time as shown in Table 2. The frequency of patients aged 75 years or older requiring packed red blood cell transfusion was significantly higher than those younger than 75 years (48% versus 35%, $p < 0.0009$).

A comparison of postoperative morbidity and mortality is shown in Table 1. Patients aged 75 years or older and those younger than 75 years had similar postoperative laboratory values except for the levels of INR (1.56 versus 1.80; $p < 0.005$). There were a total of 45 deaths within the 90-day postoperative period, for an overall mortality of 4.8%. The 90-day mortality rate for patients younger than 75 years was 3.2% (31), compared with 5% (14) for patients aged 75 years or older ($p = 0.09$). On multivariate analysis of preoperative factors associated with mortality (Table 3), age of 75 years or older was not associated with an increase in the likelihood of 90-day mortality (odds ratio 1.46; 95% confidence interval 0.74–2.87; $p = 0.272$). Despite no significant difference in 90-day mortality, postoperative complications were more significantly seen in patients aged 75 years or older as compared to patients younger than 75 years. A significantly higher proportion of patients aged 75 years or older experienced cardiac complications (17% versus 9%, $p = 0.0001$), pulmonary complications (15% versus 11%, $p = 0.027$), respiratory failure (8.5% versus 5%, $p = 0.013$), and renal insufficiency (5.5% versus 5%, $p = 0.017$).

3.2. Discussion. As the older population increases, there is an increasing demand for surgery in this older population. Outcomes of various surgical procedures, including PD, in

TABLE 1: Demographic details and postoperative morbidity.

Characteristic	Age < 75 years ($n = 737$)	Age ≥ 75 years ($n = 197$)	p value
Females (%)	54% (399)	49.2% (98)	0.26
Race			0.14
Caucasian	89% (655)	94.4% (188)	
Non-Caucasian	11% (82)	5.6% (9)	
Cardiovascular history			
Hypertension	56% (413)	66.8% (133)	0.001
Cardiac disease	40% (294)	76% (151)	0.001
Peripheral vascular disease	3.6% (27)	6% (13)	0.069
Pulmonary disease	8% (59)	11% (21)	0.23
Tobacco use			0.001
Past	41.5% (307)	53% (106)	
Active	19% (140)	6% (12)	
ECOG status			0.001
0	68.6% (517)	51.5% (103)	
1	27.7% (205)	40.5% (81)	
2	2.3% (17)	6% (12)	
Pathology			
Pancreatic ductal adenocarcinoma	31% (229)	42.6% (84)	0.002
Pancreatic cysts (IPMN, MCN, SCN)	21.9% (162)	20.3% (40)	0.61
Ampullary adenocarcinoma	6.5% (48)	11.1% (22)	0.03
Miscellaneous neoplasm (GIST, RCC, sarcoma, etc.)	2.5% (67)	8% (15)	0.51
Neuroendocrine tumors	13.7% (102)	5.5% (11)	0.002
Cholangiocarcinoma	8.5% (62)	9% (18)	0.74
Benign (pseudocyst, pancreatitis, trauma)	8.5% (67)	3.5% (7)	0.013
Postoperative morbidity and mortality			
90-day mortality	3.2% (31)	5% (14)	0.09
Mean number of ICU days	1.35 days	2.33 days	0.027
(Range)	(0–59 days)	(0–58 days)	
Clavien grade of complications (90 days)			0.56
(a) Minor (grades 1-2)	31% (227)	37% (73)	
(b) Major (grades 3–5)	21% (157)	22% (78)	
Pancreatic fistula	14.6% (108)	12% (24)	0.123
Grade A	6.3% (47)	5% (10)	
Grade B	4.2% (31)	4.5% (9)	
Grade C	4.2% (31)	2.5% (5)	
Postpancreatectomy hemorrhage	5% (38)	2.5% (5)	0.013
Grade A	1.2% (9)	0% (0)	
Grade B	1.2% (9)	1.5% (3)	
Grade C	2.7% (20)	1% (2)	

ECOG status: Eastern Cooperative Oncology Group (ECOG) performance status; IPMN: intraductal papillary mucinous neoplasm; SCN: serous cystic neoplasm; MCN: mucinous cystic neoplasms; GIST: gastrointestinal stromal tumors; RCC: renal cell cancer.

the older population, have become a subject of concern; however, limited data exist [4, 7–12, 17]. It has been well established in previous studies that PD could safely be performed for patients aged 70 years or older. However, PD becomes daunting with patients who are older than 80 years. Outcomes in octogenarians have been reported over the last few years. While some of these studies have reported age as a risk factor in postoperative morbidity after PD [6, 11, 13–16], others have shown that age does not prohibit surgery [7, 10, 12, 17, 18]. One of the most recent studies on the topic, based on the NSQIP database [3], specifically analyzed outcomes of patients older than 80 years for increased risk of complications and mortality. Even though the study had a large sample size, participation in the NSQIP database

186　　　　　　　　　　　　　　　　　　　　　　　　　　　　　　　　Recent Advances in Geriatric Medicine

TABLE 2: Operative details.

Variable	Age < 75 years (n = 737)	Age ≥ 75 years of age (n = 197)	p value
Operative procedure			0.39
(a) Pancreaticoduodenectomy	49.5% (365)	55.3% (109)	
(b) Total pancreatectomy	10% (74)	12.6% (25)	
(c) Distal pancreatectomy	37% (274)	30.9% (61)	
(d) Central Pancreatectomy/enucleation	3% (24)	1% (2)	
Operative time (minutes)	339	348	0.40
Number of patients requiring blood transfusion perioperative*	35% (260)	48% (95)	0.0009
Mean number of packed RBC transfused	1.42 units	1.75 units	0.32
Number of patients requiring blood transfusion during hospital stay in postoperative period	26% (197)	32% (64)	0.11
Mean number of packed RBC transfused	0.96 units	0.83	0.64

*up to 24 hours after surgery. RBC: red blood cells.

TABLE 3: Multivariate logistic regression analysis for preoperative factors associated with mortality.

Variable	Odds ratio (95% confidence interval)	p value
Age of 75 years or older	1.46 (0.74–2.87)	0.272
Hypertension	0.501 (0.228–1.09)	0.084
Diabetes mellitus	0.63 (0.33–1.20)	0.161
Coronary artery disease	0.479 (0.239–0.960)	0.038
Pulmonary disease	0.449 (0.196–1.02)	0.058

is voluntary, so it does not represent all of the patients in the participating institutions, and not all hospitals in the US participate. Therefore, whether age plays a role in postoperative morbidity after PD or not remains a subject of further research.

This study has a large sample size and focuses on the population aged 75 years or older undergoing pancreatic resections at our tertiary center. We evaluated postpancreatic resection outcomes for patients aged 75 years and older as inconclusive evidence has been reported for octogenarians while good outcomes for septuagenarians have been well reported [7]. The results of the study are comparable to other studies reported on the topic [7, 10, 12, 17]. Overall mortality rate was 4.5%, closer to the mean of the 0–10% reported by the majority of the studies since 2000 [3, 19–22]. The incidence of postoperative fistula and hemorrhage is also comparable to previous studies [22–24]. Even though patients aged 75 years or older were more likely to have postoperative morbidities than their younger counterparts, 90-day mortality after pancreatic resection did not differ significantly. A higher incidence of postoperative complications in patients aged 75 years or older could also be explained by the higher incidence of preoperative morbidities in the same cohort as compared to the younger group. Comparable 90-day mortality could be reflective of the optimization of medical conditions prior to the procedure, low severity of postoperative complications in the older group, better postoperative care, or selection

bias in terms of better health status prior to surgery. Despite the above, these findings suggest that age alone should not preclude patients from undergoing curative resection of pancreatic lesion.

This study is limited by its retrospective nature. By design, it spans over a time period of 20 years. Improved surgical techniques and advancements in perioperative care [4–6] have resulted in the surgeons offering PD to older patients at our tertiary center over the last 2 decades, and patients treated more recently may be doing better. Although it is well known that poor health status is associated with an increased risk of death and adverse outcomes [25, 26], this study cannot rule out selection bias as patients with overall better health status would have been selected for surgery based on ECOG scores (the included patients in the sample have ECOG scores between 0 and 2). In this study, occurrence of pancreatic ductal carcinoma (42.6% versus 31%) and solid pancreatic lesions (62.8% versus 54%) was more common in patients aged 75 years or older as compared to patients younger than 75 years, which could have influenced the outcomes as fibrotic pancreatic tissue is comparatively easier to resect. Lastly, even though the study has a large sample size, it is still underpowered for detecting minor differences between the two groups. It is also underpowered to determine preoperative risk factors in the older subgroup who have an increased number of ICU days or higher frequency of postoperative complications.

4. Conclusions

Focusing on the high-risk group of patients aged 75 years or older, this study reports that there is no significant difference in 90-day mortality despite higher postoperative complications in the subgroup. This study suggests that pancreatic resection could be a feasible option in selected older patients, and these patients should not be denied the opportunity of curative resection based on age alone.

Disclosure

Bhaumik Brahmbhatt and Abhishek Bhurwal are considered as co-first authors.

Competing Interests

The authors declare that there is no conflict of interests regarding the publication of this paper.

Authors' Contributions

B. Brahmbhatt with A. Bhurwal contributed equally to data analysis and manuscript writing. F. J. Lukens, M. A. Buchanan, J. A. Stauffer, and H. J. Asbun contributed to data gathering and editing of manuscript. All authors gave final approval of the article.

References

[1] C. A. Werner, The Older Population: 2010. 2010 Census Briefs, 2011, https://www.census.gov/prod/cen2010/briefs/c2010br-09.pdf.

[2] National Cancer Institute, "SEER stat fact sheets: pancreas cancer," http://seer.cancer.gov/statfacts/html/pancreas.html.

[3] D. Y. Lee, J. A. Schwartz, B. Wexelman, D. Kirchoff, K. C. Yang, and F. Attiyeh, "Outcomes of pancreaticoduodenectomy for pancreatic malignancy in octogenarians: an American College of Surgeons National Surgical Quality Improvement Program analysis," American Journal of Surgery, vol. 207, no. 4, pp. 540–548, 2014.

[4] J. H. Balcom, D. W. Rattner, A. L. Warshaw, Y. Chang, and C. Fernandez-del Castillo, "Ten-year experience with 733 pancreatic resections: changing indications, older patients, and decreasing length of hospitalization," Archives of Surgery, vol. 136, no. 4, pp. 391–398, 2001.

[5] A. L. Warshaw, K. D. Lillemoe, and C. Fernandez-del Castillo, "Pancreatic surgery for adenocarcinoma," Current Opinion in Gastroenterology, vol. 28, no. 5, pp. 488–493, 2012.

[6] P. J. Kneuertz, H. A. Pitt, K. Y. Bilimoria et al., "Risk of morbidity and mortality following hepato-pancreato-biliary surgery," Journal of Gastrointestinal Surgery, vol. 16, no. 9, pp. 1727–1735, 2012.

[7] V. de Franco, E. Frampas, M. Wong et al., "Safety and feasibility of pancreaticoduodenectomy in the elderly: a matched study," Pancreas, vol. 40, no. 6, pp. 920–924, 2011.

[8] T. A. Sohn, C. J. Yeo, J. L. Cameron et al., "Should pancreaticoduodenectomy be performed in octogenarians?" Journal of Gastrointestinal Surgery, vol. 2, no. 3, pp. 207–216, 1998.

[9] R. Delcore, J. H. Thomas, and A. S. Hermreck, "Pancreaticoduodenectomy for malignant pancreatic and periampullary neoplasms in elderly patients," The American Journal of Surgery, vol. 162, no. 6, pp. 532–536, 1991.

[10] A. Nanashima, T. Abo, T. Nonaka et al., "Comparison of postoperative morbidity in elderly patients who underwent pancreatic resection," Hepato-Gastroenterology, vol. 59, no. 116, pp. 1141–1146, 2012.

[11] T. S. Riall, D. M. Reddy, W. H. Nealon, and J. S. Goodwin, "The effect of age on short-term outcomes after pancreatic resection: A Population-Based Study," Annals of Surgery, vol. 248, pp. 459–467, 2008.

[12] M. A. Makary, J. M. Winter, J. L. Cameron et al., "Pancreaticoduodenectomy in the very elderly," Journal of Gastrointestinal Surgery, vol. 10, no. 3, pp. 347–356, 2006.

[13] J. S. Hill, Z. Zhou, J. P. Simons et al., "A simple risk score to predict in-hospital mortality after pancreatic resection for cancer," Annals of Surgical Oncology, vol. 17, no. 7, pp. 1802–1807, 2010.

[14] C. C. Hsu, C. L. Wolfgang, D. A. Laheru et al., "Early mortality risk score: identification of poor outcomes following upfront surgery for resectable pancreatic cancer," Journal of Gastrointestinal Surgery, vol. 16, no. 4, pp. 753–761, 2012.

[15] F. Muscari, B. Suc, S. Kirzin et al., "Risk factors for mortality and intra-abdominal complications after pancreatoduodenectomy: multivariate analysis in 300 patients," Surgery, vol. 139, no. 5, pp. 591–598, 2006.

[16] W. Pratt, S. Joseph, M. P. Callery, and C. M. Vollmer Jr., "POSSUM accurately predicts morbidity for pancreatic resection," Surgery, vol. 143, no. 1, pp. 8–19, 2008.

[17] A. S. Barbas, R. S. Turley, E. P. Ceppa et al., "Comparison of outcomes and the use of multimodality therapy in young and elderly people undergoing surgical resection of pancreatic cancer," Journal of the American Geriatrics Society, vol. 60, no. 2, pp. 344–350, 2012.

[18] V. Beltrame, M. Gruppo, D. Pastorelli, S. Pedrazzoli, S. Merigliano, and C. Sperti, "Outcome of pancreaticoduodenectomy in octogenarians: single institution's experience and review of the literature," Journal of Visceral Surgery, vol. 152, no. 5, pp. 279–284, 2015.

[19] D. J. Gouma, R. C. I. van Geenen, T. M. van Gulik et al., "Rates of complications and death after pancreaticoduodenectomy: risk factors and the impact of hospital volume," Annals of Surgery, vol. 232, no. 6, pp. 786–795, 2000.

[20] R. C. G. Martin II, M. F. Brennan, and D. P. Jaques, "Quality of complication reporting in the surgical literature," Annals of Surgery, vol. 235, no. 6, pp. 803–813, 2002.

[21] V. Ho and M. J. Heslin, "Effect of hospital volume and experience on in-hospital mortality for pancreaticoduodenectomy," Annals of Surgery, vol. 237, no. 4, pp. 509–514, 2003.

[22] M. W. Büchler, M. Wagner, B. M. Schmied et al., "Changes in morbidity after pancreatic resection: toward the end of completion pancreatectomy," Archives of Surgery, vol. 138, no. 12, pp. 1310–1315, 2003.

[23] H. Friess, H. G. Beger, U. Sulkowski et al., "Randomized controlled multicentre study of the prevention of complications by octreotide in patients undergoing surgery for chronic pancreatitis," British Journal of Surgery, vol. 82, no. 9, pp. 1270–1273, 1995.

[24] M. Büchler, H. Friess, I. Klempa et al., "Role of octreotide in the prevention of postoperative complications following pancreatic

25

Associations of Pet Ownership with Older Adults Eating Patterns and Health

Roschelle Heuberger

Department of Human Environmental Studies, Central Michigan University, Mt. Pleasant, MI, USA

Correspondence should be addressed to Roschelle Heuberger; heubelra@cmich.edu

Academic Editor: Fulvio Lauretani

Pet ownership has been shown to improve quality of life for older adults. The objective of this cross-sectional study was to compare older pet owners and older non-pet owners and assess differences between groups. This study was conducted on adults over 50 years of age, who owned either one cat or one dog versus nonowners based on age, race, gender, and education. Matched older pet owners (OPO) versus non-pet owners (NPO) pairs ($n = 84$), older cat owners (OCO) versus non-cat owners (NCO) ($n = 29$), and older dog owners (ODO) versus non-dog owners (NDO) pairs ($n = 55$) were analyzed. No differences were found between OPO and NPO for dietary, activity, or lifestyle, except OPO had fewer health conditions [$p < 0.03$]. Total OCO had greater body mass indices [BMI] ($\mu = 29.6 \pm 8.2$) than ODO ($\mu = 23.2 \pm 5.2$) [$p < 0.02$], less activity [$p < 0.02$], and shorter duration of activity [$p < 0.05$] and took fewer supplements [$p < 0.003$]. OCO and NCO differed on health conditions ($\mu = 0.8 \pm 0.9$ versus $\mu = 1.9 \pm 1.3$, [$p < 0.008$]) and ODO versus NDO differed on BMI ($\mu = 25 \pm 4$ versus $\mu = 27 \pm 6$, [$p < 0.04$]). Although there are limitations to this study, data may be useful for targeting marketing and health messages to older persons.

1. Introduction

Pet ownership is alleged to have beneficial effects on health in older adults [1]; therefore, a study of community dwelling, ill, and debilitated elderly adults was conducted. Pet ownership was evaluated against measures of health in the Netherlands. In a cross-sectional analysis of 12,297 older adults in the Netherlands, 2358 were pet owners. Older adults who owned a dog showed significantly ($p < 0.001$) increased activity and socialization. Older adults who owned a cat showed decreased activity and socialization [2]. In a study of Scandinavians older adults who owned a dog showed overall better health and health related behaviors when compared to older adult non-pet owners and cat owners. Cat ownership was associated with higher blood pressure, worse health status, and less physical activity when compared to older adult non-cat owners ($p < 0.001$) [3].

Dog ownership has been studied and found to increase activity among older adults across all seasons. Authors advocated for policies and programs that encourage walking in geographic areas with harsh seasons using dog friendly parks and neighborhoods and providing support and education to

owners [4]. Pet ownership among older adults has also been associated with the use of mental health care, but associations with loneliness or social interactions as a result of having a pet were not found [2]. Human-animal bonds are also a factor but are difficult to measure and can impact quality of life for both the owner and the pet [5]. An "ideal" dog or an educated owner that has realistic expectations of the dog increases owner satisfaction and thus quality of life [6]. Companion animal ownership or interaction has been associated with improving feelings of "wellbeing" among those with illnesses, such as HIV, long term mental illness, congestive heart failure, diabetes, end stage cancer, acute illness, chronic pain, depression, posttraumatic stress disorder, and physical disability [6–18]. However, many studies found clinical benefit, but not necessarily strong statistical significance, possibly due to the complex nature of measuring "wellbeing" and the difficulty in sampling and design in these types of studies.

In recent years, several investigators studied the attachment of people to pets and used "relational" constructs to evaluate the effects of pet ownership and the human-animal bond on overall social satisfaction and healthy aging paradigms. Pet ownership was found to be a positive influence on relationship satisfaction, empathy, social attitude, socialization, and companionship and had postulated direct effects on health, such as increasing serum levels of neurotransmitters and hormones and overriding nociception, attenuating sensory deficits, and decreasing the hemodynamic changes that occur from the stress response [19–30]. In addition, increased ambulation, physical activity (through dog walking), has been found to increase measures of cardiovascular competence, promote health aging, increase one's ability to age in place, and attenuate decrements in performing activities of daily living associated with increasing age [31–36]. Obesity, particularly central adiposity with concomitant loss of muscle and muscle function through infiltration of adipocytes into skeletal and cardiac muscle, has serious implications for morbidity and mortality in older persons. Physical activity through dog walking has also implications for the attenuation of age related sarcopenic obesity, disability, and obesity in general [37–39]. In a cross-sectional study conducted by Utz of 2,474 participants, pet ownership and overall health outcomes were assessed and analyzed. The findings of this study showed that older adults who owned a pet were in overall better health condition. Older adults who owned a pet had less arthritis, healthier weights, and decreased occurrences of congestive heart failure. One of the detriments to owning a pet was that older adults with pets did have increased allergies and asthma. This study emphasizes that pet ownership results in improved overall health [40].

There has also been some data to suggest that dementia patients may benefit from pet assisted therapies, and physical activity, nutrition, agitation, reminiscing, and increased socialization were potentially significant outcomes [41, 42]. In a 2015 study by Freidmann et al., cognitively impaired residents ($n = 22$) were randomized to 60 or 90 minutes of pet assisted therapy and statistically significant improvements were seen in physical, behavioral, and emotional function [43]. Similarly, in a study by Richeson, dementia patients ($n = 15$) who were assigned to an animal assisted therapy protocol showed decrease in agitation and greater social interactions ($p < 0.001$) from baseline [44]. Additionally research has found benefits to persons with dementia with both a robotic and a live dog. This has implications for offsetting the concerns of physical safety, zoonotic infection transmission from animal to human, and damage to property or environment, which is often cited as a rationale for restricting pet therapy in this population [45]. Further research into the cost benefit of pet ownership among older persons is required, but it appears that the benefits may outweigh the risks [46, 47].

The rural United States (US) has a greater proportion of older adults who are impoverished and exhibit greater rates of disease and disability than all other areas of the US. According to the US census, the US Centers for Disease Control and the US National Center for Health Statistics, there are more overweight and obese older persons in parts of the rural US [48]. The National Health Interview data and the Behavioral Risk Factor Surveillance System datasets have shown that a great number of older adults are impaired, are physically inactive, and meet the criteria for disability.

This study was conducted to assess older adults who reside in rural areas of the US, where insufficient descriptive data exist for the relationship between pet ownership and diet, activity, and lifestyle characteristics of the owner as well as the characteristics of their companion animals. The hypotheses included that older dog or cat owners would differ from one another or nonowners with regard to body mass index and select dietary intake variables, number of physician diagnosed diseases, and prescribed medications, related to being an older adult dog owner versus having a cat or being a nonpet owner.

2. Materials and Methods

This cross-sectional, unincentivized, convenient investigation was done to evaluate associations of pet ownership to health and weight status of older adult owners. "This study was conducted according to the guidelines laid down in the Declaration of Helsinki and all procedures involving human subjects were approved by the Institutional Review Board and Human Subjects Committee of the primary institution where the research was conducted and informed consent was obtained from all subjects." In addition, the work which involved analysis of secondary data on animals was approved by the above-mentioned board. All data was rendered anonymous and the use of ID number only in data entry, cleaning, coding, analysis, and dissemination was employed. Data were kept confidential in a secure location and were made available only to authorized researchers at the primary institution granting approval for the study.

2.1. Data. Data were not associated with any identifying information and subject confidentiality was maintained. Trained interviewers ($n = 7$), with interrater reliability ratings of Cronbach's alpha = 0.89, solicited pet owner participants from organizations known to be frequented by older adults and pet owners, using flyers, word of mouth, and ads (e.g., Senior Centers, Kiwanis, Red Hats, Pet Care Centers, Clinics, Kennel Clubs, and Guilds). Exclusion criteria consisted of the following: being <18 years of age, being unable to provide informed consent, inability to care for self or cat/dog, having >1 cat or dog/household, refusal to answer >25% of questions, or failure to reside in a rural US locale. Data were split by age >50 years, using this established cut point of the American Association of Retired Persons.

Persons who were not pet owners were continuously recruited until a match was found to a pet owner. Matching was based on age, gender, race, and education. Anyone wanting to participate in the study was allowed to do so, but persons under the age of 50 were excluded from the analyses.

Questionnaires were piloted and focus group input was used to adjust the questions in the questionnaire. Sequential focus group information was used to hone internal validity. Body Condition Scoring Charts (BCS) for pets that had a nine-point scoring system that were available without copyright were used. Scale weight was obtained when available; otherwise owner weights were self-reported, as were the data from non-pet owners. Food intake data was gathered from semiquantitative food frequency questionnaires. Data on exercise was collected using frequency, duration, and intensity scales, with respondent walking for exercise specifically

Comparison between matched cat and dog owners
and nonowners > 50 years of age

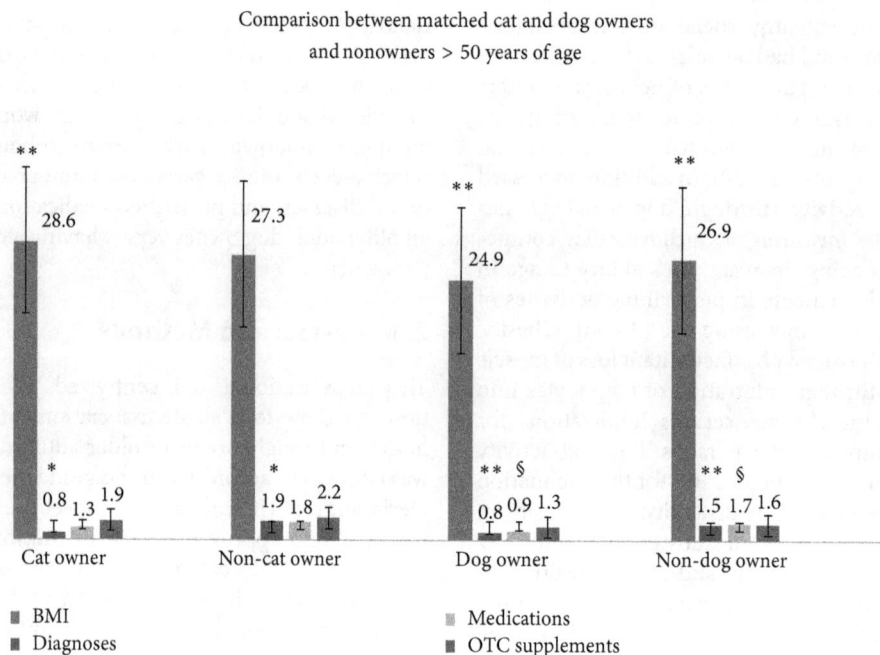

FIGURE 1: Characteristics of older pet owners versus matched nonowners >50 years residing in the rural United States (N = 168). $^*p < 0.01$, $^{**}p < 0.05$, and $^\S p < 0.004$.

excluding dog walking. Dog walking data was collected in the section devoted to the animal and its care.

2.2. Statistical Analysis. Statistical analyses were run using SPSS® v. 23, IBM Corporation, Raleigh-Durham, NC, USA, under license from Central Michigan University, Mount Pleasant, MI 48859. Descriptive statistics, such as frequencies and means, independent sample t-tests between matched owner to nonowner pairs, Chi square analysis for older owners and nonowners, and nonparametric statistics for data that were not normally distributed (such as semiquantitative food frequency intake data) were run. Analyses were run on all data with split analyses done by gender. Logistic regression models were run stepwise. Significance was determined by a p value of <0.05 for all tests. Trend was determined by a p value set at <0.075. Failure to reach statistical significance was denoted by NS.

3. Results

3.1. Older Owners versus Older Nonowners. Split analyses resulted in matched older pet owners (OPO) versus non-pet owners (NPO) usable pairs (n = 84), cat owners (OCO) versus non-cat owners (NCO) pairs (n = 29), and dog owners (ODO) versus non-dog owners (NDO) pairs (n = 55). No significant differences were found between total OPO and NPO for dietary intake, physical activity, or lifestyle characteristics, with exception of OPO having fewer numbers of documented health conditions, despite being matched for demographics using t-testing. There were differences between OCO versus NCO and ODO versus NDO on prescribed medication number and BMI (Figure 1). Older pet owners did differ from

older non-pet owners on other health related characteristics within groups.

Logistic regressions were run on all age matched owners and nonowners. Regression models showed that the largest contribution to variance in the number of physician diagnosed owner health conditions was pet ownership (Table 1). An increase in BMI was also related to number of owner diagnoses in the sample, and a trend was observed for increased intake of added fat. No other variables, either dietary or lifestyle, contributed significantly to the models.

To investigate contributions by gender, the data were split and analyzed; significant contributions were seen in number of diagnoses for males on BMI, dietary intake of added fats, and servings of whole grains, fruits, and vegetables. In females, pet ownership was found to be significantly related to decrease in disease number, but BMI ceased to be contributory. No other dietary or lifestyle variable was found to contribute significantly among females. It should be noted that there were more females than males in the sample and, thus, data from female respondents' contributed heavily to the findings from the total sample.

3.2. Older Dog Owners versus Older Non-Dog Owners. There were 110 ODO and NDO over age of 50 in the sample. Mean age was 56.8 ± 6.4 years; 97% of the sample was Caucasian and 65% female. ODO versus NDO showed significant differences between BMI, number of diagnoses, and prescribed medications using t-tests (Figure 1). The dog owners' dogs were, on average, 7.7 ± 4.3 years old and had been owned for $\mu = 7.4 \pm 4.3$ years. The most commonly owned dog was female (86%) and neutered (100%) and 27% were identified as pure bred Labrador Retriever. Respondents classified their dogs by

TABLE 1: Regression models of body mass index, dietary, and lifestyle characteristics on health in pet owners and matched nonowners over age of fifty (N = 168).

All older owners versus matched older nonowners

	Total (N = 168)					Males (n = 50)					Females (n = 118)				
	B	SE	β	t	Sig.	B	SE	β	t	Sig.	B	SE	β	t	Sig.
Owns pet	-0.75	0.19	-0.30	-3.9	0.001	-0.73	0.38	-0.27	-1.93	0.06	-0.68	0.23	-0.28	-3.04	0.003
BMI (kg/m²)	0.035	0.02	0.16	2.1	0.04	0.08	0.04	0.31	2.17	0.04	0.03	0.02	0.12	1.29	0.20
‡‡Model	‡R = 0.35; R² = 0.12; AR² = 0.11; SEE = 1.2					‡R = 0.48; R² = 0.23; AR² = 0.19; SEE = 1.2					‡R = 0.34; R² = 0.09; AR² = 0.08; SEE = 1.2				
Smoke (pack years)	0.35	0.29	0.20	1.2	0.20	0.44	0.51	0.33	0.86	0.40	0.91	0.33	0.14	0.58	0.60
Alcohol (drink/week)	0.20	0.25	0.15	0.8	0.40	0.51	0.55	0.36	0.95	0.40	0.30	0.39	0.18	0.78	0.40
†Model	R = 0.28; R² = 0.08; AR² = 0.01; SEE = 1.5					R = 0.42; R² = 0.18; AR² = -0.09; SEE = 1.6					R = 0.26; R² = 0.07; AR² = -0.03; SEE = 1.54				
Fruit, vegetable (serving/week)	-0.01	0.01	-0.06	-0.07	0.50	-0.02	0.02	-0.19	-1.13	0.30	0.001	0.01	0.001	0.001	1.00
Whole grain (serving/week)	0.02	0.02	0.12	1.4	0.20	0.05	0.02	0.39	2.42	0.02	0.01	0.02	0.06	0.55	0.60
Low fat dairy (serving/week)	-0.01	0.01	-0.06	-0.60	0.50	-0.04	0.02	-0.23	-1.50	0.10	-0.01	0.02	-0.04	-0.35	0.70
Fast food (serving/week)	0.04	0.15	0.03	0.30	0.80	-0.09	0.23	-0.06	-0.40	0.70	0.05	0.19	0.03	0.28	0.80
Added fat (serving/week)	0.20	0.11	0.16	1.83	0.07	0.58	0.19	0.44	3.13	0.003	0.001	0.13	0.001	-0.01	0.90
Fish (serving/week)	-0.03	0.13	-0.02	-0.21	0.80	-0.35	0.25	-0.20	-1.40	0.20	0.07	0.15	0.05	0.48	0.60
†Model	R = 0.21; R² = 0.04; AR² = 0.01; SEE = 1.3					‡R = 0.62; R² = 0.39; AR² = 0.28; SEE = 1.2					R = 0.08; R² = 0.01; AR² = -0.06; SEE = 1.3				

Older dog owners versus matched non-dog owners

	Total (N = 110)					Males (n = 40)					Females (n = 70)				
	B	SE	β	t	Sig.	B	SE	β	t	Sig.	B	SE	β	t	Sig.
Owns pet	-0.67	0.23	-0.27	-2.95	0.004	-0.71	0.37	-0.30	-1.94	0.06	-0.64	0.29	-0.26	-2.21	0.03
BMI (kg/m²)	0.06	0.03	0.22	2.27	0.03	0.13	0.04	0.51	3.48	0.001	0.06	0.04	0.2	1.7	0.10
†Model	‡R = 0.32; R² = 0.10; AR² = 0.09; SEE = 1.2					‡R = 0.30; R² = 0.09; AR² = 0.07; SEE = 1.2					‡R = 0.26; R² = 0.07; AR² = 0.05; SEE = 1.2				
Smoke (pack years)	0.89	0.42	0.48	2.1	0.06	0.19	0.26	0.46	0.72	0.55	1.3	0.60	0.59	2.17	0.06
Alcohol (drink/week)	0.38	0.34	0.25	1.1	0.30	0.13	0.34	0.23	0.37	0.75	0.34	0.41	0.22	0.82	0.44
†Model	R = 0.58; R² = 0.33; AR² = 0.23; SEE = 1.4					R = 0.47; R² = 0.22; AR² = -0.56; SEE = 0.56					R = 0.69; R² = 0.47; AR² = 0.34; SEE = 1.50				
Fruit, vegetable (serving/week)	-0.01	0.01	-0.12	-0.97	0.30	-0.03	0.02	-0.28	-1.40	0.17	-0.01	0.02	-0.04	-0.27	0.79

TABLE 1: Continued.

	B	SE	β	t	Sig.	B	SE	β	t	Sig.	B	SE	β	t	Sig.
Whole grain (serving/week)	0.02	0.01	0.19	1.69	0.10	0.05	0.02	0.46	2.38	0.03	0.01	0.02	0.09	0.63	0.53
Low fat dairy (serving/week)	−0.01	0.02	−0.06	−0.48	0.60	−0.03	0.03	−0.25	−1.36	0.18	−0.001	0.02	−0.01	−0.06	0.95
Fast food (serving/week)	0.03	0.17	0.02	0.15	0.90	−0.13	0.24	−0.09	−0.53	0.60	0.036	0.25	0.02	0.15	0.89
Added fat (serving/week)	0.32	0.14	0.24	2.3	0.02	0.51	0.20	0.43	2.52	0.02	0.16	0.19	0.12	0.87	0.39
Fish (serving/week)	−0.02	0.15	−0.02	−0.16	0.87	−0.23	0.26	−0.14	−0.86	0.40	0.02	0.20	0.02	0.11	0.91
‡‡Model	‡‡$R = 0.31$; $R^2 = 0.09$; $AR^2 = 0.03$; $SEE = 1.3$					‡$R = 0.63$; $R^2 = 0.40$; $AR^2 = 0.26$; $SEE = 1.09$					‡†$R = 0.14$; $R^2 = 0.02$; $AR^2 = -0.09$; $SEE = 1.32$				

Older cat owners versus matched non-cat owners

	Total (N = 58)					Males (n = 12)					Females (n = 46)				
	B	SE	β	t	Sig.	B	SE	β	t	Sig.	B	SE	β	t	Sig.
Owns pet	−1.2	0.30	−0.43	−3.57	0.001	−1.37	0.89	−0.45	−1.53	0.16	−0.99	0.316	−0.43	−3.15	0.003
BMI (kg/m²)	0.013	0.03	0.07	0.50	0.62	0.04	0.09	0.14	0.40	0.70	0.01	0.03	0.05	0.33	0.74
‡Model	‡$R = 0.43$; $R^2 = 0.19$; $AR^2 = 0.17$; $SEE = 1.1$					$R = 0.45$; $R^2 = 0.21$; $AR^2 = 0.12$; $SEE = 1.48$					‡$R = 0.43$; $R^2 = 0.18$; $AR^2 = 0.16$; $SEE = 1.08$				
Smoke (pack years)	−0.07	0.39	−0.06	−0.19	0.85	0.60	1.72	0.36	0.35	0.79	−0.24	0.42	−0.21	−0.58	0.58
Alcohol (drink/week)	0.02	0.34	0.01	0.04	0.97	0.20	1.4	0.15	0.14	0.91	−0.17	0.44	−0.14	−0.38	0.71
†Model	$R = 0.06$; $R^2 = 0.003$; $AR^2 = -0.16$; $SEE = 1.5$					$R = 0.33$; $R^2 = 0.11$; $AR^2 = -1.67$; $SEE = 3.13$					$R = 0.29$; $R^2 = 0.09$; $AR^2 = -0.14$; $SEE = 1.27$				
Fruit, vegetable (serving/week)	−0.004	0.02	−0.05	−0.23	0.82	−0.01	0.07	−0.11	−0.22	0.84	0.00	0.02	0.01	0.02	0.98
Whole grain (serving/week)	0.01	0.03	0.08	0.46	0.65	0.95	0.11	0.35	0.84	0.47	0.02	0.03	0.12	0.62	0.54
Low fat dairy (serving/week)	−0.01	0.03	−0.07	−0.43	0.67	0.14	0.15	0.41	0.93	0.42	−0.01	0.03	−0.07	−0.35	0.73
Fast food (serving/week)	0.01	0.3	0.01	0.03	0.97	−0.10	0.86	−0.04	−0.11	0.92	0.04	0.35	0.02	0.11	0.92
Added fat (serving/week)	0.03	0.21	0.02	0.14	0.89	1.20	0.55	0.75	2.17	0.12	−0.24	0.22	−0.20	−1.10	0.28
Fish (serving/week)	0.06	0.30	0.04	0.20	0.85	−0.86	1.04	−0.37	−0.82	0.47	0.25	0.30	0.16	0.83	0.41
†Model	$R = 0.11$; $R^2 = 0.01$; $AR^2 = -0.14$; $SEE = 1.39$					$R = 0.84$; $R^2 = 0.70$; $AR^2 = 0.10$; $SEE = 1.49$					$R = 0.25$; $R^2 = 0.06$; $AR^2 = -0.13$; $SEE = 1.31$				

†Constant. ‡Statistically significant at the level of $p < 0.05$.

breed. Respondents were specifically asked if the dog was a mix or pure bred, but no further investigation into lineage was made by interviewers.

In regression models for NDO matched on age to ODO, pet ownership contributed significantly to decreased number of diagnosed conditions in both males and females. In males, increased BMI was significantly related to increased number of health conditions, but the relationship did not hold for females. Smoking and alcohol use did not show statistical significance in the regression models, although a trend was seen between smoking history and increased number of diagnoses in women. In men, dietary intake of whole grain and added fat contributed significantly to model variance (Table 1).

3.3. Older Cat Owners versus Older Non-Cat Owners. There were 58 OCO and NCO in this sample. Mean age of the participants was 57.1 ± 6.2 years; 98% were Caucasian and 81% were female. Older CO and NCO differed significantly on number of diagnosed health conditions ($\mu = 0.8 \pm 0.9$ versus $\mu = 1.9 \pm 1.3$, [$p < 0.008$]) using t-tests. Older cat owners had fewer health problems than NCO despite being matched on available demographics (Figure 1). Their cats were on average 7.3 ± 4.6 years of age and had been owned for $\mu = 6.1 \pm 4.8$ years. The most commonly owned cat was female (76%), neutered (95%), and shorthaired (32%).

Regression models for diagnosed health conditions among OCO and matched NCO are shown in Table 1. Owning a cat was associated with fewer health problems in the sample, but significance was only seen in females, after the data were split by gender. There were too few males in this sample, which reduced power to detect significance. No other body habitus, lifestyle, or dietary intake variable was contributory in OCO and NCO with respect to number of health conditions in regression models.

3.4. Older Dog Owners versus Older Cat Owners. Using nonparametric testing OCO were significantly more likely to be female than ODO ($p < 0.01$). Total OCO had significantly greater body mass indices [BMI = wt.-kg/ht-m^2] ($\mu = 29.6 \pm 8.2$) than total ODO ($\mu = 23.2 \pm 5.2$) [$p < 0.02$], less physical activity [$p < 0.02$], and duration of activity [$p < 0.05$] and took fewer supplements [$p < 0.003$] in t-test analyses.

Older pet owners had senior pets, and their senior pets had veterinarian diagnosed health conditions, most commonly allergies (37%) and arthritis (21%) among ODO and allergies (27%) and hyperthyroidism (15%) among OCO. The most frequently used supplement was glucosamine for dogs and a multivitamin for cats. The most common medications were for pain control (22%) in dogs and hyperthyroidism in cats.

3.5. Matched Older Cat Owners to Dog Owners to Non-Owners. The most frequently diagnosed health conditions among ODO, OCO, and NPO were allergies followed by hypertension. The over-the-counter supplements used most commonly by OCO, ODO, and NPO were multivitamins, calcium, and fish oil/omega-3 fatty acids, in that order. Walking was the most common form of non-pet-related physical

activity reported among NPO, ODO, and OCO. Respondents were specifically asked to separate out walking for exercise without their dog from dog walking. Walking on a treadmill or track, walking in the mall, and walking with a walking group are examples of non-dog walking exercise that was classified as "walking." To decrease confounding, all three groups were matched for all available demographics yielding 22 usable triads (age $\mu = 55.4 \pm 4.5$ years). Analyses of these triads revealed no significant differences between NPO, ODO, and OCO using t-tests for dietary intake data or lifestyle characteristics. The decreased sample size diminished power to detect differences among groups. Nonowners had slightly but not significantly higher intakes of fruits, vegetables, and whole grains, but lower or equivalent servings of low fat dairy products. Multiple linear regressions for number of owner diagnoses showed significant contributions of pet ownership and BMI, but other variables were NS.

4. Discussion

Health and behaviors impacting health can be influenced by pet ownership [49]. An example is increased activity through dog walking [35–37, 50–52]. In this self-selected sample of pet owners >50 years of age matched to non-pet owners on key demographic characteristics, owning a pet was associated with fewer health problems and less prescribed medication. There were differences seen between cat versus dog owners and between those groups and nonowners on variables such as BMI, diagnoses, and health behaviors. The results point to the inherent health benefits of pet ownership for older adults, with dog ownership imparting greater health advantages. This may be due to the increased socialization, tactile stimulation, and psychological deterrent to loneliness that pets provide [53–55]. It has also been shown that companion animals may provide pain relief and stimulate oxytocin production, which increases bonding and feeling needed, which improves quality of life. These indicators are known to influence food consumption, eating patterns, body weight, and body habitus, as well as food choices, meal satisfaction, and appetite. Additionally, there are influences on neurotransmission, chemokines, and inflammation as well as hormones regulating blood pressure [56, 57].

Significant limitations to this study exist, including, but not limited to, convenience sampling, respondent bias, lack of generalizability to other populations, and lack of power to detect significant differences among the matched triads, NPO, ODO, and OCO.

Older adults owning dogs may be an inherently different population than older cat owners; they may be more mobile, active, and predisposed to socialization in the first place. In addition, subjects were only included if they had one pet per household, which is a significant limitation but was necessary to ensure that the data collection on diet and other characteristics were specifically for the one pet in the home. Multiple pets would have presented problems in collecting dietary and activity data, particularly if they were provided food ad libitum. Also, older adults keeping multiple pets in advanced age may be a very different demographic than those with a one pet household. Further research evaluating owning multiple pets among those of advanced age would be beneficial.

Owner demographics, socioeconomics, body habitus, and health are important to consider when advising older clients or marketing to older adults for themselves or their companion animals [58]. Older owners caring for older pets are a research area that should be explored, given the burgeoning older adult population in rural areas of the United States.

5. Conclusions

In this sample, rural, older pet owners differed from matched nonowners of companion animals, on several variables, including number of health conditions and BMI. Older cat owners differed from older dog owners, with higher BMIs, less physical activity, and less supplement usage. Older cat owners were much more likely to be female than dog owners and in worse condition. Differences in dietary, lifestyle, or health related characteristics between older cat, dog, and nonowners, when matched to one another on all available demographics, while not statistically significant, showed that pet ownership was indeed beneficial for older persons. Pet ownership and BMI significantly contributed to better overall health, using number of diagnosed conditions as a surrogate marker. Further research in this arena is required, particularly in light of the burgeoning older adult population and the trend towards viewing pets as family members. Older owner lifestyle, health practices, and care decisions may extend to their pet. Treatment options for either the owner or the pet should be tailored in the context of the pet as a family member for enhanced outcomes.

Additional Points

(i) Older adult pet owners have overall better health with regard to weight, health conditions, and fewer medications. (ii) Older adult dog owners have better health status than older adult cat owners. (iii) Pets help keep older adults more physically active and decrease loneliness and physical and cognitive decline, which improves quality of life and overall health.

Authors' Contributions

Roschelle Heuberger conceived, planned, and conducted the analysis of the article.

Acknowledgments

The author wishes to acknowledge Central Michigan University for ancillary services provided and the graduate students who assisted in the data collection, entry, cleaning, coding, and analysis and would like to thank the following persons for their contributions to either collecting, entering, cleaning, or coding of the data: Keirsten DeWitt, Allison Corby, and Rebecca Vander Sluis.

References

[1] G. Levine, K. Allen, L. Braun et al., "Pet ownership and cardiovascular risk: a scientific statement from the heart association," *Circulation*, vol. 127, no. 23, pp. 2353–2363, 2013.

[2] M. Rijken and S. van Beek, "About Cats and Dogs . reconsidering the relationship between pet ownership and health related outcomes in community-dwelling elderly," *Social Indicators Research*, vol. 102, no. 3, pp. 373–388, 2011.

[3] I. Enmarker, O. Hellzén, K. Ekker, and A.-G. Berg, "Health in older cat and dog owners: the nord-trondelag health study (HUNT)-3 study," *Scandinavian Journal of Public Health*, vol. 40, no. 8, pp. 718–724, 2012.

[4] P. Lail, G. R. McCormack, and M. Rock, "Does dog-ownership influence seasonal patterns of neighbourhood-based walking among adults? A longitudinal study," *BMC Public Health*, vol. 11, article 148, 2011.

[5] T. R. Schneider, J. B. Lyons, M. A. Tetrick, and E. E. Accortt, "Multidimensional quality of life and human-animal bond measures for companion dogs," *Journal of Veterinary Behavior: Clinical Applications and Research*, vol. 5, no. 6, pp. 287–301, 2010.

[6] T. King, L. C. Marston, and P. C. Bennett, "Describing the ideal Australian companion dog," *Applied Animal Behaviour Science*, vol. 120, no. 1-2, pp. 84–93, 2009.

[7] V. Hutton, "Companion animals and wellbeing when living with HIV in Australia," *Anthrozoos*, vol. 27, pp. 407–421, 2014.

[8] H. Brooks, K. Rushton, S. Walker et al., "Ontological security, and connectivity provided by pets: a study in the self-management of the everyday lives of people diagnosed with long-term mental illness," *BMC Psychiatry*, vol. 16, pp. 1–8, 2016.

[9] S. Ryan and S. Ziebland, "On interviewing people with pets: reflections from qualitative research on people with long-term conditions," *Sociology of Health and Illness*, vol. 37, no. 1, pp. 67–80, 2015.

[10] H. L. Brooks, A. Rogers, D. Kapadia, J. Pilgrim, D. Reeves, and I. Vassilev, "Creature comforts: personal communities, pets and the work of managing a long-term condition," *Chronic Illness*, vol. 9, no. 2, pp. 87–102, 2013.

[11] N. J. Rooney, S. Morant, and C. Guest, "Investigation into the value of trained glycaemia alert dogs to clients with type I diabetes," *PLoS ONE*, vol. 8, no. 8, article e69921, 2013.

[12] S. R. Engelman, "Palliative care and use of animal-assisted therapy," *Omega (United States)*, vol. 67, no. 1-2, pp. 63–67, 2013.

[13] S. Burres, N. E. Edwards, A. M. Beck, and E. Richards, "Incorporating pets into acute inpatient rehabilitation: a case study," *Rehabilitation Nursing*, vol. 41, no. 6, pp. 336–341, 2016.

[14] L. Bradley and P. C. Bennett, "Companion-Animals' effectiveness in managing chronic pain in adult community members," *Anthrozoos*, vol. 28, no. 4, pp. 635–647, 2015.

[15] S. M. Skjorestad and B. Johannessen, "The relationship between persons with mental health problems and their dogs: a qualitative study within a nursing perspective," *Journal of Nursing Education and Practice*, vol. 3, pp. 130–133, 2013.

[16] I. Enmarker, O. Hellzén, K. Ekker, and A.-G. T. Berg, "Depression in older cat and dog owners: The Nord-Trøndelag Health

Study (HUNT)-3," *Aging and Mental Health*, vol. 19, no. 4, pp. 347–352, 2015.

[17] A. L. Johnson, D. Pride, D. A. Donahue et al., "Potential benefits of canine companionship for military veterans with Posttraumatic Stress Disorder (PTSD)," *Society and Animals*, vol. 21, no. 6, pp. 568–581, 2013.

[18] D. Silcox, Y. Castillo, and B. Reed, "The human animal bond: applications for rehabilitation professionals," *Journal of Applied Rehabilitation Counseling*, vol. 45, pp. 27–37, 2014.

[19] P. Sable, "The pet connection: an attachment perspective," *Clinical Social Work Journal*, vol. 41, no. 1, pp. 93–99, 2013.

[20] J. McNicholas, "The role of pets in the lives of older people: a review," *Working with Older People*, vol. 18, no. 3, pp. 128–133, 2014.

[21] A. Cloutier and J. Peetz, "Relationships' Best Friend: Links between Pet Ownership, Empathy, and Romantic Relationship Outcomes," *Anthrozoos*, vol. 29, no. 3, pp. 395–408, 2016.

[22] M. Mueller, R. Bures, and N. Gee, "Human animal interaction and healthy aging," *Gerontologist*, vol. 56, article 261, 2016.

[23] I. H. Stanley, Y. Conwell, C. Bowen, and K. A. Van Orden, "Pet ownership may attenuate loneliness among older adult primary care patients who live alone," *Aging and Mental Health*, vol. 18, no. 3, pp. 394–399, 2014.

[24] L. Wood, K. Martin, H. Christian et al., "The pet factor—companion animals as a conduit for getting to know people, friendship formation and social support," *PLoS ONE*, vol. 10, no. 4, Article ID e0122085, 2015.

[25] J. L. Bryan, M. C. Quist, C. M. Young, M.-L. N. Steers, D. W. Foster, and Q. Lu, "Canine comfort: pet affinity buffers the negative impact of ambivalence over emotional expression on perceived social support," *Personality and Individual Differences*, vol. 68, pp. 23–27, 2014.

[26] C. G. Himsworth and M. Rock, "Pet ownership, other domestic relationships, and satisfaction with life among seniors: results from a Canadian national survey," *Anthrozoos*, vol. 26, no. 2, pp. 295–305, 2013.

[27] C. A. Krause-Parello, J. Tychowski, A. Gonzalez, and Z. Boyd, "Human-canine interaction: exploring stress indicator response patterns of salivary cortisol and immunoglobulin A," *Research and Theory for Nursing Practice*, vol. 26, no. 1, pp. 25–40, 2012.

[28] S. B. Barker, J. S. Knisely, N. L. McCain, C. M. Schubert, and A. K. Pandurangi, "Exploratory study of Stress-Buffering response patterns from interaction with a therapy dog," *Anthrozoos*, vol. 23, no. 1, pp. 79–91, 2010.

[29] E. Cherniak and A. Cherniak, "The benefit of pets and animal-assisted therapy to the health of older individuals," *Current Gerontology and Geriatrics Research*, vol. 2014, Article ID 623203, 9 pages, 2014.

[30] D. A. Marcus, C. D. Bernstein, J. M. Constantin, F. A. Kunkel, P. Breuer, and R. B. Hanlon, "Animal-assisted therapy at an outpatient pain management clinic," *Pain Medicine*, vol. 13, no. 1, pp. 45–57, 2012.

[31] C. G. Byers, C. C. Wilson, M. B. Stephens, J. L. Goodie, F. E. Netting, and C. H. Olsen, "Owners and pets exercising together: canine response to veterinarian-prescribed physical activity," *Anthrozoos*, vol. 27, no. 3, pp. 325–333, 2014.

[32] N. M. D. Antonacopoulos and T. A. Pychyl, "An examination of the possible benefits for well-being arising from the social interactions that occur while dog walking," *Society and Animals*, vol. 22, no. 5, pp. 459–480, 2014.

[33] D. O. Garcia, B. C. Wertheim, J. E. Manson et al., "Relationships between dog ownership and physical activity in postmenopausal women," *Preventive Medicine*, vol. 70, pp. 33–38, 2015.

[34] M. Gonzalez-Ramirez and R. Landero-Hernandez, "Benefits of dog ownership," *Journal of Veterinary Behavior*, vol. 9, pp. 311–315, 2014.

[35] K. Campbell, C. M. Smith, S. Tumilty, C. Cameron, and G. J. Treharne, "How does dog-walking influence perceptions of health and wellbeing in healthy adults? a qualitative dog-walk-along study," *Anthrozoos*, vol. 29, no. 2, pp. 181–192, 2016.

[36] R. J. Thorpe Jr., E. M. Simonsick, J. S. Brach et al., "Dog ownership, walking behavior, and maintained mobility in late life," *Journal of the American Geriatrics Society*, vol. 54, no. 9, pp. 1419–1424, 2006.

[37] J. A. Boisvert and W. Harrell, "Dog walking: a leisurely solution to pediatric and adult obesity," *World Leisure Journal*, no. 2, pp. 168–171, 2014.

[38] S. Holt, R. A. Johnson, H. D. Yaglom, and C. Brenner, "Animal assisted activity with older adult retirement facility residents: the PAWSitive visits program," *Activities, Adaptation and Aging*, vol. 39, no. 4, pp. 267–279, 2015.

[39] M. Perantonaki, K. Pyrga, K. Margaritis, M. Tsigga, and M. G. Grammatikopoulou, "Centrally obese adults walking their dogs benefit from improved anthropometry in selected body sites," *Obesity Medicine*, vol. 3, pp. 17–19, 2016.

[40] R. L. Utz, "Walking the dog: the effect of pet ownership on human health and health behaviors," *Social Indicators Research*, vol. 116, no. 2, pp. 327–339, 2014.

[41] N. Edwards and A. Beck, "Animal-assisted therapy and nutrition in alzheimer's disease," *Western Journal of Nursing Research*, vol. 24, no. 6, pp. 697–712, 2002.

[42] L. Nordgren and G. Engström, "Effects of dog-assisted intervention on behavioural and psychological symptoms of dementia," *Nursing Older People*, vol. 26, no. 3, pp. 31–38, 2014.

[43] E. Friedmann, E. Galik, S. A. Thomas et al., "Evaluation of a pet assisted living intervention for improving functional status in assisted living residents with mild to moderate cognitive impairment," *American Journal of Alzheimer's Disease & Other Dementias®*, vol. 30, no. 3, pp. 276–289, 2015.

[44] N. Richeson, "Effects of animal assisted therapy on agitated behaviors and social interactions of older adults with dementia," *The American Journal of Alzheimer's Disease and other Dementias*, vol. 18, no. 6, pp. 353–358, 2003.

[45] S. C. Kramer, E. Friedmann, and P. L. Bernstein, "Comparison of the effect of human interaction, animal-assisted therapy, and AIBO-assisted therapy on long-term care residents with dementia," *Anthrozoos*, vol. 22, no. 1, pp. 43–57, 2009.

[46] K. A. Anderson, L. K. Lord, L. N. Hill, and S. McCune, "Fostering the human-animal bond for older adults: challenges and opportunities," *Activities, Adaptation and Aging*, vol. 39, no. 1, pp. 32–42, 2015.

[47] K. Hodgson, L. Barton, M. Darling, V. Antao, F. A. Kim, and A. Monavvari, "Pets' impact on your patients' health: leveraging benefits and mitigating risk," *Journal of the American Board of Family Medicine*, vol. 28, no. 4, pp. 526–534, 2015.

[48] K. A. Kirtland, M. M. Zack, and C. J. Caspersen, "State-specific synthetic estimates of health status groups among inactive older adults with self-reported diabetes, 2000–2009," *Preventing Chronic Disease*, vol. 9, no. 4, Article ID 110221, 2012.

[49] V. I. Rohlf, P. C. Bennett, S. Toukhsati, and G. Coleman, "Beliefs underlying dog owners' health care behaviors: results from a

large, self-selected, internet sample," *Anthrozoos*, vol. 25, no. 2, pp. 171–185, 2012.

[50] C. Hayley, L. Wood, A. Nathan, and et al, "The association between dog walking, physical activity and owners perceptions of safety: cross sectional evidence from the US and Australia," *BMC Public Health*, vol. 16, no. 1, article 1010, 2016.

[51] E. A. Richards, "Does dog walking predict physical activity participation: results from a national survey," *American Journal of Health Promotion*, vol. 30, no. 5, pp. 323–330, 2016.

[52] N. Campbell and D. Kim, "Designing an ageless social community: adapting a new urbanist social core to suit baby boomers in later life," *Journal of Housing for the Elderly*, vol. 30, no. 2, pp. 156–174, 2016.

[53] J. M. Smith, "Toward a better understanding of loneliness in community-dwelling older adults," *Journal of Psychology: Interdisciplinary and Applied*, vol. 146, no. 3, pp. 293–311, 2012.

[54] R. Jenkins and E. Williams, "Dog visitation therapy in dementia care: a literature review," *Nursing Older People*, vol. 20, no. 8, pp. 31–40, 2008.

[55] P. Martens, M.-J. Enders-Slegers, and J. K. Walker, "The emotional lives of companion animals: attachment and subjective claims by owners of cats and dogs," *Anthrozoos*, vol. 29, no. 1, pp. 73–88, 2016.

[56] S. Branson, L. Boss, S. Cron, and D.-H. Kang, "Examining differences between homebound older adult pet owners and non-pet owners in depression, systemic inflammation, and executive function," *Anthrozoos*, vol. 29, no. 2, pp. 323–334, 2016.

[57] E. Friedmann, S. A. Thomas, H. Son, D. Chapa, and S. McCune, "Pet's presence and owner's blood pressures during the daily lives of pet owners with pre- to mild hypertension," *Anthrozoos*, vol. 26, no. 4, pp. 535–550, 2013.

[58] C. M. Martins, A. Mohamed, A. M. S. Guimarães et al., "Impact of demographic characteristics in pet ownership: modeling animal count according to owners income and age," *Preventive Veterinary Medicine*, vol. 109, no. 3-4, pp. 213–218, 2013.

26

A Study on Mortality Profile among Fifty Plus-(50+-) Population (FPP) of India: A 5-Year Retrospective Study at New Delhi District

B. L. Chaudhary,[1] **Raghvendra K. Vidua,**[2] **Arvind Kumar,**[1] **and Amrita V. Bajaj**[3]

[1]*Department of Forensic Medicine & Toxicology, Lady Hardinge Medical College, C-604, Shaheed Bhagat Singh Marg, Connaught Place, New Delhi 110001, India*
[2]*Department of Forensic Medicine & Toxicology, AIIMS, Saket Nagar, Bhopal, Madhya Pradesh 462020, India*
[3]*Department of Medicine, AIIM, Saket Nagar, Bhopal, Madhya Pradesh 462020, India*

Correspondence should be addressed to Raghvendra K. Vidua; raghvendra.fmt@aiimsbhopal.edu.in

Academic Editor: Tomasz Kostka

Objectives. To find out the mortality profile vis-a-vis different epidemiological factors at the time of autopsy among the 50+-Population. *Material and Method.* A five-year retrospective evaluation of medicolegal records between 2006 and 2010 was done at Lady Hardinge Medical College, New Delhi. *Results.* A total of 493 (17.78%) cases belonged to 50+-Population age group out of total 2773 autopsies performed. The proportion of unidentified/unknown persons among this age group was 36.51%. The unnatural and natural causes constituted 44.62% and 55.38% cases, respectively. The unspecified pneumonitis (50.18%) was reported as the commonest cause followed by coronary artery disease and respiratory tuberculosis among natural ones and the transport accident (57.27%) followed by accidental and intentional self-poisoning and exposure to noxious substances and falls among the unnatural ones. *Conclusion.* The findings reveal that this age group most commonly dies of natural causes rather than the unnatural ones even in autopsy cases. They have definite cure with timely interventions. The study also points out the need to devise the road and home safety measures to reduce mortality among the study population.

1. Introduction

As per 2011 census, 19, 20, 64,349 (50.18% males and 49.82% females) people in India were of fifty plus- (50+-) age group, which made about 15.86 percent of the total population while 39,67,805 (20,96,841 males and 18,70,964 females) and 21,773 (12,391 males and 9,382 females) persons out of total fifty plus- (50+-) population used to live in National Capital Territory of Delhi and district of New Delhi, respectively [1]. India's population aged fifty plus- (50+-) is expected to double by 2050 when nearly one-third of its total population would fall in this age group, according to a US census [2]. Fifty plus- (50+-) population (FPP) taken for the present study means the persons who are at or above the age of 50 years or the persons who have already spent their 50 years of lives. This group includes ageing population comprised of those who are already elders (60 years or above) or those who are on the verge of inclusion into this group (50+). Such type of persons

is usually on the declining phase for their body growth and general health.

Elderly or old age consists of ages nearing or surpassing the average life span of human beings. The boundary of old age cannot be defined exactly because it does not have the same meaning in all societies. Government of India adopted a National Policy on Older Persons in January, 1999; the policy defines "senior citizen" or "elderly" as a person who is of age 60 years or above (60+). This age group is inclusive in the fifty plus- (50+-) population age group taken for the present study.

As per survey conducted under National Sample Survey 60th round during January and June 2004, the survey estimated the number of aged persons (60+) as 829917, accounting for 5.49% of the total population of Delhi, and fifty plus- (50+-) population (FPP) was about 1877393 (12.42% of Delhi's population) [3]. The life expectancy of Indians has increased from 56.6 to 63.7 during the last two decades. With marginal success in control of communicable and infectious diseases along with improved standards of living, the number of elderly people has been on the increase. Consequently, people are living longer and elderly population has been increasing. Nearly 8% of Indian population belongs to 60+ years' age group [4].

2. Materials and Methods

In the present study, the medicolegal autopsy reports at Department of Forensic Medicine & Toxicology, Lady Hardinge Medical College, New Delhi (India), from 2006 to 2010, was taken into account. During this period, a total of 2773 medicolegal autopsies were performed. In the same period a total of 3,45,707 (64.43% males and 35.57% females) deaths of age group above 45 years were registered in National Capital territory of Delhi. In the same period NDMC (New Delhi Municipal Corporation) which registers all the deaths of New Delhi district has registered a total of 1,04,478 deaths (66.33% males and 33.67% females) [5]. Thus the number of cases in present study constitutes 0.80% of total registered deaths of 45+ years of age group in National Capital territory of Delhi and 2.65% of all the registered deaths of all the age groups reported by the NDMC.

Medical and other investigative data from the police requisition reports were available in each case and they provided the data about the personal details, the manner of death, and approximate time since death of the deceased while the autopsy reports provided the postmortem findings, time of death, and cause of death. The inclusion criteria were that the deceased was of 50+ years of age at the time of death. The manner of death was registered as natural, accidental, suicidal, homicidal, or unknown, after evaluation of all available information in police inquest report and post-mortem examination. All deaths were further subcategorized according to the different epidemiological factors such as age, sex, year, manner and cause of death, and whether deceased was identified/known with a valid home address available or homeless and unidentified/unknown person (HUP).

3. Results

In the present study a total 2773 medicolegal autopsies were reported during this time period. A total of 493 (17.78%) cases were belonging to 50+ population age group. Out of total cases of 50+ population age group, the males were 438 cases (88.84%) and females were 55 cases (11.16%). The male to female cases ratio was 7.96 : 1. The deaths due to unnatural and natural events constituted 220 (44.62%) and 273 (55.38%) cases, respectively (Table 1). Out of 493 cases, 180 (36.51%) cases were unidentified/unknown persons (HUPs) or persons without any valid home address whose identity could not be established at the time of autopsy. The male and female deaths in unidentified/unknown persons constituted 158 cases (87.77%) and 22 cases (12.22%), respectively.

There were 273 (55.38%) deaths due to natural causes and unspecified pneumonitis contributed to the maximum number of 137 (50.18%) of cases followed by coronary artery

TABLE 1: Year- and sex-wise distribution of natural and unnatural deaths in 50+ population.

Year	Natural deaths		Unnatural deaths		Total
	Male	Female	Male	Female	
2006	49	4	25	8	86
2007	27	0	47	11	85
2008	52	3	50	4	109
2009	41	5	27	6	79
2010	84	8	36	6	134
Total	**253**	**20**	**185**	**35**	**493**

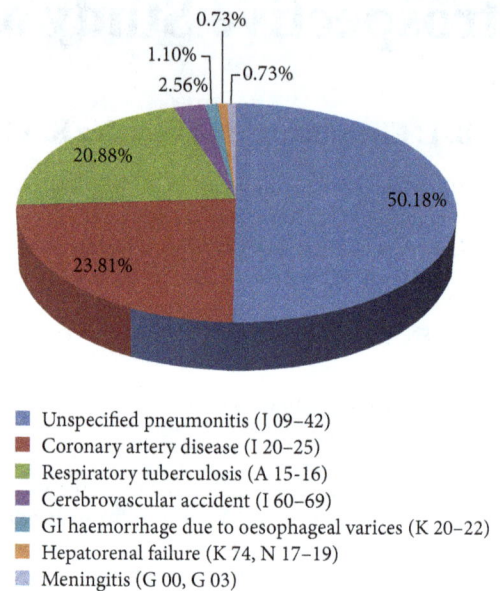

- Unspecified pneumonitis (J 09–42)
- Coronary artery disease (I 20–25)
- Respiratory tuberculosis (A 15-16)
- Cerebrovascular accident (I 60–69)
- GI haemorrhage due to oesophageal varices (K 20–22)
- Hepatorenal failure (K 74, N 17–19)
- Meningitis (G 00, G 03)

FIGURE 1: Distribution of natural causes of death among 50+ population.

disease 65 cases (23.81%) and respiratory tuberculosis 57 cases (20.88%) among them (Figure 1). Out of 273 cases, 155 (56.78%) cases were homeless unknown/unidentified persons (HUPs) and remaining 119 (43.22%) cases were identified or having a valid home addresses. Coronary artery disease was major cause of death in 60 cases (38.71%) among identified/known or persons having a valid home address but the unspecified pneumonitis was major cause of death in 105 (67.74%) cases of homeless unidentified/unknown persons (HUPs).

Respiratory tuberculosis was reported as cause of death in 40 cases (25.81%) of homeless unknown/unidentified and in 17 cases (14.29%) of identified/known persons having a valid home address. The male and female ratio among the persons who died of natural deaths was 12.65 : 1. Unspecified pneumonitis ($n = 137$, 50.18%) was the major health problem in 50+ population and was a leading cause of natural deaths. The male-to-female ratio for unspecified pneumonitis was 12.7 : 1. After unspecified pneumonitis, respiratory tuberculosis was the second leading cause of death among natural deaths in 57 (20.88%) cases.

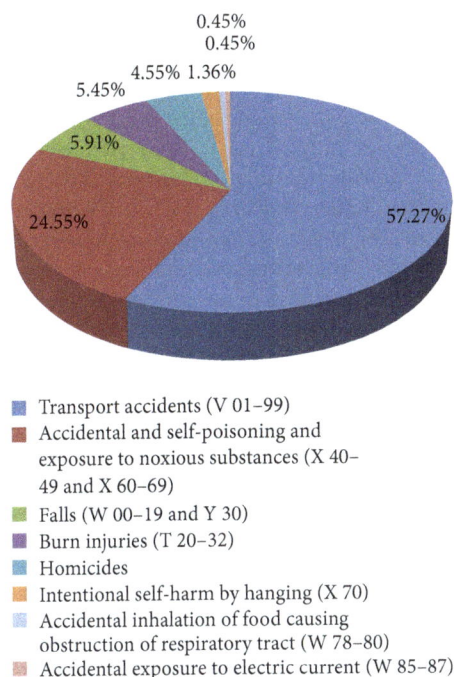

Transport accidents (V 01–99)

Accidental and self-poisoning and
exposure to noxious substances (X 40–
49 and X 60–69)

Falls (W 00–19 and Y 30)

Burn injuries (T 20–32)

Homicides

Intentional self-harm by hanging (X 70)

Accidental inhalation of food causing
obstruction of respiratory tract (W 78–80)

Accidental exposure to electric current (W 85–87)

FIGURE 2: Distribution of unnatural causes of death among 50+
population.

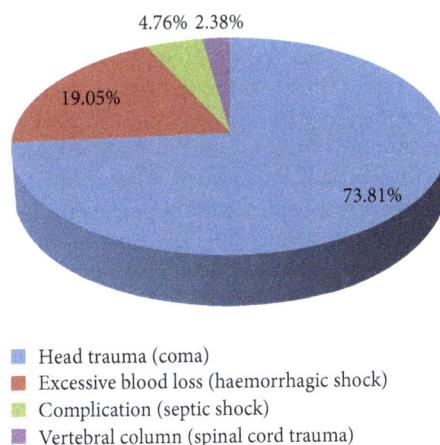

Head trauma (coma)

Excessive blood loss (haemorrhagic shock)

Complication (septic shock)

Vertebral column (spinal cord trauma)

FIGURE 3: Mode of death in transport accidents among 50+ population.

4. Discussion

In the present study, 493 (17.78%) cases were of 50+ population age group and the male-to-female ratio among them
was 7.96 : 1. As per the National Sample Survey organization,
39% of the elderly of 60+ age are likely to be suffering from
one or the other health problem [3]. It is estimated that 1.7%
and 1% suffer from visual disability, 1.5% and 1.3% hearing,
and 2.7% and 2.8% locomotor difficulties in rural and urban
areas, respectively [4]. Data from National Crime Records
Bureau–2006 [6] indicate that 34,594, 60+ individuals lost
their life due to an injury. Some epidemiological surveys on
aged population indicate that 1.7% was affected with injuries
[7]. Previous studies from NIMHANS on traumatic brain
injuries and road traffic injuries reveal that 5–8% of deaths
and hospitalisations are among 60+ people [8]. Among the
various types of injuries, road traffic injuries and falls are
found to be the leading causes of injury. One-year (2007)
data from Bengaluru injury surveillance programme showed
that 360 individuals of 60+ years age group died and 2643
of 60+ years age group are individuals suffering from various
forms of injuries brought to hospitals. Majority of those killed
or hospitalized belonged to middle-income families [9]. The
male-to-female distribution was almost equal with 198 men
and 162 women in contrast to the present study with 438 male
cases to 55 female cases.

In the 50+ population, the accidental and intentional
self-poisoning and exposure to noxious substances were
reported as the second leading cause of unnatural deaths and
responsible for deaths in 54 (34.55%) cases. The organophos-
phates which is very commonly used agricultural pesticide
in India was found as the commonest poison responsible for
deaths due to exposure of poisons and noxious substances
based upon police inquest report, postmortem examination
awaiting viscera lab analysis report. The financial burden and
family dispute were the most common reason for committing
suicide as per the police inquest report. All the cases had
occurred at home when the person was alone in absence
of immediate family members. The homicides constituted a
total of 10 deaths among the unnatural deaths and the assault
by firearm weapon (40% cases) was the commonest means
used (Figure 2).

Among 220 unnatural deaths the leading contributor to
death was the transport accidents (n = 126, 57.27%) in
50+ population and out of that, in 16 (12.70%) cases, the
identity of the person could not be established. All of the road
traffic accidents had occurred within the New Delhi district
of the city and majority (n = 41 cases, 32.54%) during the
evening hours between 6 pm and 12 midnight followed by
morning hours (n = 33 cases, 26.19%) between 6 am and 12
at noon. Pedestrians was the most commonly affected group
and nearly half of deaths were due to be hit by heavy vehicles
like buses, cars, trucks, and van/jeeps. The head injury (coma)
was found as the commonest mode of death in 93 (73.81%)
cases (Figure 3).

In the present study, 50+ population cases accounted for
17.81% (55.46% natural deaths and 44.53% unnatural deaths)
of the total medicolegal autopsies conducted in the mortuary
of Lady Hardinge Medical College (LHMC), New Delhi. In
the study by Ince et al. [10], this rate was 7.8%. Homicide and
suicide origins accounted for 18.9% which can be considered
as higher compared with the literature. In Osaka [11], during
1994–1998, this rate was 13.2%. In another study by Collins
and Presnell [12], this rate was 12.4%. In the present study,
stabbing was the most common method of homicide, while
gunshot was the most common method in other studies [13,
14]. In the present study, male/female proportion was 3 : 1 and
this was consistent with other Turkish studies [10, 15]. Psychiatric illnesses were associated with suicide tendency [11].

In the elderly, 19% of the female and 9% of the male victims had a history of previous suicide attempts [16]. In the present study, poisoning (47.1%) was the most common method of suicide unlike hanging in the study held in Aydin [17, 18]. Hanging is the most frequent suicide method used by the elderly also in Austria [19] and many other countries [10, 18]. Use of poison was very common in the present study as also in Pritchard and Hansen's study [18]. The most common wound site was the head region in road traffic accidents consistently with other studies [18, 20]. The 60+ victims had a higher rate of chest injuries and the commonest method of suicide was hanging followed by organophosphate poisoning [21].

5. Limitations of the Study

Consider

(1) There were a large number of deceased persons in this study whose identity could not be established till the time of autopsy which adversely affected the amount of reliability and details of history obtained.

(2) Authors could not find any other such type of studies conducted in this particular age group, so not much data was available for comparison. Therefore, in the present study a comparison was made with the mortality profile of age group of sixty plus- (60+-) population (SPP) as many of the studies have been conducted in this group in the past and it is also inclusive in fifty plus- (50+-) population (FPP) age group.

(3) The Lady Hardinge Medical College is located in the National Capital Territory region of the country. The demographic profile of population is much different in such type of metropolitan city compared to the other cities or villages of India so the results of the studies cannot be generalised for the similar age group population of rest of the country but of course it may be taken as a comparable reference point for similar kind of metropolitan cities.

(4) The detailed lab analysis report regarding poisoning cases was not available on time and in most of the cases of unspecified pneumonitis and respiratory tuberculosis the histopathological investigations were not done and the diagnosis was made on the basis of gross examination of lung and its cut sections.

6. Conclusion

With the growth of ageing population in almost each and every society of the world and consequent rise in their mortality, it is important to study their mortality profile to find out various reasons responsible for their untimely natural and unnatural mortality because of emergence of certain age related risk factors for devising appropriate intervention strategies. In this study the major factors responsible for mortality among them were found out as unspecified pneumonitis, coronary artery disease, and respiratory tuberculosis among natural causes and transport accidents, accidental and intentional self-exposure to poisoning, and falls among unnatural causes. The interventions need to be integrated in a comprehensive manner with the focus on provision of early diagnosis and treatment along with the modification of risk factors for natural causes and effective preventive strategies along with the timely treatment and enforcement of adequate road safety measures like use of helmet to reduce the occurrence of head injuries in transport accidents for unnatural causes. The findings clearly reveal that this age group most commonly dies of natural causes like pulmonary and cardiovascular diseases rather than the unnatural ones even in autopsy cases. They have definite cure with timely interventions and that will also be helpful to reduce the spread of communicable infections to the rest of the population. The home safety measures should also be devised to reduce their accidental and intentional self-exposure to poisoning and fall injuries to reduce the mortality in fifty plus- (50+-) population (FPP) at New Delhi district in India.

Disclaimer

The authors own full responsibility in case any conflict arises after publication of the paper.

References

[1] http://www.censusindia.gov.in/2011census/population_enumeration.html.

[2] http://www.rediff.com/news/report/india-s-50-plus-population-to-double-by-2050/20120508.htm.

[3] National Sample Survey Organization, "Morbidity, health care and the condition of the aged," NSS 60th Round, Report 507, 2006.

[4] http://www.censusindia.gov.in/Census_Data_2001/India_at_glance/broad.aspx.

[5] http://www.delhi.gov.in/wps/wcm/connect/7c47f10048e377b4a705bfb2120f29ae/B+%26+D+2010.pdf?MOD=AJPERES&lmod=1488121114&CACHEID=7c47f10048e377b4a705bfb2120f29ae&lmod=1488121114&CACHEID=7c47f10048e377b4a705bfb2120f29ae.

[6] National Crime Records Bureau, Accidental Deaths and Suicides in India, Ministry of Home Affairs, Government of India, New Delhi, India, 2006.

[7] V. Rao, Health Care of the Aged, Indian Council of Medical Research, New Delhi, India, 1990.

[8] G. Gururaj, K. V. R. Shastry, A. B. Chandramouli, D. K. Subbakrishna, and J. F. Kraus, Traumatic Brain Injury, Bengaluru Publication no. 61, National Institute of Mental Health and Neurosciences, Bengaluru, India, 2005.

[9] Bengaluru Injury Surveillance Collaborators Group, Bengaluru Injury/Road Traffic Injury Surveillance Programme: A Feasibility Study, Publication no. 68, National Institute of Mental Health and Neurosciences, Bangalore, India, 2008.

[10] H. Ince, S. Aliustaoglu, and Y. Yazici, "Deahts of the elderly exposed to violence in Turkey," Collegium Antropologicum, vol. 32, pp. 315–319, 2008.

[11] B.-L. Zhu, S. Oritani, K. Ishida et al., "Child and elderly victims in forensic autopsy during a recent 5 year period in the southern half of Osaka city and surrounding areas," Forensic Science International, vol. 113, no. 1–3, pp. 215–218, 2000.

[12] K. A. Collins and S. E. Presnell, "Elder homicide: a 20-year study," *The American Journal of Forensic Medicine and Pathology*, vol. 27, no. 2, pp. 183–187, 2006.

[13] R. W. Byard, K. A. Hanson, and J. D. Gilbert, "Suicide methods in the elderly in South Australia 1981–2000," *Journal of Clinical Forensic Medicine*, vol. 11, no. 2, pp. 71–74, 2004.

[14] H. O'Connell, A.-V. Chin, C. Cunningham, and B. A. Lawlor, "Recent developments: suicide in older people," *British Medical Journal*, vol. 329, no. 7471, pp. 895–899, 2004.

[15] Ö. Kurtaş, Ü. Biçer, İ. Demirbaş, Ü. N. Gündoğmuş, B. Çolak, and N. Etiler, "Determination of pre and elderly age deaths in Kocaeli Forensic Medicine Unit," *Journal of Forensic Medicine*, vol. 18, no. 2, pp. 67–74, 2004.

[16] H. J. Koponen, K. Viilo, H. Hakko et al., "Rates and previous disease history in old age suicide," *International Journal of Geriatric Psychiatry*, vol. 22, no. 1, pp. 38–46, 2007.

[17] A. Yafililardak, "Homicide and suicide in the elderly: data from Aydin," *Turkish Journal of Geriatrics*, vol. 14, no. 4, pp. 306–310, 2011.

[18] C. Pritchard and L. Hansen, "Comparison of suicide in people aged 65-74 and 75+ by gender in England and Wales and the major Western countries 1979–1999," *International Journal of Geriatric Psychiatry*, vol. 20, no. 1, pp. 17–25, 2005.

[19] N. D. Kapusta, E. Etzersdorfer, and G. Sonneck, "Trends in suicide rates of the elderly in Austria, 1970–2004: an analysis of changes in terms of age groups, suicide methods and gender," *International Journal of Geriatric Psychiatry*, vol. 22, no. 5, pp. 438–444, 2007.

[20] H. H. Eilertsen, P. K. Lilleng, B. O. Mæhle, and I. Morild, "Forensic examination of death in the elderly," *Scandinavian Journal of Forensic Science*, vol. 1, pp. 15–19, 2005.

[21] W. Y. Yee, P. A. Cameron, and M. J. Bailey, "Road traffic injuries in the elderly," *Emergency Medicine Journal*, vol. 23, no. 1, pp. 42–46, 2006.

Identification of Neuroprotective Factors Associated with Successful Ageing and Risk of Cognitive Impairment among Malaysia Older Adults

Huijin Lau,[1] Arimi Fitri Mat Ludin,[1] Nor Fadilah Rajab,[1] and Suzana Shahar[2]

[1]*Biomedical Science Programme, School of Diagnostic and Applied Health Sciences, Faculty of Health Sciences, Universiti Kebangsaan Malaysia, Kuala Lumpur, Malaysia*
[2]*Dietetics Programme, School of Healthcare Sciences, Faculty of Health Sciences, Universiti Kebangsaan Malaysia, Kuala Lumpur, Malaysia*

Correspondence should be addressed to Arimi Fitri Mat Ludin; arimifitri@ukm.edu.my

Academic Editor: Marco Malavolta

The increase of ageing population has raised public attention on the concept of successful ageing. Studies have shown that vitamin D, telomere length, and brain-derived neurotrophic factor (BDNF) have been associated with cognitive function. Therefore, this study aimed to identify neuroprotective factors for cognitive decline in different ageing groups. A total of 300 older adults aged 60 years and above were recruited in this population based cross-sectional study. Participants were categorized into three groups: mild cognitive impairment (MCI) ($n = 100$), usual ageing (UA) ($n = 100$), and successful ageing (SA) ($n = 100$). Dietary vitamin D intake was assessed through Diet History Questionnaire (DHQ). Out of the 300 participants, only 150 were subjected to fasting blood sample collection. These samples were used for serum vitamin D and plasma BDNF measurements. Whole blood telomere length was measured using RT-PCR method. The results show that the reduction of the risk of MCI was achieved by higher serum vitamin D level (OR: 0.96, 95% CI: 0.92–0.99, $p < 0.05$), higher plasma BDNF level (OR: 0.51, 95% CI: 0.30–0.88, $p < 0.05$), and longer telomere (OR: 0.97, 95% CI: 0.95–0.99, $p < 0.001$). In conclusion, participants with higher vitamin D level, higher BDNF level, and longer telomere length were more likely to age successfully.

1. Introduction

Ageing population in Malaysia is expected to reach 15% of the total population in year 2030 [1]. This can burden a nation especially that a significant percentage of healthcare budget is channelled to the elderly population. Recently, neurodegenerative diseases such as dementia and Alzheimer's diseases have become a major concern. The rapid growth of ageing population has raised much attention and awareness on the concept of successful ageing. The main goal of successful ageing is to maintain or improve emotional well-being and quality of life [2]. Therefore, discovery of potential noninvasive and easily accessible neuroprotective factors for cognitive impairment is needed to delay or prevent the onset of dementia and Alzheimer's disease. These would also promote successful ageing.

Balanced dietary intake is a well-established lifestyle factor in maintaining cognition during ageing. However, vitamin D deficiency is a very common problem in geriatric population. Previous animal study showed that vitamin D supplementation may reverse age-related cognitive decline in ageing rats [3]. In addition, cross-sectional study by Annweiler et al. [4] revealed that there is a significant association between vitamin D and cognitive function. Therefore, vitamin D has been suggested as a potential neuroprotective agent in ageing process.

Ageing is also often related to telomere shortening and decrease in BDNF level. Ageing increased oxidative stress, which leads to DNA damage characterized by telomere shortening [5]. Ma et al. [6] reported a significant correlation between telomere length and cognitive function and suggested that telomere length may serve as a biomarker for

TABLE 1: Classification criteria for ageing groups.

Successful ageing	Usual ageing	Mild cognitive impairment
(1) Free from diabetes, hypertension, cancer, heart diseases, chronic lung diseases, and stroke	(1) Participants with average performance in most of the cognitive test administered (scores above MCI but below SA)	(1) Subjective memory complaint by participants or caregivers
(2) No functional limitations as indicated by full score in ADL	(2) No dementia	(2) Objective memory impairment [poor performance in one or more cognitive tests (Digit span and RAVLT) with score of at least 1.5 SD below the mean average]
(3) Normal global function as indicated by MMSE score ≥ 22	(3) No or very minimal functional limitations	(3) No dementia
(4) No depression by having a score of ≤4 in the GDS-15 item		(4) No limitations in basic activities of daily living (ADL)
(5) Good quality of life		(5) No or very minimal difficulties in instrumental activities of daily living by having a score of ≤1.5 SD from mean norm
(6) Good self-perceived health		(6) Preserved global function by having MMSE score of ≥19

ADL: activities of daily living; MMSE: Mini-Mental State Examination; GDS: Geriatric Depression Scale.

cognitive decline. BDNF level has been found to decrease with increasing age. High level of BDNF is believed to protect neurons from damage and maintain cognitive function in the elderly [7]. Therefore, reduction of BDNF could also be a risk factor for cognitive decline.

Although previous studies showed significant associations between the vitamin D level, telomere length, and BDNF level with cognitive function, their relationships with SA, UA, and MCI have not fully been explored. Therefore, this study aimed to identify the neuroprotective factors and their relationship with successful ageing and risk of MCI.

2. Method

This comparative cross-sectional study is a part of the large-scale community based longitudinal study which investigates neuroprotection model for the purpose of healthy longevity among Malaysian older adults (TUA) [8]. The study protocol was approved by Research and Medical Research Ethics Committee of Universiti Kebangsaan Malaysia (UKM) and informed consent was obtained from all the participants.

2.1. Participants and Cognitive Ageing Groups Classification. Participants in the previous large-scale study were divided into three different cognitive ageing groups, namely, mild cognitive impairment (MCI), usual ageing (UA), and successful ageing (SA). The classification of cognitive status was done based on multidimensional domains including physical function, subjective and objective memory impairments, psychocognitive functioning, major diseases, health status, and quality of life by using pretested questionnaires. The details of cognitive ageing groups classification protocol were described in Table 1 [8]. The present study involved a total of 300 community-dwelling older adults aged 60 years and above recruited from the previous study using multistage

random sampling. A total of 100 participants with MCI were randomly drawn from the large population in the community based longitudinal study reported earlier [8]. Age- and gender-matched participants with UA ($n = 100$) and SA ($n = 100$) were randomly drawn from the same cohort. Sociodemographic information and dietary intake were obtained using questionnaire at this stage. Biological samples were randomly collected from 50 participants from each group.

2.1.1. Sociodemographic Information and Dietary Intake of Vitamin D. Sociodemographic information including age, ethnicity, years of education, marriage, and living status, as well as alcohol intake and smoking habit, was recorded. Vitamin D intake was also recorded using Diet History Questionnaire (DHQ) among the total of 300 elderly. Standardised pictures were provided to guide the participants in filling the questionnaire. They were asked to recall all the foods and beverages consumed in the past 7 days from the day the questionnaire was administered. The obtained data were then analysed using Nutritionist ProTM diet analysis software (Axxya Systems, USA) to calculate the total vitamin D intake.

2.1.2. Blood Samples Collection. A total of 150 age- and gender-matched subsamples were randomly chosen for laboratory analysis including serum vitamin D level, buccal micronucleus assay, absolute telomere length, and plasma BDNF level. A total of 5 ml of fasting blood sample was collected through venipuncture procedure by trained phlebotomist into three separate vacutainers. Total of 2 ml of blood samples was centrifuged for 10 minutes at 3500 r.p.m. to obtain plasma. Plasma and another 2 ml of whole blood were then stored at −80°C prior to analysis. The remaining 1 ml of whole blood was immediately sent to clinical lab for serum vitamin D level determination.

2.1.3. Serum Vitamin D Level. The serum vitamin D level was measured using validated ARCHITECT 25-OH Vitamin D assay by BP clinical lab (BP Healthcare, Kuala Lumpur, Malaysia). It is a delayed one-step immunoassay including a sample pretreatment for the quantitative determination of vitamin D in human serum based on Chemiflex (CMIA technology with flexible) assay protocols. The resulting chemiluminescent reaction is measured as relative light units (RLUs). ARCHITECT i System optics (Abbott Laboratories, Wiesbaden, Germany) was used to detect an indirect relationship between the amount of vitamin D in the sample and the RLUs [9].

2.1.4. Absolute Telomere Length. DNA extraction from whole blood was done using commercially available kit (QIAamp® Blood Mini Kit, QIAGEN, Netherlands). Absolute telomere length measurement was carried out based on method adopted from O'Callaghan and Fenech [10] using iQ5 Real-Time Polymerase Chain Reaction (RT-PCR) detection system (Bio-Rad, CA, USA). The standard oligomers used in this assay were as follows:

(1) Telomere (TTAGGG)14

(2) Single copy gene (SCG) 36B4 (CAGCAAGTGGG-AAGGTGTAATCCGTCTCCACAGACAAGGCC-AGGACTCGTTTGTACCCGTTGATGATAGAA-TGGG) (Bio Basics, Canada Inc.)

PCR primers included the following:

(1) teloF (CGGTTTGTTTGGGTTTGGGTTTGGGTT-TGGGTTTGGGTT),

(2) teloR (GGCTTGCCTTACCCTTACCCTTACCCT-TACCCTTACCCT),

(3) 36B4F (CAGCAAGTGGGAAGGTGTAATCC)

(4) 36B4R (CCCATTCTATCATCAACGGGTACAA) (Bio Basic, Canada Inc.)

Absolute telomere length was calculated by dividing kb/telomere reaction with copies/diploid genome of 36B4.

2.1.5. Plasma Brain-Derived Neurotrophic Factor (BDNF). Plasma concentration of BDNF was quantified using commercially available enzyme-linked immunoassay (ELISA) kit (Sigma Aldrich, USA) based on manufacturer's instructions. Duplicates of BDNF levels were determined at an absorbance of 450 nm. The coefficient of variation between the standards and duplicates was less than 5% [11].

3. Data Analysis

All data were analysed using Statistical Package for Social Science (SPSS) version 22. Significant value was set at $p < 0.05$. Comparison of sociodemographic factors and potential neuroprotective factors between SA, UA, and MCI groups were analysed using χ^2 tests for categorical variables and one-way Analysis of Variance (ANOVA) test for continuous variables. Results are presented as mean ± standard deviation for normally distributed data and median (quartile range) for

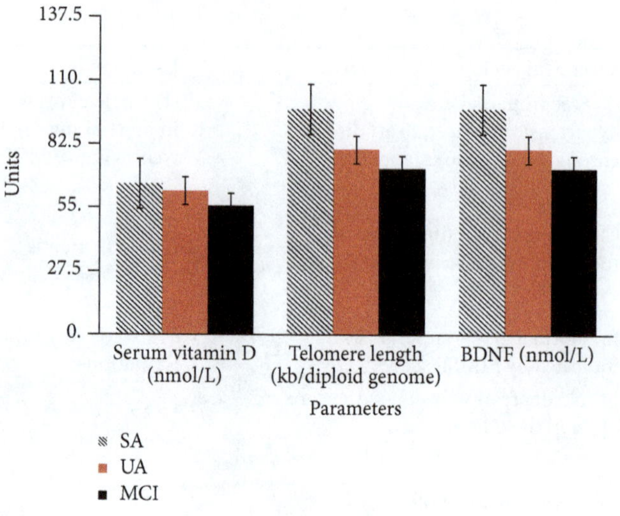

FIGURE 1: Comparison of selected neuroprotective factors between ageing groups. BDNF: brain-derived neurotrophic factor; SA: successful ageing; UA: usual ageing; MCI: mild cognitive impairment. One-way ANOVA and post hoc test LSD. Serum vitamin D and BDNF significant between MCI and SA; telomere length significant between UA and SA.

data that were not normally distributed. LSD post hoc test was used to compare the significant difference of continuous variables between groups. Multinomial Logistic Regression was performed to determine the significant neuroprotective factors related to successful ageing and cognitive impairment.

4. Results

Table 2 summarizes the sociodemographic characteristics of the 300 participants. The mean age of participants was 68.04 ± 5.56 years old, and there was no significant difference between ageing groups ($p > 0.05$). The majority of the participants in this study were Malays (61.3%), followed by Chinese (35.7%) and Indians (3.0%). A total of 67.7% participants received education less than 6 years and the rest received education more than 6 years. The difference between ageing groups is significant ($p < 0.001$). Cognitive performances, physical function, and depressive scale also showed significant difference between groups ($p < 0.05$). However, smoking habit and ethnicity among participants did not show significant difference in the three ageing groups.

Figure 1 shows the comparison of selected neuroprotective factors between different ageing groups. Vitamin D intake was significantly higher in SA group ($0.33 \pm 0.77\,\mu g$) compared to MCI group ($0.13 \pm 0.33\,\mu g$) ($p < 0.05$). Participants in SA group also showed significantly higher serum vitamin D level (65.11 ± 17.08 nmol/L) than those in MCI group (55.71 ± 19.97 nmol/L) ($p < 0.05$). Telomere length was also reported to be significantly different between SA (97.52 ± 35.49 kb/genome diploid) with UA (80.07 ± 32.78 kb/genome diploid) and MCI (71.84 ± 30.97 kb/genome diploid) ($p < 0.05$). Plasma BDNF was reported to be higher in SA group (14.24 ± 1.26 nmol/L) than MCI group (13.38 ± 26.2 nmol/L) ($p < 0.05$).

TABLE 2: Sociodemographic characteristics.

Parameter	SA ($n = 100$)	UA ($n = 100$)	MCI ($n = 100$)	Total ($N = 300$)	p
Age[a]	67.99 ± 5.52	68.00 ± 5.57	68.14 ± 5.64	68.04 ± 5.56	>0.05
Ethnic					
Malay	61 (33.2)	61 (33.2)	62 (33.7)	184 (61.3)	
Chinese	36 (33.6)	36 (33.6)	35 (32.7)	107 (35.7)	>0.05
Indian	3 (33.3)	3 (33.3)	3 (33.3)	9 (3.0)	
Marriage status					
Single/widow/widower/divorced	17 (17.0)	19 (19.0)	25 (25.0)	61 (20.3)	>0.05
Married	83 (83.0)	81 (81.0)	75 (75.0)	239 (79.7)	
Educational year					
≤6 years	44 (44.0)	78 (78.0)	81 (81.0)	203 (67.7)	<0.001
>6 years	56 (56.0)	22 (22.0)	19 (19.0)	97 (32.3)	
Smoking habit					
Smoking	20 (20.0)	20 (20.0)	26 (26.0)	66 (22.0)	>0.05
Past or nonsmokers	80 (80.0)	80 (80.0)	74 (74.0)	234 (78.0)	
Cognitive measures[a]					
MMSE	26.34 ± 0.22	23.24 ± 0.40	22.18 ± 0.48		<0.001*
Digit Span	13.88 ± 0.34	11.96 ± 0.37	10.72 ± 0.39		<0.001**
RAVLT	8.82 ± 0.29	7.28 ± 0.30	1.68 ± 0.13		<0.001**
Physical function[a]					
ADL	14.00 ± 0.00	12.42 ± 0.25	12.17 ± 0.17		<0.001***
Depressive symptoms[a]					
GDS	1.98 ± 0.14	2.07 ± 0.13	1.76 ± 0.13		>0.05
Vitamin D intake (µg)[a]	0.33 ± 0.77	0.25 ± 0.21	0.13 ± 0.33		<0.05

SA: successful ageing; UA: usual ageing; MCI: mild cognitive impairment; MMSE: Mini-Mental State Examination; ADL: activities of daily living; GDS: Geriatric Depression Scale. Chi-squared test, significant at $p < 0.001$. [a]One-way ANOVA (mean ± standard deviation). *Significant at $p < 0.05$ between SA and MCI. **Significant at $p < 0.001$ between SA, UA, and MCI. ***Significant at $p < 0.001$ between SA and UA, SA, and MCI.

TABLE 3: Determination of significant neuroprotective factors associated with risk of cognitive impairment.

	Selected neuroprotective factors	B	exp(B)	95% confidence interval Upper	95% confidence interval Lower	p
MCI	Serum Vitamin D (nmol/L)	−0.05	0.96	0.92	0.99	<0.05[a]
	Telomere Length (kb/diploid genome)	−0.03	0.97	0.95	0.99	<0.001[a]
	BDNF (nmol/L)	−0.67	0.51	0.30	0.88	<0.05[b]
UA	Serum Vitamin D (nmol/L)	−0.02	0.98	0.94	1.02	>0.05
	Telomere Length (kb/diploid genome)	−0.03	0.98	0.96	0.99	<0.01[a]
	BDNF (nmol/L)	−0.59	0.56	0.33	0.93	<0.05[b]

BDNF: brain-derived neurotrophic factor; SA: successful ageing; UA: usual ageing; MCI: mild cognitive impairment. Multinomial Logistic Regression with reference group is successful ageing. [a]Significant at $p < 0.05$ after being controlled for age, gender, educational level, and smoking status. [b]Significant at $p < 0.05$ after being controlled for confounding factors: age, gender, educational level, smoking, physical function, and depressive symptoms.

The selected neuroprotective factors that were found to be significantly different ($p < 0.05$) were further analysed by Multinomial Logistic Regression model for the identification of significant neuroprotective factors associated with successful ageing and the risk of cognitive impairment. Table 3 demonstrates the significant neuroprotective factors associated with the risk of cognitive impairment. After controlling the age, gender, educational years, and smoking status, it was

found that every one nmol/L increased in serum vitamin D level could reduce the risk of MCI by 4% (OR: 0.96, 95% CI: 0.92–0.99, $p < 0.05$). The risk of getting MCI and UA can also be lowered by 3% (OR: 0.97, 95% CI: 0.95–0.99, $p < 0.001$) and 2% (OR: 0.98, 95% CI: 0.96–0.99, $p < 0.01$), respectively, with an increase of one kb/genome diploid in telomere length when compared to SA group. In addition, increase in one nmol/L in plasma BDNF level may also reduce the risk of MCI (OR: 0.51, 95% CI: 0.30–0.88, $p <$ 0.05) and UA (OR: 0.56, 95% CI: 0.33–0.93, $p < 0.05$) by 49% and 44%, respectively.

5. Discussion

Malnutrition such as vitamin D and protein deficiency accompanying the ageing process and living a sedentary lifestyle could accelerate muscle weakness. Increased prevalence of disability, falls, fractures, and even mortality among older adults is often related to frailty and sarcopenia. In a systematic review, most cross-sectional and longitudinal studies also demonstrate significant relationships between frailty and cognitive performance and impairment [12]. Therefore, a link between vitamin D deficiency and cognitive impairment could be hypothesized. Our results revealed that dietary intake and serum vitamin D levels were significantly higher in SA group than MCI group. In addition, the findings also showed that increased vitamin D level was associated with the risk of MCI. The wide distribution of vitamin D receptors (VDR) in central nervous system (CNS) has suggested that vitamin D plays a role in neurogenesis [13]. This finding is in line with previous study which reported that increased serum vitamin D could reduce the risk of MCI among the elderly [4]. Ahn and Kang [14] also stated in their study that serum vitamin D could be the predictor for cognitive decline based on MMSE score among the elderly. However, there was no significant association between serum vitamin D with MMSE score in the study conducted by Lapid et al. [15]. The optimum level of vitamin D to prevent bone fractures is between 50 and 80 nmol/L [16]. However, its optimum level to maintain cognitive function has not been identified.

In this study, the telomere length was found to be significantly longer in SA group as compared to MCI group. The significant association between longer telomere length and reduced risk of MCI among older adults is novel. Our finding corroborates Roberts et al. [17] which reported that shorter telomere length was significantly associated with MCI. In contrary, Hochstrasser et al. [18] did not observe any significant difference in telomere length between control and MCI group among older adults aged 70 years and above. Their finding was also confirmed by Arai et al. [19]. The inconsistency across studies might be attributed by several reasons. This includes narrow age range in the previous studies [5], wide inter- and intraindividual variability in telomere lengths, unmeasured confounding, and the use of different cognitive assessment tools (Mather et al. 2011). Nevertheless, the underlying mechanisms are still unclear even though the significant association was observed in this study. One possible explanation is that oxidative stress is a common cause of both telomere shortening and cognitive decline [20].

Serum contains large amount of platelets and has a longer lifespan of turnover, which is approximately 10 days. Plasma was chosen over serum in measuring BDNF in this study as it has a shorter lifespan of turnover as compared to serum due to minimal influence of the amount of platelets. In addition, vascular endothelial cells and the brain secrete the circulating BDNF in plasma [21]. Peripheral BDNF level could represent the BDNF brain level. These reasons suggested that plasma BDNF is more suitable to indicate the BDNF levels in the brain. Several animal studies demonstrated positive association between BDNF levels in frontal cortex and hippocampus with plasma BDNF levels. Positive correlation was also found between serum and cortical levels of BDNF [22]. It is thus suggested that BDNF in the central nervous system (CNS) may change along with the changes of in peripheral BDNF levels.

Higher plasma BDNF level was significantly associated with reduced risk of MCI in this study. Our finding is consistent with studies by Shimada et al. [23] and Turana et al. [24]. Generally, decreased BDNF levels in MCI may contribute to the development of neurodegenerative diseases such as dementia and Alzheimer's disease. These diseases may be due to lack of neurotrophic support. Although peripheral BDNF level was found to potentially act as protective factor for cognitive decline, the optimum level of peripheral BDNF is yet to be determined. Several studies have identified significant contrasting differences in BDNF levels between healthy and MCI/dementia/Alzheimer's disease (AD) participants. Lee et al. [25] observed an increased BDNF levels with MCI and Alzheimer's disease. However, Borba et al. [26] reported a decrease BDNF levels in MCI and dementia participants when compared to healthy controls. Decreased plasma BDNF levels were related to depression, bipolar disorder, and anxiety [27], whereas increased BDNF levels were found to be associated with smoking [28]. Therefore, factors such as depression, smoking, and alcohol intake should be taken into consideration as these could affect the BDNF levels and contribute to contrasting findings.

This study has several limitations. Firstly, the division of the ageing groups (SA, UA, and MCI) may raise conflict on the merging between social and clinical concepts of ageing. This is because, to date, there is no standard clinical diagnostic procedure to determine successful ageing or normal ageing. Achievement of successful ageing presented here may not be realistic for most people as stated by Bowling and Dieppe [29]. Some older people who do not have any diseases or impairments may not consider themselves as successful agers. However, there is also evidence that many older adults consider themselves to be happy and satisfied with life, despite the illness or physical function decline that they have. Secondly, it is possible that some of the potential confounders for vitamin D level determination were not measured in this study. These include parathyroid hormone, hours of sunlight exposure, the use of sunscreen products, and outdoor activities. Despite all the limitations, our findings provide substantial insights into the potential of vitamin D, telomere length, and BDNF as neuroprotective factors for MCI and their relationships with successful ageing.

6. Conclusion

In conclusion, vitamin D level, telomere length, and BDNF could act as neuroprotective factors for mild cognitive impairment. However, future prospective studies are warranted to determine the cut-off value of these factors in maintaining cognitive function among older adults. Besides, the relevant professionals should also establish a more balanced and interdisciplinary perspective on ageing due to the great heterogeneity that exists among the older adults.

Acknowledgments

This study was funded by Ministry of Higher Education Malaysia under the Long-term Research Grant Scheme (LRGS) LRGS/BU/2012/UKM-UKM/K/01. The authors express utmost gratitude to all the participants, field workers, and coresearchers involved in this study. The authors also wish to thank Dr. Mohamad Sham Othman who assisted in proofreading of the manuscript.

References

[1] S. A. Samad, "Population ageing and social protection in Malaysia," *Malaysian Journal of Economic Studies*, vol. 50, no. 2, pp. 139–156, 2013.

[2] K. R. Daffner, "Promoting successful cognitive aging: a comprehensive review," *Journal of Alzheimer's Disease*, vol. 19, no. 4, pp. 1101–1122, 2010.

[3] T. L. Briones and H. Darwish, "Vitamin D mitigates age-related cognitive decline through the modulation of pro-inflammatory state and decrease in amyloid burden," *Journal of Neuroinflammation*, vol. 9, article 244, 2012.

[4] C. Annweiler, B. Fantino, A. M. Schott, P. Krolak-Salmon, G. Allali, and O. Beauchet, "Vitamin D insufficiency and mild cognitive impairment: cross-sectional association," *European Journal of Neurology*, vol. 19, no. 7, pp. 1023–1029, 2012.

[5] K. A. Mather, A. F. Jorm, P. J. Milburn, X. Tan, S. Easteal, and H. Christensen, "No associations between telomere length and age-sensitive indicators of physical function in mid and later life," *Journals of Gerontology - Series A Biological Sciences and Medical Sciences*, vol. 65A, no. 8, pp. 792–799, 2010.

[6] S. L. Ma, E. S. S. Lau, E. W. C. Suen et al., "Telomere length and cognitive function in southern Chinese community-dwelling male elders," *Age and Ageing*, vol. 42, no. 4, pp. 450–455, 2013.

[7] S. L. Patterson, "Immune dysregulation and cognitive vulnerability in the aging brain: interactions of microglia, IL-1β, BDNF and synaptic plasticity," *Neuropharmacology*, vol. 96, part A, pp. 11–18, 2015.

[8] S. Shahar, A. Omar, D. Vanoh et al., "Approaches in methodology for population-based longitudinal study on neuroprotective model for healthy longevity (TUA) among Malaysian Older Adults," *Aging Clinical and Experimental Research*, vol. 28, no. 6, pp. 1089–1104, 2016.

[9] E. Cavalier, A. Carlisi, A.-C. Bekaert, O. Rousselle, J.-P. Chapelle, and J.-C. Souberbielle, "Analytical evaluation of the new Abbott Architect 25-OH vitamin D assay," *Clinical Biochemistry*, vol. 45, no. 6, pp. 505–508, 2012.

[10] N. J. O'Callaghan and M. Fenech, "A quantitative PCR method for measuring absolute telomere length," *Biological Procedures Online*, vol. 13, no. 1, article 3, 2011.

[11] C. M. C. Nascimento, J. R. Pereira, L. Pires de Andrade et al., "Physical exercise improves peripheral BDNF levels and cognitive function in mild cognitive impairment elderly with different bndf Val66Met genotypes," *Journal of Alzheimer's Disease*, vol. 43, no. 1, pp. 81–91, 2015.

[12] A. G. Brigola, E. S. Rossetti, B. R. dos Santos et al., "Relationship between cognition and frailty in elderly: a systematic review," *Dementia & Neuropsychologia*, vol. 9, no. 2, pp. 110–119, 2015.

[13] D. W. Eyles, P. Y. Liu, P. Josh, and X. Cui, "Intracellular distribution of the vitamin D receptor in the brain: Comparison with classic target tissues and redistribution with development," *Neuroscience*, vol. 268, pp. 1–9, 2014.

[14] J. D. Ahn and H. Kang, "Physical fitness and serum vitamin D and cognition in elderly Koreans," *Journal of Sports Science and Medicine*, vol. 14, no. 4, pp. 740–746, 2015.

[15] M. I. Lapid, M. T. Drake, J. R. Geske et al., "Hypovitaminosis D in psychogeriatric inpatients," *Journal of Nutrition, Health and Aging*, vol. 17, no. 3, pp. 231–234, 2013.

[16] B. Dawson-Hughes, R. P. Heaney, M. F. Holick, P. Lips, P. J. Meunier, and R. Vieth, "Estimates of optimal vitamin D status," *Osteoporosis International*, vol. 16, no. 7, pp. 713–716, 2005.

[17] R. O. Roberts, L. A. Boardman, R. H. Cha et al., "Short and long telomeres increase risk of amnestic mild cognitive impairment," *Mechanisms of Ageing and Development*, vol. 141-142, pp. 64–69, 2014.

[18] T. Hochstrasser, J. Marksteiner, and C. Humpel, "Telomere length is age-dependent and reduced in monocytes of Alzheimer patients," *Experimental Gerontology*, vol. 47, no. 2, pp. 160–163, 2012.

[19] Y. Arai, C. M. Martin-Ruiz, M. Takayama et al., "Inflammation, but not telomere length, predicts successful ageing at extreme old age: a longitudinal study of semi-supercentenarians," *EBioMedicine*, vol. 2, no. 10, pp. 1549–1558, 2015.

[20] E. E. Devore, J. Prescott, I. De Vivo, and F. Grodstein, "Relative telomere length and cognitive decline in the Nurses' Health Study," *Neuroscience Letters*, vol. 492, no. 1, pp. 15–18, 2011.

[21] R. Yoshimura, A. Sugita-Ikenouchi, H. Hori et al., "A close correlation between plasma and serum levels of brain-derived neurotrophic factor (BDNF) in healthy volunteers," *International Journal of Psychiatry in Clinical Practice*, vol. 14, no. 3, pp. 220–222, 2010.

[22] T. Seifert, P. Brassard, M. Wissenberg et al., "Endurance training enhances BDNF release from the human brain," *American Journal of Physiology - Regulatory Integrative and Comparative Physiology*, vol. 298, no. 2, pp. R372–R377, 2010.

[23] H. Shimada, H. Makizako, T. Doi et al., "A large, cross-sectional observational study of serum BDNF, cognitive function, and mild cognitive impairment in the elderly," *Frontiers in Aging Neuroscience*, vol. 6, article 69, 2014.

[24] Y. Turana, T. A. S. Ranakusuma, J. S. Purba et al., "Enhancing diagnostic accuracy of aMCI in the elderly: combination of olfactory test, pupillary response test, BDNF plasma level, and APOE genotype," *International Journal of Alzheimer's Disease*, vol. 2014, Article ID 912586, 9 pages, 2014.

[25] S. J. Lee, J. H. Baek, and Y. H. Kim, "Brain-derived Neurotrophic Factor is associated with cognitive impairment in elderly Korean individuals," *Clinical Psychopharmacology and Neuroscience*, vol. 13, no. 3, pp. 283–287, 2015.

[26] E. M. Borba, J. A. Duarte, G. Bristot, E. Scotton, A. L. Camozzato, and M. L. F. Chaves, "Brain-Derived Neurotrophic Factor Serum Levels and Hippocampal Volume in Mild Cognitive Impairment and Dementia due to Alzheimer Disease," *Dementia and Geriatric Cognitive Disorders Extra*, vol. 6, no. 3, pp. 559–567, 2016.

[27] H. Yu and Z. Chen, "The role of BDNF in depression on the basis of its location in the neural circuity," *Acta Pharmacologica Sinica*, vol. 32, no. 1, pp. 3–11, 2011.

[28] M. Jamal, W. Van der Does, B. M. Elzinga, M. L. Molendijk, and B. W. J. H. Penninx, "Association between smoking, nicotine dependence, and BDNF Val66Met polymorphism with BDNF concentrations in serum," *Nicotine and Tobacco Research*, vol. 17, no. 3, pp. 323–329, 2015.

[29] A. Bowling and P. Dieppe, "What is successful ageing and who should define it?" *British Medical Journal*, vol. 331, no. 7531, pp. 1548–1551, 2005.

Associations between Tactile Sensory Threshold and Postural Performance and Effects of Healthy Aging and Subthreshold Vibrotactile Stimulation on Postural Outcomes in a Simple Dual Task

Marius Dettmer,[1,2] Amir Pourmoghaddam,[1,2] Beom-Chan Lee,[2] and Charles S. Layne[2]

[1]Memorial Bone & Joint Research Foundation, 1140 Business Center Drive, Suite 101, Houston, TX 77043-2740, USA
[2]Center for Neuromotor and Biomechanics Research, John P. McGovern Campus, 2450 Holcombe Boulevard, Houston, TX 77021-2040, USA

Correspondence should be addressed to Marius Dettmer; marius.dettmer@uth.tmc.edu

Academic Editor: Abebaw Yohannes

Specific activities that require concurrent processing of postural and cognitive tasks may increase the risk for falls in older adults. We investigated whether peripheral receptor sensitivity was associated with postural performance in a dual-task and whether an intervention in form of subthreshold vibration could affect performance. Ten younger (age: 20–35 years) and ten older adults (70–85 years) performed repeated auditory-verbal 1-back tasks while standing quietly on a force platform. Foot sole vibration was randomly added during several trials. Several postural control and performance measures were assessed and statistically analyzed (significance set to α-levels of .05). There were moderate correlations between peripheral sensitivity and several postural performance and control measures ($r = .45$ to .59). Several postural performance measures differed significantly between older and younger adults ($p < 0.05$); addition of vibration did not affect outcome measures. Aging affects healthy older adults' performance in dual-tasks, and peripheral sensitivity may be a contributor to the observed differences. A vibration intervention may only be useful when there are more severe impairments of the sensorimotor system. Hence, future research regarding the efficacy of sensorimotor interventions in the form of vibrotactile stimulation should focus on older adults whose balance is significantly affected.

1. Introduction

Aging is known to cause multiple changes in anatomy and physiology of the human body. One significant modification is observed in sensory systems that provide information about body configurations and properties of the external environment. In general, there is a constant decline of sensory functioning and associated sensitivity to stimuli, which begins around the 4th to 5th decade of life with a more rapid decline during the 7th decade. This decline, in addition to loss of cognitive/executive function, leads to problems in sensorimotor processing [1]. Aging of the sensorimotor systems involved in assuring postural stability is a main contributor to the increased prevalence of balance impairments and

associated falls in older adults [2–4]. In 2007, there were approximately 1.5 million falls of older citizens (75 years of age and older) reported in the US and approximately 400.000 patients required hospitalization after falls [5]. It is believed that progressive decline of sensory systems function (e.g., plantar mechanoreceptors, vestibular system, muscle spindle afferents, vision) and impairments in proprioceptive-spinal circuits lead to issues regarding the detection of small fluctuations in postural orientation during upright stance [6], which in turn increases the risk for postural balance performance decline and falls [7].

Such deterioration of function often interacts with the affordances posed by specific tasks: Among the major challenges to postural stability is the simultaneous processing of both motor and cognitive tasks. Concurrent postural and cognitive tasking, as often experienced in activities of daily living, may pose a major challenge to older adults, who often exhibit less cognitive capacity (meaning there are fewer available cognitive resources that can be allocated to either of the two tasks) and exhibit generally lower sensorimotor and postural performance. The deterioration in either the cognitive or postural compartment (or both) of such dual-tasks can be interpreted as changes of task processing strategies or prioritization modification.

The modalities of dual-task processing in older adults have been the focus of numerous research endeavors, with major aims being the investigation of executive mechanisms, like concurrent processing modalities, prioritization, and altered behavior patterns due to aging or pathologies [3, 8–14]. Postural control may require cognitive resource itself, and it becomes more difficult at older age and is cognitively more demanding for older people than for younger people [15]. Empirical evidence suggests that aging has a significant effect on processing of attention mechanisms and attention capacity, which is reflected in experimental results showing differences between younger and older participants [6, 14, 16, 17].

Mainly, aging seems to require more attention focused towards the motor control/postural task at hand, whereas complex secondary tasks may lead to increased postural sway compared to younger adults. The specific attention allocation patterns inherent in older adults during sensorimotor/cognitive task processing are based on the complex morphological and functional effects of aging in humans [18, 19]. A common phenomenon related to aging and dual-tasking is the prioritized division of attention and concurrent processing in specific task situations. As an example, older adults more often tend to stop walking when initiating a conversation with a walking companion [3]. Alternatively, often there is a shifting towards more of a motor prioritization that becomes more prominent in demanding postural perturbation tasks and balance threatening situations. Experimental results support the theory of a "posture-first" strategy when facing balance threats, which describes a focus of attention on the postural task in order to prevent falls in older adults, specifically those who are prone to falls [20]. Experiments exposing older adults to postural balance or gait stability threats, like heavy sway, obstacles, or sudden change of surface rigidity, showed a significant prioritization of postural control over cognitive processing either independent of aging or specifically in older adults [21, 22]. Modification of prioritization in specific postural situations can be seen as a plasticity mechanism [3] that is observable in healthy aging and patients suffering from sensory impairments [23].

Results from a number of studies highlight the significance of aging-related degeneration in central and peripheral sensorimotor processing and its effects on postural control [1, 2, 24–28]. Deterioration of the sensory system therefore affects postural control and in turn interacts with attention requirements and modified postural strategies in older adults, specifically in dual-task situations. Younger adults are able to adapt and to compensate for changes of sensory conditions [29]. However, it is also possible to modify and to improve sensory detection and processing, which may assist balance performance in older individuals and patients with neuropathies. A promising approach to achieve augmentation and better function of the somatosensory system is the utilization of interventions based on stochastic resonance (SR). SR is a phenomenon associated with induction of noise into a nonlinear system that is applicable to natural and man-made systems [30]. The term describes the enhancement of neural information transmission and weak stimuli detection when optimal noise is added to the system. The positive impact of SR on system functioning has been observed in a variety of sensory entities and over a wide range of tasks. Hence, tactile receptors and associated touch perception exhibit the beneficial features of SR enhancement. For instance, Well et al. showed that random vibration enhances the detection of weak touch, which has been observed for the foot soles as well [31]. If detection and processing of information can be enhanced via SR, this has significant implications for control of human motion and specifically for human postural control; hence, several studies have investigated the effects of tactile vibration to elicit SR effects on postural and gait performance [7, 32–37]. Considering the potential to enhance peripheral sensory detection and information transmission, it may be possible that a SR-based intervention may have effects on performance dual-task performance. This augmentation of feedback emerging from the foot soles could improve postural control efficiency, which would be associated with less cognitive demand, as potentially expressed either in better cognitive or postural performance in concurrent tasks. An improvement of postural performance in a dual-task has been observed in younger adults [35] but has not yet been investigated for older adults. Such investigations are important since older adults may benefit the most from a potentially balance-enhancing intervention; additionally, the effects of SR may be greater for older adults and those with lower baseline performance [38] or patients suffering from neuropathies [34].

It is still unclear to what extent this improvement of sensory afferent functioning might assist older individuals in performing postural tasks when additional cognitive processing load is added. To our knowledge, no study yet has methodologically investigated whether augmentation of somatosensory feedback does improve dual-task performance in older individuals or whether this intervention could lead to modifications of postural strategies in dual-task conditions.

We designed a study to investigate associations between postural performance and peripheral sensitivity and to investigate effects of aging and SR on healthy adults' postural control and performance. We hypothesized that there would be correlations between sensitivity and postural outcomes and that older adults and younger adults' postural outcomes would differ significantly. We further hypothesized that an SR intervention would affect participants' postural characteristics.

TABLE 1: Anthropometric characteristics of younger and older participants and sensory threshold expressed as fraction of potential maximum amplitude output of the vibrotactile device.

	N	Gender	Height	Weight	Age	Foot length	% of vibration
Younger	10	f 5 m 5	165.6 ± 9.2	148.3 ± 27.2	25.1 ± 2.3	25.4 ± 2.3	2.1 ± 0.6
Older	10	f 8 m 2	165.6 ± 10.6	151.1 ± 35.2	78.6 ± 5.4	25.4 ± 1.6	23.2 ± 21.8

2. Methods

This study was conducted according to University of Houston policies concerning the protection of participants in human research. The protocol was approved by the University of Houston Committee for the Protection of Human Subjects (CPHS). All participants in the study provided informed written consent before participation.

2.1. Participants. Two groups of participants were recruited for this study, one healthy younger control group and one older experimental group (see Table 1).

Participants were included in the study if they were between the ages of either 20–35 years or 70–85 years. Physical health and cognitive function were initially evaluated based on a modified version of the Physical Activity Readiness Questionnaire and Mini Mental State Exam [39]. Participants were only included if they scored a minimum of 27 on the MMSE and did not report any significant impairments that could put them at risk during the experiment or may affect results. Only those with a BMI below 30 were included in the study. Additionally, participants were only included if they did (at the time of study participation) not use any medication that could interfere with their balance performance. An initial sensory detection test was administered to ensure that older adults displayed an increased tactile threshold at the foot sole, according to criteria described before [7]. Only those individuals who exhibited lower tactile sensitivity were included in the study. Foot length was measured as a requirement for the analysis of limits of stability (time-to-boundary). Demographics of the recruited participant groups are summarized in Table 1.

2.2. Equipment. A custom-made silicone insole was built (Hardness shore 50a) to integrate vibrotactile stimulators (C-2; Engineering Acoustics, FL) that have been used in earlier SR studies [7, 34, 38, 40]. The stimulators were integrated in the insole under the heel, the 1st and 5th metatarsal-phalangeal joint region. The stimulators are magnet motor devices (diameter 30.5 mm, height 7.9 mm, and maximum displacement amplitude of about 0.635 mm) that are connected to a control box including amplifiers and the power supply. In our study, the control box was connected to a PC via a USB cable. A computer-generated white-noise vibration signal band-limited from 1 Hz to about 500 Hz was used as the main mechanoreceptor stimulus. Customized software allowed the modulation of vibration amplitude to adapt it to individually required levels (Figure 1).

To pose a dual-task to participants, custom-made software was used to present verbal cues to the participants during each trial of the experiment via a headset. Verbal responses of the participants were recorded via the headset's microphone, whereas the software used speech recognition to compute both response latency and response accuracy (right/wrong answer).

2.2.1. Center-of-Pressure Data Collection. Center-of-pressure data was assessed using a force plate system (NeuroCom EquiTest, NeuroCom Intl., Clackamas, OR). Force plate data was collected at 100 Hz and processed via software on a connected computer (NeuroCom software version 8.0, NeuroCom Intl., Clackamas, OR).

2.3. Procedures. An initial test was conducted to determine if older participants were exhibiting different sensitivity levels related to mechanoreceptors of the foot sole. The testing was based on Semmes-Weinstein filament stimulation according to procedures described elsewhere [7].

After initial testing, participants were accustomed to the vibrating soles, which were adjusted to each participant's shoe size (several silicone strips in the mid-foot section could be added or removed to adjust size). After it was confirmed that the sole fitted well and all stimulators were in place, an initial vibration threshold test was performed. A stimulus intensity level of 90% of perception threshold (100%) has been shown to be effective in SR stimulation experiments, so each participant's threshold was evaluated based on a method of levels [41], to gradually achieve an estimate of each individual's sensory threshold (ST).

In the following experimental trials, participants stood on the force plate for six 20 s trials, with 30 s breaks between each trial (and a two-minute break after three trials). They were instructed to stand quietly during each trial. Vibration conditions were randomized, so that there were three trials including vibration and three without. Due to the vibration amplitude set at 90%, participants were not aware of the current vibration condition.

During each 20 s trial, participants were presented with a series of words via headphones (first word was presented at beginning of each trial, each subsequent word was presented in intervals of 4 seconds). The sequence of words was randomized by the software prior to each trial. Participants were asked to remember and then verbally repeat each word that was presented before the current one (1-back task). They were also asked to try to respond quickly and to speak clearly. Words consisted of the International Radiotelephony Spelling

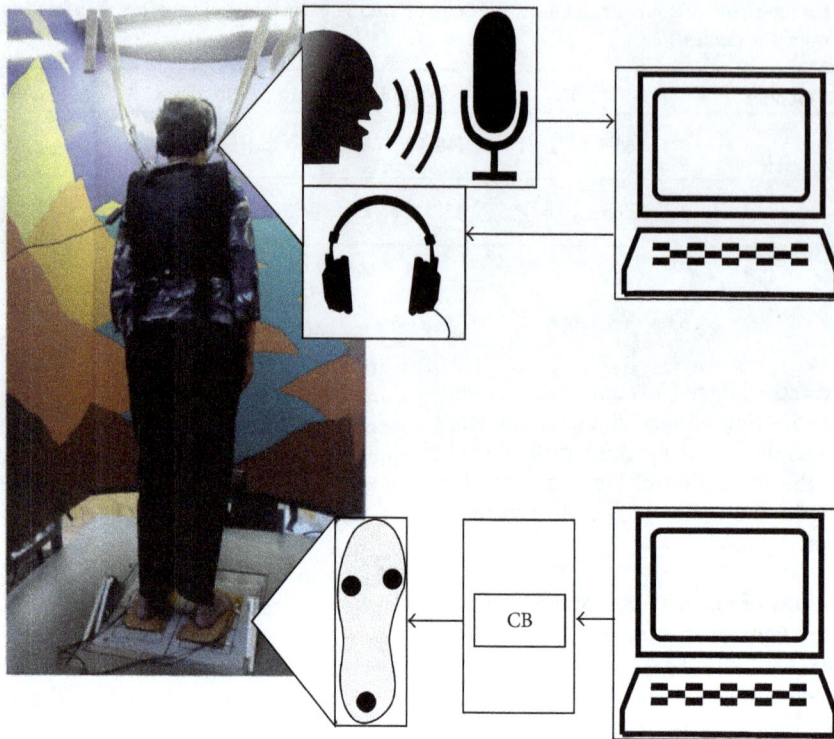

FIGURE 1: Schematic overview of the experimental setup. Participants received verbal cues to memorize and to recall (1-back task). Custom-made software was used to provide cues and to analyze responses. Vibration was provided via tactor devices embedded in a silicone rubber sole. The soles were connected to a control box (CB) containing the power supply. The control box received commands from custom-made software on a connected computer. Not pictured: A trigger signal from the NeuroCom system was used to initiate stimulus presentation and data collection for the cognitive task.

Alphabet, whereas only polysyllabic items were included (24 different items). Initially, participants performed three trials (of 20 s each) of the task in standing position without force plate data collection. These training trials were performed to minimize adaptation to the cognitive task within the experimental trials.

2.4. Data Reduction.

All outcome measures were computed using customized MATLAB (MATLAB 2012b, The Math-Works, Inc., Natick, MA) scripts and NeuroCom 8.0 software (NeuroCom, Clackamas, OR). Cognitive performance (error rate and reaction time) were assessed via customized software. Outcome measures were averaged for each subject over one block of trials (vibration on or vibration off).

2.4.1. Integrated Time-to-Boundary.

Time-to-boundary (TTB) values were generated based on force plate data (measured at 100 Hz). Velocity of the COP in anterior-posterior direction was first calculated based on earlier work [42]. Stability boundaries in the anterior-posterior direction were estimated based on the anterior-posterior limits of a rectangle involving the foot support base and initial foot length measurements. TTB was computed using the formula

$$TTB = \frac{d}{v},\qquad(1)$$

whereas d is the distance to boundary (d), estimated as the distance between the instantaneous COM location and the defined stability limits (boundary) in either given anterior-posterior direction at any moment and v is velocity. An integrated area of TTB (iTTB) below a 10 s threshold was then computed for each trial to estimate general stability [42].

2.4.2. Root Mean Square (RMSAP) of COP.

RMSAP as a measure of the magnitude of varying quantity was calculated from COP in anterior-posterior plane over the course of each trial of 20 seconds.

2.4.3. Approximate Entropy (ApEn).

ApEn is a nonlinear measure that provides information about the regularity of a time series and has been applied to COP data in a number of different postural studies [43–46]. ApEn calculation was based on computations found elsewhere [47]. ApEn measures were generated using a customized MATLAB code and anterior-posterior COP displacement data for each trial. The data was processed with the following settings in the MAT-LAB analysis: A series length of 2 ($m = 2$ data points), an error tolerance window of 0.2 times the standard deviation of the respective time series ($r = 0.2$), and a lag value of 10 [48]. A single ApEn value for each trial was generated, which was then used for further statistical analysis and for surrogate analysis (as a necessary precursor to nonlinear/ApEn analysis).

2.4.4. Equilibrium Score (ES).
ES is a measure of postural stability based on hypothetical limits of stability. The formula to calculate ES is

$$ES = \frac{12.5 - [\theta_{max} - \theta_{min}]}{12.5} * 100, \qquad (2)$$

where θ are sway angles and 12.5 is the estimated limit of sway (in degrees) for postural control [49]. The score ranges from 0 (a fall) to 100 (no sway).

2.4.5. Anterior-Posterior and Mediolateral Path Length (APPlength and MLPlength).
The summation of all COP displacements over the course of each individual trial was calculated and is expressed through APPlength and MLPlength.

2.4.6. Anterior-Posterior and Mediolateral Maximal COP Excursion ($COPmax_A$ and $COPmax_P$).
The maximal excursion of the COP within each individual trial in both anterior and posterior direction was assessed as an indicator of instability; additionally, the combined maximal excursion in both directions was assessed.

2.4.7. Strategy Score (SS).
SS evaluates movements around the upper body and hips and the lower body (ankles) that are generated for maintenance of postural stability.

The score is based on the formula

$$1 - \frac{SH_{max} - SH_{min}}{25} * 100, \qquad (3)$$

where SH_{max} and SH_{min} are the shear forces exerted to the force platform. A score of about 100 indicates a strategy based solely on an ankle strategy, and 0 would represent a strategy solely based on hip movements.

2.4.8. N-Back Cognitive Task: Response Time.
For evaluation of cognitive performance in the experiment, participants' responses in each trial were analyzed. Data was collected using custom-made software that provided timed presentation of words. The software used Windows-based speech recognition to record both reaction time and correctness of responses during each trial. Correctness was evaluated by the software and defined by the participant correctly verbalizing the earlier (memorized) word right after the presentation of the currently presented one. Correctness was also evaluated by the investigators, who checked each response and noted incorrect responses in an Excel file during each trial. Responses that were incorrect but were corrected immediately by the participants were omitted from the data analysis. The main outcome of the cognitive portion of the experiment was a response time measure (timed at end of response), with response times averaged over all four responses of each trial.

2.5. Data Analysis.
Statistical analyses of outcome measures were performed using SPSS v. 20 (IBM Corp., Somers, NY). Data are presented as group mean values ± standard deviations (SD). Pearson product-moment correlation coefficients (Pearson's r) were computed to investigate associations between tactile sensitivity and postural measures. Mixed-model ANOVA was used to investigate group differences and effects of SR. There was one between-groups factor (age) and one within-group factor (vibration). Analysis was conducted to investigate main effects (vibration and age) and potential interactions (age by vibration). Prior to computation of ANOVA statistics, data were analyzed to evaluate whether all required assumptions (for mixed ANOVA analysis) were fulfilled. Nonnormal distribution of data (as evaluated using Shapiro-Wilk tests with α-levels set at 0.05) warranted the use of alternative, nonparametric statistical analysis. Mann-Whitney U tests were used for comparisons of pairs of independent samples in this case. Bonferroni adjustment was used to account for multiple comparisons. Significance of statistical comparisons was set at $\alpha < .05$ level.

3. Results

Statistical analysis of the initial vibration threshold test revealed that the required vibration amplitude (to achieve 90% of the individual threshold) was significantly larger for the older group than for the younger group, $t(9.012)$, $p = 0.013$.

A Pearson product-moment correlation coefficient was computed to assess the relationship between the tactile sensitivity as measured in the beginning of the experiment and different outcomes assessed during dual-tasking. There were several moderate to strong relationships, such as between sensory threshold (ST) and SS ($r = -.59$, $n = 20$, $p = 0.006$), ST and iTTB ($r = .45$, $n = 20$, $p = 0.047$), ST and $COPmax_A$ ($r = .54$, $n = 20$, $p = 0.015$), ST and RMSAP ($r = .57$, $n = 20$, $p = 0.01$), ST and APPlength ($r = .49$, $n = 20$, $p = 0.042$), and ST and MLPlength ($r = .56$, $n = 20$, $p = 0.008$).

Results from the dual-task experiment are summarized in Table 2. Older and younger participants differed regarding several outcome measures during dual-tasking, that is, $COPmax_A$, $F(1, 18) = 17.658$, $p = 0.001$ (Figure 2), $\eta_p^2 = .50$, $COPmax_P$, $F(1, 18) = 12.349$, $p = 0.002$, $\eta_p^2 = .41$ (Figure 3), RMSAP, $F(1, 18) = 5.956$, $p = 0.025$ (Figure 4), $\eta_p^2 = .25$, and MLPlength, $F(1, 18) = 5.473$, $p = 0.031$, $\eta_p^2 = .233$.

Nonparametric testing showed group differences for APPlength, which differed between older and younger adults both without vibration, $U = 18$, $p = 0.015$, $\eta_p^2 = .29$, and with vibration, $U = 15$, $p = 0.007$, $\eta_p^2 = .35$. Response time was also significantly different between groups without vibration, $U = 1.5$, $p < 0.001$, $\eta_p^2 = .67$, and with vibration, $U = 6$, $p = 0.001$, $\eta_p^2 = .55$ (Figure 5). There was no statistical significance for the main factor vibration, and there were no vibration-by-group interactions.

4. Discussion

The current experiment was designed to investigate the effects of aging and vibration on dual-task performance and control characteristics. We hypothesized that age and age-dependent

TABLE 2: Means and standard deviations of postural performance, control, and cognitive response time of younger adults (YA) and older adults (OA) with and without vibration.

	ITTB		APPlength (in cm)		MLPlength (in cm)		COPmax$_A$ (in cm)		COPmax$_P$ (in cm)	
	YA	OA	YA	OA	YA	OA	YA	OA	YA	OA
No vibration	1.4 ± 1.8	2.6 ± 4.2	10.2 ± 2.8	17 ± 7.9	4.1 ± 1.6	6.2 ± 2.1	4.7 ± 1.4	7.1 ± 1.0	3.3 ± 1.2	5.2 ± 1.3
Vibration	1.6 ± 3.1	2.4 ± 3.6	10.3 ± 3.9	16.9 ± 6.8	4.27 ± 2.3	1.6 ± 3.1	4.7 ± 1.3	6.8 ± 1.1	3.4 ± 1.0	5.0 ± 1.1
	RMSAP (in cm)		Strategy score		ES		ApEn		Response time	
	YA	OA	YA	OA	YA	OA	YA	OA	YA	OA
No vibration	.42 ± .2	.58 ± .1	98.5 ± .7	98.0 ± 1.0	92.0 ± 5.8	92.0 ± 2.3	0.62 ± .1	0.68 ± .2	1.7 ± .1	2.1 ± .3
Vibration	.41 ± .2	.59 ± .2	98.5 ± .7	98.0 ± 1.1	93.0 ± 3.0	92.6 ± 1.4	0.62 ± .1	0.69 ± .1	1.8 ± .1	2.2 ± .3

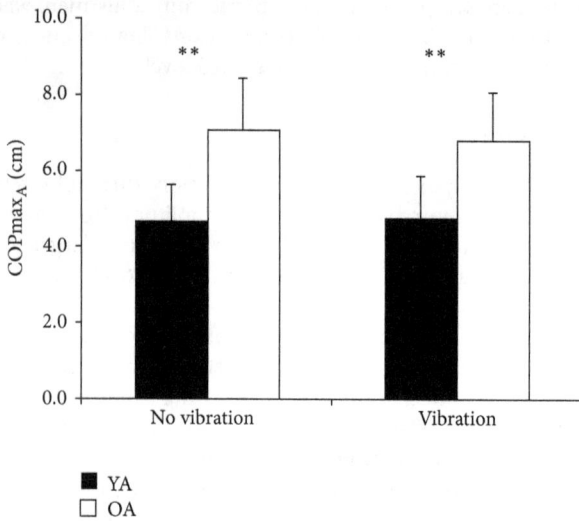

FIGURE 2: COPmax$_A$ means and SD of younger age group (YA) and older age group (OA) without vibration and with vibration. ∗∗ = $p < 0.01$.

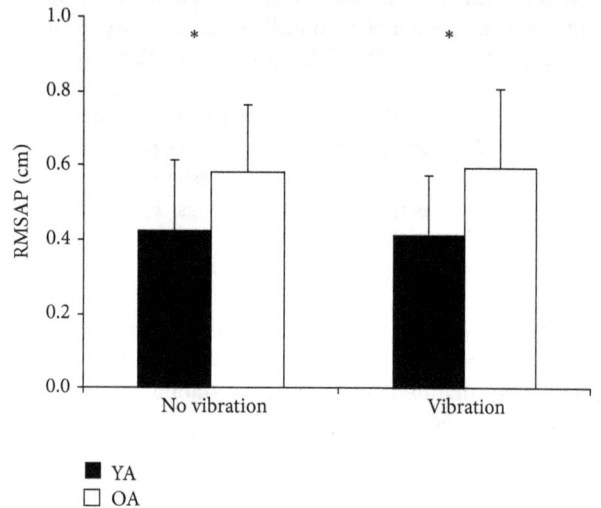

FIGURE 4: RMSAP means and SD of younger age group (YA) and older age group (OA) without vibration and with vibration. ∗ = $p < 0.05$.

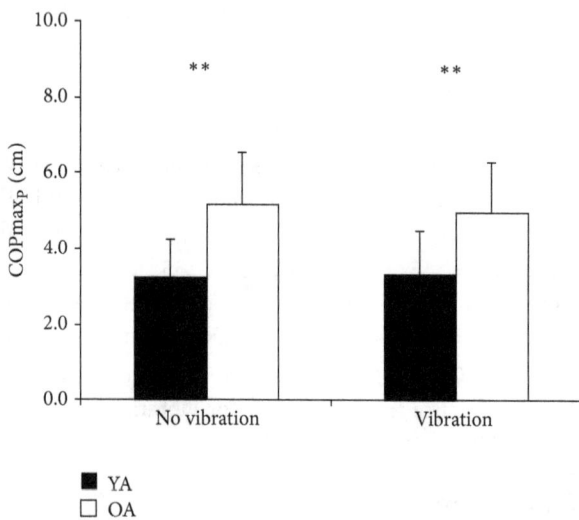

FIGURE 3: COPmax$_P$ means and SD of younger age group (YA) and older age group (OA) without vibration and with vibration. ∗∗ = $p < 0.01$.

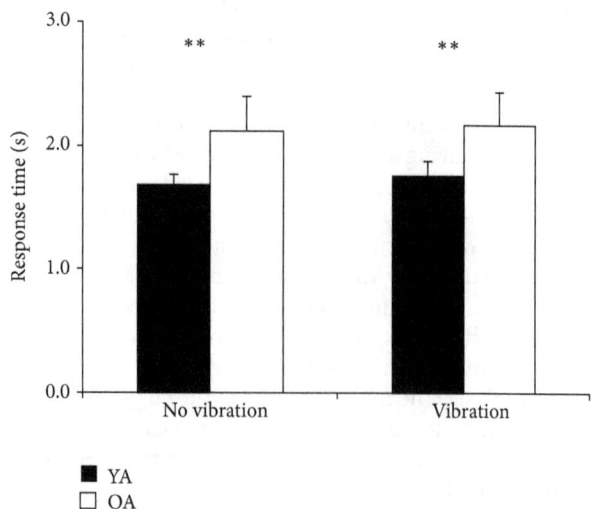

FIGURE 5: Response time means and SD of younger age group (YA) and older age group (OA) without vibration and with vibration. ∗∗ = $p < 0.01$.

loss of peripheral sensory function would be associated with performance and motor control in a dual-task situation and that outcomes would differ between conditions where vibration was either applied or not. We expected that the effects of aging on mental capacity and the sensorimotor decline observed with aging would affect outcomes related to one or both components of the dual-task.

Our hypothesis regarding associations between sensitivity of the foot sole and postural characteristics was confirmed, since several outcomes exhibited moderate to strong correlations with results from initial sensory testing. These findings confirm earlier results regarding the importance of tactile receptor feedback for postural tasks [50–53]. It has been postulated that deterioration of central integrative processes and peripheral sensitivity are contributors to postural control decline [54], and the current experiment provides evidence for this association in a dual-task situation. Additionally, the correlation observed between SS and sensitivity could be interpreted as an expression of sensorimotor adaptation that is required to maintain high levels of balance performance, as those participants who have less sensory feedback are known to adopt a strategy that includes more agonist-antagonist coactivation on the lower leg for higher stiffness with more reliance on hip movements and less ankle movement. Deterioration of sensitivity at the foot soles may be a valuable predictor for balance issues; however, in the current experiment, older adults performed very well regarding the postural task despite increased sensory thresholds. This is remarkable, since older adults exhibiting high function regarding balance tasks or dual-tasking are also affected by sensory decline but potentially adapt to the deterioration by applying different movement strategies, for example, by using different multiple muscle activation patterns [55]. Alternatively, high-functioning older individuals may also have better control through postural reflexes, based on better function of the neuromuscular system in comparison to low-balance performance individuals.

4.1. Aging Effects on Balance Control and Performance. Older and younger adults' balance performance differed regarding several but not all postural performance and control measures. This highlights the significance of assessing a number of different COP-based balance parameters, whereas such analyses can assist in the exploration of subtle changes of postural control due to aging, even in individuals whose balance performance is high.

APPlength/MLPlength, maximal COP excursion, and RMS of COP displacement are considered potential indicators of elevated postural instability, so the observed results regarding effects of aging on these outcomes could be interpreted as evidence for less stability in the older group when facing a dual-task challenge. However, considering the otherwise high performance levels of the specific group of older adults in this study, it is possible that path length and COP displacement increases in older adults were based on strategy modification, whereas participants allow for more sway to gather more sensory cues from the lower legs. This exploratory strategy may support the gathering of information [56] and ultimately would improve postural stability.

Results from iTTB and ES analysis did not reveal any group differences. The fact that older adults performed at similar levels to younger adults is unexpected but may be based on the specific task and the group of older adults that served as participants in the study. The *n*-back task performed concurrently in this experiment was designed to divert attention from postural control processes. It has been shown in younger adults that a fairly simple cognitive task (as is the 1-back task applied in our study) can actually lead to improved posture, associated with even less sway than when performing a single-task. The underlying idea is that an internal focus in an overlearned, mostly automatic, and self-organized task like quiet standing (e.g., based on the instruction "stand as quiet as possible") could interfere with the motor system [57–59]. The cognitive task in our experiment may have shifted the participants' focus towards an external cue, and automatic postural processes ensured maintenance of postural stability. This could explain why our results are contrary to earlier findings that suggested that older adults allowed about 40% increase of instability in favor of maintaining high performance in a concurrent cognitive task [8]. Doumas and colleagues administered a cognitive task that was more demanding than the task applied in the current study. It is likely that increased difficulty of the cognitive task would have shown pronounced age differences, based on increased resource competition. Additionally, the recall task that was applied in the current study differs from some of the tasks used in earlier studies, specifically regarding existing input-output modality pairings. In the current study, a verbal-vocal task was used, which is considered a "compatible" pairing, and which has been shown to be less demanding than dual-tasks including "incompatible" modality pairings [60, 61]. Hence, these tasks require less cognitive effort, which may then be reflected in the postural performance component of an experiment. This highlights the need to consider aspects of modality compatibility in the design of future dual-task studies.

Participants in both groups were able to maintain overall high levels of stability, as evidenced by ES in the range of 90–95, and iTTB values indicating that COP-velocity and overall excursion towards the limits of stability were kept low.

However, we observed a potential trade-off in the cognitive domain. The response times in the *n*-back task administered in this experiment were different between older and younger adults. Older adults required more time to respond in the simple 1-back test compared to younger adults. It is possible that this observation indicates a trade-off between posture and cognitive processing, whereas longer response times were necessary to maintain high levels of postural performance. Alternatively, the trade-off may be a reflection of general aging processes between cognitive features, whereas older adults maintain accuracy of their responses (as observed in our study) while allowing for greater response times. This phenomenon has been observed before whereas, in certain tasks, reaction times are greater in older adults, but response accuracy is the same in comparison to younger adults [62]. This finding was accompanied by higher prefrontal cortex activity in older adults, potentially as a countermeasure to aging processes in the cognitive system [63]. It is possible that this increased cortical activity could make a difference when postural tasks (the primary task) become more difficult, for example, when the visual surrounding or the support surface is sway-referenced. Those tasks would require more conscious control of posture, and aging effects become more pronounced, as has been shown with more demanding secondary tasks [62]. The current results indicate that the older group accepted a trade-off regarding response time in favor of accuracy, a phenomenon that can occur when investigating both measures of accuracy and reaction time [64]. An alternative explanation is that the longer response latency in older adults could stem from prioritization differences due to aging. Participants were given the instruction to respond as quickly as possible, while standing as quiet as possible. Potentially, a higher prioritization was given to the postural task, affecting response times in this group. It is known that older adults have the ability to reallocate cognitive resources according to either instructions or due to strategic decisions, for example, postural stability over cognitive performance [15, 65]. There were no wrong responses in either of the two groups, but it is possible that this would have changed if participants would have focused more on response time than on accuracy. Alternatively, a more demanding 2-back test would have probably caused incorrect responses [62].

In contrast to our initial hypothesis, measures of postural control were not different between younger and older adults, as indicated by similar ApEn and strategy scores. This means that older and younger adults mainly used the same strategic approach to perform the dual-task. Concurrent processing of a cognitive task did not affect older adults in a manner that required them to change the strategy of attention sharing in comparison to younger adults. There arguably was no need for the older group to change the postural strategy compared to younger adults, as would have been evidenced by differences in strategy scores. For more demanding postural/cognitive tasks, more of a top-down strategy, including increased stiffness of the lower-leg musculature [66] and less ankle/more hip rotation, is expected, which is more pronounced in older adults. However, considering the nature of the experimental task in the current study, the need to adopt a top-down approach to postural control was not required.

This idea was supported by results from ApEn analysis. In the current task, temporal dynamics of COP variability were unaffected by age. ApEn seems to be dependent on amount of attention invested in postural control or a secondary task [43, 44]. It can be concluded that the group of older adults included in this study did not adjust postural control to accommodate the requirements posed by the secondary cognitive task, as would have been indicated by changes of our entropy measure. Although ApEn has been shown to detect effects of the addition of a secondary task, even when initial postural sway was minimal [43], it may not be possible to detect age differences when highly functioning older adults are recruited.

4.2. Effects of Subthreshold Vibration. We had hypothesized that subthreshold vibration would alter postural performance, control characteristics, or cognitive performance, specifically in the older group. Our initial hypotheses concerning potential effects of subthreshold vibration on dual-tasking, specifically in the elderly, were not confirmed.

Aging requires the allocation of more mental capacity or cognitive resources directed towards postural control or gait [3, 10, 12]. The enhancement of sensory feedback, especially about small excursions of the COP, could have effects on postural stability. This was not the case in the current experiment. The lack of any effects of vibration on either postural or cognitive measures indicates that the subtle enhancement of sensory feedback was not sufficient to affect outcomes. However, the overall high performance levels of the older adults group indicate that there was little necessity for improvement since performance mainly did not differ from the arguably near-optimal performance in the younger group (without vibration). It is unclear if the intervention used in this study could have positive effects if performance levels were lower, for example, in patient populations and recurrent fallers, specifically since SR effects are more pronounced when baseline levels are lower, which has been shown regarding the observed decreases of variability through SR in walking [38]. Additionally, it would be valuable to investigate if the intervention does have an effect in those individuals that suffer from mild or more severe cognitive impairments (and on their cognitive or postural performance).

The connection between postural stability, dual-tasking, and cognitive impairments has been previously identified. As has been concluded from findings in a recent study including a large number of older adults ($n = 717$), it is possible that dual-tasking performance correlates more with fall risk among individuals that suffer from pathological conditions than those who are healthy [66]. The older group recruited for the current study consisted of high-functioning individuals, who live mostly independently and who did not have any cognitive impairment. Earlier research has shown an age-dependent increase in the correlation between cognitive/intellectual abilities and sensorimotor function [19], with an increasingly negative age-dependent correlation between sensorimotor fluctuation and cognitive abilities [67]. The group in our study exhibited higher sensory thresholds but were very similar to the younger group concerning performance and postural control measures. Therefore, the high levels of cognitive function and sensorimotor function retained by this recruited group allowed for performance and control that was similar regarding some performance outcomes, with vibration having no effects on outcomes in either group.

The participant group in this study probably affected results, and considering the exclusion and inclusion criteria that we established, only healthy older adults with high levels of function were recruited. Although those individuals may exhibit higher sensory thresholds and slight decline regarding postural performance compared to younger individuals, differences were relatively small. Further research could aim at investigating the effects of the presented intervention in individuals suffering from mild or more severe cognitive impairment, which could interfere with postural control in dual-tasks. It would be valuable to evaluate whether the intervention can affect performance in those individuals, compared to the current results in healthy older adults.

5. Conclusions

Results from the current study indicate specific correlations between tactile sensitivity and postural performance and control in a simple dual-task. The evaluation of tactile sensitivity in older adults for the purpose of prediction of fall risk or postural performance may not be adequate for otherwise high-functioning individuals. Healthy aging affects several postural outcomes in dual-tasking, but the nature of the dual-task and associated modality compatibility may affect results. This has implications for future study designs and the interpretability of results regarding a translation to real-life situations.

A tactile SR intervention may not improve performance if the task is simple, or when participants exhibit high-baseline performance. The application of the technology in a clinical setting may therefore benefit from extensive initial testing, whereas SR-based interventions may be only valuable for certain individuals. Future research should investigate effects of SR in more demanding tasks, in a number of dual-tasks using different sets of modality-mappings, and in individuals suffering from severe sensorimotor impairments.

Competing Interests

The authors declare that they have no competing interests.

References

[1] D. L. Sturnieks, R. St George, and S. R. Lord, "Balance disorders in the elderly," *Clinical Neurophysiology*, vol. 38, no. 6, pp. 467–478, 2008.

[2] F. B. Horak, C. L. Shupert, and A. Mirka, "Components of postural dyscontrol in the elderly: a review," *Neurobiology of Aging*, vol. 10, no. 6, pp. 727–738, 1989.

[3] M. Lacour, L. Bernard-Demanze, and M. Dumitrescu, "Posture control, aging, and attention resources: models and posture-analysis methods," *Neurophysiologie Clinique*, vol. 38, no. 6, pp. 411–421, 2008.

[4] M. H. Woollacott and A. Shumway-Cook, "Changes in posture control across the life span—a systems approach," *Physical Therapy*, vol. 70, no. 12, pp. 799–807, 1990.

[5] J. J. Siracuse, D. D. Odell, S. P. Gondek et al., "Health care and socioeconomic impact of falls in the elderly," *American Journal of Surgery*, vol. 203, no. 3, pp. 335–338, 2012.

[6] L. Berger and L. Bernard-Demanze, "Age-related effects of a memorizing spatial task in the adults and elderly postural control," *Gait and Posture*, vol. 33, no. 2, pp. 300–302, 2011.

[7] M. Dettmer, A. Pourmoghaddam, B.-C. Lee, and C. S. Layne, "Effects of aging and tactile stochastic resonance on postural performance and postural control in a sensory conflict task," *Somatosensory and Motor Research*, vol. 32, no. 2, pp. 128–135, 2015.

[8] M. Doumas, C. Smolders, and R. T. Krampe, "Task prioritization in aging: effects of sensory information on concurrent posture and memory performance," *Experimental Brain Research*, vol. 187, no. 2, pp. 275–281, 2008.

[9] M. Doumas, M. A. Rapp, and R. T. Krampe, "Working memory and postural control: adult age differences in potential for improvement, task priority, and dual tasking," *Journals of Gerontology B. Psychological Sciences and Social Sciences*, vol. 64, no. 2, pp. 193–201, 2009.

[10] R. T. Krampe, M. A. Rapp, A. Bondar, and P. B. Baltes, "Allocation of cognitive resources during the simultaneous performance of cognitive and sensorimotor tasks," *Nervenarzt*, vol. 74, no. 3, pp. 211–218, 2003.

[11] A. P. Marsh and S. E. Geel, "The effect of age on the attentional demands of postural control," *Gait and Posture*, vol. 12, no. 2, pp. 105–113, 2000.

[12] Y. Lajoie, N. Teasdale, C. Bard, and M. Fleury, "Upright standing and gait: are there changes in attentional requirements related to normal aging?" *Experimental Aging Research*, vol. 22, no. 2, pp. 185–198, 1996.

[13] I. Melzer, N. Benjuya, and J. Kaplanski, "Age-related changes of postural control: effect of cognitive tasks," *Gerontology*, vol. 47, no. 4, pp. 189–194, 2001.

[14] I. Olivier, R. Cuisinier, M. Vaugoyeau, V. Nougier, and C. Assaiante, "Age-related differences in cognitive and postural dual-task performance," *Gait and Posture*, vol. 32, no. 4, pp. 494–499, 2010.

[15] K. Z. H. Li, R. T. Krampe, and A. Bondar, "An ecological approach to studying aging and dual-task performance," in *Cognitive Limitations in Aging and Psychopathology*, R. W. Engle, G. Sedek, U. von Hecker, and D. N. McIntosh, Eds., pp. 190–218, Cambridge University Press, New York, NY, USA, 2005.

[16] L. A. Brown, A. Shumway-Cook, and M. H. Woollacott, "Attentional demands and postural recovery: the effects of aging," *The Journals of Gerontology—Series A*, vol. 54, no. 4, pp. M165–M171, 1999.

[17] N. Teasdale and M. Simoneau, "Attentional demands for postural control: the effects of aging and sensory reintegration," *Gait and Posture*, vol. 14, no. 3, pp. 203–210, 2001.

[18] S.-C. Li and H. R. Dinse, "Aging of the brain, sensorimotor, and cognitive processes," *Neuroscience and Biobehavioral Reviews*, vol. 26, no. 7, pp. 729–732, 2002.

[19] K. Z. H. Li and U. Lindenberger, "Relations between aging sensory/sensorimotor and cognitive functions," *Neuroscience and Biobehavioral Reviews*, vol. 26, no. 7, pp. 777–783, 2002.

[20] A. Shumway-Cook and M. Woollacott, "Attentional demands and postural control: the effect of sensory context," *Journals of Gerontology, Series A: Biological Sciences and Medical Sciences*, vol. 55, no. 1, pp. M10–M16, 2000.

[21] F. Mersmann, S. Bohm, S. Bierbaum, R. Dietrich, and A. Arampatzis, "Young and old adults prioritize dynamic stability control following gait perturbations when performing a concurrent cognitive task," *Gait and Posture*, vol. 37, no. 3, pp. 373–377, 2013.

[22] A. Shumway-Cook, M. Woollacott, K. A. Kerns, and M. Baldwin, "The effects of two types of cognitive tasks on postural stability in older adults with and without a history of falls," *Journals of Gerontology A. Biological Sciences and Medical Sciences*, vol. 52, no. 4, pp. M232–M240, 1997.

[23] M. Lacour, "Restoration of vestibular function: basic aspects and practical advances for rehabilitation," *Current Medical Research and Opinion*, vol. 22, no. 9, pp. 1651–1659, 2006.

[24] I. Amiridis, V. Hatzitaki, and F. Arabatzi, "Age-induced modifications of static postural control in humans," *Neuroscience Letters*, vol. 350, no. 3, pp. 137–140, 2003.

[25] D. Abrahamová and F. Hlavacka, "Age-related changes of human balance during quiet stance," *Physiological Research/ Academia Scientiarum Bohemoslovaca*, vol. 57, no. 6, pp. 957–964, 2008.

[26] M. Bosek, B. Grzegorzewski, A. Kowalczyk, and I. Lubiński, "Degradation of postural control system as a consequence of Parkinson's disease and ageing," *Neuroscience Letters*, vol. 376, no. 3, pp. 215–220, 2005.

[27] R. D. Seidler, J. A. Bernard, T. B. Burutolu et al., "Motor control and aging: links to age-related brain structural, functional, and biochemical effects," *Neuroscience and Biobehavioral Reviews*, vol. 34, no. 5, pp. 721–733, 2010.

[28] S. W. Shaffer and A. L. Harrison, "Aging of the somatosensory system: a translational perspective," *Physical Therapy*, vol. 87, no. 2, pp. 193–207, 2007.

[29] M. Dettmer, A. Pourmoghaddam, D. P. O'Connor, and C. S. Layne, "Interaction of support surface stability and Achilles tendon vibration during a postural adaptation task," *Human Movement Science*, vol. 32, no. 1, pp. 214–227, 2013.

[30] F. Moss, L. M. Ward, and W. G. Sannita, "Stochastic resonance and sensory information processing: a tutorial and review of application," *Clinical Neurophysiology*, vol. 115, no. 2, pp. 267–281, 2004.

[31] C. Well, L. M. Ward, R. Chua, and J. Timothy Inglis, "Touch noise increases vibrotactile sensitivity in old and young," *Psychological Science*, vol. 16, no. 4, pp. 313–320, 2005.

[32] M. Costa, A. A. Priplata, L. A. Lipsitz et al., "Noise and poise: enhancement of postural complexity in the elderly with a stochastic-resonance-based therapy," *Europhysics Letters*, vol. 77, no. 6, Article ID 68008, 2007.

[33] J. J. Collins, A. A. Priplata, D. C. Gravelle, J. Niemi, J. Harry, and L. A. Lipsitz, "Noise-enhanced human sensorimotor function," *IEEE Engineering in Medicine and Biology Magazine*, vol. 22, no. 2, pp. 76–83, 2003.

[34] A. A. Priplata, B. L. Patritti, J. B. Niemi et al., "Noise-enhanced balance control in patients with diabetes and patients with stroke," *Annals of Neurology*, vol. 59, no. 1, pp. 4–12, 2006.

[35] E. A. Keshner, J. C. Slaboda, L. L. Day, and K. Darvish, "Visual conflict and cognitive load modify postural responses to vibrotactile noise," *Journal of NeuroEngineering and Rehabilitation*, vol. 11, article 6, 2014.

[36] J. M. Hijmans, J. H. B. Geertzen, W. Zijlstra, A. L. Hof, and K. Postema, "Effects of vibrating insoles on standing balance in diabetic neuropathy," *Journal of Rehabilitation Research and Development*, vol. 45, no. 9, pp. 1441–1450, 2008.

[37] L. A. Lipsitz, M. Lough, J. Niemi, T. Travison, H. Howlett, and B. Manor, "A shoe insole delivering subsensory vibratory noise improves balance and gait in healthy elderly people," *Archives of Physical Medicine and Rehabilitation*, vol. 96, no. 3, pp. 432–439, 2015.

[38] D. G. Stephen, B. J. Wilcox, J. B. Niemi, J. Franz, D. Casey Kerrigan, and S. E. D'Andrea, "Baseline-dependent effect of noise-enhanced insoles on gait variability in healthy elderly walkers," *Gait and Posture*, vol. 36, no. 3, pp. 537–540, 2012.

[39] M. F. Folstein, S. E. Folstein, and P. R. McHugh, "'Mini-mental state'. A practical method for grading the cognitive state of patients for the clinician," *Journal of Psychiatric Research*, vol. 12, no. 3, pp. 189–198, 1975.

[40] A. M. Galica, H. G. Kang, A. A. Priplata et al., "Subsensory vibrations to the feet reduce gait variability in elderly fallers," *Gait and Posture*, vol. 30, no. 3, pp. 383–387, 2009.

[41] M. E. Shy, E. M. Frohman, Y. T. So et al., "Quantitative sensory testing: report of the therapeutics and technology assessment subcommittee of the American academy of neurology," *Neurology*, vol. 60, no. 6, pp. 898–904, 2003.

[42] R. A. Ozdemir, A. Pourmoghaddam, and W. H. Paloski, "Sensorimotor posture control in the blind: superior ankle proprioceptive acuity does not compensate for vision loss," *Gait and Posture*, vol. 38, no. 4, pp. 603–608, 2013.

[43] J. T. Cavanaugh, V. S. Mercer, and N. Stergiou, "Approximate entropy detects the effect of a secondary cognitive task on postural control in healthy young adults: a methodological report," *Journal of NeuroEngineering and Rehabilitation*, vol. 4, article 42, 2007.

[44] S. F. Donker, M. Roerdink, A. J. Greven, and P. J. Beek, "Regularity of center-of-pressure trajectories depends on the amount of attention invested in postural control," *Experimental Brain Research*, vol. 181, no. 1, pp. 1–11, 2007.

[45] S. L. Hong, B. Manor, and L. Li, "Stance and sensory feedback influence on postural dynamics," *Neuroscience Letters*, vol. 423, no. 2, pp. 104–108, 2007.

[46] C. K. Rhea, T. A. Silver, S. L. Hong et al., "Noise and complexity in human postural control: interpreting the different estimations of entropy," *PLoS ONE*, vol. 6, no. 3, Article ID e17696, 2011.

[47] H. Ocak, "Automatic detection of epileptic seizures in EEG using discrete wavelet transform and approximate entropy," *Expert Systems with Applications*, vol. 36, no. 2, pp. 2027–2036, 2009.

[48] J. T. Cavanaugh, K. M. Guskiewicz, C. Giuliani, S. Marshall, V. S. Mercer, and N. Stergiou, "Recovery of postural control after cerebral concussion: new insights using approximate entropy," *Journal of Athletic Training*, vol. 41, no. 3, pp. 305–313, 2006.

[49] H. Chaudhry, B. Bukiet, Z. Ji, and T. Findley, "Measurement of balance in computer posturography: comparison of methods—a brief review," *Journal of Bodywork and Movement Therapies*, vol. 15, no. 1, pp. 82–91, 2011.

[50] S. R. Lord, R. D. Clark, and I. W. Webster, "Postural stability and associated physiological factors in a population of aged persons," *Journals of Gerontology*, vol. 46, no. 3, pp. M69–76, 1991.

[51] B. E. Maki, S. D. Perry, R. G. Nome, and W. E. McIlroy, "Effect of facilitation of sensation from plantar foot-surface boundaries on postural stabilization in young and older adults," *Journals of Gerontology A. Biological Sciences and Medical Sciences*, vol. 54, no. 6, pp. M281–M287, 1999.

[52] P. F. Meyer, L. I. E. Oddsson, and C. J. De Luca, "The role of plantar cutaneous sensation in unperturbed stance," *Experimental Brain Research*, vol. 156, no. 4, pp. 505–512, 2004.

[53] M. Patel, M. Magnusson, E. Kristinsdottir, and P.-A. Fransson, "The contribution of mechanoreceptive sensation on stability and adaptation in the young and elderly," *European Journal of Applied Physiology*, vol. 105, no. 2, pp. 167–173, 2009.

[54] E. Palluel, I. Olivier, and V. Nougier, "The lasting effects of spike insoles on postural control in the elderly," *Behavioral Neuroscience*, vol. 123, no. 5, pp. 1141–1147, 2009.

[55] A. Pourmoghaddam, M. Dettmer, D. P. O'Connor, W. H. Paloski, and C. S. Layne, "Identification of changing lower limb neuromuscular activation in Parkinson's disease during treadmill gait with and without levodopa using a nonlinear analysis index," *Parkinson's Disease*, vol. 2015, Article ID 497825, 8 pages, 2015.

[56] M. A. Riley, R. Balasubramaniam, and M. T. Turvey, "Recurrence quantification analysis of postural fluctuations," *Gait and Posture*, vol. 9, no. 1, pp. 65–78, 1999.

[57] O. Huxhold, S.-C. Li, F. Schmiedek, and U. Lindenberger, "Dual-tasking postural control: aging and the effects of cognitive demand in conjunction with focus of attention," *Brain Research Bulletin*, vol. 69, no. 3, pp. 294–305, 2006.

[58] J. Verrel, M. Lövdén, M. Schellenbach, S. Schaefer, and U. Lindenberger, "Interacting effects of cognitive load and adult age on the regularity of whole-body motion during treadmill walking," *Psychology and Aging*, vol. 24, no. 1, pp. 75–81, 2009.

[59] R. C. O'Reilly, "Biologically based computational models of high-level cognition," *Science*, vol. 314, no. 5796, pp. 91–94, 2006.

[60] E. Hazeltine, E. Ruthruff, and R. W. Remington, "The role of input and output modality pairings in dual-task performance: evidence for content-dependent central interference," *Cognitive Psychology*, vol. 52, no. 4, pp. 291–345, 2006.

[61] C. Stelzel, E. H. Schumacher, T. Schubert, and M. D'Esposito, "The neural effect of stimulus-response modality compatibility on dual-task performance: an fMRI study," *Psychological Research*, vol. 70, no. 6, pp. 514–525, 2006.

[62] V. S. Mattay, F. Fera, A. Tessitore et al., "Neurophysiological correlates of age-related changes in working memory capacity," *Neuroscience Letters*, vol. 392, no. 1-2, pp. 32–37, 2006.

[63] C. L. Grady, "Cognitive neuroscience of aging," *Annals of the New York Academy of Sciences*, vol. 1124, pp. 127–144, 2008.

[64] A. Remaud, S. Boyas, G. A. Caron, and M. Bilodeau, "Attentional demands associated with postural control depend on task difficulty and visual condition," *Journal of Motor Behavior*, vol. 44, no. 5, pp. 329–340, 2012.

[65] M. Riediger, S.-C. Li, and U. Lindenberger, "Selection, optimization, and compensation as developmental mechanisms of adaptive resource allocation: review and preview," in *Handbook of the Psychology of Aging*, J. E. Birren, K. W. Schaie, R. P. Abeles, M. Gatz, and T. A. Salthouse, Eds., pp. 289–313, Elsevier, Burlington, Mass, USA, 6th edition, 2006.

[66] H. G. Kang, L. Quach, W. Li, and L. A. Lipsitz, "Stiffness control of balance during dual task and prospective falls in older adults: the MOBILIZE Boston Study," *Gait and Posture*, vol. 38, no. 4, pp. 757–763, 2013.

[67] S.-C. Li, U. Lindenberger, and S. Sikström, "Aging cognition: from neuromodulation to representation," *Trends in Cognitive Sciences*, vol. 5, no. 11, pp. 479–486, 2001.

29

Does Frailty Predict Health Care Utilization in Community-Living Older Romanians?

Marinela Olaroiu,[1] Minerva Ghinescu,[2] Viorica Naumov,[3] Ileana Brinza,[4] and Wim van den Heuvel[5]

[1]Foundation Research and Advice on Elderly, Heggerweg 2a, 6176 RB Spaubeek, Netherlands
[2]Department of Family Medicine, University Titu Maiorescu, Street Pictor Petraşcu 67A, Sector 3, Bucharest, Romania
[3]Office General Practitioner, Boulevard Dorobantilor, No. 15, Bloc A14, Braila, Romania
[4]College of Physicians, Street Scolilor, No. 42, Bloc BPP, Sector 5, Braila, Romania
[5]Research School SHARE, University of Groningen, Heggerweg 2a, 6176 RB Spaubeek, Netherlands

Correspondence should be addressed to Wim van den Heuvel; heuvelwim@hotmail.com

Academic Editor: Yong-Fang Kuo

Background. The predictive value of frailty assessment is still debated. We analyzed the predictive value of frailty of independent living elderly. The outcomes variables were visits to the general practitioner, hospital admission, and occurrence of new health problems. *Methods.* A one-year follow-up study was executed among 215 community-living old Romanians. General practitioners reported the outcome variables of patients, whose frailty was assessed one year before, using the Groningen Frailty Indicator. The predictive validity is analyzed by descriptive and regression analysis. *Results.* Three-quarters of all participants visited their general practitioner three times more last year and one-third were at least once admitted to a hospital. Patients who scored frail one year before were more often admitted to a hospital. Visits to the general practitioner and occurrence of new health problems were not statistically significant related to frailty scores. The frailty items polypharmacy, social support, and activities in daily living were associated with adverse outcomes. *Conclusions.* The predictive value of frailty instruments as the Groningen Frailty Indicator is still limited. More research is needed to predict health outcomes, health care utilization, and quality of life of frailty self-assessment instruments. Validation research on frailty in different "environments" is recommended to answer the question to what extent contextual characteristics influence the predictive value.

1. Introduction

Frailty is considered as common in old age [1]. Frailty indicates a loss of resources on physical, cognitive, and social domains, but a uniform definition does not exist [2]. Frailty is associated with a higher risk for dependence, falls, decreasing quality of life, utilization of care services, depressive symptoms, and mortality in frail old [3–8]. In clinical, inpatient studies frailty indexes are related to various adverse health outcomes [3, 8, 9]. In outpatient adults with cardiovascular diseases frailty is a predictor for disability and mortality [10]. In primary health care screening on frailty may discover unrecognized health problems [11], and geriatric intervention based on identified frail old through screening in primary health care may reduce risks of hospitalization [4, 5, 11]. Kiely et al. showed that frailty in community-living elderly had a predictive value for the incidence of recurrent falls, overnight hospitalization, emergency room visit, and the prevalence of disability, chronic diseases, self-reported health, and cognitive functioning [12].

Frailty is very common in older people. The overall weighted prevalence of frailty in community-dwelling old citizens is 10.7%, but it varies between countries from 4.0% to 59.1% [13, 14]. In Europe, the highest mean frailty index scores are found in Italy, Spain, and Poland and the lowest in Denmark, Switzerland, and Ireland [14]. The prevalence of frailty is strongly related to national economic indicators, showing that the prevalence of frailty is lower in higher-income countries [15].

Screening on frailty is important [11, 12]. An overview study identified 11 instruments with the potential to be used to assess frailty in primary health care settings [2]. Only six of these were validated. However, the validity of the same instrument varies between different studies, which may be related to the study design. Although they all are based on community-dwelling elderly, the age, context, and country/region do vary [8, 11, 12, 16, 17]. Despite the variety in assessment instruments, consensus is growing that simply and easily executing screening on frailty might allow physicians to objectively recognize frail persons [18]. The predictive value of these instruments is still a matter of debate. The value of frailty to predict adverse health outcomes is defined as a major research question in the European Union, related to the aging of its population [19].

Our research is executed in Romania, which is interesting for various reasons, while most studies on predictive validity are executed in well-structured health care systems [2, 4, 17, 19–22]. The context of the health care system and the role of the GP may affect the predictive value of frailty assessment instruments. The Romanian context differs considerably in infrastructural facilities, health status of old people, and health care arrangements as compared to the studies published so far [22].

The Romanian population is one of the fastest aging populations in Europe, whereas the total population is simultaneously decreasing. This number will increase by 5.4% in the coming decade, while the total population will decrease by 3.1% [22]. Long-term care facilities are lacking, which would necessitate interventions to prevent dependency. During the last decade, health policy has been directed to strengthening the role of primary health care, to reducing (unnecessary) hospitalization, and to encouraging preventive screening programs [22]. Simultaneously, the Romanian elderly population has been confronted with dramatic changes in social security (reductions in pension plans and in free access to health care) as well as in the quality of health care (waiting lists, a lack of personnel and facilities, copayments). Research showed that such measures have affected negatively the health status of old Romanians [22]. Because personal and environmental conditions may affect frailty self-assessment, considering these factors is needed also in studying the predictive value of self-assessed frailty instruments [23].

2. Material and Methods

2.1. Design and Sampling. This study used a prospective design to analyze the predictive value of frailty in primary health care. We used, as outcomes, the number of general practitioner (GP) visits and hospital admissions and the occurrence of new health problems. These outcomes are easy to register and reliable because they are part of the GPs registration system.

This study is executed in the Braila district, situated in eastern Romania, which has 230.000 inhabitants. All 145 general practitioners (GPs) received an invitation letter by the Regional College of Physicians to participate in a study to assess frailty in community-living old Romanians [24]. Twenty-two GPs expressed their willingness and did participate in the research. They were asked to send a frailty self-assessment questionnaire, the Groningen Frailty Indicator (GFI), to 10 randomly selected patients of 65 years and over in their practice. The 10 patients were selected from the patients list of all patients of 65 years and over by randomly selecting one patient and then every tenth till 10. The letter asked for informed consent and requested to complete and return the questionnaire. To assess frailty the Groningen Frailty Indicator (GFI) was used. In total 215 questionnaires were returned.

One year after frailty was assessed, the GPs were asked for information on the health care utilization of the participating patients. Three indicators were used for health care utilization: did the patient consult the GP in the year after the frailty was assessed (and if so how often), was the patient admitted to a hospital in the year after the frailty was assessed (and if so how often), and/or did the patient develop a new health problem in the year after the frailty was assessed (no/yes and if yes what kind of problem) and if so what kind of problem. All but two GPs send back this information, so 20 patients were lost in follow-up. The data of five patients were incomplete and therefore had to be excluded for further analysis. In total we included 190 patients. No statistically significant differences were found between the sociodemographic characteristics and frailty scores of the 25 excluded patients as compared to the 190 patients.

2.2. Measures. The GFI has been identified as a well-validated instrument to assess frailty and tested in multiple settings [2, 4, 18, 20, 24, 25]. It is a 15-item screening instrument assessing four domains of functioning and resources: physical, cognitive, social, and psychological [2, 5]. The GFI is a 15-item self-assessment screening instrument assessing functioning and resources in the domains: physical (9 items, e.g., shopping, dressing, and toileting), cognitive (1 item, i.e., memory), social (3 items, e.g., network and getting attention), and psychological (2 items, i.e., feeling sad and being calm). The items and answer categories are variably positive or negative formulated, and the answer categories vary from yes/no to a 0–10 scale (for details see [20]). The designers of the GFI recommend dichotomizing the answer categories by 0-1, with 1 indicating a dependency problem. The total score may vary between 0 and 15, and a score of 4 or higher is considered to indicate "moderate" or "severe" frailty by the designers of the GFI [20]. A validation study of the GFI in Romania recommended to use a score >5 as indication for frailty [24]. In addition to the GFI we asked participants for age (in years), gender (female-male), marital status (married, divorced, widowed, never married, and other), and whether they lived in an urban or rural area.

2.3. Data Analysis. We used SPSS-20 to analyze the data. We presented the frequencies of sociodemographic data (in categories) and frailty scores according to the GFI. As dependent variables we used frequency of visits to the GP in

TABLE 1: Frequencies of sociodemographic data, visits to the general practitioner (GP), hospital admission, and occurrence of new health problems by frailty scores on Groningen Frailty Indicator (GFI), in %; $n = 190$.

Variable	Score	Frailty score GFI		Percentages (total 100%)
		Not frail	Frail	
Age	65–69 years	23.5%	20.6%	22.1%
	70–74 years	31.6%	26.1%	29.0%
	75–79 years	30.6%	28.3%	29.4%
	80 years or >	14.3%	25.0%	19.5%
Gender	Women	60.2%	70.7%	65.3%
	Men	39.8%	29.3%	34.7%
Marital status	Married	60.2%	55.4%	57.9%
	Widowed	39.8%	43.4%	41.6%
	Not married	0.0%	1.2%	0.5%
Urban-rural living	Urban	78.6%	72.5%	75.3%
	Rural	21.4%	27.5%	24.7%
Frequency of visits to GP in the last 12 month	No visit	7.1%	12.1%	9.5%
	1 visit	6.1%	6.5%	6.3%
	2 visits	10.2%	9.7%	10.0%
	>2 visits	76.5%	71.7%	74.2%
Hospital admission in the last 12 months	None	73.5%	60.9%	67.4%
	1 admission	19.4%	31.5%	25.3%
	2 admissions+	7.1%	7.6%	7.4%
Occurrence of a new health care problem	No	67.3%	63.1%	65.2%
	Do not know	9.2%	9.5%	7.9%
	Yes	23.5%	30.4%	26.9%

the last year (number of visits, scores 1 to 4), frequency of hospital admission in the last year (number of admissions, scores 1 to 3), and occurrence of new health problem in the last year (scores 1 to 3 and type of problems) (Table 1).

First we described the sociodemographic variables, frailty score, and outcome variables and the statistically significant bivariate relationships. We analyzed the relationship between sociodemographic data and GFI frailty scores and the three dependent variables by stepwise linear regression analysis. Regression model solutions were checked for collinearity. Also we explored the role of individual items of the GFI in outcome variables through bivariate analysis and report the statistically significant correlations.

3. Results

The sociodemographic variables showed a representative picture of the older Romanians in the region, with the exception of urban living: older Romanians living in the city were overrepresented in the sample. Frailty scores were relatively high: 48% was assessed as frail, following the recommended cut-off point of a frailty score of 6 points or more.

Older Romanians visited their GP frequently, that is, three-quarters went for consultation or control three times of more during the last year, while 9.5% did not visit their GP during the last year.

One-third of the participants were at least once admitted to a hospital during the last year and three out of ten older Romanians developed a new health problem during the last year. The following health problems were most frequently mentioned: psychogeriatric problems (4.3%), heart diseases (3.1%), and stroke (2.5%).

Older old citizens scored higher on the GFI than younger ones. However, older citizens did not visit their GP more frequently as compared to younger ones; on the contrary: young-old patients did visit their GP more frequently as old-old patients (Pearson's $r = -0.194$, $p < 0.01$).

GFI frailty scores correlated statistically significant to frequency of hospital admission (Pearson's $r = 0.163$, $p < 0.05$), but not to GP visits or the occurrence of new health problems in the last year. Old Romanians, who were admitted to the hospital in the last year, had been more frequently scored as frail by the GFI one year before.

Hospital admission was strongly related to the occurrence of new health problems (Pearson's $r = 0.367$, $p < 0.01$). The occurrence of new health problems was also statistically significant related to visits to the GP (Pearson's $r = 0.233$, $p < 0.01$).

Multivariate analysis showed low predictive value of sociodemographic data on GP visits, hospital admission, and new morbidity with the exception of age, which was significantly related to GP visits.

TABLE 2: Final models of stepwise linear regression analysis with frailty scores by Groningen Frailty Indicator (GFI) as predictive variable and visits to the general practitioner (GP) and hospital admission over the last year as outcome variables (standardized coefficients beta are presented).

Variables	GP visits	Hospital admission	New health problem
Age	−0.175*	0.002	0.149
Gender	0.096	0.074	−0.022
Marital status	−0.076	0.053	−0.114
Urban/rural living	−0.019	0.031	−0.145
GFI score	−0.076	0.146*	0.107
Adjusted R squared	0.043	0.002	0.027

*Statistically significant at < 0.05 level.

The GFI forecasted hospital admission also when sociodemographic data were taken into account (see Table 2). Persons with high GFI scores, that is, frail one year ago, were more frequently admitted to the hospital in the last year.

Visits to the GP and occurrence of new health problems in the last year were not statistically significant related to GFI frailty scores one year before in the regression analysis.

At item level we looked for statistically significant associations between each GFI item and health care utilization. Various statistically significant associations were found. The use of more medicines (polypharmacy as assessed by the GFI) was strongly related to both more GP visits and more hospital admissions (Pearson's $r = -0.275$, $p < 0.01$, and $r = -0.232$, $p < 0.01$, resp.).

Receiving social support was significantly related to GP visits, hospital admission, and the occurrence of new health problems (Pearson's $r = 0.168$, $p < 0.05$, $r = -0.174$, $p < 0.05$, and $r = -0.152$, $p < 0.05$, resp.): well supported old citizens did visit the GP more frequently, while less supported old citizens were admitted more frequently to the hospital and developed a new health problem during the last year.

Older Romanians without problems in activities of daily living did visit their GP more frequently, while those with problems in daily activities were admitted more frequently to the hospital and developed more frequently new health problems (Pearson's $r = -0.195$, $p < 0.01$, $r = -0.148$, $p < 0.05$, and $r = -0.172$, $p < 0.05$, resp.).

4. Discussion

The findings of this prospective study indicated a predictive value of the GFI for hospital admission, which is confirmed in other studies [4, 20]. The occurrence of new health problems had also an important effect on care utilization. In the literature it is recommended to take into account (new) morbidity in explaining care utilization [26]. Indeed, when we additionally analyzed the bivariate correlation (Pearson's $r = 0.287$, $p < 0.01$ and $n = 124$) between GFI scores and hospital admission for elderly who had developed a new health care problem the predictive value was stronger.

The *absence* of a significant relationship between frailty and GP visits in our study was remarkable as was the direction of the relationship. Most studies found a positive association between frailty scores and GP visits [4, 20]. However, our study showed that *less* frail elderly did visit their GP more frequently. Also we found that old Romanians without problems in activities of daily living did visit their GP more frequently. This could be explained by difficulties frail patients experience to reach their GP for consultation, which may be specific to the Romanian context, due to absence of appointment consultation, transportation difficulties, and copayment. This underlines the importance of taking into account the role of contextual characteristics (infrastructure, social support and security systems, and economic development) in the predictive value of frailty scores.

Thirty percent of older Romanians developed a new health problem during the last year, but no significant association was found with the frailty score one year before. This could be explained in relation to the finding that more frail old Romanians visited their GP less frequently, because they could not visit their GP by themselves. The GP might not be aware of new health problems in these patients.

Various items of the GFI had a significant correlation with health care utilization. The relationship between more medicines and both more GP visits and more hospital admissions indicates the risks of polypharmacy and underlines the importance of polypharmacy control. Maybe the frequent visit to the GP of polypharmacy patients may be seen as a control visit to check for side effects of polypharmacy. Although patients with polypharmacy often have multiple comorbidities, which affects their risk on health complications, polypharmacy itself is also related to various health complications as weight loss and reduced walking speed [27].

Interesting is the finding that old citizens with sufficient social support did visit their GP more frequently, while less supported old citizens were admitted more frequently to the hospital and had developed new health problems. Could it be that old citizens with sufficient support are "advised" to visit their GP "in time," while less supported elderly stayed at home till they were admitted to the hospital? Other studies showed that GP visits by patients were significantly and positively related to *activities of daily living* (ADL) problems [4, 12]. However, this study showed that in the Romanian context community-living elderly with *no* ADL problems did visit their GP more frequently. This finding is in line with what we mentioned before; that is, less frail old did visit their GP more often. Is it because they still were mobile and active and/or were stimulated by their partner or "social environment" to see their doctor? And on the other hand, we have to realize that Romanian patients are rarely visited at home by the GO patients at home.

The findings about the relationship between individual GFI items and outcome variables indicated that looking at these items may be worthwhile, especially in clinical practice, which raises the question whether individual items in frailty scales should be weighted to assess an overall frailty score [12, 28, 29].

As all studies this one had some strong and weak points. Strong points included the longitudinal design and the Romanian context. Validity studies were executed until now in health care systems and cultural context which were alike. As explained in Section 1, the Romanian context differed in various ways, which indicates that health care system and cultural context affect the prevalence of frailty as well as its predictive value [14, 22]. Another strong point is the willingness of patients to participate in health studies as is found in various studies in central-eastern European countries. A point of consideration is the representativeness of the sample because the sample was taken indirectly (through GPs patient lists) and from one district. We do not believe that the Braila district differs significantly from the other Romanian districts, but still we would recommend a national study on frailty, sampled on population base (65 years and over). The more because the number of elderly living in rural areas maybe underrepresented in our study. In rural areas less GPs are available.

A weak point of the study was that we could not assess changes in frailty or disability during the last year. Changes in frailty scores in the last year could be related to higher health care utilization. Another aspect to be mentioned is the loss of 25 patients in our follow-up. However, as we mentioned, no significant differences were found between the characteristics of the 25 and 190 participants, respectively.

5. Conclusions

We conclude that the predictive value of the GFI in primary health care is limited, which is in line with other findings [1, 2, 4, 25]. More research is needed to predict health outcomes, health care utilization, and quality of life of frailty self-assessment instruments in primary health care [19].

We recommend to execute validation research on frailty in different "environments" to answer the question to what extent contextual characteristics influence the predictive value of frailty. Validated and simple self-assessment screening tests allow health care workers to recognize frail elderly [18]. In primary health care such recognition opens possibilities for (preventive) actions as well as the identification of treatable health problems [16, 25, 30].

Ethical Approval

The study design and research protocol were approved by the Medical Ethical Committee of the Faculty of Medicine, University Titu Maiorescu, Bucharest, Romania.

Competing Interests

The authors declare that they have no competing interests.

Authors' Contributions

All authors contributed to the research project as well as to writing of the paper. All authors approve the paper.

References

[1] T. Pialoux, J. Goyard, and B. Lesourd, "Screening tools for frailty in primary health care: a systematic review," *Geriatrics and Gerontology International*, vol. 12, no. 2, pp. 189–197, 2012.

[2] Diagnostic Technology, "Screening instruments for frailty in primary health care," Horizon Scan Report 0026, Diagnostic Technology, Oxford, UK, 2012.

[3] A. Pilotto, F. Rengo, N. Marchionni et al., "Comparing the prognostic accuracy for all-cause mortality of frailty instruments: a multicentre 1-year follow-up in hospitalized older patients," *PLoS ONE*, vol. 7, no. 1, Article ID e29090, 2012.

[4] R. J. Gobbens, M. A. Van Assen, K. G. Luijkx, and J. M. Schols, "The predictive validity of the tilburg frailty indicator: disability, health care utilization, and quality of life in a population at risk," *Gerontologist*, vol. 52, no. 5, pp. 619–631, 2012.

[5] A. Clegg, J. Young, S. Iliffe, M. Olde Rikkert, and K. Rockwood, "Frailty in elderly people," *The Lancet*, vol. 381, no. 9868, pp. 752–762, 2013.

[6] R. Samper-Ternent, A. Karmarkar, J. E. Graham, T. A. Reistetter, and K. J. Ottenbacher, "Frailty as a predictor of falls in older Mexican Americans," *Journal of Aging and Health*, vol. 24, no. 4, pp. 641–653, 2012.

[7] L. Feng, M. S. Z. Nyunt, L. Feng, K. B. Yap, and T. P. Ng, "Frailty predicts new and persistent depressive symptoms among community-dwelling older adults: findings from Singapore longitudinal aging study," *Journal of the American Medical Directors Association*, vol. 15, no. 1, pp. 76.e7–76.e12, 2014.

[8] E. Joosten, M. Demuynck, E. Detroyer, and K. Milisen, "Prevalence of frailty and its ability to predict in hospital delirium, falls, and 6-month mortality in hospitalized older patients," *BMC Geriatrics*, vol. 14, no. 1, article 1, 2014.

[9] D. Basic and C. Shanley, "Frailty in an older inpatient population: using the clinical frailty scale to predict patient outcomes," *Journal of Aging and Health*, vol. 27, no. 4, pp. 670–685, 2015.

[10] A. Frisoli, S. J. McNeill Ingham, Â. T. Paes et al., "Frailty predictors and outcomes among older patients with cardiovascular disease: data from Fragicor," *Archives of Gerontology and Geriatrics*, vol. 61, no. 1, pp. 1–7, 2015.

[11] Y. van Mourik, L. C. M. Bertens, M. J. M. Cramer et al., "Unrecognized heart failure and chronic obstructive pulmonary disease (COPD) in frail elderly detected through a near-home targeted screening strategy," *Journal of the American Board of Family Medicine*, vol. 27, no. 6, pp. 811–821, 2014.

[12] D. K. Kiely, L. A. Cupples, and L. A. Lipsitz, "Validation and comparison of two frailty indexes: The MOBILIZE Boston study," *Journal of the American Geriatrics Society*, vol. 57, no. 9, pp. 1532–1539, 2009.

[13] R. M. Collard, H. Boter, R. A. Schoevers, and R. C. Oude Voshaar, "Prevalence of frailty in community-dwelling older persons: a systematic review," *Journal of the American Geriatrics Society*, vol. 60, no. 8, pp. 1487–1492, 2012.

[14] K. Harttgen, P. Kowal, H. Strulik, S. Chatterji, and S. Vollmer, "Patterns of Frailty in older adults: comparing results from higher and lower income countries using the survey of health, ageing and retirement in Europe (SHARE) and the study on global ageing and adult health (SAGE)," *PloS ONE*, vol. 8, no. 10, Article ID e75847, 2013.

[15] O. Theou, T. D. Brothers, M. R. Rockwood, D. Haardt, and A. Mitnitski, "Exploring the relationship between national

economic indicators and relative fitness and frailty in middle-aged and older europeans," *Age and Ageing*, vol. 42, no. 5, Article ID aft010, pp. 614–619, 2013.

[16] J. Vermeulen, J. C. L. Neyens, E. van Rossum, M. D. Spreeuwenberg, and L. P. de Witte, "Predicting ADL disability in community-dwelling elderly people using physical frailty indicators: a systematic review," *BMC Geriatrics*, vol. 11, article 33, 2011.

[17] T. Nguyen, R. G. Cumming, and S. N. Hilmer, "A review of frailty in developing countries," *Journal of Nutrition, Health and Aging*, vol. 19, no. 9, pp. 941–946, 2015.

[18] J. E. Morley, B. Vellas, G. Abellan van Kan et al., "Frailty consensus: a call to action," *Journal of the American Medical Directors Association*, vol. 14, no. 6, pp. 392–397, 2013.

[19] L. R. Manas, E. Grundy, and T. Grodzicki, "Frailty: defining variables for preventing disabilities," Discussion Paper for the Working Group 'Health and Performance', Brussels, Belgium, 2014.

[20] L. L. Peters, H. Boter, E. Buskens, and J. P. J. Slaets, "Measurement properties of the groningen frailty indicator in home-dwelling and institutionalized elderly people," *Journal of the American Medical Directors Association*, vol. 13, no. 6, pp. 546–551, 2012.

[21] K. Bouillon, M. Kivimaki, M. Hamer et al., "Measures of frailty in population-based studies: an overview," *BMC Geriatrics*, vol. 13, article 64, 2013.

[22] M. Ghinescu, M. Olaroiu, J. P. van Dijk, T. Olteanu, and W. J. A. van den Heuvel, "Health status of independently living older adults in Romania," *Geriatrics and Gerontology International*, vol. 14, no. 4, pp. 926–933, 2014.

[23] N. de Witte, R. Gobbens, L. de Donder et al., "The comprehensive frailty assessment instrument: development, validity and reliability," *Geriatric Nursing*, vol. 34, no. 4, pp. 274–281, 2013.

[24] M. Olaroiu, M. Ghinescu, V. Naumov, I. Brinza, and W. van den Heuvel, "The psychometric qualities of the Groningen Frailty Indicator in Romanian community-dwelling old citizens," *Family Practice*, vol. 31, no. 4, pp. 490–495, 2014.

[25] R. Daniels, E. van Rossum, A. Beurskens, W. van den Heuvel, and L. de Witte, "The predictive validity of three self-report screening instruments for identifying frail older people in the community," *BMC Public Health*, vol. 12, article 69, 2012.

[26] A. McNamara, C. Normand, and B. Whelan, *Patterns and Determinants of Health Care Utilisation in Ireland*, Trinity College, Dublin, Ireland, 2013.

[27] Y. Rolland, J. E. Morley, and B. Vellas, "Frailty and polypharmacy," *The Journal of Nutrition Health and Aging*, vol. 15, pp. 1–3, 2014.

[28] I. Drubbel, M. E. Numans, G. Kranenburg, N. Bleijenberg, N. J. De Wit, and M. J. Schuurmans, "Screening for frailty in primary care: a systematic review of the psychometric properties of the frailty index in community-dwelling older people," *BMC Geriatrics*, vol. 14, article 27, 2014.

[29] O. Theou, T. D. Brothers, A. Mitnitski, and K. Rockwood, "Operationalization of frailty using eight commonly used scales and comparison of their ability to predict all-cause mortality," *Journal of the American Geriatrics Society*, vol. 61, no. 9, pp. 1537–1551, 2013.

[30] J. E. Morley, "Frailty screening comes of age," *Journal of Nutrition, Health and Aging*, vol. 18, no. 5, pp. 453–454, 2014.

30

In Their Voices: Client and Staff Perceptions of the Physical and Social Environments of Adult Day Services Centers in Taiwan

Chih-ling Liou ⓘ[1] and Shannon Jarrott[2]

[1]Department of Human Development and Family Studies, Kent State University at Stark, North Canton, OH 44721, USA
[2]College of Social Work, Ohio State University, Columbus, OH 43210, USA

Correspondence should be addressed to Chih-ling Liou; cliou@kent.edu

Academic Editor: Jacek Witkowski

Studies have examined the impact of environments on long-term care residents' quality of life; however, environment gets little attention in adult day services (ADS). The current study gives voice to clients and staff by capturing their perceptions of the physical and social environments of their ADS centers. Data were collected from 23 interviews with staff and clients and 270 hours of participant observations at two ADS centers in Taiwan. The authors triangulated field notes with interview transcriptions and analyzed them with the Grounded Theory coding procedure method. Findings reveal clients' and staff members' perceptions of appropriate and inappropriate physical and social environmental features affecting quality of life at the center and reflecting Taiwanese culture. We address how perceived appropriate features can be sustained or replicated and how perceived inappropriate influences can be remedied. Results can be translated into action research by implementing supportive environments for both staff and clients at ADS centers.

1. Introduction

Adult day service (ADS) is a popular community-based service designed to provide respite to family caregivers by offering long-term care (LTC) services during the day to adults with physical and/or cognitive impairment who need supervised care [1]. ADS programs have rapidly grown in the United States as families and researchers find them beneficial, cost-effective alternatives to nursing homes [1, 2]. ADS programs in Taiwan are largely informed by American models and have also grown drastically because of the government's promotion and planning to develop more centers for the rapid growth of people aged 65 and over: from 10.9% in 2010 to 41.6% by 2060 [3].

ADS researchers have focused primarily on caregiver outcomes of ADS use [4]; attention should now turn to ADS clients and staff who spend most of their day in the care environment. The environment in which LTC is provided consists of a physical and a social environment. The physical environment encompasses the setting, décor, and private

spaces, while facility regulations, activities, culture, and interpersonal interactions comprise the social environment [5]. Both the physical and social environments have been closely associated with client well-being [6]. As a "partial institution" where clients do not live together but receive care services similar to those provided at LTC, researchers, practitioners, and families should be concerned with the impact of the ADS environment as well.

ADS clients are particularly susceptible to environmental influences given associated decline in physical and cognitive functioning [7]. The environment can be a therapeutic resource to reduce need-driven behaviors and promote the well-being of persons with dementia [8]. However, it can also contribute to ill-being [5, 9]. Among the limited research on the ADS environment, Lyman [10] discovered that ADS staff responded to increased caregiving demands by exerting increasing control over clients within a physical environment characterized by architectural barriers (e.g., no wheelchair accessibility) and space limitations (e.g., no separate activity rooms). Salari and Rich [9] found that a classroom-like environment encouraged a teacher-student relationship that supported staff tendencies to control clients' behavior. Liou and Jarrott [11] reported that staff working in a hospital-like environment used a nurse-patient style of interaction that focused on physical care and ignored clients' social care. In contrast, a person-centered approach has frequently achieved a therapeutic environment for persons with dementia [6]. Examining the care environment from the perspective of ADS clients can support achievement of a therapeutic physical and social environment.

While models of environmental influence on function, such as Lawton's environmental press model [12], have been developed for elders in LTC, they can also be applied to staff members working in these environments. Staff have intimate interactions with clients and both influence and are influenced by the environments in which these interactions occur [7]. If staff experience demands exceeding their capabilities, such as working with a high client load or low supervision, they may engage in maladaptive behaviors, such as making derogatory comments about clients' abilities [13].

The current study was part of a larger project named "Examination of Social and Physical Environments in Two Centers in Taiwan" possessing two unique features. First, the lead author collected the data at two ADS centers in her native country of Taiwan; her familiarity with the culture and tradition of Taiwan provided a nonwestern cultural lens to data interpretation. Second, we gave voice to both ADS clients and staff who were observed and interviewed for their experiences and perceptions of the centers' physical and social environments. We sought to answer the question: *How do staff and clients at ADS centers in Taiwan perceive the centers' physical and social environments?* We will address those physical and social features perceived as appropriate or inappropriate by ADS staff and clients and recommend strategies for the ADS environment to enhance the quality of life and quality of care at centers.

2. Method

We utilized focused ethnography to elicit the perceptions, meanings, and experiences of participants and to provide rich descriptions [14]. Focused ethnographic studies, which are common in nursing research [15], are shorter in nature in comparison to traditional ethnographic study design; however, they still provide in-depth understanding of specific groups and places through interviews and intensive participant observations [14]. Ethnographic studies normally focus on one setting or a small number of settings that are geographically close to the researcher [16]. We had the advantage of doing research at the first author's hometown to develop understanding of the ADS environments' impact reflected in participants' voices [17].

2.1. Settings. According to Taiwanese governing regulations, the Department of Social Affairs (DSA) oversees community-based services, and the Department of Health (DOH) oversees institutional services providing medical treatment, located primarily in hospitals and nursing homes [18]. Two centers were selected because they were well known within their respective systems. Center A was supervised by the DSA; it was designed for people with dementia (33% mild, 56% moderate, and 11% severe) with physical features that elicit a sense of clients' past. Center B was operated by a university hospital and regulated by the DOH. Most Center B clients (83%) had cognitive impairment. Both centers, regulated by different departments, were promoted by the government as providing community-based services meeting the clients and family caregiver needs.

2.2. Participants. Participants included ADS clients, staff, and volunteers. There were between 28 and 34 clients in Center A when this study was conducted. Most of the clients attended the center every weekday, and five or so came two to three times a week. The female clients were the majority, accounting for 65% of the total group. The average age of clients in Center A was 80. More than half of the clients were widows or widowers and lived with their adult children, particularly their sons.

There were between 17 and 19 clients who attended Center B daily. The number of female and male clients was almost even in Center B, where 58% were female and 42% were male. The average age of the clients in Center B was 80. Like Center A, more than half of the clients were widows or widowers and lived with their adult children, with sons in particular.

Including both full- and part-time staff, there were 11 employees in Center A: one director, one nurse, five nurse aides, one social worker, two bus drivers, and one cook.

Staff members in Center B were one director, one nurse, three nurse aides, one bus driver, and one housekeeper. There were two to three regular volunteers at Center B every weekday, whereas no volunteers attended Center A regularly. Volunteers were included because they also contributed to the social environments and influenced clients' behavior.

2.3. Data Collection. Data were collected through participant observation, interviews, and examination of related documents, which characterize most ethnographic research [19]. After Institutional Review Board approval, the first author made participant observations at both centers for eight hours a day, five days per week for a total of 240 hours. The observer also served as a volunteer to support staff and clients during programming. Volunteering allowed the observer to build a close relationship with clients and staff. Clients and staff became more open over time and shared their thoughts with the observer, enabling her to critically compare individuals' statements with her observations.

The first author conducted semistructured interviews with eight clients, one volunteer, and 14 staff. For the clients, they were asked about their lives in the center, feelings about the activities, circumstances surrounding their attendance, and relationships with staff. Staff and one volunteer were interviewed on their perceptions of clients, their views on their own roles at center, and what they think about the environment of the center. All interviews were conducted and audio-recorded in private space at the centers and lasted from 40 to 90 minutes. Clients and staff described their thoughts on the physical and social environments at the center. Interviews were conducted in Mandarin Chinese,

TABLE 1: Initial themes and subcategories reflecting participants' views on ADS environment.

Subcategories	Themes
Clients' perceptions of the physical environment	
Appropriate physical features	Old style setting (Center A)
	Cleanliness (Center A)
Inappropriate physical feature	Small, hospital-like space (Center B)
Staff's perceptions of the physical environment	
Appropriate physical features	Old style setting matches the clients' life experiences (Center A)
	Open-space layout (Center A)
Inappropriate physical feature	Open-space layout (Center A)
	Limited seating in the living room (Center A)
	Hospital-like environment (Center B)
	Small space with confusing floor patterns (Center B)
Clients' perceptions of the social environment	
Appropriate social features	Being treated with respect (Center A)
	Being treated like family (Center A)
	Having someone to watch over me (Center B)
Inappropriate social features	Collectivist orientation neglects individual choice (Center A) (Center B)
	Being at the center is like being at school (Center A)
Staff's perceptions of the social environment	
Appropriate social features	A sense of collective life (Center A) (Center B)
	Emotional suppression when working with elders (Center A)
Inappropriate social features	Confining clients in wheelchairs (Center B)
	Labelling the clients (Center A) (Center B)

transcribed in Mandarin Chinese, and then translated to English by the first author.

2.4. Data Analysis. We selected the Grounded Theory (GT) coding method because it takes researchers into the real world so that findings emerge from participants' voices [20]. GT analysis began when all of the interviews and field notes were concluded and completely transcribed. The first author independently open-coded all transcriptions line-by-line, which Charmaz [21] recommended for ethnographic research. Altlas.ti Version 7 was utilized to facilitate data coding. The initial open coding was followed by focused coding to select some initial codes, which make the most analytical sense based on our research questions. Next, 1062 initial codes were combined into 17 themes (see Table 1); axial coding involved a process of reviewing the themes and placing them into subcategories around the phenomena of care environment. Previous ADS ethnographic studies examining the environment used structured subcategories to do the axial coding [5, 22, 23]. To bring coherence to the analysis and identify patterns to inform environment-enhancing strategies, we structured subcategories with a simple distinction between appropriate and inappropriate physical and social features (see Table 1). Appropriate features reflected a positive evaluation of the feature or its impact on participants or staff in the center. Inappropriate features were evaluated negatively for their impact on center occupants.

3. Results

3.1. Clients' Perceptions of the Physical Environment. During the interviews, clients were asked about their opinions on the setting, décor, and other physical characteristics of the center that comprise the physical environment. Overall, they either expressed little interest in talking about the physical environment or indicated that the physical environment exerted little influence on them.

Clients responded, "I have nothing to share," or "We human beings will get used to a new [physical] environment if we stay there for a while, so we have gotten used to everything within this [physical] environment." Although the clients did not want to directly comment on the physical features during the interview, they talked more about their preferences and dislikes of this environment during informal conversations.

3.1.1. Appropriate Physical Features. Information from the informal conversations revealed that the clients in Center A liked its *old-style setting* and *cleanliness*. Center A was originally designed and built for people with dementia to elicit a sense of their past. It created an atmosphere of an old-fashioned Taiwanese living space familiar to people who are now in their 70s to 90s. From the main entrance to the restrooms and the décor in the living room, interior features were designed with a reminiscent orientation to a 1960s and 1970s' Taiwanese home or community. More than half of the clients at Center A shared the fact that "the old style design helps us to talk more and creates a feeling of belonging in the center." "Here it is just like the place I grew up. I feel secure here." They rated the physical environment as "very clean" so they "feel safe here." One male client interpreted cleanliness as a sign that "it is not for people who are insane or poor," which reflects a Taiwanese stereotype that houses for poor, homeless, or mentally disabled people are unclean. Therefore, clients appreciated feeling safe in a clean center because they did not encounter people who are mentally ill or poor.

3.1.2. Inappropriate Physical Feature.

Center B's clients complained the *center's small size* so they could not find a place to rest privately or "cannot walk easily in the center." Interestingly, by the end of the conversation, they all told the first author that it is not their business to talk about the physical environment at the center because "this is not my home" or "we are here as the guests not the masters."

Lawton [12] stated that sometimes people do not pay attention to their physical environment or are unaware of its influence on them. In contrast, clients in this study not only paid attention to the physical environment but also were aware of its influence on their lives at the center. They might have hesitated to speak directly about the inappropriate physical features because they felt powerless to change them. Our data suggest that caretakers should not automatically assume that the physical environment meets all the clients' needs if they do not voice complaints.

3.2. Staff Members' Perceptions of the Physical Environment.

Unlike the clients, the staff at both centers willingly shared their opinions of the influence of the physical environment on them and their clients during both formal interviews and informal conversations. Staff identified appropriate and inappropriate physical environmental characteristics that affected clients and their ability to care for them.

3.2.1. Appropriate Physical Features.

Staff perceived that appropriate physical features reflected *a client-centered interior design* and *open space layout*. Center A staff described the old-style design as client-centered because "this old-style setting is copied from the environment in which they [the clients] grew up. When they [the clients] are in this old-style environment, they feel familiar and safe, and easily accept staff directions." That is, the interior design created a therapeutic atmosphere to help clients remember and talk more about the past. Moreover, the familiarity relieved clients' anxiety, leading to fewer behavioral problems. Additionally, the open design kept sight lines clear so staff could easily find where the clients were at the center. If the center was not designed as an open space, it would have had partitions blocking staff members' view of clients, thereby increasing supervision demands. As a result, staff workload and stress were low, and staff were able to concentrate on activities and positive interactions with the clients.

The open space design offered advantages but also had unwanted effects. Staff reported one downside of the open space design: "the clients with moderate or severe dementia are easily distracted because the noise from other groups travels across the center and influences the clients." To solve this problem, staff suggested curtains at the center would absorb sound and create the perception of closed space.

3.2.2. Inappropriate Physical Features.

Inappropriate physical features perceived by staff included features of *a non-client-centered interior design*, *small size*, and *limited seating*. The first two features presented in Center B, which was designed as an emergency room. Because of its appearance, staff reported that "the newcomers with moderate/severe dementia feel insecure at the center and repeatedly ask to go home." Repeated efforts by staff to convey that clients were not in a hospital failed; newcomers still associated Center B with a hospital and continued to search for an exit. The physical space of Center B further challenged staff work because wall placement created blind spots where the staff and clients could not see each other. The combination of wandering clients and blind spots required high staff supervision. In response, staff restrained clients at risk of falling in wheelchairs.

Like the clients at Center B, staff also complained about its small space. The nurse described the dining area as it "is barely able to accommodate half of the clients - the small dining room increases the risk of falling." The director shared that three clients had fallen in the previous month; consequently, she required the staff to supervise the clients at all times. Staff agreed that Center B requires remodeling, such as removing some walls and painting the walls with a warm color to make the space more accessible, safe, and inviting. Unfortunately, staff expressed little hope of remodeling: "It is hard to make any changes here...the administrators do not pay attention to the physical environment."

Although Center A staff and clients alike complimented the physical environment, there is one inappropriate element; insufficient seating in the living room led clients to fight for a seat. The social worker at Center A suggested that clients claimed chairs as theirs to form a sense of belonging. When clients could not find a chair in the living room, a disrupted sense of belonging might have contributed to restless behavior.

3.3. Clients' Perceptions of the Social Environment

3.3.1. Appropriate Social Features.

Appropriate social features described by all clients in the interviews encompassed *being treated with respect*, *being treated like family*, and *having someone to watch over them*. Based on Confucianism, which emphasizes respect for age and seniority, the appropriate treatment of old clients involves showing them respect [3]. Participants in this study were happy to be greeted as "grandma" or "grandpa" with a sincere manner. In Taiwan, calling someone aged 65 and over "grandpa" or "grandma" is a way to respect and honor their life experiences even though they are not biologically related.

During activities, staff at Center A did not view clients as passive participants but as contributors or teachers, telling the clients, "I learned a lot from you and will remember what you taught me today." Responding to client feedback was another common form of showing respect to clients. Most of the time, staff responded to clients' questions promptly, just as clients expected to be treated at home.

In addition to being treated with respect, clients valued kin-like relationships with staff members. One female client stated that "the staff here are thoughtful and concerned about me and treat me just like family." The majority of clients said that they were alone and bored at home and enjoyed being at the center, including one client who "wished to stay at the center 24 hours each day." Although staff were perceived occasionally as "bossy," clients tolerated directives when they felt that the staff treated them like family. A good quality of life for Taiwanese ADS clients includes respectful treatment reflecting family dynamics common among Taiwanese families.

Some clients, however, did not care whether they were treated like family but were merely contented with having someone to care for them while their adult children worked. One female client shared the fact that "after falling at home several times…my daughter brought me here to have more people watch over me. The best thing about coming here is having someone to take care of me." Some clients tolerated staff's inappropriate treatment so long as they received supervision, which eased their adult children's worries.

3.3.2. Inappropriate Social Features.
Inappropriate social features named by the clients at both centers were embodied by the *collective life at the center*. Clients were aware of the bureaucratic management that shaped their lives at the centers. When asked about invitations from staff to join the activity, one client responded passively: "I am not "invited" but assembled. They just announce, 'Go to the tea shop,' so I know where to go and what to do." Such a response echoes Goffman's [24] characterization of the total institution in which individuals were forced to forego self-determination, autonomy, and freedom of action to meet staff expectations.

Some clients, however, embraced the uniformity: "Here [The center] is for a group of people to do the same things together for the same goal." According to Goffman [24], when institutional goals did not match individual needs, most individuals might find a way to justify their compliance with institutional rules. One client, a veteran, described during the interview, "I just follow whatever they [the staff] tell us…. I have been used to this kind of life since I was in the army." The army is an example of a total institution in which people follow all orders, live the same schedules, and give up self-authority in order to increase technical skills [24].

Other clients shared the fact that "being at the center is just like being at school. The staff are the teachers so we have to ask them where to go and what to do if we do not know." The Taiwanese cultural tradition stresses hierarchical relationships and collectivism in which individuals surrender autonomy to a higher authority in order to reach a group goal [25]. In Taiwan, four types of occupations have authority over others, and teachers are one of them. Therefore, some clients did not just passively tolerate the staff's direction but believed that they as "students" were supposed to obey staff as "teachers."

3.4. Staff Members' Perception of the Social Environment

3.4.1. Appropriate Social Features. Staff identified *a sense of collective life* and *emotional suppression* as appropriate social features. Staff agreed that collectivism is the best way to orient the facility because "if the clients just do whatever they want at the center, they will break the rules and make things difficult." Following a practice of collectivism, similar to total institutions, means that "they [clients] have to follow our directions while doing things. Freedom might be the thing that elders here do not have." The collectivist approach applied to staff as well as clients. One staff member shared the fact that "everyone here has to follow a schedule of things to do, and that is same for the staff who also follow the schedule to lead the activities."

The collective life at Center A was evident during activities, when staff provided one-way, call-and-response instruction. Every client had to follow the staff member's direction; even sleep was prohibited during the activity. Staff believed that their responsibilities included leading group activities that engaged every client. The Center A director indicated that effective activities "keep their [clients'] attention and reduce their dementia-related behaviors. Because of participating in the activities, the elders here have fewer behavior problems than they have at home." In order to lead a successful group activity, Center A staff treated clients like school students, for example, asking them to answer questions with a loud voice or to study hard at home for activities at the center. Staff believed that this hierarchical, teacher-student communication style promoted engagement and helped clients use their brain to slow cognitive decline.

To "protect" the clients, staff at Center B compelled all clients to exercise and directed them on how to eat their food. One afternoon, a nurse's aide led exercises. She scolded a female client for not doing the exercises, explaining to the group that the woman's illness resulted from inactivity. Volunteers followed suit, directing the woman to perform the exercises; one said "some clients are really lazy so we have to push them to do some exercise to move their body to keep them healthy." The staff and volunteers did not ask the client why she did not participate but concluded that she was lazy. This conclusion reflected a collectivist approach because the client did not follow the group.

Directing the clients on how and what to eat was viewed as another way to "keep clients healthy" at Center B. During lunch time, aides and volunteers walked around the dining tables pushing clients to finish their food. The director of Center B claimed that the clients would not otherwise eat vegetables. When staff help clients put the vegetables in their bowls and "tell them that the vegetable is good for their health, the elders eat them all." Aides also controlled clients' pace of eating. To have all clients napping at the same time, aides rushed clients to finish, saying "you have to eat fast and finish your food as soon as possible. Otherwise, it will be too late for you to use the restroom, so you may pee your pants again." The staff explained that they cared more about clients' physical health because if they did not take good care of the clients physically, they would not be able care for them psychologically.

Consistent with family caregiver studies [4], staff reported that caring for clients with dementia was emotionally demanding and that they had to suppress their emotional reactions. Despite their efforts to hide emotions, staff admitted that their emotions were sometimes affected by the clients. One staff member confessed that she easily lost patience; when that happened, other staff members reminded her to calm down and helped her distract the clients: "I have worked here for two years and been asked those same questions million times. Even though I know that their behavior is driven by their disease, I am still influenced by their behavior and feel frustrated and lose patience." If the staff sensed themselves being negatively influenced by the clients, the appropriate response was leaving the situation and having other staff assume responsibility. To maintain good mental health, one staff member reported "we have to know how to adjust our minds and release our tensions. If we accumulate too many negative emotions, it will lead to bad interactions with the elders."

3.4.2. Inappropriate Social Features. Staff did not directly recognize the inappropriate social features at center, but the lead author observed some included *confining clients in wheelchairs* and *labeling them*. Staff at Center B admitted they knew confinement was inappropriate, but they "do not know other ways to deal with clients' challenging behavior." One female client with severe dementia was capable of walking alone yet was strapped in a wheelchair every day. The nurse explained: "That client has a risk of falling due to her medication [to control her aggressive behavior]. In order to prevent her falling, we have to confine her." However, the female client was not satisfied with being confined in a wheelchair and struggled to get out of the wheelchair by taking off all her clothes. The confinement intended to reduce one undesirable behavior actually triggered another behavior, but staff preferred she struggle in a wheelchair than let her move around freely and risk of falling.

Staff at both centers labeled the clients with their diagnosis and attributed the clients' challenging behaviors to their understanding of the diagnosis, which was not always accurate, as illustrated by the staff member who said, "We do not know when they [the clients] will go crazy.... The only thing I can do is to tell myself that they are sick." Staff members associated clients' challenging behavior with a medical label rather than linking the behavior to a need that staff members might be able to address. The clients at both centers responded to staff's labeling by colonizing the idea and labeling themselves or other clients as persons who "will become senile," "have a childish mind," and "are similar to children." According to labeling theory, clients' self-labeling and the staff's labeling gave staff members power to control client behavior [26].

Reflecting the power dynamic of the two ADS centers, staff members forced rules upon clients who were expected to be physically and cognitively incompetent. Client acceptance of staff labeling or peer self-labeling can be understood through a cultural lens. Clients recognized the staff as authority figures in Taiwanese society and submitted to caregiving

practices that detracted from client personhood even when treated like family.

4. Discussion

Environment gets little attention in LTC outside nursing homes, though studies highlight its influence on the behavior and attitudes of staff and clients [12]. Little is known about clients' and staff members' perceptions of the ADS environment, which is unfortunate as clients with cognitive and functional impairment associated with dementia are especially vulnerable to environmental influences [7]. Our study provides an in-depth understanding of two ADS centers from both staff and client perspectives with a cultural consideration.

Previous research demonstrated that appropriate physical environmental settings reduced accidents and problem behaviors and enhanced occupants' wellness [7]. In contrast, poorly designed environments limit clients' mobility and independence, negatively affecting their health and behavior. In the United States, a home-like interior design has been promoted to benefit nursing home residents [27]. In Taiwan, we demonstrated that the client-centered interior design is much more than a place that looks like home with non-institutional furniture; rather, its features matching clients' temporal experiences. Clients receiving care in this matched environment quickly adapted to its physical environment, experienced belonging and security, conversed comfortably with peers, and engaged in fewer aggressive behaviors. Staff also benefited from working in the client-centered physical environment of Center A, reporting low levels of stress managing client behaviors and high levels of energy for personal interactions with clients. The physical features enhanced both clients' and staff members' quality of life at the center, which aligns with Kitwood's [28] conceptualization of person-centered care that creates a more positive experience of life for staff and clients.

In contrast, the interior of Center B, reflecting its past use as an emergency room, made new clients uncomfortable and led to challenging behaviors, such as wandering. The staff faced significant demand supervising wandering clients, even confining some to wheelchairs to keep them stationery. The effect of the unsupportive physical environment at the center contributed to a restless social environment, as Altman [29] argued in his social systems model depicting bidirection influence between behavior and environment. In the present study, this model is illustrated by a feedback loop in which the physical environment influenced staff care practices, which shaped client response to the care setting and, ultimately, affected staff response to clients.

A home-like physical environment is most valuable to occupants when it corresponds to a home-like social environment [8]. A home-like physical environment promotes clients' desire for independence. However, if the social environment entails strict schedules and inflexible practices that silence clients' independence, the therapeutic potential is undermined, and maladaptive behaviors are common. In the current study, we found that the supportive physical environment at Center A led to both positive and negative outcomes. On the one hand, the client-centered interior design created a home-like atmosphere to encourage the clients to exercise control, which could enhance their self-esteem [27]. Clients in Center A cared about their rights and benefits and fought with staff and other clients to exercise their authority. On the other hand, the home-like atmosphere fostered a close, quasi-kin relationship where staff viewed the clients as their parents or grandparents. This kin-like relationship eroded the clients' autonomy when staff demonstrated their respect to clients by doing things or making decisions for them, as they would serve their aging parents at home [11]. Staff members' respectful intentions actually infantilized the clients, fostered learned helplessness, and contributed to a negative self-image.

In contrast, within Center B, clients usually claimed that they were hospitalized rather than in a "home." Staff shared in interviews that clients' families also associated the ADS with a hospital. The perception of Center B as a hospital may be interpreted through the cultural lens of the traditional Confucian value of filial piety. Fifteen elements comprise classical Chinese Confucianism; four of them emphasize how to serve, treat, and look after one's parents [30]. Accordingly, adult children are responsible for providing good care to their aging parents at home with a spirit of true caring [31]. Leaving a parent at ADS may feel like a violation of a child's duty [32]. To protect themselves from feeling guilty, adult children may adopt the idea that Center B is like a hospital; they can then justify their decision to seek ADS services as a treatment for their parents, rather than a failure to practice filial piety.

The notion of being in a hospital led new clients to feel insecure, while long-term clients possessed low expectations for social and emotional support from the staff. Most Center B clients limited their requests or complaints. They silently accepted their care and attributed their tolerance of inappropriate treatment to a value for compromising one's needs for a common good. Compromise is embedded in Taiwanese culture where harmony and collectivism are emphasized. Taiwanese people are taught that self-suppression is valued over self-expression, especially in institutional settings [32]. If something or someone might damage the harmony of the institution, the Taiwanese will compromise to maintain a calm collective. The institutional physical setting of Center B fostered harmony by suppressing the voices of clients seeking to avoid conflict with providers respected as medical professionals [31]. Professional caregivers can benefit from knowing if their clients grew up in a collectivist culture. These clients may be appreciated as "good" clients with few complaints who are easy to care for. Culturally appropriate techniques may be needed to elicit clients' preferences if they diverge from the collective. Further, these clients may face greater risk of mistreatment in semi-institutional care settings as they have learned to sacrifice their preferences for a predominant group good.

Collective life was the dominant theme in our study. The lives of both clients and staff were dictated almost entirely by a fixed schedule with frequently repeated activities that limited choices or control for either group. Caregiving focused heavily on the group as individual needs were put aside. Without any choice or control over everyday matters

at the center, some clients, particularly those at Center B, felt unvalued and expressed low self-esteem. Staff at such sites can learn to offer clients more decision-making opportunities while maintaining their safety and respecting their cultural backgrounds [32].

Just as direct care staff are advised to support a positive social environment among clients, their administrators should also foster a social environment that promotes staff well-being [13]. Staff choices at both centers were limited as they enforced collectivism at the behest of care management; studies in Taiwanese nursing homes yielded similar results [32, 33]. Though our data were gathered in Taiwan, other studies suggest that ADS in other countries without collectivist traditions also often hold expectations that participants will join programming in a collectivist fashion [5]. Future care professionals at ADS centers may find value in attending to clients' expectations of the program. They may consider shifting from traditional, collectivist attitudes and behaviors to a person-centered model with participant-driven programming, as well as incorporating clients' interests, preference, and abilities into care delivery to optimally support individuals' autonomy, competence, and relatedness.

5. Limitations and Future Directions

We based our study on rich data from observations and interviews with the clients and staff (including volunteers) at two ADS centers in Taiwan. This study is one of the few ADS studies that derived findings directly from the clients' and staff's perception. Our findings reflect how deeply the physical and social environments affected clients' quality of life and staff's care delivery centers in care settings. Although data gathered at two centers cannot be considered representative of all Taiwanese ADS environments, the results can inform future research on other ADS centers. To capture a holistic view of individual differences, future research should include a third group of informants [34]—clients' family caregivers—to more fully understand individuals' experiences.

We conducted interviews with those able to hold coherent conversations; clients with advanced dementia were observed but excluded from interviews. Future studies of the ADS environment may seek additional methods to represent the experiences of ADS clients with greater cognitive impairment. For example, Carroll and colleagues [34] posed closed-ended questions to cognitively impaired clients on topics such as environment, food, safety, activities, autonomy, and socializing. Dementia Care Mapping yields a detailed behavioral map of participants' behavior and affect, including staff behaviors that support and detract from personhood [35]. Efforts to gather information directly from clients can inform practice as well as convey to clients that their opinions are valued. Assessments of occupants' experiences in a built environment can be integrated with architectural assessments of physical features to inform design and remodeling of care facilities [36]. Future aging services providers collaborating with ADS practitioners have the moral and ethical responsibility to provide quality care, in part by ensuring that clients' voices are heard.

6. Conclusion

The goal of the current study was to listen directly to ADS clients and staff about their perceptions of the impact of the center's environments. Clients and staff at different environments experienced different daily lives at the centers. At Center A, clients felt secure because the physical environment reflected their life experiences and produced a sense of belonging like what they experienced at home. The home-like environment, however, had both positive and negative impacts on clients. At Center B, both clients and staff disliked the institution-like physical and social environments, which contributed to inappropriate treatment by the staff of the clients. This study revealed important implications on how clients and staff were positively and negatively affected by the physical and social features at ADS centers. Our findings showed that both clients and staff were well aware of the physical environment's influence on their lives at the center but believed they were powerless to change the problematic physical features at their center. The social environment of practicing collectivist traditions at both centers led to the mistreatment of clients by prohibiting them from exercising their autonomy. Previous research has emphasized providing a home-like environment at LTC settings; however, supporting clients' quality of life and improving the center's quality of care, care providers must also consider the social environment as a means to amplify positive outcomes. This study, therefore, lays the foundation for future research focused on enhancing the ADS environment and supporting the quality of life of ADS clients through a cultural lens.

References

[1] N. L. Fields, K. A. Anderson, and H. Dabelko-Schoeny, "The effectiveness of adult day services for older adults: a review of the literature from 2000 to 2011," *Journal of Applied Gerontology*, vol. 33, no. 2, pp. 130–163, 2014.

[2] B. J. Kim, "Mediating Effect of Adult Day Health Care (ADHC) and Family Network on Quality of Life Among Low-Income Older Korean Immigrants," *Research on Aging*, vol. 36, no. 3, pp. 343–363, 2014.

[3] C. Chen, "Advertising Representations of Older People in the United Kingdom and Taiwan," *The International Journal of Aging and Human Development*, vol. 80, no. 2, pp. 140–183, 2015.

[4] S. H. Zarit, K. Kim, E. E. Femia, D. M. Almeida, J. Savla, and P. C. M. Molenaar, "Effects of adult day care on daily stress of caregivers: A within-person approach," in *The Journals of Gerontology: Series B, Psychological Sciences and Social Sciences*, vol. 66, pp. 538–546, 2011.

[5] S. M. Salari, "Infantilization as elder mistreatment: Evidence from five adult day centers," *Journal of Elder Abuse & Neglect*, vol. 17, no. 4, pp. 53–91, 2006.

[6] P. S. Sparks Stein, M. J. Steffen, C. Smith et al., "Serum antibodies to periodontal pathogens are a risk factor for Alzheimer's disease," *Alzheimer's & Dementia*, vol. 8, no. 3, pp. 196–203, 2012.

[7] S. Y. Lee, H. Chaudhury, and L. Hung, "Exploring staff perceptions on the role of physical environment in dementia care setting," *Dementia*, vol. 15, no. 4, pp. 743–755, 2016.

[8] K. Day, D. Carreon, and C. Stump, "The therapeutic design of environments for people with dementia: A review of the empirical research," *The Gerontologist*, vol. 40, no. 4, pp. 397–416, 2000.

[9] S. M. Salari and M. Rich, "Social and environmental infantilization of aged persons: Observations in two adult day care centers," in *Proceedings of the International Journal of Aging and Human Development*, vol. 52, pp. 115–134, 2001.

[10] K. A. Lyman and L. P. Gwyther, "Day care for persons with dementia: The impact of the physical environment on staff stress and quality of care," *The Gerontologist*, vol. 29, no. 4, pp. 557–560, 1989.

[11] C.-L. Liou and S. E. Jarrott, "Experiences of Taiwanese elders in two different dementia day care environment," *Aging and Mental Health*, vol. 17, pp. 942—951, 2013.

[12] M. P. Lawton, "Environment and other determinants of well-being in older people.," *The Gerontologist*, vol. 23, no. 4, pp. 349–357, 1983.

[13] B. C. Yang, "A half-discrete Hilbert's inequality," *Journal of Guangdong University of Education*, vol. 31, no. 3, pp. 1–7, 2011.

[14] J. Roper and J. Shapira, *Ethnography in nursing research*, Sage, Thousand Oaks, CA, 2000.

[15] R. Coatsworth-Puspoky, C. Forchuk, and C. Ward-Griffin, "Nurse-client processes in mental health: Recipients' perspectives," *Journal of Psychiatric and Mental Health Nursing*, vol. 13, no. 3, pp. 347–355, 2006.

[16] M. Hammersley and P. Atkinson, *Ethnography, Principles in practice*, Tavistok, London, UK, 1995.

[17] H. Dabelko-Schoeny and S. King, "In their own words: Participants' perceptions of the impact of adult day services," *Journal of Gerontological Social Work*, vol. 53, no. 2, pp. 176–192, 2010.

[18] "The Ten Year Long-term Care Project," https://1966.gov.tw/LTC/cp-3636-38462-201.html.

[19] T. Schwandt, *The SAGE Dictionary of Qualitative Inquiry*, SAGE Publications, Inc., 2455 Teller Road, Thousand Oaks California 91320 United States of America , 2007.

[20] M. Q. Patton, *Qualitative research evaluation methods*, Sage, Thousand Oaks, CA, 2002.

[21] K. Charmaz, *Constructing grounded theory: A practical guide through qualitative analysis*, Sage, Thousand Oak, CA, USA, 2006.

[22] K. D. Moore, "Interpreting the "hidden program" of a place: An example from dementia day care," *Journal of Aging Studies*, vol. 18, no. 3, pp. 297–320, 2004.

[23] S. M. Salari, "Intergenerational partnerships in adult day centers: Importance of age-appropriate environments and behaviors," *The Gerontologist*, vol. 42, no. 3, pp. 321–333, 2002.

[24] E. Goffman, *Asylums: Essays on The Social Situation of Mental Patients And Other Inmates*, Aldine, Chicago, IL, USA, 2017.

[25] L. J. Lee, "Adults perceived images of life experience and personality traits of middle-aged and older adults," *Bulletin of National Chengchi University*, vol. 78, p. 54, 1999.

[26] R. A. Triplett and G. R. Jarjoura, "Theoretical and empirical specification of a model of informal labeling," *Journal of Quantitative Criminology*, vol. 10, no. 3, pp. 241–276, 1994.

[27] M. P. Calkins, "The physical and social environment of the person with Alzheimers disease," *Aging & Mental Health*, vol. 5, no. 1, Article ID 713650003, pp. 74–78, 2001.

[28] T. Kitwood, *Dementia reconsidered: The person comes first*, Open University Press., Buckingham, UK, 1997.

[29] I. Altman, "Some perspectives on the study of man-environment phenomenon," *Representative Research in Social Psychology*, vol. 4, no. 1, pp. 109–126, 1973.

[30] K. K. Kwan, "Counseling Chinese people: perspectives of filial piety," *Asian Journal of Counselling*, vol. 7, pp. 23–41, 2002.

[31] S. Chen, "A model to assess perceptions of need for nursing homes in community settings," *Journal of Advanced Nursing*, vol. 52, pp. 609–619, 2001.

[32] Y. Chuang and J. Abbey, "The culture of a Taiwanese nursing home," *Journal of Clinical Nursing*, vol. 18, no. 11, pp. 1640–1648, 2009.

[33] S. H. Chang and M. C. Fang, "The elderly living in nursing homes: Cross-culture comparison," *Tzu Chi Nursing Journal*, pp. 41–49, 2004.

[34] A. M. Carroll, S. Holmes, and K. P. Supiano, "Ask the consumer: An innovative approach to dementia-related adult day service evaluation," *American Journal of Alzheimers Disease Other Dementias*, vol. 20, no. 5, pp. 290–294, 2005.

[35] D. Brooker and I. Latham, *Person-centered dementia care*, Jessica Kingsley Publishers, London, UK, 2016.

[36] N. Norouzi, "Intergenerational architectural place-making through human development theories," in *Proceedings of the Workshop presented at the annual meetings of the Gerontological Society of America*, vol. Nov 2016.

31

Reaching 100 in the Countryside: Health Profile and Living Circumstances of Portuguese Centenarians from the Beira Interior Region

Rosa Marina Afonso (ID),[1,2] Oscar Ribeiro,[2,3,4] Maria Vaz Patto,[1,5] Marli Loureiro,[6] Manuel Joaquim Loureiro,[1,7] Miguel Castelo-Branco,[1,5] Susana Patrício,[1] Sara Alvarinhas,[1] Tatiana Tomáz,[1] Clara Rocha,[1] Ana Margarida Jerónimo,[1] Fátima Gouveia,[1] and Ana Paula Amaral[1,5]

[1]University of Beira Interior, Rua Marquês d'Ávila e Bolama, 6201-001 Covilhã, Portugal
[2]Center for Health Technology and Services Research (CINTESIS), Faculty of Medicine, University of Porto, Rua Dr. Plácido da Costa, 4200-450 Porto, Portugal
[3]Abel Salazar Biomedical Sciences Institute, University of Porto, Rua Jorge de Viterbo Ferreira 228, 4050-313 Porto, Portugal
[4]University of Aveiro, Campus Universitário de Santiago, 3810-193 Aveiro, Portugal
[5]Health Sciences Research Centre (CICS), Avenida Infante D. Henrique, 6200-506 Covilhã, Portugal
[6]Cluster of Cova da Beira Health Centers (ACeS Cova da Beira), Av. 25 de Abril, 6200-090 Covilhã, Portugal
[7]Research Center in Sport Sciences, Health Sciences and Human Development (CIDESD), Quinta de Prados, Edifício de Ciências do Desporto, 5001-801 Vila Real, Portugal

Correspondence should be addressed to Rosa Marina Afonso; rmafonso@ubi.pt

Academic Editor: Gjumrakch Aliev

The interest in studying a specific population of centenarians who lives in the country's interior region (PT100-BI) emerged during the first Portuguese systematic study about centenarians (PT100 Oporto Centenarian Study). This region of Portugal is predominantly rural and is one of the regions with the largest number of aged people. The aim of this study is to provide information on the centenarians who live in the Beira Interior region, specifically in terms of their health status and the health services they use. A total of 101 centenarians (mean age: 101.1 years; SD = 1.5 years), 14 males and 87 females, were considered. Most centenarians lived in the community, and 47.6% lived in nursing homes. Nearly half (47.5%) presented cognitive functioning without deficits. A noteworthy percentage presented conditioned mobility and sensory problems. The most common self-reported diseases include urinary incontinence (31.7%), high blood pressure (23.8%), and heart conditions (19.8%). Despite these health and functional characteristics, formal support services and technical assistance were found to be scarcely used. Further research is needed to understand how the role of contextual variables and the countryside environment contribute to the centenarians' adaptation to advanced longevity.

1. Introduction

It is estimated that more than 50% of babies born in developed countries since 2000 will live to be more than 100 years old [1]. This is a controversial perspective, however, as it is opposed by several authors who have a less optimistic view [2]. Nonetheless, it is known that a growing number of people in the most developed countries are living up to the age of 100.

Globally, considering the total world population, the estimated number of centenarians in 2013 was 441,000; 3.4 million are expected in 2050, and 20.1 million are expected in 2100 [3]. In Portugal, the centenarian population was 589 in 2001 [4] and 1,526 in 2011 [5]. These data show that this age group has almost tripled within a decade. Although centenarians still represent a small proportion of the world's total population, the remarkable growth of this age group has generated different studies worldwide.

Centenarian studies and research about longevity have increased considerably in recent decades [6] and are currently recognized as providing important contributions to the understanding of what can be "successful aging." Through a review of the results of international centenarians' studies, it is possible to determine their main sociodemographic characteristics, health, functionality, and psychosocial features. Within the range of these studies, we can highlight an extensive number of countries that have already profiled their centenarian population, such as Denmark [7, 8], Greece [9], Italy [10], USA [11, 12], Japan [13], Germany [14], Sweden [15], and Australia [16].

Research about centenarians and exceptional longevity contemplates variables pertaining to the aging process, such as its genetic, environmental, biomedical, and psychosocial dimensions [17]; however, aging has assumed a more biomedical perspective rather than a psychosocial one [18]. Centenarians constitute a very heterogeneous age group comprising, on one hand, individuals who live in the community by themselves or with family members and who are cognitively intact and autonomous and, on the other hand, centenarians who have some kind of cognitive impairment and/or are functionally dependent [12, 19–21]. Concerning health and functional capacity, a pronounced variability is also observed [21], but the great majority of studies that compare centenarians with younger groups show an increasing number of difficulties [19] and reveal that physical frailty and chronic conditions are more common at the age of 100+ than in other age groups [20].

In Portugal, the first systematic study about centenarians started in 2015, the PT100 Oporto Centenarian Study [22]. This is a population-based study developed in the metropolitan area of Porto, a seaside area in Northern Portugal, where the main urban centers are located. The well-documented role of the environmental and contextual resources in the aging (e.g., [23, 24]), namely, the distinguishing characteristics of urban versus rural or inland versus seaside environments [25, 26], motivated the development of the present satellite study, the Beira Interior Centenarian Study (PT100-BI). This study closely follows the same study design and methodology of the PT100 [22] and was conducted in the inner part of the country, around the city of Covilhã, in an area with similar geographical extension to that of the Porto metropolitan area.

There is a consensus in literature about the asymmetric socioeconomic reality in Portugal, accentuating the contrast in life conditions and public equipment available in the countryside versus seaside [27]. The concentration of major decision centers and the progressive shutting down of public services in inland Portugal, such as schools, health centers, maternities, and train lines, have accentuated these differences over the years [27]. Inland Portugal is therefore far from the centers of production, consumption, and larger institutions (particularly large hospital centers), being one of the areas with the most aged populations of Portugal, with a low population density, high rate of migration, and small towns and several villages. Most villages do not have any health services or trade and the public transport network to the centers where these services exist is scarce or even nonexistent.

The Portuguese scenario on aging corresponds with the demand for a high level of social and health services specifically designed for elderly people, since Portugal is a country that has only recently incorporated aging questions into its political, social, professional, and scientific agendas. For instance, Portugal is one of a reduced number of European countries where there is not a geriatric specialty among physicians. Profiling the oldest old population and their specific use of services has been a recent concern among Portuguese researchers (e.g., [28, 29]), but further insights are needed from deprived regions like rural areas, which are indicated as areas of increased risk of poor health [25, 30, 31]. According to Santana [32], fragile rural communities had higher mortality rates, higher levels of aging population, lower levels of education, poorer geographical accessibility to health care, and higher alcohol consumption. On the other hand, areas of intensive urbanization, such as Porto, present higher levels of education, geographical proximity to health care, higher incidence rates of AIDS and tuberculosis, and unfavorable general health conditions.

Geographic disparities on the availability of health services are the main obstacle to the unmet medical needs in Portugal, namely, the fact that hospitals located outside large metropolitan areas tend not to offer all medical specialties [33]. Regarding gender differences, in Portugal, it is observed that the avoidable mortality rate through the provision of quality and timely health care is higher in men than in women [33]. Although access to health care is formally identical for both men and women, due to the process of gender typing, women continue to benefit more from formal health care.

Profiling Portuguese individuals who have reached 100 years of age in rural places is thought to be an important step forward in understanding the longevity process in our country, as it can also improve service delivery and programming, particularly when becoming a centenarian may not be a rarity. Furthermore, studying the health status of centenarians from a rural area is important for longevity research as it allows the characterization of a group where the access to the services and health care can be more limited, as is the case in Portugal. This study aims to present sociodemographic information, health conditions, and centenarians' use of services among those who live in Beira Interior and add to the available knowledge in Portugal about this population.

2. Participants and Methods

2.1. Study Design and Sampling. The participants included in this study were centenarians from Beira Interior, Portugal, and come from a geographical area that includes Beira Interior Norte, Beira Interior Sul, Cova da Beira, and Serra da Estrela (comprising 19 municipalities in total) with an area involving around 9,000 km^2. This region has 311,051 inhabitants, 27.72% aged 65 and older, and 100 centenarians, according the last National Census. As the data collection reported on centenarians in 2013/14 and the last available census was from 2011, there was a query and search for the location of potential centenarians that, in 2011, were older than 96 years. No exclusion criteria to participate in the study were established other than not being 100 years old (accomplished by age validation procedures, i.e., via confirmation with identity card or birth certificate). This was the only criterion used, as our aim was to have a descriptive profile of all the centenarians in this geographical area. Different levels of participation were, therefore, expected: (i) a basic level (total number of centenarians identified); (ii) those who were not able to participate owing to physical/mental status and/or those who did not want to participate (providing only elementary data); (iii) those who had a partial protocol assessment; (iv) and those who were able to have a full assessment.

The first step for recruiting centenarians was to identify and locate all potential participants in each municipality and parish. This was made based on the census information and through contacting parish councils, local churches, nursing homes, institutions, and health care centers. Then, in the case of centenarians residing in nursing homes, a contact was initially made with the institution's technical director to introduce the study and request collaboration with the research, followed by contacting the centenarians and/or their proxy. As for the centenarians who lived in the community, researchers contacted the centenarians and/or their relatives directly (in some cases the contact was mediated by local research partners who were enrolled in the identification of centenarians: doctors, nurses, social workers, or parish council).

The presentation of the study was always implemented, being guaranteed the understanding of the study and its implications. Informed consent for participating in the study was fully applied. All centenarians (and/or their proxies in case of cognitive impairment) signed a written informed consent form. The study followed all ethical procedures in accordance with the Declaration of Helsinki and was approved by the Ethics Committee of Hospital Sousa Martins, Guarda, Portugal.

A total of 130 potential centenarians were contacted, and of these 29 were excluded. Eight centenarians died between the first contact and the interview, four centenarians refused collaboration due to serious health problems, and five centenarians did not show interest in participating in the study. In four cases, the centenarians or their relatives refused to participate in the study. In eight cases, the reported age could not be proven by the documents/registration. The final sample comprised 101 centenarians.

Information was collected during interviews in one, two, or more sequential sessions. Two researchers of the PT100 Beira Interior team who had been trained with the PT100 Porto team conducted the interviews. Most information was directly obtained from the centenarians. In case of cognitive impairment or in the cases where the centenarian, despite the fact that he/she did not have cognitive impairment, expressed doubts regarding the questions asked (e.g., related to diseases, medication, and use of health services), the information was obtained from the proxies (or complemented with a reference professional in those situations where the centenarian lived in a nursing home).

2.2. Instruments. The interview included the use of an extended protocol especially developed in the context of the Oporto Centenarian Study [22]. This protocol covered a wide range of measures and instruments: sociodemographic characteristics of the respondents, overall health status, lifestyle, relationships, psychological variables (e.g., personality and wellbeing), anthropometric measures, and service use. For this particular study, we have only considered sociodemographic information, health status (functionality and cognition), and health and social services use.

Regarding sociodemographic data, information was obtained on age, sex, marital status, schooling, type of accommodation, and whether the centenarian had ever lived outside Portugal. Information about centenarians' income was also collected, namely, the main source of income, monthly value, income management, and whether it was enough to cover regular and health related expenses (i.e., income adequacy).

The morbidity profile was assessed using a self-report checklist of diseases provided by OARS—the Multidimensional Functional Assessment Questionnaire [34] adapted for Portuguese population [35]. The checklist included the following health conditions: high blood pressure, heart condition, diabetes, chronic lung disease, stomach ulcers, irritable bowel syndrome or other serious problems with stomach or bowels, cirrhosis or any other serious liver problems, problems with kidneys, frequent urinary infections, urinary incontinence, prostate problems (for men), problems with vision, problems with hearing, arthritis (hands, knee, hip, shoulder, and spine), and osteoporosis at the time of the interview.

As for cognitive status, the Global Deterioration Scale (GDS) [36] provided an overview of the stages of cognitive function for those suffering from a primary degenerative dementia, such as Alzheimer's disease. GDS is an interviewer rating of subjective memory complaints, orientation, and functional ability covering seven stages of deterioration. The interviewers according to the information collected and the observation of the centenarians' behavioral characteristics completed this scale. Each participant was rated according to seven distinct stages: (1) no subjective complaints of memory deficit; (2) subjective complaints of memory deficit; (3) earliest clear-cut deficits, with evidence of memory deficit in an intensive interview; (4) clear-cut deficit on clinical interview with decreased knowledge of current and recent events; (5) patient being no longer able to survive without assistance and being unable to recall major relevant aspects of their current lives; (6) occasionally forgetting the name of the spouse upon whom they are dependent, retaining some knowledge of their past lives, and requiring some assistance with activities of daily living; and (7) very poor cognitive skills with all verbal abilities being lost. Stage 1 (no cognitive decline) and stage 2 (very mild cognitive decline) were considered as indicative of good cognitive functioning.

The use of the health services was assessed by self-report questions on the number of visits to the family doctor, number of visits to the emergency service, and number of hospitalizations during the preceding year. The number of drugs that centenarians took per day was also considered. The use of support services was assessed by a self-report list on which it was marked if the centenarian did or did not use each service. The list included day center, social center, house support service, outpatient care nursing, nursing, physiotherapy, speech therapy, and occupational therapy. There was the possibility to indicate other types of services. The use of technical aids was explored by means of a list of the most frequently used technical aids by older population: walking stick, hiker, wheelchair, hearing aid, glasses, and the possibility to indicate other types of services. Interviewers complementarily classified the centenarians' mobility in one of three categories: (1) limited to a wheelchair or bed; (2) able to get out of the chair or the bed but does not; and (3) gets out.

2.3. Statistical Analysis. The statistical analysis was conducted using the Statistical Package for the Social Sciences (SPSS) version 21. Descriptive analysis included assessment of frequency distributions and the calculation of measures of central tendency and dispersion. Sex differences were considered based on their clinical and psychosocial relevance. Statistical significance of the observed sex differences was carried out using the *chi-square test* and *Student's t-test*. The level of statistical significance used was $p < 0.05$.

3. Results

A total of 101 centenarians participated in this study: 14 (13.9%) males and 87 (86.1%) females. The mean age of the centenarians was 101.1 years (SD = 1.5), and the median age was 101. The age range was 100–108 years. Most centenarians were widows (91.1%); 5.9% of the participants, all women, were single, and 3% of the participants (two men and one woman) had partners who were still alive. The differences between men and women concerning marital status are statistically significant, with more widowers and never-married women and fewer women who had married when compared to men.

More than half of the centenarians never attended school (53.4%), and the mean of school years attended was 1.45 (SD = 1.97). Men reported significantly more years of education than women. As for the type of accommodation, 50 centenarians (49.5%) lived in institutions, 47 (46.6%) lived in houses/flats, and 4 (4%) lived in other kinds of accommodation (such as pensions, religious institutions, or house annexes). More women (51.7%) than men (35.7%) were found to be living in nursing homes; however, this difference was not statistically significant. Of the participants, 86 (85.1%) always lived in the same region they currently live in, showing no significant geographical mobility. Only the centenarians who reported having been emigrants (15, 11.5%) lived in a different region than Beira Interior. More men than women reported having been emigrants and this difference was statistically significant (see Table 1).

Concerning monthly income, the main resource of 68 centenarians (67.3%) was a state pension, followed by social security for 30 centenarians (29.7%). Statistically significant differences were observed on this aspect, with more women (71.3%) than men (42.9%) reporting that their main source of income was their pension and more men (50%) than women (26.4%) being dependent on social security. The income per month for 18 centenarians (17.8%) was less than €250; for 66 centenarians (71%), it was between €250 and €500 and for nine (9.7%) of them it was more than €500 per month. 40 centenarians (39.6%) had difficulties in paying their expenses, and 43 centenarians (42.6%) could only cover the most essential needs.

We observed statistically significant differences between women and men regarding income management: there was a higher percentage of women (45.9%) than men (21.4%) who considered the income just manageable to get by on and a higher percentage of men (42.9%) than women (39%) who struggled to make ends meet. Only five male centenarians (35.7%) and seven female centenarians (8%) stated that not only was the money enough but also they could save a little extra. Concerning income adequacy for medical expenses specifically, 17 (16.8%) did not report difficulties, 33 (32.7%) indicated it was not very difficult, and 46 (45.5%) reported difficulties. No statistically significant differences were observed between men and women (see Table 2).

Table 3 presents the prevalence of self-reported health problems. More than half of the centenarians reported not having had health problems related to high blood pressure, a heart condition, diabetes, chronic lung disease, stomach ulcers, irritable bowel syndrome, or other serious problems with stomach or bowels, cirrhosis or any other serious liver problem, problems with kidneys, frequent urinary infections, urinary incontinence, prostate problems, arthritis, or osteoporosis. In the diseases checklist, the most prevalent diseases were urinary incontinence (32 cases, 31.7%) followed by high blood pressure (24 cases, 23.8%) and heart conditions (20 cases, 19.8%). Vision and hearing impairments presented a much higher incidence compared to the other health problems. There were 61 cases (50 women and 11 men) that reported suffering from problems with vision and 74 cases (11 men and 63 women) that reported hearing problems. The analysis of sex differences only indicates statistically significant differences with respect to arthritis, with 19 women (21.8%) and no men having this health problem. It is worth mentioning that 39 centenarians (38.6%) reported never having had a serious health problem throughout their lives.

Concerning the general cognitive status of the centenarians, 48 participants (47.5%) presented no cognitive impairment, 32 (10.9%) presented earlier clear-cut deficits, and 40 (39.5%) had a level of cognitive impairment that invalidated their functioning. There are no statistically significant sex differences (see Table 4). As for the centenarians' mobility, 39 (38.6%) were confined to a wheelchair or bed, 11 (10.9%) were able to get out of the chair or bed but did not do so, and 51 (50.5%) had clear autonomy of movement.

With regard to the use of health services, several centenarians had no assisting doctor (see Table 5). For those who did, the annual average use was 1.09 (±1.655). On average,

TABLE 1: Sociodemographic profile of the Beira Interior Portuguese centenarians ($N = 101$) by sex.

		Male	Female	Total	p
Sex	Female	14 (13.9%)	87 (86.1%)	101	
Age (in years)	Mean (±SD)	100.93 ± 1.439	101.17 ± 1.519	101.14 ± 1.504	0.576
	Median	100.50	101	101	
	Range (min/max)	100–105	100–108	100–108	
Marital status	Never married	0	6 (6.9%)	6 (5.9%)	0.018
	Married	2 (14.3%)	1 (1.1%)	3 (3%)	
	Widowed	12 (85.7%)	80 (92%)	92 (91.1%)	
Did you attend school?	No	5 (35.7%)	42 (48.3%)	47 (46.5%)	0.617
	No, but can read and write	1 (7.1%)	6 (6.9%)	7 (6.9%)	
	Yes	8 (57,1%)	37 (42.5%)	45 (44.6%)	
	N/A	-	2 (2.3%)	2 (2%)	
Years of education	Mean (±SD)	2.46 (± 2.757)	1.28 (± 1.775)	1.45 (± 1.969)	0.044
	Median	3	0	0	
	Range (min/max)	0/9	0/7	0/9	
Type of accommodation	House/flat	8 (57.1%)	39 (44.8%)	47 (46.6%)	0.637
	Nursing home	5 (35.7%)	45 (51.7%)	50 (49.5%)	
	Other	1 (7.1%)	3 (3.4%)	4 (4%)	
Residence outside Portugal	No	9 (64.3%)	77 (88.5%)	86 (85.1%)	0.033
	Yes	5 (35.7%)	10 (11.5%)	15 (14.9%)	

TABLE 2: Income of the Beira Interior Portuguese centenarians ($N = 101$).

		Male (n = 14)	Female (n = 87)	Total	p
Main source of income	Pension	6 (42.9%)	62 (71.3%)	68 (67.3%)	0.008
	Social security	7 (50%)	23 (26.4%)	30 (29.7%)	
	Financial aid by children	1 (7.1%)	0	1 (1%)	
	N/A	-	2 (2.3%)	2 (2%)	
Income per month	<€250	1 (7.1%)	17 (19.5%)	18 (17.8%)	0.243
	€250–500	10 (71.4%)	56 (64.4%)	66 (65.3%)	
	€500–750	2 (14.3%)	5 (5.8%)	7 (6.9%)	
	€750–1,000	1 (7.1%)	1 (1.1%)	2 (2%)	
	N/A	-	8 (9.2%)	8 (7.9%)	
Income management	You cannot make ends meet	6 (42.9%)	34 (39%)	40 (39.6%)	0.021
	You just manage to get by	3 (21.4%)	40 (45.9%)	43 (42.6%)	
	You have enough money with a little extra	5 (35.7%)	7 (8%)	12 (11.9%)	
	Money is not a problem	0	3 (3.4%)	3 (3%)	
	N/A	-	3 (3.4%)	3 (3%)	
Cover medical expenses	Not difficult at all	4 (28.6%)	13 (14.9%)	17 (16.8%)	0.566
	Not very difficult	5 (35.7%)	28 (32.2%)	33 (32.7%)	
	Somewhat difficult	4 (28.6%)	26 (29.9%)	30 (29.7%)	
	Very difficult	1 (7.1%)	15 (17.2%)	16 (15.8%)	
	N/A	-	5 (5.7%)	5 (5%)	

TABLE 3: Current health problems of the centenarians of Beira Interior ($N = 101$).

	Male (n = 14)	Female (n = 87)	Total	p
High blood pressure	5 (35.7%)	19 (21.8%)	24 (23.8%)	0.209
Heart condition	5 (35.7%)	15 (17.2%)	20 (19.8%)	0.109
Diabetes	1 (7.1%)	3 (3.4%)	4 (4%)	0.455
Chronic lung disease	3 (21.4%)	11 (12.6%)	14 (13.9%)	0.301
Stomach ulcers, irritable bowel syndrome, or other serious problems with stomach or bowels	4 (28.6%)	7 (8%)	11 (36,6%)	0.044
Cirrhosis or any other serious liver problems	0	1	1 (1%)	0.861
Problems with kidneys	0	2 (2.3%)	2 (2%)	0.741
Frequent urinary infections	0	4 (4.6%)	4 (4%)	0.545
Urinary incontinence	5 (35.7%)	27 (31%)	32 (31.7%)	0.473
Prostate problems (for men)	3 (21.4%)	-	-	
Problems with vision	11 (78.6%)	50 (57.5%)	61 (60.4%)	0.113
Problems with hearing	11 (78.6%)	63 (72.4%)	74 (73.3%)	0.452
Arthritis (hands, knee, hip, shoulder, and spine)	0	19 (21.8%)	19 (18.2%)	0.043
Osteoporosis	0	8 (9.2%)	8 (7.9%)	0.289
Other medical conditions	1 (7.1%)	8 (9.1%)	9 (9.9%)	0.637

TABLE 4: Global Deterioration Scale of the Portuguese centenarians from Beira Interior ($N = 101$).

	Male (n =14)	Female (n = 87)	Total	p
No subjective complaints of memory deficit	2 (14.3%)	8 (9.2%)	10 (9.9%)	0.446
Subjective complaints of memory deficit	5 (35.7%)	33 (37.9%)	38 (37.6%)	
Earlier clear-cut deficits	3 (21.4%)	8 (9.2%)	11 (10.9%)	
Clear-cut deficit in clinical interview	2 (14.3%)	6 (6.9%)	8 (7.9%)	
Patient can no longer survive without assistance	0	7 (8%)	7 (6.9%)	
Occasionally forgets the name of the spouse upon whom they are dependent	0	12 (13.8%)	12 (11.8%)	
All verbal abilities are lost	2 (14.3%)	11 (12.6%)	13 (12.9%)	
N/A	0	2 (2.3%)	2 (2%)	

women go to the doctor more often (1.13 ± 1.731) than men (0.86 ± 1.167); however, this difference was not statistically significant. Concerning the use of the emergency service, 67 centenarians (66.3%) had not used this service in the last year. Men had a statistically significant higher mean use of this service (0.71 ± 0.825) than women (0.31 ± 0.562). Concerning hospitalizations, 90 centenarians (89.1%) reported not having been hospitalized. The mean of these centenarians' hospitalizations in the last year was 0.33 (±1.891), and there were no statistically significant sex differences.

The mean number of daily drugs taken was 2.87 (±2.455). There were 16 centenarians (2 males and 14 females) taking no medication, 44 (43.5%) taking between 1 and 3 drugs, and 35 (34.7%) taking more than 3 drugs. There were no sex differences concerning the mean number of drugs and the number of drugs used by these centenarians per day.

The support services for elder people are scarcely used by the centenarians from Beira Interior (see Table 6). The most widely used service was nursing ($n = 29$, 28.7%), followed by house support services ($n = 13$, 12.8%) and day centers ($n = 8$, 7.9%). Social centers, speech therapy, outpatient nursing care, physiotherapy, speech therapy, occupational therapy, and other kinds of services had a percentage of use equal to or less than 4%. There were no sex differences concerning the use of support services by centenarians in this geographical area.

Among the available technical aids, 29 centenarians (28.7%) used walking sticks, 13 (12.9%) used hikers, and 37 (36.6%) used wheelchairs. The use of glasses stands out, as they are the most used technical aid: 38 centenarians (37.6%) need them. Hearing aids were used by only 3 (3%) of the centenarians (see Table 6).

4. Discussion and Conclusions

This is one of the few studies about Portuguese centenarians and it focuses on a specific geographic population living in the

Reaching 100 in the Countryside: Health Profile and Living Circumstances of Portuguese Centenarians...

241

TABLE 5: Use of health services/support by the Portuguese centenarians from Beira Interior throughout the last year ($N = 101$).

	Male	Female	Total	p
Family doctor				0.575
Mean (±SD)	0.86 (±1.167)	1.13 (±1.731)	1.09 (±1.655)	
Median	0.50	0.00	0.00	
Range (min/max)	0/4	0/9	0/9	
Emergency services				0.023
Mean (±SD)	0.71 (±0.825)	0.31 (±0.562)	0.37 (±0.620)	
Median	0.50	0.00	0.00	
Range (min/max)	0/2	0/2	0/2	
Hospital/continuous care				0.925
Mean (±SD)	0.29 (±0.611)	0.34 (±2.032)	0.33 (±1.891)	
Median	0.00	0.00	0.00	
Range (min/max)	0/2	0/15	0/15	

countryside. It provides information about the sociodemographic profile of 101 centenarians living in one of the regions with the largest aging population in Portugal, and it provides valuable information about their health profiles and their use of the health support system, services, and technical aids.

With regard to the sociodemographic profile of this group, as expected, women outnumber men and the male/female ratio was 6.1:1 (87 women/14 men). Women represented 86.1% of the centenarians, which is in accordance with the values reported by other studies on centenarians (e.g., [30]) and with the profile of the overall Portuguese centenarian population [29] and of the Oporto centenarian study [22]. More than half of the centenarians (53.4%) never attended school. This is a surprisingly positive number if we take into account the fact that, in 1900, about ten years before most of the centenarians enrolled in this study were born, 75% of the population was illiterate [37], so it could be expected that a higher rate of centenarians would similarly be illiterate, especially in a rural area, where traditionally people had fewer chances of attending school due to restrictions to education access and demanding agricultural chores in childhood.

In the current study, sex differences were found in some sociodemographic characteristics. There are more widowers and never-married women than men, which may be related to the much higher survival rate of women in older age compared to that of men and to the fact that women tend to marry men who are older [38]. Concerning education, men reported a significantly higher average number of years of education than women. This is expected and reflects the dominant position of men in general Portuguese society from 100 years ago. In these centenarians' generation, especially in rural areas, the illiteracy rate was higher and more prevalent among women, as their social roles were mainly connected to the family and home caring [37]. Sex differences are also apparent in the higher number of men having been emigrants, which could be related to the fact that a man's role was essentially that of a provider. Portugal has a long and important history of emigration to different countries in the world, more evident in rural and inland areas of the country,

where living conditions were worse, compelling men to leave the country first. This fact was also confirmed in our study.

Concerning centenarians' income, the majority had a monthly income between €250 and 500. This value is rooted in the Portuguese sociohistorical background of a dictatorship that was characterized by a global poverty [22] and in the fact that most of these centenarians worked in agriculture with low earnings. With these incomes, the majority showed difficulties in paying their expenses, namely, health treatments that imply costly travel arrangements to hospital centers located away for their living geographical area. This can help to explain the reduced use of health care services and technical aids among these centenarians.

With regard to the type of accommodation, the number of centenarians living in private households (50.6%) is lower than the national rate of 71% [29]. This may be due to the fact that most of them live in very small isolated areas with a very reduced number of inhabitants, without proper housing conditions, and with a reduced use of technical support and assistance services (e.g., domiciliary care) to enable them to live in their homes. Another explanation is that the rural areas of inland Portugal had in the 1960s and 1970s a strong migratory movement to other European countries [37]. For this reason, many of these centenarians' children live abroad and therefore cannot be their caregivers, which, in turn, has led them to recur to nursing homes.

Regarding diseases, back in the beginning of last century, about the time the people in this study were born, the rate of Portuguese infant mortality was 140‰ [32]. During their childhood and adult life, there were no vaccinations or health care support for diseases that are now treatable, which means that many of these centenarians resisted several pathologies in very adverse circumstances, rendering them survivors and the most resistant of their generation. This high percentage of healthy centenarians supports Evert et al.'s perspective that exceptional longevity can be related to one's ability to escape all major age-related diseases [37]. According to this perspective, this group of centenarians could be labelled as "escapers" (i.e., individuals with no diagnosis of major age-related diseases up to 100 years of age), which could suggest

TABLE 6: Use of elder support services and technical aids by the Portuguese centenarians from Beira Interior ($N = 101$).

		Male (N = 14)	Female (N = 87)	Total	p
Day center	No	14 (100%)	77 (88.5%)	91 (90.1%)	0.281
	Yes	0	8 (9.2%)	8 (7.9%)	
	N/A	0	2 (2.3%)	2 (2%)	
Social center	No	14 (100%)	80 (91.9%)	94 (93.1%)	0.623
	Yes	0	3 (3.4%)	3 (3%)	
	N/A	0	4 (4.6%)	4 (4%)	
House support service	No	12 (85.7%)	85 (97.7%)	85 (84.2%)	0.589
	Yes	2 (14.3%)	13 (14.9%)	13 (12.8%)	
	N/A	0	3 (3.4%)	3 (3%)	
Outpatient nursing care	No	14 (100%)	81 (93.1%)	95 (94.1%)	0.731
	Yes	0	2 (2.3%)	2 (2%)	
	N/A	0	4 (4.6%)	4 (4%)	
Nursing	No	10 (71.4%)	59 (67.8%)	69 (68.3%)	0.601
	Yes	4 (4.6%)	25 (28.7%)	29 (28.7%)	
	N/A	0	3 (3.4%)	3 (3%)	
Physiotherapy	No	14 (100%)	76 (87.4%)	90 (89.1%)	0.323
	Yes	0	7 (8%)	7 (6.9%)	
	N/A	0	4 (4.6%)	4 (4%)	
Speech therapy	No	14 (100%)	83 (95.4%)	97 (96%)	-
	Yes	0	0	0	
	N/A	0	4 (4.6%)	4 (4%)	
Occupational therapy	No	14 (100%)	82 (94.2%)	96 (95%)	0.733
	Yes	0	2 (2.3%)	2 (2%)	
	N/A	0	3 (3.4%)	3 (3%)	
Other services	No	13 (92.8%)	74 (85%)	87 (86.1%)	0.402
	Yes	1 (7.2%)	2 (2.3%)	3 (3%)	
	N/A	0	11 (12.6%)	11 (10.9%)	
Technical aids					
Walking stick	No	6 (42.8%)	60 (69%)	66 (65.3%)	0.111
	Yes	6 (42.8%)	23 (26.4%)	29 (28.7%)	
	N/A	2 (14.3%)	4 (4.6%)	6 (5.9%)	
Hiker	No	12 (85.7%)	71 (81.6%)	83 (82.2%)	0.155
	Yes	0	13 (14.9%)	13 (12.9%)	
	N/A	2 (14.3%)	3 (3.5%)	5 (4.9%)	
Wheelchair	No	9 (64.3%)	52 (59.8%)	61 (60.4%)	0.409
	Yes	4 (28.6%)	33 (33.9%)	37 (36.6%)	
	N/A	1 (7.1%)	2 (2.3%)	3 (3%)	
Hearing aids	No	12 (85.7%)	80 (91.9%)	92 (91.1%)	0.360
	Yes	1 (7.1%)	2 (2.3%)	3 (3%)	
	N/A	1 (7.1%)	5 (5.7%)	6 (5.9%)	
Glasses	No	6 (42.8%)	52 (59.8%)	58 (57.4%)	0.203
	Yes	7 (50%)	31 (35.6%)	38 (37.6%)	
	N/A	1 (7.1%)	4 (4.6%)	5 (5%)	

the existence of specific conditions that allowed the survival of the most robust individuals [39]. On the other hand, we can also hypothesize that better health care access in inner part of the country can lead to a higher number of centenarians in this rural area, probably, with increased levels of morbidity, according to Robine et al.'s (2010) perspective about the trade-off between the level of mortality selection and the functional health status of the oldest old survivors. This perspective could explain the fact that centenarians from Beira Interior show lower prevalence of diseases when compared to global results of age-related illnesses for the centenarians from Porto (with easier access to health care).

In the context of reported diseases, the high rate of sensory problems connected to vision (60.4%) must be highlighted: while glasses are the most used technical aid mentioned by centenarians, only 38 (37.6%) used them. Similarly, problems with hearing are mentioned by 73% of the centenarians; nevertheless, hearing aids were used by only 3%. This data indicates a low use of technical aids by this group, a finding that can be connected to lack of information, low incomes, and difficulties in income management or, eventually, ageist attitudes in the potential treatment of these sensorial gaps with technical aids, in line with findings observed in the Oporto Centenarian Study [40]. On the other side, this data indicates that there is a possibility for compensation or attenuation of part of the potential sensorial gaps of these centenarians, which could have important implications for cognitive performance, interpersonal relationships, and overall quality of life.

As for the general cognitive status of the centenarians, nearly a half (47.5%) presented no cognitive impairment (GDS1 and GDS2), which is slightly above the values observed in the Oporto Centenarians (30,3%) [22]. It is very difficult to compare these results with results from other international studies because the cognitive status was differently evaluated. Even considering this important methodological limitation, some assumptions can be made. For instance, it is possible to relate Beira Interior centenarians' cognitive status with their isolation, as this may have enhanced their ability to adapt and to find solutions. Comparing the prevalence of dementia obtained in this study with values observed in a review on cognition in centenarians made by Ishioka and Gondo [41], it is in the range found, which is from 33% to 100% (average was 62%, 48,5% for males and 66,1% for females). Comparing our results to specific centenarian studies, we can cautiously conclude that, due to the mentioned methodological concerns, the centenarians of Beira Interior present lower prevalence of dementia than in Canadian centenarians [42], Danish centenarians [19], Dutch centenarians [43, 44], Korean Centenarian [45], Italian centenarians [46], Japanese centenarians [47–49], and centenarians from the Georgia Centenarian Study [12]. On the other hand, the prevalence of dementia in Portuguese centenarians of Beira Interior is higher than that in Finish centenarians [50]. In this specific group of Portuguese centenarians from Beira Interior, there are no statistically significant differences between men and women in cognition, which contradicts results from other centenarians studies (e.g., [46, 48]) that pointed out dementia prevalence rates as being higher among women than among men.

With regard to the use of the health services, the annual average use of the assistant doctor is notably under the values observed in other centenarian studies (e.g., [9, 19, 42, 51]) and also below the average of consultations of the Portuguese population, which is near 4 consultations per year [52]. Nonetheless, the data confirms the importance of a primary health care physician for this group, to whom most Portuguese centenarians have access, even though the number of appointments is reduced. The data does not include information about access and the number of appointments with medical specialists, which would have been important in order to discuss and analyze their role in centenarian caretaking. Considering the rural context the centenarians are living in and the difficulty in accessing health services, home care and other strategies would mean a significant improvement in the use of primary health care and avoiding emergency services.

Finally, with regard to hospitalizations, 90% of centenarians reported not having been hospitalized. This result is specifically the reverse of that found in other studies, such as Andersen-Ranberg et al.'s [19] in Denmark, which refers to 94% hospitalizations. On the other hand, it is a very similar result to that of Rochon et al. [42], in Canada, which indicates 18.2% hospitalizations in the last year. In fact, there are contradictory facts in the literature concerning the higher rates of hospitalizations in advanced age. There is evidence that the oldest old have higher rates of hospitalizations [53], although hospital admissions are higher in nonagenarians than in centenarians [54] and there are a lower number of hospital admissions in centenarians than in persons who died before this age [8].

Concerning support services to elderly people, these were scarcely used by these centenarians from rural areas. Data reveal a very low use of services and equipment needs other than technical interventions. The very low level of use of interventions like psychological support or physiotherapy may be associated with the reduced offer of such services in the geographical area and/or with low (health) literacy levels that could be constraining the recognition of their benefits to the centenarians. Moreover, ageist attitudes towards such benefits should also be appointed as potential justifications. Nevertheless, referring this group to the health services mentioned could make up for the deficits and problems identified and improve their dignity and life quality.

This study has several limitations, namely, as mentioned before, the fact that it was mostly based on self-reporting measures, which may have led to an underestimation of diseases and service uses. Though important, self-reported data should be crosschecked with objective health measures and data connected to the use of health services. The most important contribution of this study consists in the description of a centenarian Portuguese population resident in a rural environment. The profile obtained will help to better understand health care service use (and needs) by this population in order to promote life quality of centenarians in contexts with low population density and sparse health care services. Further research is needed to understand the role of contextual variables in the Beira Interior centenarians' adaptive process to advanced longevity. The comparative analysis of this group with other centenarian groups will also be an important step in understanding the aspects that differentiate centenarians living in a region that is predominantly rural.

Acknowledgments

This article was supported by ERDF through the operation POCI-01-0145-FEDER-007746 funded by Programa Operacional Competitividade e Internacionalização-COMPETE2020 and by National Funds through Fundação para a Ciência e a Tecnologia (FCT) within CINTESIS, R&D

Unit (reference UID/IC/4255/2013). The authors would like to thank the team of PT100-Oporto Centenarian Project (funded by FCT-C/SAU/UI0688/2011 and C/SAU/UI0688/2014) and the team of PT100-Beira Interior Centenarian Project (promoted by the University of Beira Interior) and collaborators. A special recognition is to be made to Dr. Laetitia Teixeira (ICBAS.UP) for her support in the database management and to Professor Henrique Pereira (UBI) for his extraordinary support in the implementation of this project and writing correction.

References

[1] K. Christensen, G. Doblhammer, R. Rau, and J. W. Vaupel, "Ageing populations: the challenges ahead," *The Lancet*, vol. 374, no. 9696, pp. 1196–1208, 2009.

[2] S. J. Olshansky, D. J. Passaro, R. C. Hershow et al., "A potential decline in life expectancy in the United States in the 21st century," *The New England Journal of Medicine*, vol. 352, no. 11, pp. 1138–1145, 2005.

[3] *United Nations, Department of Economic and Social Affairs, Population Division*, World Population Ageing, New York, NY, USA, 2013.

[4] Instituto Nacional de Estatística, "População residente por Local de residência, Sexo e Grupo etário (Decenal)," http://www.ine.pt/xportal/xmain?xpid=INE&xpgid=ine_indicadores&indOcorrCod=0002192&contexto=bd&selTab=tab2.

[5] Instituto Nacional de Estatística, "População residente por Local de residência, Sexo e Grupo etário (Decenal)," http://www.ine.pt/xportal/xmain?xpid=INE&xpgid=ine_indicadores&indOcorrCod=0006368&contexto=bd&selTab=tab2.

[6] L. Poon and S. Cheung, "Centenarian research in the past two Decades," *Asian Journal of Gerontology & Geriatrics*, vol. 7, p. 13, 2012.

[7] K. Andersen-Ranberg, K. Christensen, B. Jeune, A. Skytthe, L. Vasegaard, and J. W. Vaupel, "Declining physical abilities with age: A cross-sectional study of older twins and centenarians in Denmark," *Age and Ageing*, vol. 28, no. 4, pp. 373–377, 1999.

[8] H. Engberg, A. Oksuzyan, B. Jeune, J. W. Vaupel, and K. Christensen, "Centenarians - A useful model for healthy aging? A 29-year follow-up of hospitalizations among 40000 Danes born in 1905," *Aging Cell*, vol. 8, no. 3, pp. 270–276, 2009.

[9] C. Darviri, P. Demakakos, F. Charizani et al., "Assessment of the health status of Greek centenarians," *Archives of Gerontology and Geriatrics*, vol. 46, no. 1, pp. 67–78, 2008.

[10] M. Motta, L. Ferlito, S. U. Magnolfi et al., "Cognitive and functional status in the extreme longevity," *Archives of Gerontology and Geriatrics*, vol. 46, no. 2, pp. 245–252, 2008.

[11] T. T. Perls, K. Bochen, M. Freeman, L. Alpert, and M. H. Silver, "Validity of reported age and centenarian prevalence in New England," *Age and Ageing*, vol. 28, no. 2, pp. 193–197, 1999.

[12] L. W. Poon, G. M. Clayton, P. Martin et al., "The Georgia Centenarian Study," *International Journal of Aging and Human Development*, vol. 34, no. 1, pp. 1–17, 1992.

[13] B. J. Willcox, D. C. Willcox, and L. Ferrucci, "Secrets of healthy aging and longevity from exceptional survivors around the globe: Lessons from octogenarians to supercentenarians," *The Journals of Gerontology. Series A, Biological Sciences and Medical Sciences*, vol. 63, no. 11, pp. 1181–1185, 2008.

[14] D. Jopp and C. Rott, "Adaptation in very old age: Exploring the role of resources, beliefs, and attitudes for centenarians' happiness," *Psychology and Aging*, vol. 21, no. 2, pp. 266–280, 2006.

[15] S. M. Samuelsson, B. Bauer Alfredson, B. Hagberg et al., "The Swedish Centenarian Study: A multidisciplinary study of five consecutive cohorts at the age of 100," *International Journal of Aging and Human Development*, vol. 45, no. 3, pp. 223–253, 1997.

[16] T. Koch, R. Turner, P. Smith, and N. Hutnik, "Storytelling reveals the active, positive lives of centenarians," *Nursing Older People*, vol. 22, no. 8, pp. 31–36, 2010.

[17] P. Martin, L. W. Poon, E. Kim, and M. A. Johnson, "Social and Psychological Resources in the Oldest Old," *Experimental Aging Research*, vol. 22, no. 2, pp. 121–139, 1996.

[18] L. W. Poon, P. Martin, A. Bishop et al., "Understanding centenarians' psychosocial dynamics and their contributions to health and quality of life," *Current Gerontology and Geriatrics Research*, vol. 2010, 2010.

[19] K. Andersen-Ranberg, M. Schroll, and B. Jeune, "Healthy centenarians do not exist, but autonomous centenarians do: A population-based study of morbidity among danish centenarians," *Journal of the American Geriatrics Society*, vol. 49, no. 7, pp. 900–908, 2001.

[20] B. Jeune, "Living longer - But better?" *Aging Clinical and Experimental Research*, vol. 14, no. 2, pp. 72–93, 2002.

[21] C. Pa and C. Paúl, "Centenários: o novo desafio para a medicina e as ciências sociais," in *Jornadas de Gerontopsiquiatria*, L. Fernandes, M. Gonçalves-Pereira, L. Pinto, H. Firmino, and A. Leuschner, Eds., pp. 9–12, 2011.

[22] O. Ribeiro, L. Araújo, L. Teixeira, D. Brandão, N. Duarte, and C. Paúl, "PT100 Oporto Centenarian Study," in *Encyclopedia of Geropsychology*, N. Pachana, Ed., 2015.

[23] R. J. Gobbens and M. A. van Assen, "Associations of Environmental Factors With Quality of Life in Older Adults," *The Gerontologist*, vol. 58, no. 1, pp. 101–110, 2018.

[24] H.-W. Wahl, S. Iwarsson, and F. Oswald, "Aging well and the environment: Toward an integrative model and research agenda for the future," *The Gerontologist*, vol. 52, no. 3, pp. 306–316, 2012.

[25] K. A. Greiner, C. Li, I. Kwachi, D. C. Hunt, and J. S. Ahlwaia, "The relationships of social participation and community ratings to health and health behaviours in areas with high and low population density," *Social Science Medicine*, vol. 59, pp. 2303–2312, 2004.

[26] O. P. Nummela, T. T. Sulander, H. S. Heinonen, and A. K. Uutela, "Self-rated health and indicators of SES among the ageing in three types of communities," *Scandinavian Journal of Public Health*, vol. 35, no. 1, pp. 39–47, 2007.

[27] J. F. Silva and C. Ribeiro, *As Assimetrias Regionais em Portugal: análise da convergência versus divergência ao nível dos municípios*, Working Paper Series, Núcleo de Investigação em Políticas Económicas Universidade do Minho, 2013.

[28] D. Brandão, O. Ribeiro, A. Freitas, and C. Paúl, "Hospital admissions by the oldest old: Past trends in one of the most ageing countries in the world," *Geriatrics & Gerontology International*, vol. 17, no. 11, pp. 2255–2265, 2017.

[29] O. Ribeiro, L. Teixeira, L. Araújo, and C. Paúl, "Health profile of centenarians in Portugal: A census-based approach," *Population Health Metrics*, vol. 14, no. 1, 2016.

[30] R. T. Goins, K. A. Williams, M. W. Carter, S. M. Spencer, and T. Solovieva, "Perceived barriers to health care access among rural older adults: A Qualitative Study," *The Journal of Rural Health*, vol. 21, no. 3, pp. 206–213, 2005.

[31] C. N. Bull, J. A. Krout, E. Rathbone-McCuan, and M. J. Shreffler, "Access and issues of equity in remote/rural areas," *The Journal of Rural Health*, vol. 17, no. 4, pp. 356–359, 2001.

[32] P. Santana, *A Geografia da Saúde da População. Evolução nos últimos 20 anos em Portugal Continental.*, Centro de Estudos em Geografia e Ordenamento do Território (CEGOT), 2015.

[33] OECD/European Observatory on Health Systems and Policies (OHSP), *Portugal: Perfil de Saúde do País 2017, State of Health in the EU*, OECD Publishing, Paris/European Observatory on Health Systems and Policies, Brussels, Belgium, 2017.

[34] G. G. Fillenbaum and M. A. Smyer, "The development, validity, and reliability of the OARS multidimensional functional assessment questionnaire," *The Journals of Gerontology. Series A, Biological Sciences and Medical Sciences*, vol. 36, no. 4, pp. 428–434, 1981.

[35] R. M. Rodrigues, "Validação da versão em português europeu de questionário de avaliação funcional multidimensional de idosos," *Revista Panamericana de Salud Pública/Pan American Journal of Public Health*, vol. 23, no. 2, pp. 109–115, 2008.

[36] B. Reisberg, S. H. Ferris, M. J. De Leon, and T. Crook, "The global deterioration scale for assessment of primary degenerative dementia," *The American Journal of Psychiatry*, vol. 139, no. 9, pp. 1136–1139, 1982.

[37] M. J. G. Moreira and F. D. C. Henriques, "Demographic and health changes in Portugal (1900–2013)," *Hygiea Internationalis*, vol. 12, no. 1, pp. 9–39, 2016.

[38] P. A. Rochon, S. E. Bronskill, A. Gruneir et al., *Older Women's Health. Project for an Ontario Women's Health Evidence- Based Report*, St. Michael's Hospital and the Institute for Clinical Evaluative Sciences, Toronto, ON, USA, 2011.

[39] J.-M. Robine, S. L. K. Cheung, Y. Saito, B. Jeune, M. G. Parker, and F. R. Herrmann, "Centenarians today: New insights on selection from the 5-COOP study," *Current Gerontology and Geriatrics Research*, vol. 2010, 2010.

[40] O. Ribeiro, L. Araújo, L. Teixeira et al., "Health Status, Living Arrangements, and Service Use at 100: Findings From the Oporto Centenarian Study," *Journal of Aging & Social Policy*, vol. 28, no. 3, pp. 148–164, 2016.

[41] Y. L. Ishioka and Y. Gondo, "Cognition," in *Encyclopedia of Geropsychology*, N. Pachana, Ed., 2015.

[42] P. A. Rochon, A. Gruneir, W. Wu et al., "Demographic characteristics and healthcare use of centenarians: A population-based cohort study," *Journal of the American Geriatrics Society*, vol. 62, no. 1, pp. 86–93, 2014.

[43] B. A. Blansjaar, R. Thomassen, and H. W. Van Schaick, "Prevalence of dementia in centenarians," *International Journal of Geriatric Psychiatry*, vol. 15, pp. 219–225, 2000.

[44] M. Kliegel and M. Sliwinski, "MMSE cross-domain variability predicts cognitive decline in centenarians," *Gerontology*, vol. 50, no. 1, pp. 39–43, 2004.

[45] Y.-H. Choi, J.-H. Kim, D. K. Kim et al., "Distributions of ACE and APOE polymorphisms and their relations with dementia status in Korean centenarians," *The Journals of Gerontology. Series A, Biological Sciences and Medical Sciences*, vol. 58, no. 3, pp. 227–231, 2003.

[46] G. Ravaglia, P. Forti, D. De Ronchi et al., "Prevalence and severity of dementia among northern Italian centenarians," *Neurology*, vol. 53, no. 2, pp. 416–418, 1999.

[47] T. Asada, Z. Yamagata, T. Kinoshita et al., "Prevalence of dementia and distribution of ApoE alleles in Japanese centenarians: An almost-complete survey in Yamanashi Prefecture, Japan," *Journal of the American Geriatrics Society*, vol. 44, no. 2, pp. 151–155, 1996.

[48] Y. Gondo, N. Hirose, Y. Arai et al., "Functional Status of Centenarians in Tokyo, Japan: Developing Better Phenotypes of Exceptional Longevity," *The Journals of Gerontology. Series A, Biological Sciences and Medical Sciences*, vol. 61, no. 3, pp. 305–310, 2006.

[49] A. Homma, Y. Shimonaka, and K. Nakazato, "Psychosomatic state of centenarians," *Japanese Journal of Geriatrics*, vol. 29, no. 12, pp. 922–930, 1992.

[50] E. Sobel, J. Louhija, R. Sulkava et al., "Lack of association of apolipoprotein E allele ε4 with late-onset alzheimer's disease among finnish centenarians," *Neurology*, vol. 45, no. 5, pp. 903–907, 1995.

[51] E. E. Roughead, L. M. Kalisch, E. N. Ramsay, P. Ryan, and A. L. Gilbert, "Use of health services and medicines amongst Australian war veterans: A comparison of young elderly, near centenarians and centenarians," *BMC Geriatrics*, vol. 10, article no. 83, 2010.

[52] OECD, *Health at a Glance 2017: OECD Indicators*, OECD Publishing, Paris, France, 2017.

[53] F. Aminzadeh and W. B. Dalziel, "Older adults in the emergency department: a systematic review of patterns of use, adverse outcomes, and effectiveness of interventions," *Annals of Emergency Medicine*, vol. 39, no. 3, pp. 238–247, 2002.

[54] T. J. Wilkinson, "Reasons for Hospital Admission in New Zealand's Oldest Old," *Australasian Journal on Ageing*, vol. 18, no. 2, pp. 93–97, 1999.

32

Clinical Screening Tools for Sarcopenia and Its Management

Solomon C. Y. Yu, [1,2,3] **Kareeann S. F. Khow,** [1,2,3]
Agathe D. Jadczak, [1,2,3] **and Renuka Visvanathan** [1,2,3]

[1] *Aged and Extended Care Services, The Queen Elizabeth Hospital, Central Adelaide Local Health Network, 28 Woodville Road, Woodville South, Adelaide, SA 5011, Australia*
[2] *Adelaide Geriatrics Training and Research with Aged Care (G-TRAC) Centre, School of Medicine and Faculty of Health Science, University of Adelaide, Adelaide, SA 5000, Australia*
[3] *Centre of Research Excellence: Frailty Trans-Disciplinary Research to Achieve Healthy Aging, University of Adelaide, Adelaide, SA 5000, Australia*

Correspondence should be addressed to Solomon C. Y. Yu; solomon.yu@adelaide.edu.au

Academic Editor: Marco Malavolta

Sarcopenia, an age-related decline in muscle mass and function, is affecting the older population worldwide. Sarcopenia is associated with poor health outcomes, such as falls, disability, loss of independence, and mortality; however it is potentially treatable if recognized and intervened early. Over the last two decades, there has been significant expansion of research in this area. Currently there is international recognition of a need to identify the condition early for intervention and prevention of the disastrous consequences of sarcopenia if left untreated. There are currently various screening tools proposed. As yet, there is no consensus on the best tool. Effective interventions of sarcopenia include physical exercise and nutrition supplementation. This review paper examined the screening tools and interventions for sarcopenia.

1. Introduction

Physiological changes to body composition with aging are well known [1]. Muscle mass is lost at a rate of approximately 8% per decade from the age of 50 years until the age of 70 years, after which weight loss is coupled with an accelerated loss of muscle mass, reaching a rate of 15% per decade [2]. There is now general agreement that sarcopenia includes loss of muscle mass, strength, and function. However, ongoing debate continues in relation to the optimal cutoff values for diagnosing sarcopenia and, more practically, the most appropriate clinical tool to use for screening [3].

Sarcopenia is common and its prevalence will rise with population aging. The prevalence of sarcopenia is said to range between 5% and 13% in community-dwelling older people aged 65 years and over. This prevalence is higher in those 80 years and older (e.g., one in five) and those who reside in residential care or in hospital setting [3]. Sarcopenia is important clinically because of the harm related to it. It has been described that sarcopenia is an independent predictor of falls

[4], disability [5], loss of independence [5], and increased mortality [6–8]. In one study conducted in the United States in 2000, it was estimated that 1.5% of the total health care expenditure was attributable to sarcopenia [9]. The authors concluded that a 10% reduction in sarcopenia could potentially save US$1.1 billion in health-related costs.

According to the operational definition by European Working Group on Sarcopenia in Older People (EWGSOP), the diagnosis of sarcopenia requires the presence of low muscle mass, with either the presence of low grip strength or low physical performance [10]. Current diagnostic methods for sarcopenia include measuring muscle mass using either dual-energy X-ray absorptiometry (DXA) or bioelectrical impedance analysis (BIA) [3]. However, these tools are not practical for clinical practice because they are costly and require burdensome trips to a health facility. Other methods such as computed tomography (CT) or magnetic resonance imaging (MRI), whilst accurate, are not practical and expensive and expose patient to radiation. Therefore, using a diagnostic approach to detect presence of sarcopenia will be time consuming and expensive and requires highly specialized equipment.

Sarcopenia is very often not noticeable in earlier phases but becomes more apparent once a critical event such as a fall has occurred or disability has set in [11]. While it is possible to preserve skeletal muscle mass in older age, it is extremely challenging to regain substantial quantities once the loss has occurred. Therefore, a screening strategy to a larger population in the community that allows for early detection is important. An ideal screening test that is clinically useful should be safe, have a reasonable cutoff level defined, be cost-effective and is both valid and reliable, easily performed in clinical setting that does not require further training, with reasonable accurate sensitivity and specificity [12]. It is currently a prevalent view that screening approach is to target those who are screen "positive" or "high risk" of sarcopenia with a multidisciplinary intervention, so that prescriptive intervention by optimizing nutrition and exercise could reduce the rate of muscle loss, thus preventing sarcopenia.

This review aims to examine the literature on screening tools and interventions for sarcopenia. With this information, clinicians will hopefully be better able to make an earlier diagnosis and intervene to prevent a decline in physical health.

2. Screening Method for Sarcopenia

Despite increasing research into sarcopenia, there appears to be a dearth of practical and implementable clinical screening tool to support the early identification of sarcopenia in primary care. In general, current screening methods have taken the approach of either developing a screening questionnaire, a diagnostic grid, or prediction equations. Screening test is defined by sensitivity, specificity, positive predictive value (PPV), and negative predictive value (NPV). As a general rule, a "rule-out" screening test is one that has high sensitivity and high NPV, whilst a "rule-in" screening test would have high specificity and high PPV [13]. Current screening methods are mostly "rule-out" tests identifying those not at-risk of sarcopenia in the community. It is currently unknown if any one tool is superior to the others because no head-to-head comparison study has been performed to evaluate these different screening tools for sarcopenia. Table 1 summarises all the screening tools currently available.

In 2010, the first screening method for sarcopenia was described by the EWGSOP and a two-step algorithm using gait speed assessment and handgrip strength was recommended [10]. Patients with a gait speed cutoff of ≤0.8 m/s should have their muscle mass measured to confirm presence of sarcopenia. On the other hand, those with gait speed of >0.8 m/s undergo measurement of their handgrip strength. Those with low handgrip strength will then be recommended to have muscle mass tested. The gait speed cutoff was derived from the study by Abellan van Kan et al. which found that adverse outcomes were associated with cutoff <0.8 m/s [19]. This algorithm was intended as a rule-out test. However no derivation or validation study has been reported on the development of this two-step screening algorithm. In one study of 3260 community-dwelling older people from Brazil, Mexico, and Spain, 83.4% of the total participants were suspected to

have sarcopenia either by gait speed or by handgrip strength below the cutoff as suggested above [14]. Therefore this algorithm is of limited clinical utility in screening older adults for sarcopenia due to the high proportion of subjects selected to further undergo muscle mass assessment. However, this study did not establish the proportion of positively screened subjects who are actually sarcopenic. These findings indicate that the EWGSOP proposed cutoff values for gait speed and handgrip strength may not be widely usable across different populations.

Working on the principles that clinicians prefer simple questionnaires, Malmstrom and Morley developed the SARC-F where the following five domains were assessed: strength, ambulation (walking independence), rising from a chair, stair climbing, and history of falls [20]. The total score was 10 points with each domain scoring two. A score of 4 or more indicates a risk of sarcopenia and has been demonstrated to be associated with poor outcomes in older adults [20] (Table 1). This tool is intended to identify older people who require diagnostic evaluation for sarcopenia. Woo and colleagues have demonstrated the comparability of the SARC-F to three major consensus definitions for sarcopenia (American, European, and Asian) in 4000 community-dwelling older people in Hong Kong [21]. This questionnaire was found to be a suitable tool to exclude older people without sarcopenia, hence avoiding unnecessary and inconvenient investigations for those not at-risk [21]. Furthermore, Cao et al. showed that a score of SARC-F ≥ 4 is associated with poor physical function and hospitalization of falls in the previous 2 years adds to the strength and usefulness of this tool [22]. The strength of this screening tool is that the questions are very simple and it does not require complex measurements of strength or gait speed (Table 2). In addition, this tool has been linked to predicting clinical outcome and therefore has clinical relevance when the result screen is positive using this screening tool. However, the ability of this screening tool to monitor for improvement or deterioration is not known and, also, this tool has mainly been investigated in the community setting. Its efficacy in hospitals or residential aged care is not known.

Goodman et al. on the other hand have proposed a screening grid for low muscle mass by age and body mass index (BMI) [15]. The grid was derived from the National Health and Nutrition Examination Surveys (NHANES) 1999–2004 data where appendicular skeletal mass (ASM) was calculated from DXA measurements. The older person was classified as having low muscle mass if their skeletal muscle index (SMI) [ASM/height^2] was one standard deviation (SD) below the mean SMI of young adults (20–40 years old). It should be noted that this cutoff is different to the less than two SD SMI recommended by EWSGOP to diagnose low muscle mass. This grid has been validated in a cohort of patients aged 65 years and above who attended the University of Utah Health Care System. However, this screening grid has not been externally validated or evaluated in a wider population.

Ishii et al. developed a simple screening test to identify older adults at high risk for sarcopenia based on the EWGSOP criteria of ASM, grip strength, and usual gait speed [16]. They found that the probability of sarcopenia could be estimated

TABLE 1: Summary of currently available screening tools for sarcopenia.

	EWGSOP algorithm [10]	SARC-F questionnaire [14]	Goodman et al. [15]	Ishii et al. [16]	Anthropometric PE [17, 18]
Description	Two-step algorithm: First step: gait speed. Second step: handgrip strength if gait speed >0.8 m/s. If hand grip is low, proceed to muscle mass. Muscle mass measurement if gait speed ≤0.8 m/s	Assessed 5 domains: Strength, independence walking, rising from a chair, climbing stairs, and history of falls. Total score is 10 points (2 for each domain). A score of ≥4 indicates a risk for sarcopenia	Grid based on age and BMI is used to generate probability of sarcopenia which can be <0.20, 0.20–0.49 and ≥0.50	To estimate probability of sarcopenia with a score chart using age, handgrip strength, and calf circumference	$PE = 10.05 + 0.35$ (weight) $- 0.62$ (BMI) $- 0.02$ (age) $+ 5.10$ (if male)
Definition of sarcopenia	EWGSOP	EWGSOP IWGS AWGS	Sarcopenia defined as low skeletal muscle index (SMI) [ASM/height^2] <1 SD below the mean SMI of young adults (20–40 years)	EWGSOP	Sarcopenia as defined by ASM and low grip strength. Men: ASM_{DXA} <7.36 kg/m^2 Grip strength < 30 kg. Women: ASM_{DXA} 5.81 kg/m^2 Grip strength < 20 kg
Development model	NA	Not published in a peer-reviewed journal	Development model from NHANES, USA. Aged ≥ 65 years. M = 3538, F = 5272	Development model from Japanese community-dwellers. Aged ≥ 65 years. M = 977, F = 994	Derived from healthy subject (age 18 to 83 years), Australia. $n = 195$
Validation study	NA	Two studies: (a) Community dwellers in Hong Kong $n = 4000$ (b) Chinese older adults aged >65 years in various settings (i.e., community dwellers and nursing home residents) $n = 230$	Independent sample from patients in the University of Utah Health Care System, USA. Aged ≥65 years. M = 103, F = 103	Internal validation using bootstrapping procedure and final models were derived by correcting regression coefficient for over optimism	Independent sample from NWAHS and FAMAS community dwelling population adults ≥65 years. M = 611, F = 375

Clinical Screening Tools for Sarcopenia and Its Management

TABLE 1: Continued.

	EWGSOP algorithm [10]	SARC-F questionnaire [14]	Goodman et al. [15]	Ishii et al. [16]	Anthropometric PE [17, 18]
Sensitivity (%)	NA	*EWGSOP* M 4.2 W 9.9 *IWGS* M 3.8 W 8.2 *AWGS* M 4.8 W 9.4	M 81.2 W 90.6	M 84.9 W 75.5	M 88.2 W 100.0
Specificity (%)	NA	*EWGSOP* M 98.7 W 94.4 *IWGS* M 99.1 W 94.6 *AWGS* M 98.8 W 94.2	M 66.2 W 66.2	M 88.2 W 92	M 95.5 W 83.0
PPV (%)	NA	*EWGSOP* M 25.8 W 14.3 *IWGS* M 54.8 W 25.2 *AWGS* M 29.0 W 8.4	M 58.5 W 54.7	M 54.4 W 72.8	M 65.2 W 29.2
NPV (%)	NA	*EWGSOP* M 90.8 W 91.8 *IWGS* M 78.4 W 82.2 *AWGS* M 91.0 W 94.4	M 86 W 94	M 97.2 W 93.0	M 98.8 W 100.0

BMI: body mass index; EWGSOP: European Working Group on Sarcopenia in Older People; IWGS: International Working Group on Sarcopenia; AWGS: Asian Working Group for Sarcopenia; FAMAS: Florey Adelaide Male Aging Study; SARC-F: slowness, independence walking, rising from chair, climbing stairs, and history of falls questionnaire; NHANES: National Health and Nutrition Examination Surveys; NWAHS: Northwestern Adelaide Healthy Study; PE: prediction equation; ASM$_{PE}$: appendicular skeletal muscle mass as measured by anthropometric prediction equation; PPV: positive predictive value; NPV: negative predictive value; M: men; W: women.

TABLE 2: Strengths and weaknesses of sarcopenia screening tools.

	Strengths/advantages	Limitations/disadvantages
EWGSOP algorithm [10]	Simple two-step algorithm	No validation studies evaluated this tool Sensitivity, specificity, PPV, and NPV of this tool are unknown Limited clinical utility in screening older adults for sarcopenia due to the high proportion of subjects selected to further undergo muscle assessment
Goodman et al. [15]	Uses two simple variable	Age range limited to 65–85 years Adults with morbid obesity and significant disability were excluded from the derivation study Screening for only probability of low muscle mass
Ishii et al. [16]	Simple tool requiring three variables	External validity is unknown Calf circumference is not currently a routine measurement in clinical practice and therefore may require training to measure this accurately
SARC-F questionnaire [20]	Uses 5 questions without requiring measurements involving cutoff values They have comparable specificity and predictive power for adverse outcomes when validated against criteria requiring measurements developed by consensus panels (American, European, and Asian). Rapid screening and cost-effective	Low sensitivity may miss out people who are sarcopenic but classified as "not sarcopenic" according to SARC-F questionnaire not currently used in clinical practice
Anthropometric PE [17, 18]	Good discriminatory tool as a "rule-out" screening test Variables are already a routine clinical practice such as measurement of weight, height, and gender Can be used as screening tool in primary care setting	Not yet validated in care facility residents or hospital inpatients Not yet validated in non-Caucasian population.

EWGSOP: European Working Group on Sarcopenia in Older People; NPV: negative predictive value; SARC-F: slowness, assistance with walking, rising from chair, climbing stairs, and falls questionnaire; PE: prediction equation; PPV: positive predictive value.

using a score chart, which includes three variables: age, grip strength, and calf circumference (Table 1). The sensitivity, specificity, and positive and negative predictive values of this tool are shown in Table 1 but essentially this tool worked best to rule-out those at-risk of sarcopenia. This tool was developed in a Japanese population and has not undergone external validation or been tested with other ethnic populations (Table 2).

Yu and colleagues in Australia have developed a screening method incorporating the use of an anthropometric prediction equation for appendicular skeletal muscle mass (ASM_{PE}) [17, 18]. With this study, the researchers demonstrated that when the anthropometric PE was combined with a measure of muscle function such as grip strength, that screening method was able to "rule-out" those not at-risk of sarcopenia (Table 1). There is a further need to research this method with gait speed. There is also the opportunity to improve the accuracy of this method by improving the performance of the ASM_{PE}.

Other anthropometric measurements such as calf circumference have been proposed as a screening tool for sarcopenia. Although calf circumference correlated with ASM

in 1458 community-dwelling French women aged above 70 years, it was unable to predict sarcopenia defined by the ASM estimated with DXA [23]. Despite its low cost and ability to predict physical function, calf circumference is not a good screening tool for sarcopenia. Furthermore, this measurement has also not been studied in male participants [23].

3. Interventions

It is better to prevent progressive loss of skeletal muscle mass, strength, and function rather than try to restore it at older age. Preventive strategies go along with treatment interventions and should be initiated as early as possible before the loss of skeletal muscle mass, strength, and function will occur. Exercise interventions and nutritional approach play a significant role in the management of sarcopenia. The literature indicates that exercise interventions have the most significant improvement on sarcopenia [24]. Other evidence goes further to suggest that the combination of exercise and nutrition is the key intervention to prevent, treat, and slow down the progress of sarcopenia [25]. Pharmaceutical agents are still under investigation with no clear evidence of benefit yet.

4. Physical Activity and Exercise Intervention

Physical activity is defined as any movement produced by the contraction of skeletal muscles that increases energy expenditure [26]. The term "physical activity" comprises all kinds of activities (e.g., daily activities) while exercise is characterized as a planned, structured, and repetitive movement to improve or maintain components of physical function and fitness [27]. Therefore, exercise is a form of physical activity with a specific purpose and is typically described by type, intensity, frequency, and duration. Exercise increases muscle strength and muscle mass and improves physical performance. Evidence shows that progressive resistance and aerobic exercises are most beneficial for the prevention and treatment of sarcopenia [28].

Muscular strength is the ability to generate maximal force by a single muscle or a muscle group but this decreases with aging [10]. Muscular hypertrophy is the enhancement of muscle size through mechanical, metabolic, and hormonal processes [29]. Muscular power is a product of force and speed and it is a significant predictor of performing activities of daily living [30]. Muscular power declines more steeply with age compared to muscular strength but appears to be amenable to intervention in older people with sarcopenia [31].

4.1. Progressive Resistance Exercise. Resistance exercise comprises dynamic and static contractions against an external resistance with a progressive increase over time [32]. Resistant training can be executed on resistance machines in the gymnasium, by lifting weights, stretching bands, or using the individual's body weight. Resistant training improves muscle strength and mass by improving protein synthesis in skeletal muscle cells [24]. This leads to muscle hypertrophy and increases muscle power [30]. Resistance training is a safe, feasible, and effective intervention for older people and it is strongly recommended for people with sarcopenia [11, 33].

In older people, resistance exercise should be performed on two or three nonconsecutive days per week with at least one set of 8–12 repetitions (experts recommend 10–15) of the major muscle groups [34]. The load can be increased by 2–10% when two sets can be performed over the desired number on two consecutive training sessions [33].

A 2009 Cochrane review of 121 trials with 6,700 participants assessed the effects of progressive resistance training on physical function of older people [35]. In most trials, resistance exercise was performed 2-3 times a week at a high intensity. Resistance exercise had a large positive effect on muscle strength and a small but significant improvement in physical ability. There was a modest improvement in gait speed but a larger effect on getting up from a chair. The review concluded that resistance exercise is an effective intervention for improving strength and physical functioning in older people. However adverse events were not adequately reported in many studies and translation of these findings into clinical practice has to be approached cautiously.

4.2. Aerobic Exercise. Aerobic exercise is a form of structured physical activity using oxygen to meet the energy demands during exercise [36]. Examples of aerobic exercise are swimming, brisk walking, cycling, jogging, dancing or water aerobics. Aerobic exercise improves metabolic control, reduces oxidative stress, and optimizes exercise capacity [33]. It has also beneficial impact on sarcopenia by improving skeletal muscle insulin sensitivity; stimulating skeletal muscle hypertrophy; and increasing skeletal muscle mass [24, 37]. However, it does not produce the same magnitude of improvement in muscle mass and strength as resistance exercise, but it is still recommended for patients with sarcopenia [11, 33]. Table 3 summarises the recommendation of aerobic exercise in sarcopenic individuals.

A recent systematic review on exercise interventions for sarcopenia determined that aerobic and resistance exercise can improve muscle strength and physical function although it seems not consistently to increase muscle mass [28]. The presented recommendations illustrate a first step in the standardization of exercise interventions for sarcopenic people. However, further research is needed to determine optimal and significant exercise conditions for older sarcopenic people.

5. Nutritional Interventions

5.1. Protein Supplements. Nutrition also plays an important role in preventing and reversing sarcopenia. Daily muscle protein turnover is regulated in large part by nutrition, especially dietary protein [41]. Increasing age is associated with reduced appetite and early satiety resulting in many older people failing to meet the recommended daily dietary allowance (RDA) for protein which has important implications for skeletal muscles [11]. The current RDA in Australia for protein in an adult is 0.75 g/kg/day [42]. However, new evidence has shown that older adults will require higher dietary protein (up to 1.2 g/kg/day) to counteract age-related changes in protein metabolism and higher catabolic state associated with chronic or acute diseases [38]. Table 3 summarises the amount, type, and timing of protein ingestion. The table also included the adjusted amount of dietary protein intake in the setting of renal failure.

5.2. Essential Amino Acid Supplements. Branched chain amino acids (BCAA), such as leucine, at daily amount of either 2.5 g or 2.8 g in combination with resistance exercise may affect muscle protein synthesis, muscle recovery following illness, and muscle mass (Table 3) [38]. BCAA has shown beneficial effects on sarcopenic patients who are severely ill [43]. However, the number of studies using this supplement in older people is still limited and not all have shown beneficial results.

5.3. Beta-Hydroxy-Beta-Methylbutyrate (HMB). HMB used alone or with combination of resistance exercise or lysine and arginine has shown some effects on improved muscle strength and physical performance in some studies (Table 3) [39, 40]. However, these studies were limited by small sample size.

5.4. Vitamin D. Low serum vitamin D levels (<50 nmol/L) are associated with reduced muscle strength and frailty [44].

TABLE 3: Exercise and nutritional interventions for sarcopenia.

Exercise [33]			
Type of training	Frequency	Intensity	Duration/set
Aerobic exercise	Minimum 5 days/week for moderate intensity or 3 days/week for vigorous intensity	Moderate intensity at 5-6 on a 10-point scale Vigorous intensity at 7-8 on a 10-point scale	Accumulate at least 30 min/day of moderate intensity activity in bouts of at least 10 min each continuous vigorous activity for at least 20 min/day
Resistance exercise (for major muscle groups using free weights and machines)	At least 2 days/week	Slow-to-moderate velocity 60–80% of 1 RM	8–10 exercises 1–3 sets per exercise 8–12 repetitions 1–3 min rest
Power training (to practice only after the resistance training)	Two days a week	High repetition velocity Light-to-moderate loading 30–60% of 1 RM	1–3 sets 6–10 repetitions

Nutritional supplementation [38–40]			
Intervention	Evidence or recommendation		
	Amount of protein	Type of protein	Timing
Protein supplement	At least 1.0–1.2 g/kg/day in people aged 65 years and above GFR 30–60—0.8 g/kg/day GFR <30—between 0.6 and 0.8 g/kg/day	"Fast" proteins are thought to be more beneficial compared to "slow" proteins but lacks robust evidence.	Even distribution of protein intake in main meals through the day
Vitamin D	Replace depleted serum vitamin D level and maintain adequate intake at 700 to 1000 IU/day of cholecalciferol		
*Essential amino acid supplementation	Daily leucine 2.5 g or 2.8 g with combination of resistance exercise (benefits only shown in a small number of studies)		
*Beta-hydroxy-beta-methylbutyrate (HMB)	HMB alone, or with combination of resistance exercise or arginine and lysine (evidence not consistently positive and only shown in a small number of studies)		

GFR: glomerular filtration rate, mL/min/1.73 m^2. *Not currently incorporated into mainstream of treatment.

Hence, it is paramount that a depleted serum vitamin D level be replaced and adequate intake is maintained according to current recommendations (i.e., 700 to 1000 IU/day of cholecalciferol) in all older people with sarcopenia [45]. Cholecalciferol in doses of 800 IU/day has been shown to decrease the risk of falls and this reduction is partly related to improved muscle strength [46].

6. Combination of Exercise and Nutrition

Regularly performed exercise, including resistance training, combined with an adequate nutritional intake seems to be the best way to prevent and treat sarcopenia [25]. There is evidence that resistance exercise combined with protein supplementation leads to greater muscle mass gain compared to resistance exercise or protein supplementation alone [47]. Other evidence suggests that the combination of exercise and amino acid supplementations can be effective in enhancing muscle strength, muscle mass, and walking speed in sarcopenia [48]. Also the dose of protein supplementation seems to play a significant role in the enhancement of resistance exercise and muscle protein synthesis. Evidence shows that

resistance exercise increases muscle protein synthesis in the elderly at all protein doses, but to a greater extent with higher protein doses of 40 g [49]. Therefore, exercise and nutrition in combination should be always considered as a significant and important strategy in the prevention and treatment of sarcopenic patients.

7. Pharmacological Treatment

Many pharmacological agents such as myostatin inhibitor, testosterone, and angiotensin converting enzyme inhibitors and ghrelin-modulating agents are being investigated to treat sarcopenia but there is inadequate evidence to support their use in mainstream practice [50]. A recent proof-of-concept randomized-controlled phase 2 study has found that a humanized monoclonal antibody LY2495655, a myostatin inhibitor, increased lean mass and might improve functional measures of muscle power [51]. There are other pharmacological agents such as proteasome inhibitors and cyclophilin inhibitor, which are currently being evaluated in terms of their effects on skeletal muscles, but studies have so far been restricted to animal models [52, 53].

8. Challenges in Preventing Sarcopenia

While the idea of sarcopenia prevention and early management makes sense, the actual clinical detection and implementation of management remain a challenge, two main areas that require further research.

Firstly, a robust screening tool for sarcopenia is needed for clinical practice. Although anthropometric measurements are easy to obtain in clinical practice, their ability to predict sarcopenia is still limited. Several biological markers have been shown to be associated with skeletal muscle mass, strength, and function. However, these biomarkers may not be specific to skeletal muscle and are likely to be only weakly associated with clinically relevant outcomes [54]. For example, a recent study has found that copper and zinc ratio is associated with decline in physical function and development of disability [55]. The use of biomarkers in screening for sarcopenia requires further investigation.

Secondly, the implementation of interventions for sarcopenia comes with several challenges and barriers in older people. The awareness of the benefits of exercise and diet needs to be raised among older people. A recent systematic review confirmed that older people still believe that exercise is unnecessary or even potentially harmful [56]. Others recognize the benefits of exercise but report a range of barriers to participate in exercise interventions. Raising awareness is one of the most important strategies to enhance exercise participation among older people and to prevent sarcopenia on a long-term scale. Evidence shows that older people would be more active if they were advised to do so by their general practitioner [57].

It is more challenging for older people with activity limitations to engage in physical activity or exercises. In this situation, more targeted exercise plans will need to be designed. Another barrier in older people is the financial ability to attend exercise programs [27]. This barrier needs to be considered in planning long-term strategies to prevent and treat people with sarcopenia. From a dietary point of view, factors such as access to food, finances, and social isolation may all impact on an older person's ability to obtain optimal food intake. Furthermore many older people have difficulties with swallowing and loss of taste and smell which can lead to decrease in oral intake [11].

9. Conclusion

Strategies are needed to screen for sarcopenia and identify effective ways for preventive and therapeutic interventions. Several tools are currently available to screen older people for sarcopenia and further research is needed to determine which is most effective for use in the general population. Exercise and nutrition remain the cornerstone for good health and prevention of sarcopenia. Adequate dietary protein intake is an important measure to prevent or delay sarcopenia in the elderly. It is currently difficult to recommend any pharmacological agents as part of routine treatment of sarcopenia until larger long-term studies have found evidence to support their safe and effective use.

References

[1] B. Steen, "Body composition and aging," *Nutrition Reviews*, vol. 46, no. 2, pp. 45–51, 1988.

[2] G. Grimby and B. Saltin, "The ageing muscle," *Clinical Physiology*, vol. 3, no. 3, pp. 209–218, 1983.

[3] S. Yu, K. Umapathysivam, and R. Visvanathan, "Sarcopenia in older people," *International Journal of Evidence-Based Healthcare*, vol. 12, no. 4, pp. 227–243, 2014.

[4] F. Landi, R. Liperoti, A. Russo et al., "Sarcopenia as a risk factor for falls in elderly individuals: results from the ilSIRENTE study," *Clinical Nutrition*, vol. 31, no. 5, pp. 652–658, 2012.

[5] T. da Silva Alexandre, Y. A. de Oliveira Duarte, J. L. Ferreira Santos, R. Wong, and M. L. Lebrao, "Sarcopenia according to the European working group on sarcopenia in older people (EWGSOP) versus dynapenia as a risk factor for disability in the elderly," *The Journal of Nutrition, Health & Aging*, vol. 18, no. 5, pp. 547–553, 2014.

[6] F. Landi, R. Liperoti, D. Fusco et al., "Sarcopenia and mortality among older nursing home residents," *Journal of the American Medical Directors Association*, vol. 13, no. 2, pp. 121–126, 2012.

[7] J. H. E. Kim, S. Lim, S. H. Choi et al., "Sarcopenia: an independent predictor of mortality in community-dwelling older Korean men," *The Journals of Gerontology Series A, Biological Sciences and Medical Sciences*, vol. 69, no. 10, pp. 1244–1252, 2014.

[8] D. L. Vetrano, F. Landi, S. Volpato et al., "Association of sarcopenia with short- and long-term mortality in older adults admitted to acute care wards: results from the CRIME study," *The Journals of Gerontology Series A: Biological Sciences and Medical Sciences*, vol. 69, no. 9, pp. 1154–1161, 2014.

[9] I. Janssen, D. S. Shepard, P. T. Katzmarzyk, and R. Roubenoff, "The healthcare costs of sarcopenia in the United States," *Journal of the American Geriatrics Society*, vol. 52, no. 1, pp. 80–85, 2004.

[10] A. J. Cruz-Jentoft, J. P. Baeyens, J. M. Bauer et al., "Sarcopenia: European consensus on definition and diagnosis," *Age and Ageing*, vol. 39, no. 4, Article ID afq034, pp. 412–423, 2010.

[11] R. Visvanathan and I. Chapman, "Preventing sarcopaenia in older people," *Maturitas*, vol. 66, no. 4, pp. 383–388, 2010.

[12] D. A. Grimes and K. F. Schulz, "Uses and abuses of screening tests," *The Lancet*, vol. 359, no. 9309, pp. 881–884, 2002.

[13] C. M. Florkowski, "Sensitivity, specificity, Receiver-Operating Characteristic (ROC) curves and likelihood ratios: communicating the performance of diagnostic tests," *The Clinical Biochemist Reviews*, vol. 29, supplement 1, pp. S83–S87, 2008.

[14] R. A. Lourenco, M. Perez-Zepeda, L. Gutierrez-Robledo, F. J. Garcia-Garcia, and L. R. Manas, "Performance of the European Working Group on Sarcopenia in Older People algorithm in screening older adults for muscle mass assessment," *Age and Ageing*, vol. 44, no. 2, pp. 334–338, 2015.

[15] M. J. Goodman, S. R. Ghate, P. Mavros et al., "Development of a practical screening tool to predict low muscle mass using NHANES 1999–2004," *Journal of Cachexia, Sarcopenia and Muscle*, vol. 4, no. 3, pp. 187–197, 2013.

[16] S. Ishii, T. Tanaka, K. Shibasaki et al., "Development of a simple screening test for sarcopenia in older adults," *Geriatrics & Gerontology International*, vol. 14, supplement 1, pp. 93–101, 2014.

[17] R. Visvanathan, S. Yu, J. Field et al., "Appendicular skeletal muscle mass: development and validation of anthropometric prediction equations," *The Journal of Frailty & Aging*, vol. 1, no. 4, pp. 147–151, 2012.

[18] S. Yu, S. Appleton, I. Chapman et al., "An anthropometric prediction equation for appendicular skeletal muscle mass in combination with a measure of muscle function to screen for sarcopenia in primary and aged care," *Journal of the American Medical Directors Association*, vol. 16, no. 1, pp. 25–30, 2015.

[19] G. Abellan van Kan, M. Cesari, S. Gillette-Guyonnet et al., "Sarcopenia and cognitive impairment in elderly women: results from the EPIDOS cohort," *Age and Ageing*, vol. 42, no. 2, pp. 196–202, 2013.

[20] T. K. Malmstrom and J. E. Morley, "SARC-F: a simple questionnaire to rapidly diagnose sarcopenia," *Journal of the American Medical Directors Association*, vol. 14, no. 8, pp. 531–532, 2013.

[21] J. Woo, J. Leung, and J. E. Morley, "Validating the SARC-F: a suitable community screening tool for sarcopenia?" *Journal of the American Medical Directors Association*, vol. 15, no. 9, pp. 630–634, 2014.

[22] L. Cao, S. Chen, C. Zou et al., "A pilot study of the SARC-F scale on screening sarcopenia and physical disability in the Chinese older people," *The Journal of Nutrition, Health & Aging*, vol. 18, no. 3, pp. 277–283, 2014.

[23] Y. Rolland, V. Lauwers-Cances, M. Cournot et al., "Sarcopenia, calf circumference, and physical function of elderly women: a cross-sectional study," *Journal of the American Geriatrics Society*, vol. 51, no. 8, pp. 1120–1124, 2003.

[24] A. M. Martone, F. Lattanzio, A. M. Abbatecola et al., "Treating sarcopenia in older and oldest old," *Current Pharmaceutical Design*, vol. 21, no. 13, pp. 1715–1722, 2015.

[25] N. E. P. Deutz, J. M. Bauer, R. Barazzoni et al., "Protein intake and exercise for optimal muscle function with aging: recommendations from the ESPEN Expert Group," *Clinical Nutrition*, vol. 33, no. 6, pp. 929–936, 2014.

[26] N. Montero-Fernández and J. A. Serra-Rexach, "Role of exercise on sarcopenia in the elderly," *European Journal of Physical and Rehabilitation Medicine*, vol. 49, no. 1, pp. 131–143, 2013.

[27] E. Freiberger, C. Sieber, and K. Pfeifer, "Physical activity, exercise, and sarcopenia—future challenges," *Wiener Medizinische Wochenschrift*, vol. 161, no. 17-18, pp. 416–425, 2011.

[28] A. J. Cruz-Jentoft, F. Landi, S. M. Schneider et al., "Prevalence of and interventions for sarcopenia in ageing adults: a systematic review. Report of the International Sarcopenia Initiative (EWGSOP and IWGS)," *Age and Ageing*, vol. 43, no. 6, pp. 748–759, 2014.

[29] N. A. Ratamess, B. A. Alvar, T. K. Evetoch et al., "American College of Sports Medicine position stand. Progression models in resistance training for healthy adults," *Medicine and Science in Sports and Exercise*, vol. 41, no. 3, pp. 687–708, 2009.

[30] M. L. Puthoff and D. H. Nielsen, "Relationships among impairments in lower-extremity strength and power, functional limitations, and disability in older adults," *Physical Therapy*, vol. 87, no. 10, pp. 1334–1347, 2007.

[31] E. J. Metter, R. Conwit, J. Tobin, and J. L. Fozard, "Age-associated loss of power and strength in the upper extremities in women and men," *The Journals of Gerontology—Series A: Biological Sciences and Medical Sciences*, vol. 52, no. 5, pp. B267–B276, 1997.

[32] S. M. Phillips, "Resistance exercise: good for more than just Grandma and Grandpa's muscles," *Applied Physiology, Nutrition, and Metabolism*, vol. 32, no. 6, pp. 1198–1205, 2007.

[33] G. Iolascon, G. Di Pietro, F. Gimigliano et al., "Physical exercise and sarcopenia in older people: position paper of the Italian Society of Orthopaedics and Medicine (OrtoMed)," *Clinical Cases in Mineral and Bone Metabolism*, vol. 11, no. 3, pp. 215–221, 2014.

[34] M. E. Nelson, W. J. Rejeski, S. N. Blair et al., "Physical activity and public health in older adults: recommendation from the American College of Sports Medicine and the American Heart Association," *Medicine & Science in Sports & Exercise*, vol. 39, no. 8, pp. 1435–1445, 2007.

[35] C.-J. Liu and N. K. Latham, "Progressive resistance strength training for improving physical function in older adults," *Cochrane Database of Systematic Reviews*, no. 3, Article ID CD002759, 2009.

[36] W. L. Haskell, I.-M. Lee, R. R. Pate et al., "Physical activity and public health: updated recommendation for adults from the American College of Sports Medicine and the American Heart Association," *Medicine and Science in Sports and Exercise*, vol. 39, no. 8, pp. 1423–1434, 2007.

[37] A. R. Konopka and M. P. Harber, "Skeletal muscle hypertrophy after aerobic exercise training," *Exercise and Sport Sciences Reviews*, vol. 42, no. 2, pp. 53–61, 2014.

[38] J. Bauer, G. Biolo, T. Cederholm et al., "Evidence-based recommendations for optimal dietary protein intake in older people: a position paper from the PROT-AGE study group," *Journal of the American Medical Directors Association*, vol. 14, no. 8, pp. 542–559, 2013.

[39] P. Flakoll, R. Sharp, S. Baier, D. Levenhagen, C. Carr, and S. Nissen, "Effect of β-hydroxy-β-methylbutyrate, arginine, and lysine supplementation on strength, functionality, body composition, and protein metabolism in elderly women," *Nutrition*, vol. 20, no. 5, pp. 445–451, 2004.

[40] J. R. Stout, A. E. Smith-Ryan, D. H. Fukuda et al., "Effect of calcium β-hydroxy-β-methylbutyrate (CaHMB) with and without resistance training in men and women 65$^+$yrs: a randomized, double-blind pilot trial," *Experimental Gerontology*, vol. 48, no. 11, pp. 1303–1310, 2013.

[41] M. J. Rennie, H. Wackerhage, E. E. Spangenburg, and F. W. Booth, "Control of the size of the human muscle mass," *Annual Review of Physiology*, vol. 66, pp. 799–828, 2004.

[42] A. Truswell, I. Cole-Ruthishauser, I. Dresoti, and R. English, *Recommended Dietary Allowance*, Australian Government Publishing Service, 1991.

[43] G. Biolo, M. De Cicco, V. Dal Mas et al., "Response of muscle protein and glutamine kinetics to branched-chain-enriched amino acids in intensive care patients after radical cancer surgery," *Nutrition*, vol. 22, no. 5, pp. 475–482, 2006.

[44] C. Beaudart, F. Buckinx, V. Rabenda et al., "The effects of vitamin D on skeletal muscle strength, muscle mass, and muscle power: a systematic review and meta-analysis of randomized controlled trials," *The Journal of Clinical Endocrinology & Metabolism*, vol. 99, no. 11, pp. 4336–4345, 2014.

[45] J. E. Morley, J. M. Argiles, W. J. Evans et al., "Nutritional recommendations for the management of sarcopenia," *Journal of the American Medical Directors Association*, vol. 11, no. 6, pp. 391–396, 2010.

[46] H. A. Bischoff-Ferrari, B. Dawson-Hughes, H. B. Staehelin et al., "Fall prevention with supplemental and active forms of

vitamin D: a meta-analysis of randomised controlled trials," *British Medical Journal*, vol. 339, no. 7725, Article ID b3692, 2009.

[47] M. Tieland, M. L. Dirks, N. van der Zwaluw et al., "Protein supplementation increases muscle mass gain during prolonged resistance-type exercise training in frail elderly people: a randomized, double-blind, placebo-controlled trial," *Journal of the American Medical Directors Association*, vol. 13, no. 8, pp. 713–719, 2012.

[48] H. K. Kim, T. Suzuki, K. Saito et al., "Effects of exercise and amino acid supplementation on body composition and physical function in community-dwelling elderly Japanese sarcopenic women: a randomized controlled trial," *Journal of the American Geriatrics Society*, vol. 60, no. 1, pp. 16–23, 2012.

[49] Y. Yang, L. Breen, N. A. Burd et al., "Resistance exercise enhances myofibrillar protein synthesis with graded intakes of whey protein in older men," *The British Journal of Nutrition*, vol. 108, no. 10, pp. 1780–1788, 2012.

[50] K. Sakuma and A. Yamaguchi, "Novel intriguing strategies attenuating to sarcopenia," *Journal of Aging Research*, vol. 2012, Article ID 251217, 11 pages, 2012.

[51] C. Becker, S. R. Lord, S. A. Studenski et al., "Myostatin antibody (LY2495655) in older weak fallers: a proof-of-concept, randomised, phase 2 trial," *The Lancet Diabetes & Endocrinology*, vol. 3, no. 12, pp. 948–957, 2015.

[52] B. C. Beehler, P. G. Sleph, L. Benmassaoud, and G. J. Grover, "Reduction of skeletal muscle atrophy by a proteasome inhibitor in a rat model of denervation," *Experimental Biology and Medicine*, vol. 231, no. 3, pp. 335–341, 2006.

[53] T. Tiepolo, A. Angelin, E. Palma et al., "The cyclophilin inhibitor Debio 025 normalizes mitochondrial function, muscle apoptosis and ultrastructural defects in Col6a1$^{-/-}$ myopathic mice," *British Journal of Pharmacology*, vol. 157, no. 6, pp. 1045–1052, 2009.

[54] M. Cesari, R. A. Fielding, M. Pahor et al., "Biomarkers of sarcopenia in clinical trials–recommendations from the International Working Group on Sarcopenia," *Journal of Cachexia, Sarcopenia and Muscle*, vol. 3, no. 3, pp. 181–190, 2012.

[55] E. Mocchegiani, M. Malavolta, F. Lattanzio et al., "Cu to Zn ratio, physical function, disability, and mortality risk in older elderly (ilSIRENTE study)," *Age*, vol. 34, no. 3, pp. 539–552, 2012.

[56] M. R. Franco, A. Tong, K. Howard, C. Sherrington, P. H. Ferreira, R. Z. Pinto et al., "Older people's perspectives on participation in physical activity: a systematic review and thematic synthesis of qualitative literature," *British Journal of Sports Medicine*, vol. 49, no. 19, pp. 1262–1267, 2015.

[57] J. W. Keogh, J. Rice, D. Taylor, and A. Kilding, "Objective benefits, participant perceptions and retention rates of a New Zealand community-based, older-adult exercise programme," *Journal of Primary Health Care*, vol. 6, no. 2, pp. 114–122, 2014.

33

Elderly Stroke Rehabilitation: Overcoming the Complications and Its Associated Challenges

Siew Kwaon Lui [ID][1] **and Minh Ha Nguyen**[2]

[1]*Department of Rehabilitation Medicine, Singapore General Hospital, 20 College Road, Academia Level 4, Singapore 169856*
[2]*Department of Geriatric Medicine, Singapore General Hospital, 20 College Road, Academia Level 3, Singapore 169856*

Correspondence should be addressed to Siew Kwaon Lui; lui.siew.kwaon@sgh.com.sg

Academic Editor: Carlos Fernandez-Viadero

There have been many advances in management of cerebrovascular diseases. However, stroke is still one of the leading causes of disabilities and mortality worldwide with significant socioeconomic burden. This review summarizes the consequences of stroke in the elderly, predictors of stroke rehabilitation outcomes, role of rehabilitation in neuronal recovery, importance of stroke rehabilitation units, and types of rehabilitation resources and services available in Singapore. We also present the challenges faced by the elderly stroke survivors in the local setting and propose strategies to overcome the barriers to rehabilitation in this aging population.

1. Background

Despite advances in modern medicine, medications, and medical technology, stroke diseases impose a substantial mortality and morbidity risk to the individual with increased economic burden to the society. Globally, stroke is the second leading cause of death after ischemic heart disease, with approximately 6.7 million stroke deaths in 2015 [1]. In Singapore, despite decreasing trend, cerebrovascular diseases are still the fourth leading cause of death, with a prevalence of 6.6% in 2016 [2]. As the population rapidly ages, the burden of stroke is expected to increase significantly, posing challenges to limited healthcare resources.

As such, there is an urgent need to develop an optimal stroke disease management plan, incorporating a comprehensive stroke rehabilitation program.

2. Consequences of Stroke in Elderly Stroke Survivors

The incidence of stroke disease increases with age, in both men and women with approximately 50% of all strokes occurring in people over age 75 and 30% over age 85 [1, 3, 4]. Stroke is among the top leading causes of disability and reduced quality of life [5]. Elderly patients are at higher risk of mortality, poorer functional outcomes, prolonged length of hospital stay, and institutionalization [6].

Motor impairment is the most common deficit after stroke, which either happens as a direct consequence of the lack of signal transmission from cerebral cortex or as a slowly accumulating process of the cerebral injuries or muscle atrophy due to learned disuse [7, 8]. Divani et al. reported the risk of falling and fall-related injuries were higher in stroke elders [9]. Risk factors associated with increased fall risks in stroke survivors include poor general health, time from first stroke, psychiatric problems, urinary incontinence, pain, motor impairment, and a history of recurrent falls [9]. Risk factors associated with fall-related injuries are female gender, poor general health, past injury from fall, psychiatric problems, urinary incontinence, impaired hearing, pain, motor impairment, and presence of multiple strokes [9]. Motor function deficits, increased fall risks, and fall-related injuries can significantly affect the patients' mobility, and their daily living activities which limit their participation in social events and other professional activities.

Poststroke cognitive impairment is common and can affect up to one-third of stroke survivors [10, 11]. However, subtle cognitive impairment may not appear apparent, especially when the stroke survivor seems to have recovered functionally in other aspects [10, 11]. In most cases, these deficits are persistent and usually have progressively worsened [12]. Poststroke cognitive impairment is also more common in those with recurrent strokes [13]. It often coexists with other neuropsychological problems including language disorders, fatigue, depression, and apathy [13]. The mechanisms of poststroke cognitive impairment could be either directly due to cerebral vascular injury or indirectly due to an associated asymptomatic Alzheimer pathology or white matter changes from small vessel disease [14]. Factors independently associated with dementia in stroke survivors include atrial fibrillation, previous stroke, myocardial infarction, hypertension, diabetes mellitus, and previous transient ischemic attack [15]. The combined motor and cognitive impairments significantly increase risks of long term functional disability and increase healthcare cost as reflected by an increase in hospital readmission rates and mortality rates [16].

Bladder and bowel dysfunction are common and cause significant distress to stroke survivors. Poststroke urinary incontinence or retention has been shown to affect about 30% of stroke survivors [17]. Urinary incontinence is an important marker of stroke severity and has been linked with functional dependency, increased risk of institutionalization, and mortality [17]. Risk factors for poststroke urinary retention include cognitive impairment, diabetes mellitus, aphasia, poor functional status on admission, and urinary tract infection [18]. Common gastrointestinal symptoms after stroke include dysphagia, heartburn, abdominal pain, fecal incontinence, bleeding gastrointestinal tract, and constipation [19]. Among these, constipation is the most common bowel dysfunction with the incidence ranging from 29% to 79% in stroke survivors and more prevalent in hemorrhagic stroke patients [20]. Although fecal incontinence is less common with a prevalence of 11% at 1 year after stroke, it is associated with increased risk of nursing home admission and 1-year mortality rate [21].

Infection is a serious complication after a stroke despite optimal management. The reported prevalence of poststroke infection ranges from 5% to 65%, depending on the study population, study design, and the definition of infection [22]. Mortality rate is higher in stroke patients with any type of infection, particularly higher in patients with pneumonia and patients with urinary tract infection [23]. Among the survivors, stroke-associated infection is also an independent risk factor for poor outcome at discharge and at 1 year [23]. The association between poststroke infection and poor outcome is likely related to a delay in rehabilitation due to prolonged hospital stay and immobilization as well as general frailty [22]. More importantly, evidence from experimental studies suggests that infection also promotes antigen presentation and autoimmunity against the brain which worsens the outcome [24].

Following a stroke, patients may have impaired mobility which predisposes them to pressure sores and deep vein thrombosis (DVT). Pressure ulcer results from an imbalance between external mechanical forces acting on skin and soft tissue and the internal susceptibility of skin and its underlying soft tissue to injury. Pressure ulcer is associated with increased poststroke mortality in both genders and patients aged 60 years or older [25]. Stroke patients also have an increased risk of developing deep DVT and pulmonary embolism due to immobility and raised prothrombotic activity [26]. The major risk factors of poststroke DVT include advanced age, male gender, congestive heart failure, malignancy, and fluid and electrolyte disorders [27, 28].

Pain is a frequent but often neglected complication of stroke [29, 30]. It can happen immediately, weeks, or months after a stroke event and can span a spectrum from irritating headache to debilitating limb pain secondary to complex regional pain syndrome, spasticity or joint subluxation, and /or contractures [29]. Pain, together with depression and fatigue, is associated with increased risk of cognitive impairment, functional dependence, and reduced quality of life in stroke survivors [30, 31]. Reported risk factors for the development of poststroke pain include female gender, older age at stroke onset, history of alcohol use and depression, anatomical location of stroke and presence of clinical features such as spasticity, reduced upper extremity movement, and sensory deficits [32].

3. Predictors of Good Rehabilitation Outcome in Elderly Stroke Survivors

Due to the medical complications after stroke, many patients are markedly functionally disabled when they are discharged from acute care. Functional recovery is based on the restitution of brain tissue and on the relearning of and compensation for lost functions [33]. Therefore, understanding and identification of predictors of good rehabilitation outcomes in addition to institution of early rehabilitation are essential in the recovery phase after an acute stroke event.

There are several commonly used tools for measurement of rehabilitation outcomes in stroke patients, including Functional Independence Measure (FIM), Modified Rankin Scale (mRS), and the Barthel Index (BI) [34]. The FIM is the most sensitive and has been widely accepted with good validity and reliability in assessment of the patient's degree of disability and burden of care [34]. It consists of 18 items, 13 items on motor disability, and 5 items on cognitive disability. The FIM is commonly performed on admission and at discharge, with the score range from 18 to 126. Similarly, the BI is a tool used to measure functional ability, consisting of 10 items on mobility, activity of daily living (ADL), bowel, and bladder function. Its scores range from 0 to 100, with a higher score indicating higher functional ability. On the other hand, the mRS is a scale from 0 to 6 that measures the level of a patient's disability.

Age has been well established as a strong predictor of functional outcome and discharge destination in stroke patients in multiple studies across the world in both young and elderly stroke survivors [35–39]. A large community-based cohort study in Denmark reported more than 58% of the very elderly (85 years old and above) were discharged to nursing homes or died during hospital stay poststroke [40]. In a multicenter prospective cohort study of over 300 patients of at least 75 years of age with a first stroke, age was both significantly related to low FIM score upon discharge and independently and inversely related to rehabilitation efficacy (Montebello Rehabilitation Factor Score) [36]. Despite the likelihood of higher comorbidities in older patients, a multicenter cohort study showed that rehabilitation outcomes of elderly patients admitted into skilled nursing facilities (SNFs) were not associated with multimorbidity [41].

Cognitive impairment which occurs either as a prestroke condition or a poststroke is often significantly correlated with reduced functional gains and poor rehabilitation outcomes in elderly patients. A local study by Kong et al. showed that 45% of elderly stroke patients (≥75 years old) admitted to a rehabilitation facility had cognitive impairment and cognition scores strongly predicted functional outcomes [42]. Studies reported evidence of significant impairment of basic and instrumental ADLs in poststroke cognitively impaired elderly survivors [43, 44]. Another study by Pasquini et al. concluded that cognitive impairment (preexisting or new) together with age was the most important predictor of institutionalization 3 years after stroke [45]. Prestroke dementia has been shown to increase risk of 6-month and delayed poststroke mortality [46]. However, elderly stroke patients with cognitive impairments could still benefit from rehabilitation. Rabadi et al. found similar change in total FIM score and FIM efficiency in both cognitively intact and the cognitively impaired groups of stroke patients [47]. Hence, cognitive impairment should be screened for and has to be taken into consideration when rehabilitation goals are formulated and rehabilitation program ought to be individualized according to the stroke survivor's learning ability [48].

ADL dependency on admission, defined as either low FIM score or low BI score, significantly predicts functional dependency outcome in stroke survivors [39, 43, 49, 50]. Elderly stroke patients with poorer preadmission functional status also have longer length of stay and are less likely discharged to an independent or assisted living situation [39, 50, 51]. Similarly, stroke severity, measured by National Institute of Health Stroke Scale, is also another important rehabilitation outcome predictor [49–51]. Furthermore, a recent review by Lazar et al. revealed that aphasia arising from stroke was associated with worse outcomes in both the acute and chronic stroke periods with poorer functional recovery and increased length of rehabilitation and mortality risk [52].

Urinary incontinence is predictive of poor stroke outcome [53]. Mortality at 6 months has been shown to increase in stroke patients with initial urinary incontinence [53, 54]. Ween et al. reported that 64% of incontinent poststroke patients were discharged to nursing homes compared to 18% for continent poststroke patients [55]. The link between urinary incontinence and poor outcomes could be related to incontinence associated with severe hemiparesis, larger stroke lesions, stroke lesion location, and a disruption of the neuromicturition pathways [55–58].

4. Role of Rehabilitation Process in Neuronal Recovery

Rehabilitation aims to enhance and augment natural mechanisms of recovery. At the time of ischemic injury, immediate mechanisms of repair are initiated, which include resolution of poststroke edema, variation of function, and reversal of diaschisis. Vicariation refers to neighboring tissues taking over a function lost by the stroke-affected tissue [59]. Diaschisis is based on the mechanism of reduction in metabolism and blood flow of intact brain regions which are distant away from the ischemic core but are still functionally and structurally connected with the ischemic core. It is thought that at least some of the improvement observed after a stroke could be due to the reversal of diaschisis [60, 61]. Such processes lead to "unmasking" of latent networks which can be as rapid as several hours within ischemic injury [62].

Evidence suggests that, within days of stroke, the injured brain has the ability for limited neuronal regeneration by angiogenesis and is coupled with neurogenesis. The ability to self-repair has been shown to happen in aged brains [63]. The repair processes are initially intense and then slow down. Most of the spontaneous stroke recovery occurs in the first 3-6 months after the acute neurological event [64–66]. Generally, patients make 70% of their recovery in the first 3 months after a stroke [67–71]. Despite variations in therapy, such observations of proportional recovery have remained consistent which means that a minimum amount of spontaneous activity and therapy is enough for proportional recovery to happen [72]. An exception to this proportional recovery rule includes damage to the corticospinal tract which results in poorer recovery from impairment [69, 73].

In order to achieve a greater proportion of recovery, a much higher intensity of therapy has to be considered [72]. Greater intensity of stroke rehabilitation has been associated with improved outcomes [74–76]. Skill learning and active participation help to promote plasticity and network activation in stroke recovery [77, 78]. Motor retraining not only enables somatotopic reorganization to happen in perilesional areas and in distant areas connected to the infarct site but also negate the inhibitory effects of myelin associated proteins and ephrins which suppress axonal sprouting [79, 80]. An "enriched environment" in addition to motor retraining has been shown to facilitate motor recovery and neural plasticity in animal studies due to the numerous associated cellular and molecular effects [81–84]. Rehabilitation facilities are ideal enriched environments as they are often situated in stimulating and specialized centers managed by a multidisciplinary team of medical professionals.

5. Stroke Rehabilitation Units and Practitioners Involved

Several guidelines recommend all patients admitted with an acute stroke should receive an assessment by a rehabilitation professional [85, 86]. Specialized stroke rehabilitation units have been shown to improve functional outcomes, decrease mortality and reduce length of hospital stay in moderate to severe stroke patients [87]. Combining an enriched environment with skill retraining, stroke rehabilitation units are made up of a multidisciplinary team of medical professionals who offer realistic goal setting and engage in multimodal disability and impairment assessment, medical management, and functional training. The team consists of rehabilitation nurses, occupational therapists, physiotherapists, and speech therapists under the leadership of physicians specialized in rehabilitation medicine. The work of these groups is further supported by dieticians, neuropsychologists, social workers, and recreational therapists such as music therapists. The rehabilitation team addresses the many challenges stroke patients could face such as sensorimotor and balance impairments, dysphagia, cognitive-communication impairments, mood disorders, visual and hearing impairments, and hemispatial neglect. Regular multidisciplinary meetings are conducted to discuss the rehabilitation goals, rehabilitation intervention, functional improvement, discharge planning, and arrangement of outpatient rehabilitation. These structured meetings have been shown to improve functional outcomes [88, 89]. Such collaborative teamwork involves communication among the team members, working towards a common goal and accepting responsibility as a group for the final outcome of the patients [90, 91]. Recommended realistic goals are also planned together with the patients and their caregivers to prepare them for a smooth transition to outpatient rehabilitation and discharge destination with the eventual aim to achieve maximum independence as possible [92].

The hours of therapy vary across different inpatient rehabilitation settings. Generally, most guidelines advocate minimum 45 minutes of each relevant therapy for at least 5 days a week [85, 86, 93]. In United States, inpatient rehabilitation facilities (IRFs) are mandated to provide at least 3 hours of therapy per day for minimum 5 days in a week. Rehabilitation in an IRF improves functional outcomes, independence, and mortality compared to a SNF (subacute rehabilitation), given the interprofessional team of providers, advanced treatment strategies, and the requirement that patients participate in therapy at least three hours daily [86]. Patient's ability to tolerate such level of intensity has to be taken into account when considered for an acute intensive inpatient rehabilitation placement. When the stroke patient is admitted to inpatient rehabilitation, the rehabilitation team would assess the patient and determine an individualized rehabilitation program of suitable intensity and duration to suit the needs for favorable stroke recovery [85].

It is generally recommended to commence stroke rehabilitation as soon as patients are medically stable, to maximize their functional gains and to take advantage of the period of early stroke recovery [85]. However, caution and individualized clinical judgement are indicated especially in older patients and patients with intracerebral hemorrhage [94]. The large multicenter AVERT trial showed that very early, more frequent, and increased dose of mobilization (VEM) intervention reduced the odds of a favorable outcome at 3 months after stroke when compared with usual care (UC) group [95]. However, the median time to first mobilization in both groups was within 24 hours (22.4 hours in UC group versus 18.5 hours in VEM group) [95]. Further analyses from the AVERT study suggested that shorter but more frequent

mobilization early after stroke increased the odds of favorable outcome at 3 months when age and stroke severity were controlled [96]. Earlier access to rehabilitation seems to favor better functional outcomes, shorten length of hospital stay, and increase likelihood of discharge to home [97, 98].

6. Transitional Care of Poststroke Survivors

Due to residual functional disability and associated medical complications, poststroke elderly survivors and their caregivers often experience significant physical, mental, and social challenges after being discharged home. In most cases, caregivers are usually poorly understood and ill-prepared for their roles and responsibilities they must face at home [99]. As elderly stroke survivors require substantial care demands at home, their caregivers often feel overwhelmed and exhausted, which eventually lead to depression and deterioration of physical health [99].

Definition of transitional care (TC) is widely accepted as "a set of actions designed to ensure the coordination and continuity of healthcare as patients transfer between different locations or different levels of care within the same location" [100]. TC can happen within same setting (e.g., primary care to specialty care); between different settings (e.g., hospital to subacute care); across health states (e.g., acute care to palliative care), or between providers (e.g., generalist to specialist). The different types of TC models for poststroke patients include hospital-initiated support; home-visiting programs; structured telephone support; outpatient setting-based support; lastly, primary patient and caregiver education. A recent meta-analysis by Wang Y et al. reported insufficient evidence to support the role of TC interventions in reduction of mortality and functional improvement after stroke [101]. However, among all the TC interventions, home-visiting programs which focus on patients and caregivers' needs and preferences in addition to well-established rehabilitation goals via multidisciplinary approach seem to be associated with positive outcomes [101]. More research regarding TC interventions needs to be conducted before any further conclusions can be made.

7. Rehabilitation Resources and Services in Singapore in addition to the Challenges Faced

In Singapore, elderly stroke survivors after being medically stabilized at the acute hospitals will be transferred to receive inpatient rehabilitation either at rehabilitation units situated within acute hospitals or in community hospitals which are situated as stand-alone units. When the patients are ready for discharge from inpatient rehabilitation, arrangements are made for them to receive outpatient rehabilitation either at hospital outpatient clinic or at day rehabilitation center. Home therapy can be arranged for patients with difficulties to get out of their house. Government subsidies for day rehabilitation centers are available for patients who satisfy certain financial criteria [102].

However, the compliance rate of our local stroke survivors attending outpatient day rehabilitation has been dismal. Two local studies showed the attendance rates of outpatient rehabilitation at 1 year after discharge from community hospitals were 28% and 4.3%, respectively [102, 103]. Reasons for noncompliance to outpatient rehabilitation revolved around the patient's functional, social, financial, medical, and perceptual factors [103]. Firstly, stroke survivors who require ongoing rehabilitation will likely have difficulties in mobility. They also face challenges in stairs and transportation access. Secondly, some elderly live alone and have no caregiver to assist them to the outpatient rehabilitation center [103, 104]. For those with caregivers, the elderly stroke survivors often do not wish to inconvenience them [103]. Thirdly, financial constraint is also commonly cited by the elderly for noncompliance to poststroke medical care and rehabilitation after hospital discharge [103–107]. Although Singaporean residents are eligible for the public healthcare system with significant subsidies from the government, much of the outpatient rehabilitation cannot be paid for with the use of medical savings account (Medicine) or national medical insurance (Medishield) [103]. For those who are qualified for government medical subsidies, the transportation cost and cumulative cost of multiple sessions of outpatient rehabilitation often put them off from continuing rehabilitation [103]. Fourthly, the elderly stroke survivors often suffer from comorbidities which may limit their ability to fully participate in rehabilitation [103, 108]. Cardiovascular and pulmonary diseases such as ischemic heart disease, congestive heart failure, arrhythmias, and chronic obstructive pulmonary disease which are more common in the elderly can result in reduced activity tolerance and restrict them from fully participating in rehabilitation [108]. Vascular-related cognitive impairment which is more common in older stroke survivors could also pose as a barrier to successful rehabilitation [108]. Lastly, although Singapore is one of the most urbanized, modernized, and prosperous countries in Asia, a strong influence of Eastern culture is still present on the local societal perceptions, especially in the elderly. The elderly in the Asian culture are inclined to rely on their children and would perceive rehabilitation as the equivalent of doing exercises at home without the guidance of a therapist and rehabilitation physician. As such, the patients do not see the need to attend outpatient rehabilitation and follow-up [104].

Home rehabilitation could potentially overcome some of the above challenges associated with outpatient rehabilitation. A local study by Tay et al. found most of the stroke patients in an inpatient rehabilitation unit would consider home rehabilitation program (HRP) [109]. As for the minority who declined HRP, reasons given included financial constraint, unsupportive family members, privacy issues, and preference for a hospital-based rehabilitation [109]. As the cost of each home rehabilitation session in Singapore is at least twice as expensive as each outpatient rehabilitation session, most of the patients would be more inclined to undergo HRP if it is Medisave deductible [109].

8. Discussion and Conclusions

With the rapidly aging population, several initiatives have been undertaken by the local government to provide better access for the elderly which could overcome the mobility issues faced by elderly stroke survivors. Examples include installation of ramps and additional lifts at local subway stations, introduction of wheelchair-accessible public buses, lift upgrading program to provide lift access on every level of the public housing blocks, and a heavily subsidized public housing home improvement program which includes ramp installation at the entrances of the housing units with steps. As for those elderly stroke survivors who do not have caregivers to assist them to the outpatient rehabilitation center, we propose implementation of an affordable HRP or low cost telerehabilitation. An ongoing local trial looking at telerehabilitation in the first 3 months after stroke perhaps would shed more light on the potential benefit and cost-effectiveness of telerehabilitation in the Singapore poststroke population [110]. The use of home-based robot therapy (HBRT) could also be considered for those who had difficulty in accessing outpatient rehabilitation. Housley et al. found that HBRT reduced costs and increased access of rehabilitation to stroke survivors [111]. In order to rectify the misconception of rehabilitation is the equivalent of doing exercises at home without the guidance of the rehabilitation team, education on stroke rehabilitation should be provided to all stroke patients and caregivers during the acute admission. It has been shown that the use of evidence-based educational guidelines have helped stroke survivors and their families to better understand the importance of stroke rehabilitation, control their comorbidities and cardiovascular risk factors, and reduce their risk of recurrent strokes [112].

In conclusion, stroke in elderly patients poses a major public health concern, due to its strong association with multiple medical complications, poorer functional outcomes, and substantial healthcare cost. For stroke survivors and their families, a good and comprehensive rehabilitation program is the key to recovery and to enable them to reach their highest level of independence as possible. The success of a stroke rehabilitation unit depends on the effective utilization of its resources and seamless coordination between different healthcare professionals as well as the ongoing support from the caregivers and other community services. Provision of evidence-based and culturally relevant stroke rehabilitation will help to effectively manage limited local healthcare resources and improve quality of life in our aging population.

References

[1] E. J. Benjamin, M. J. Blaha, S. E. Chiuve et al., "Heart Disease and Stroke Statistics'2017 Update: A Report from the American Heart Association," *Circulation*, vol. 135, no. 10, pp. e146–e603, 2017.

[2] Ministry of Health, "Singapore Health Facts," https://www.moh.gov.sg/content/moh_web/home/statistics/Health_Facts_Singapore.html.

[3] T. Engstad, T. T. Engstad, M. Viitanen, and H. Ellekjær, "Epidemiology of stroke in the elderly in the Nordic countries.

Incidence, survival, prevalence and risk factors," *Norsk epidemiologi*, vol. 22, no. 2, pp. 121–126, 2012.

[4] N. Venketasubramanian, L. C. S. Tan, S. Sahadevan et al., "Prevalence of stroke among Chinese, Malay, and Indian Singaporeans: A community-based tri-racial cross-sectional survey," *Stroke*, vol. 36, no. 3, pp. 551–556, 2005.

[5] Disease GBD, Injury I, and Prevalence C, "Global, regional, and national incidence, prevalence, and years lived with disability for 310 diseases and injuries, 1990-2015: a systematic analysis for the Global Burden of Disease Study," *Lancet*, vol. 388, pp. 1545–1602, 2016.

[6] G. Saposnik, R. Cote, S. Phillips et al., "Stroke outcome in those over 80: A multicenter cohort study across Canada," *Stroke*, vol. 39, no. 8, pp. 2310–2317, 2008.

[7] A. A. Divani, S. Majidi, A. M. Barrett, S. Noorbaloochi, and A. R. Luft, "Consequences of stroke in community-dwelling elderly: The health and retirement study, 1998 to 2008," *Stroke*, vol. 42, no. 7, pp. 1821–1825, 2011.

[8] S. M. Hatem, G. Saussez, M. della Faille et al., "Rehabilitation of motor function after stroke: A multiple systematic review focused on techniques to stimulate upper extremity recovery," *Frontiers in Human Neuroscience*, vol. 10, no. 2016, article no. 442, 2016.

[9] A. A. Divani, G. Vazquez, A. M. Barrett, M. Asadollahi, and A. R. Luft, "Risk factors associated with injury attributable to falling among elderly population with history of stroke," *Stroke*, vol. 40, no. 10, pp. 3286–3292, 2009.

[10] M. Planton, S. Peiffer, J. F. Albucher et al., "Neuropsychological outcome after a first symptomatic ischaemic stroke with 'good recovery'," *European Journal of Neurology*, vol. 19, no. 2, pp. 212–219, 2012.

[11] S. M. C. Rasquin, J. Lodder, R. W. H. M. Ponds, I. Winkens, J. Jolles, and F. R. J. Verhey, "Cognitive functioning after stroke: A one-year follow-up study," *Dementia and Geriatric Cognitive Disorders*, vol. 18, no. 2, pp. 138–144, 2004.

[12] M. Leśniak, T. Bak, W. Czepiel, J. Seniów, and A. Członkowska, "Frequency and prognostic value of cognitive disorders in stroke patients," *Dementia and Geriatric Cognitive Disorders*, vol. 26, no. 4, pp. 356–363, 2008.

[13] S. T. Pendlebury and P. M. Rothwell, "Prevalence, incidence, and factors associated with pre-stroke and post-stroke dementia: a systematic review and meta-analysis," *The Lancet Neurology*, vol. 8, no. 11, pp. 1006–1018, 2009.

[14] F. Pasquier and D. Leys, "Why are stroke patients prone to develop dementia?" *Journal of Neurology*, vol. 244, no. 3, pp. 135–142, 1997.

[15] J. Surawan, S. Areemit, S. Tiamkao, T. Sirithanawuthichai, and S. Saensak, "Risk factors associated with post-stroke dementia: A systematic review and meta-analysis," *Neurology International*, vol. 9, no. 3, pp. 63–68, 2017.

[16] D. L. Coco, G. Lopez, and S. Corrao, "Cognitive impairment and stroke in elderly patients," *Vascular Health and Risk Management*, vol. 12, pp. 105–116, 2016.

[17] Z. Mehdi, J. Birns, and A. Bhalla, "Post-stroke urinary incontinence," *International Journal of Clinical Practice*, vol. 67, no. 11, pp. 1128–1137, 2013.

[18] K.-H. Kong and S. Young, "Incidence and outcome of poststroke urinary retention: A prospective study," *Archives of Physical Medicine and Rehabilitation*, vol. 81, no. 11, pp. 1464–1467, 2000.

[19] G. Scivoletto, U. Fuoco, D. Badiali et al., "3-07-43 Gastrointestinal dysfunction following stroke," *Journal of the Neurological Sciences*, vol. 150, p. S151, 1997.

[20] J. Li, M. Yuan, Y. Liu et al., "Incidence of constipation in stroke patients: A systematic review and meta-analysis," *Medicine (United States)*, vol. 96, no. 25, Article ID e7225, 2017.

[21] D. Harari, C. Coshall, A. G. Rudd, and C. D. A. Wolfe, "New-onset fecal incontinence after stroke: Prevalence, natural history, risk factors, and impact," *Stroke*, vol. 34, no. 1, pp. 144–150, 2003.

[22] W. F. Westendorp, P. J. Nederkoorn, J.-D. Vermeij, M. G. Dijkgraaf, and D. van de Beek, "Post-stroke infection: A systematic review and meta-analysis," *BMC Neurology*, vol. 11, article no. 110, 2011.

[23] F. H. Vermeij, W. J. M. Scholte Op Reimer, P. De Man et al., "Stroke-associated infection is an independent risk factor for poor outcome after acute ischemic stroke: Data from the netherlands stroke survey," *Cerebrovascular Disease*, vol. 27, no. 5, pp. 465–471, 2009.

[24] C. Iadecola and J. Anrather, "The immunology of stroke: from mechanisms to translation," *Nature Medicine*, vol. 17, no. 7, pp. 796–808, 2011.

[25] S.-Y. Lee, C.-L. Chou, S. P. C. Hsu et al., "Outcomes after Stroke in Patients with Previous Pressure Ulcer: A Nationwide Matched Retrospective Cohort Study," *Journal of Stroke and Cerebrovascular Diseases*, vol. 25, no. 1, pp. 220–227, 2016.

[26] E. Skaf, P. D. Stein, A. Beemath, J. Sanchez, M. A. Bustamante, and R. E. Olson, "Venous thromboembolism in patients with ischemic and hemorrhagic stroke," *American Journal of Cardiology*, vol. 96, no. 12, pp. 1731–1733, 2005.

[27] V. R. Kshettry, B. P. Rosenbaum, A. Seicean, M. L. Kelly, N. K. Schiltz, and R. J. Weil, "Incidence and risk factors associated with in-hospital venous thromboembolism after aneurysmal subarachnoid hemorrhage," *Journal of Clinical Neuroscience*, vol. 21, no. 2, pp. 282–286, 2014.

[28] J. Pongmoragot, A. A. Rabinstein, Y. Nilanont, R. H. Swartz, L. Zhou, and G. Saposnik, "Pulmonary embolism in ischemic stroke: clinical presentation, risk factors, and outcome." *Journal of the American Heart Association*, vol. 2, no. 6, p. e000372, 2013.

[29] A. Jonsson, I. Lindgren, B. Hallstrom, B. Norrving, and A. Lindgren, "Prevalence and intensity of pain after stroke: a population based study focusing on patients' perspectives," *Journal of Neurology, Neurosurgery & Psychiatry*, vol. 77, no. 5, pp. 590–595, 2006.

[30] H. Naess, L. Lunde, and J. Brogger, "The effects of fatigue, pain, and depression on quality of life in ischemic stroke patients: the Bergen Stroke Study," *Vascular Health and Risk Management*, vol. 8, no. 1, pp. 407–413, 2012.

[31] M. J. O'Donnell, H.-C. Diener, R. L. Sacco, A. A. Panju, R. Vinisko, and S. Yusuf, "Chronic pain syndromes after ischemic stroke: PRoFESS trial," *Stroke*, vol. 44, no. 5, pp. 1238–1243, 2013.

[32] R. A. Harrison and T. S. Field, "Post stroke pain: Identification, assessment, and therapy," *Cerebrovascular Disease*, vol. 39, no. 3-4, pp. 190–201, 2015.

[33] S. C. Cramer and J. D. Riley, "Neuroplasticity and brain repair after stroke," *Current Opinion in Neurology*, vol. 21, no. 1, pp. 76–82, 2008.

[34] A. W. Dromerick, D. F. Edwards, and M. N. Diringer, "Sensitivity to changes in disability after stroke: a comparison of four scales useful in clinical trials," *Journal of Rehabilitation Research and Development*, vol. 40, no. 1, pp. 1–8, 2003.

[35] S. K. Ostwald, P. R. Swank, and M. M. Khan, "Predictors of functional independence and stress level of stroke survivors at discharge from inpatient rehabilitation," *Journal of Cardiovascular Nursing*, vol. 23, no. 4, pp. 371–377, 2008.

[36] L. Denti, M. Agosti, and M. Franceschini, "Outcome predictors of rehabilitation for first stroke in the elderly," *European Journal of Physical and Rehabilitation Medicine*, vol. 44, no. 1, pp. 3–11, 2008.

[37] P. S. Pohl, S. A. Billinger, A. Lentz, and B. Gajewski, "The role of patient demographics and clinical presentation in predicting discharge placement after inpatient stroke rehabilitation: Analysis of a large, US data base," *Disability and Rehabilitation*, vol. 35, no. 12, pp. 990–994, 2013.

[38] P. J. Kelly, K. L. Furie, S. Shafqat, N. Rallis, Y. Chang, and J. Stein, "Functional recovery following rehabilitation after hemorrhagic and ischemic stroke," *Archives of Physical Medicine and Rehabilitation*, vol. 84, no. 7, pp. 968–972, 2003.

[39] H. Mutai, T. Furukawa, K. Araki, K. Misawa, and T. Hanihara, "Factors associated with functional recovery and home discharge in stroke patients admitted to a convalescent rehabilitation ward," *Geriatrics & Gerontology International*, vol. 12, no. 2, pp. 215–222, 2012.

[40] L. P. Kammersgaard, H. S. Jørgensen, J. Reith, H. Nakayama, P. M. Pedersen, and T. S. Olsen, "Short- and long-term prognosis for every old stroke patients. The Copenhagen Stroke Study," *Age and Ageing*, vol. 33, no. 2, pp. 149–154, 2004.

[41] M. Spruit-van Eijk, S. U. Zuidema, B. I. Buijck, R. T. C. M. Koopmans, and A. C. H. Geurts, "Determinants of rehabilitation outcome in geriatric patients admitted to skilled nursing facilities after stroke: A Dutch multi-centre cohort study," *Age and Ageing*, vol. 41, no. 6, Article ID afs105, pp. 746–752, 2012.

[42] K.-H. Kong, K. S. G. Chua, and A. P. Tow, "Clinical characteristics and functional outcome of stroke patients 75 years old and older," *Archives of Physical Medicine and Rehabilitation*, vol. 79, no. 12, pp. 1535–1539, 1998.

[43] S. Stephens, R. A. Kenny, E. Rowan et al., "Association between mild vascular cognitive impairment and impaired activities of daily living in older stroke survivors without dementia," *Journal of the American Geriatrics Society*, vol. 53, no. 1, pp. 103–107, 2005.

[44] S. Zinn, T. K. Dudley, H. B. Bosworth, H. M. Hoenig, P. W. Duncan, and R. D. Horner, "The effect of poststroke cognitive impairment on rehabilitation process and functional outcome," *Archives of Physical Medicine and Rehabilitation*, vol. 85, no. 7, pp. 1084–1090, 2004.

[45] M. Pasquini, D. Leys, M. Rousseaux, F. Pasquier, and H. Hénon, "Influence of cognitive impairment on the institutionalisation rate 3 years after a stroke," *Journal of Neurology, Neurosurgery & Psychiatry*, vol. 78, no. 1, pp. 56–59, 2007.

[46] H. Hénon, I. Durieu, F. Lebert, F. Pasquier, and D. Leys, "Influence of prestroke dementia on early and delayed mortality in stroke patients," *Journal of Neurology*, vol. 250, no. 1, pp. 10–16, 2003.

[47] M. H. Rabadi, F. M. Rabadi, L. Edelstein, and M. Peterson, "Cognitively Impaired Stroke Patients Do Benefit From Admission to an Acute Rehabilitation Unit," *Archives of Physical Medicine and Rehabilitation*, vol. 89, no. 3, pp. 441–448, 2008.

[48] J. S. Luxenberg and L. Z. Feigenbaum, "Cognitive impairment on a rehabilitation service," *Archives of Physical Medicine and Rehabilitation*, vol. 67, no. 11, pp. 796–798, 1986.

[49] B. Gialanella, R. Santoro, and C. Ferlucci, "Predicting outcome after stroke: The role of basic activities of daily living," *European Journal of Physical and Rehabilitation Medicine*, vol. 49, no. 5, pp. 629–637, 2013.

[50] J. M. Veerbeek, G. Kwakkel, E. E. H. Van Wegen, J. C. F. Ket, and M. W. Heymans, "Early prediction of outcome of activities of daily living after stroke: A systematic review," *Stroke*, vol. 42, no. 5, pp. 1482–1488, 2011.

[51] Y. S. Ng, K. H. X. Tan, C. Chen, G. C. Senolos, E. Chew, and G. C. Koh, "Predictors of acute, rehabilitation and total length of stay in acute stroke: A prospective cohort study," *Annals Academy of Medicine, Singapore*, vol. 45, no. 9, pp. 394–403, 2016.

[52] R. M. Lazar and A. K. Boehme, "Aphasia As a Predictor of Stroke Outcome," *Current Neurology and Neuroscience Reports*, vol. 17, no. 11, 2017.

[53] D. H. Barer, "Continence after stroke: Useful predictor or goal of therapy?" *Age and Ageing*, vol. 18, no. 3, pp. 183–191, 1989.

[54] D. T. Wade and R. L. Hewer, "Outlook after an acute stroke: Urinary incontinence and loss of consciousness compared in 532 patients," *QJM: An International Journal of Medicine*, vol. 56, no. 3-4, pp. 601–608, 1985.

[55] J. E. Ween, M. P. Alexander, M. D'Esposito, and M. Roberts, "Incontinence after stroke in a rehabilitation setting: Outcome associations and predictive factors," *Neurology*, vol. 47, no. 3, pp. 659–663, 1996.

[56] H. Nakayama, H. S. Jørgensen, P. M. Pedersen, H. O. Raaschou, and T. S. Olsen, "Prevalence and risk factors of incontinence after stroke: The Copenhagen Stroke Study," *Stroke*, vol. 28, no. 1, pp. 58–62, 1997.

[57] M. Patel, C. Coshall, A. G. Rudd, and C. D. A. Wolfe, "Natural history and effects on 2-year outcomes of urinary incontinence after stroke," *Stroke*, vol. 32, no. 1, pp. 122–127, 2001.

[58] B. Thommessen, E. Bautz-Holter, and K. Laake, "Predictors of outcome of rehabilitation of elderly stroke patients in a geriatric ward," *Clinical Rehabilitation*, vol. 13, no. 2, pp. 123–128, 1999.

[59] N. Dancause, "Vicarious function of remote cortex following stroke: recent evidence from human and animal studies," *The Neuroscientist*, vol. 12, no. 6, pp. 489–499, 2006.

[60] R. J. Nudo, "Neural bases of recovery after brain injury," *Journal of Communication Disorders*, vol. 44, no. 5, pp. 515–520, 2011.

[61] E. Carrera and G. Tononi, "Diaschisis: Past, present, future," *Brain*, vol. 137, no. 9, pp. 2408–2422, 2014.

[62] H. Duffau, "Acute functional reorganisation of the human motor cortex during resection of central lesions: a study using intraoperative brain mapping," *Journal of Neurology, Neurosurgery & Psychiatry*, vol. 70, no. 4, pp. 506–513, 2001.

[63] S. Li and S. T. Carmichael, "Growth-associated gene and protein expression in the region of axonal sprouting in the aged brain after stroke," *Neurobiology of Disease*, vol. 23, no. 2, pp. 362–373, 2006.

[64] H. S. Jorgensen, H. Nakayama, H. O. Raaschou, and T. S. Olsen, "Neurologic and functional recovery the Copenhagen Stroke Study," *Physical Medicine & Rehabilitation Clinics of North America*, vol. 10, no. 4, pp. 887–906, 1999.

[65] P. Langhorne, J. Bernhardt, and G. Kwakkel, "Stroke rehabilitation," *The Lancet*, vol. 377, no. 9778, pp. 1693–1702, 2011.

[66] C. E. Skilbeck, D. T. Wade, R. L. Hewer, and V. A. Wood, "Recovery after stroke," *Journal of Neurology, Neurosurgery & Psychiatry*, vol. 46, no. 1, pp. 5–8, 1983.

[67] C. Winters, E. E. H. Van Wegen, A. Daffertshofer, and G. Kwakkel, "Generalizability of the Proportional Recovery Model for the Upper Extremity After an Ischemic Stroke," *Neurorehabilitation and Neural Repair*, vol. 29, no. 7, pp. 614–622, 2015.

[68] E. R. Buch, S. Rizk, P. Nicolo, L. G. Cohen, A. Schnider, and A. G. Guggisberg, "Predicting motor improvement after stroke with clinical assessment and diffusion tensor imaging," *Neurology*, vol. 86, no. 20, pp. 1924-1925, 2016.

[69] W. D. Byblow, C. M. Stinear, P. A. Barber, M. A. Petoe, and S. J. Ackerley, "Proportional recovery after stroke depends on corticomotor integrity," *Annals of Neurology*, vol. 78, no. 6, pp. 848–859, 2015.

[70] W. Feng, J. Wang, P. Y. Chhatbar et al., "Corticospinal tract lesion load: an imaging biomarker for stroke motor outcomes," *Annals of Neurology*, vol. 78, no. 6, pp. 860–870, 2015.

[71] C. M. Stinear, W. D. Byblow, S. J. Ackerley, M.-C. Smith, V. M. Borges, and P. A. Barber, "Proportional Motor Recovery after Stroke: Implications for Trial Design," *Stroke*, vol. 48, no. 3, pp. 795–798, 2017.

[72] J. W. Krakauer, S. T. Carmichael, D. Corbett, and G. F. Wittenberg, "Getting neurorehabilitation right: what can be learned from animal models?" *Neurorehabilitation and Neural Repair*, vol. 26, no. 8, pp. 923–931, 2012.

[73] S. Prabhakaran, E. Zarahn, C. Riley et al., "Inter-individual variability in the capacity for motor recovery after ischemic stroke," *Neurorehabilitation and Neural Repair*, vol. 22, no. 1, pp. 64–71, 2008.

[74] R. Teasell, J. Bitensky, K. Salter, and N. A. Bayona, "The role of timing and intensity of rehabilitation therapies," *Topics in Stroke Rehabilitation*, vol. 12, no. 3, pp. 46–57, 2005.

[75] G. Kwakkel, R. C. Wagenaar, T. W. Koelman, G. J. Lankhorst, and J. C. Koetsier, "Effects of intensity of rehabilitation after stroke: A research synthesis," *Stroke*, vol. 28, no. 8, pp. 1550–1556, 1997.

[76] P. Langhorne, R. Wagenaar, and C. Partridge, "Physiotherapy after stroke: more is better?" *Physiotherapy Research International: The Journal for Researchers and Clinicians in Physical Therapy*, vol. 1, no. 2, pp. 75–88, 1996.

[77] M. Lotze, C. Braun, N. Birbaumer, S. Anders, and L. G. Cohen, "Motor learning elicited by voluntary drive," *Brain*, vol. 126, no. 4, pp. 866–872, 2003.

[78] P. Zhuang, N. Dang, A. Warzeri, C. Gerloff, L. G. Cohen, and M. Hallett, "Implicit and explicit learning in an auditory serial reaction time task," *Acta Neurologica Scandinavica*, vol. 97, no. 2, pp. 131–137, 1998.

[79] P.-C. Fang, S. Barbay, E. J. Plautz, E. Hoover, S. M. Strittmatter, and R. J. Nudo, "Combination of NEP 1-40 treatment and motor training enhances behavioral recovery after a focal cortical infarct in rats," *Stroke*, vol. 41, no. 3, pp. 544–549, 2010.

[80] L. Zai, C. Ferrari, S. Subbaiah et al., "Inosine alters gene expression and axonal projections in neurons contralateral to a cortical infarct and improves skilled use of the impaired limb," *The Journal of Neuroscience*, vol. 29, no. 25, pp. 8187–8197, 2009.

[81] J. Nithianantharajah and A. J. Hannan, "Enriched environments, experience-dependent plasticity and disorders of the nervous system," *Nature Reviews Neuroscience*, vol. 7, no. 9, pp. 697–709, 2006.

[82] B. B. Johansson and A.-L. Ohlsson, "Environment, social interaction, and physical activity as determinants of functional outcome after cerebral infarction in the rat," *Experimental Neurology*, vol. 139, no. 2, pp. 322–327, 1996.

[83] B. Kolb, M. Forgie, R. Gibb, G. Gorny, and S. Rowntree, "Age, experience and the changing brain," *Neuroscience & Biobehavioral Reviews*, vol. 22, no. 2, pp. 143–159, 1998.

[84] B. Will, R. Galani, C. Kelche, and M. R. Rosenzweig, "Recovery from brain injury in animals: Relative efficacy of environmental enrichment, physical exercise or formal training (1990-2002)," *Progress in Neurobiology*, vol. 72, no. 3, pp. 167–182, 2004.

[85] D. Hebert, M. P. Lindsay, A. McIntyre et al., "Canadian stroke best practice recommendations: Stroke rehabilitation practice guidelines, update 2015," *International Journal of Stroke*, vol. 11, no. 4, pp. 459–484, 2016.

[86] C. J. Winstein, J. Stein, R. Arena et al., "Guidelines for Adult Stroke Rehabilitation and Recovery: A Guideline for Healthcare Professionals from the American Heart Association/American Stroke Association," *Stroke*, vol. 47, no. 6, pp. e98–e169, 2016.

[87] Stroke Unit Trialists' Collaboration, "Organised inpatient (stroke unit) care for stroke," *Cochrane Database of Systematic Reviews*, vol. 9, Article ID CD000197, 2013.

[88] D. J. Clarke, "The role of multidisciplinary team care in stroke rehabilitation," *Progress in Neurology and Psychiatry*, vol. 17, no. 4, pp. 5–8, 2013.

[89] S. F. Tyson, L. Burton, and A. McGovern, "The effect of a structured model for stroke rehabilitation multi-disciplinary team meetings on functional recovery and productivity: A Phase I/II proof of concept study," *Clinical Rehabilitation*, vol. 29, no. 9, pp. 920–925, 2015.

[90] P. Mandy, "Interdisciplinary rather than multidisciplinary or generic practice," *International Journal of Therapy and Rehabilitation*, vol. 3, no. 2, pp. 110–112, 1996.

[91] D. J. Clarke, "Achieving teamwork in stroke units: The contribution of opportunistic dialogue," *Journal of Interprofessional Care*, vol. 24, no. 3, pp. 285–297, 2010.

[92] A. L. Conneeley, "Interdisciplinary collaborative goal planning in a post-acute neurological setting: A qualitative study," *The British Journal of Occupational Therapy*, vol. 67, no. 6, pp. 248–255, 2004.

[93] K. Dworzynski, G. Ritchie, and D. Playford, "Stroke rehabilitation: Long-term rehabilitation after stroke," *Clinical Medicine*, vol. 15, no. 5, pp. 461–464, 2015.

[94] P. Langhorne, O. Wu, H. Rodgers, A. Ashburn, and J. Bernhardt, "A very early rehabilitation trial after stroke (AVERT): a Phase III, multicentre, randomised controlled trial," *Health Technology Assessment*, vol. 21, no. 54, pp. 1–119, 2017.

[95] "Efficacy and safety of very early mobilisation within 24 h of stroke onset (AVERT): a randomised controlled trial," *The Lancet*, vol. 386, no. 9988, pp. 46–55, 2015.

[96] J. Bernhardt, L. Churilov, F. Ellery et al., "Prespecified dose-response analysis for A Very Early Rehabilitation Trial (AVERT)," *Neurology*, vol. 86, no. 23, pp. 2138–2145, 2016.

[97] K. Salter, J. Jutai, M. Hartley et al., "Impact of early vs delayed admission to rehabilitation on functional outcomes in persons with stroke," *Journal of Rehabilitation Medicine*, vol. 38, no. 2, pp. 113–117, 2006.

[98] S. Paolucci, G. Antonucci, M. G. Grasso et al., "Early versus delayed inpatient stroke rehabilitation: A matched comparison conducted in Italy," *Archives of Physical Medicine and Rehabilitation*, vol. 81, no. 6, pp. 695–700, 2000.

[99] B. J. Lutz, M. Young, K. J. Cox, C. Martz, and K. R. Creasy, "The crisis of stroke: Experiences of patients and their family caregivers," *Topics in Stroke Rehabilitation*, vol. 18, no. 6, pp. 786–797, 2011.

[100] E. A. Coleman, "Falling through the cracks: challenges and opportunities for improving transitional care for persons with continuous complex care needs," *Journal of the American Geriatrics Society*, vol. 51, no. 4, pp. 549–555, 2003.

[101] Y. Wang, F. Yang, H. Shi, C. Yang, and H. Hu, "What type of transitional care effectively reduced mortality and improved ADL of stroke patients? A meta-analysis," *International Journal*

of Environmental Research and Public Health, vol. 14, no. 5, article no. 510, 2017.

[102] G. C.-H. Koh, S. K. Saxena, T.-P. Ng, D. Yong, and N.-P. Fong, "Effect of duration, participation rate, and supervision during community rehabilitation on functional outcomes in the first poststroke year in Singapore," *Archives of Physical Medicine and Rehabilitation*, vol. 93, no. 2, pp. 279–286, 2012.

[103] A. W. Chen, Y. T. Koh, S. W. Leong, N. g. LW, P. S. Lee, and Koh. G. C., "Post community hospital discharge rehabilitation attendance: Self-perceived barriers and participation over time," *Annals of the Academy of Medicine, Singapore*, vol. 43, no. 3, pp. 136–144, 2014.

[104] K. Wei, C. Barr, and S. George, "Factors influencing post-stroke rehabilitation participation after discharge from hospital," *International Journal of Therapy & Rehabilitation*, vol. 21, no. 6, pp. 260–267, 2014.

[105] A. L. Fitzpatrick, N. R. Powe, L. S. Cooper, D. G. Ives, J. A. Robbins, and E. Enright, "Barriers to health care access among the elderly and who perceives them," *American Journal of Public Health*, vol. 94, no. 10, pp. 1788–1794, 2004.

[106] C. A. Okoro, T. W. Strine, S. L. Young, L. S. Balluz, and A. H. Mokdad, "Access to health care among older adults and receipt of preventive services. Results from the Behavioral Risk Factor Surveillance System, 2002," *Preventive Medicine*, vol. 40, no. 3, pp. 337–343, 2005.

[107] C. A. Okoro, S. L. Young, T. W. Strine, L. S. Balluz, and A. H. Mokdad, "Uninsured adults aged 65 years and older: Is their health at risk?" *Journal of Health Care for the Poor and Underserved*, vol. 16, no. 3, pp. 453–463, 2005.

[108] M. Shaughnessy and K. Michael, "Stroke in Older Adults," in *Stroke Recovery and Rehabilitation*, J. Stein, R. L. Harvey, C. J. Winstein, R. D. Zorowitz, and G. F. Wittenberg, Eds., pp. 753–766, demosMEDICAL, USA, 2 edition, 2015.

[109] S. S. Tay, T. C. Wee, S. Mohamed Noor, and N. Hassan, "View towards Rehabilitation in the Home - A Survey of Patient's Mindset towards a Home Rehabilitation Programme," *Annals of the Academy of Medicine, Singapore*, vol. 45, no. 12, pp. 560–562, 2016.

[110] G. C.-H. Koh, S. C. Yen, A. Tay et al., "Singapore Tele-technology Aided Rehabilitation in Stroke (STARS) trial: Protocol of a randomized clinical trial on tele-rehabilitation for stroke patients," *BMC Neurology*, vol. 15, no. 1, article no. 161, 2015.

[111] S. N. Housley, A. R. Garlow, K. Ducote et al., "Increasing Access to Cost Effective Home-Based Rehabilitation for Rural Veteran Stroke Survivors," *Austin Journal of Cerebrovascular Disease & Stroke*, vol. 3, no. 2, pp. 1–11, 2016.

[112] S. K. Ostwald, S. Davis, G. Hersch, C. Kelley, and K. M. Godwin, "Evidence-based educational guidelines for stroke survivors after discharge home," *Journal of Neuroscience Nursing*, vol. 40, no. 3, pp. 173–191, 2008.

34

Magnitude of Anemia in Geriatric Population Visiting Outpatient Department at the University of Gondar Referral Hospital, Northwest Ethiopia: Implication for Community-Based Screening

Mulugeta Melku ⓘ,[1] Wondimu Asefa,[2] Ahmed Mohamednur,[2] Tesfahun Getachew,[2] Bayechish Bazezew,[2] Meseret Workineh ⓘ,[3] Bamlaku Enawgaw ⓘ,[1] Belete Biadgo ⓘ,[4] Zegeye Getaneh,[1] Debasu Damtie ⓘ,[3] and Betelihem Terefe ⓘ[1]

[1]*Department of Hematology and Immunohematology, School of Biomedical and Laboratory Sciences, College of Medicine and Health Sciences, University of Gondar, 6200 Gondar, Ethiopia*
[2]*Department of Medical Laboratory Sciences, School of Biomedical and Laboratory Sciences, College of Medicine and Health Sciences, University of Gondar, Gondar, Ethiopia*
[3]*Department of Immunology and Molecular Biology, School of Biomedical and Laboratory Sciences, College of Medicine and Health Sciences, University of Gondar, Gondar, Ethiopia*
[4]*Department of Clinical Chemistry, School of Biomedical and Laboratory Sciences, College of Medicine and Health Sciences, University of Gondar, Gondar, Ethiopia*

Correspondence should be addressed to Mulugeta Melku; mulugeta.melku@gmail.com

Academic Editor: Fulvio Lauretani

Objective. This study is aimed at assessing the magnitude and its associated factors of anemia in geriatric population visiting outpatient department at the University of Gondar referral hospital, northwest Ethiopia. *Method*. A cross-sectional study was conducted among elder patients in Gondar town, North Gondar District, in May 2013. A total of 200 randomly selected geriatric population participated in the study. Summary statistics were computed and presented in tables and figure. Both bivariate and multivariable binary logistic regression were fitted to identify associated factors. A P value < 0.05 was considered as statistically significant. *Result*. The median age of the study participants was 65 years (Interquartile range (IQR): 8 years). The prevalence of anemia in the geriatric patients was 54.5% ($n = 109$), of which 61.5% ($n = 67$) were males. Mild type anemia was predominant, 55.96% ($n = 61$). Geriatric patients with an elevated erythrocyte sedimentation rate (AOR = 9.04, 95% CI: 4.2–19.7) and who are vegetarians (AOR = 2.2, 95% CI: 1.03–4.71) were at high risk of developing anemia. *Conclusion*. The magnitude of anemia was high in geriatrics. Mild anemia was the predominant type. Vegetarians and geriatrics with elevated erythrocyte sedimentation rate were more likely to develop anemia. Hence, early diagnosis and management of anemia have paramount importance to prevent adverse outcomes in geriatrics.

1. Background

Anemia is a decrease in the number of red blood cells or hemoglobin (Hb), resulting in a lower ability for the blood to carry oxygen to body tissues. As to World Health Organization (WHO) recommendation, anemia as Hb level $< 12.0\,g/dL$ for women and $<13.0\,g/L$ for men is most frequently used, even though the appropriateness in older populations may be questioned [1]. Anemia is a worldwide public health problem, with global prevalence estimated to be 24.8% (95% CI: 22.9–26.7). The majority of the global disease burden of anemia is shouldered by the developing world, with high prevalence in Africa and southeast Asia [2].

In geriatric age group, anemia is a common concern and public health problem [3–6]. It is frequently underdiagnosed and often not reported to the patient because it is mostly perceived as a mere consequence of aging or as a disease marker [7]. However, anemia has been implicated with severe complications. It can greatly hamper the quality of life and, consequently, it can have an impact on healthcare requirements and expenditure. Thus, it is becoming a significant healthcare burden [8, 9].

Evidences showed that anemia in elderly has been strongly linked with severe complications, including impaired physical functioning [10], decreased functionality [11], multidimensional loss of function [12], increased risk of frailty [13–15], depression [16], cognitive impairment [17], obstructive sleeping apnea [18], frequent comorbidity and hospitalization [19–21], and increased risk of death [20, 22, 23]. Despite old age being a major risk factor for anemia which threatens the quality of elderly life and has a substantial social and economic effects, anemia, however, should not be accepted as an inevitable consequence of aging, as it does reflect poor health and increased vulnerability to adverse outcomes in older persons [24, 25].

Anemia in elderly is multifactorial in etiology and a complex interaction of many factors. Causes of anemia in the elderly are divided into three groups: anemia of chronic disease, nutritional deficiency, and unexplained anemia [26]. These groups are not, however, mutually exclusive. In most of the cases, several of these causes may coexist and may each contribute independently to the anemia. The most common causes of anemia in the elderly are chronic diseases and iron deficiency [24]. Approximately, one-third of anemia in elderly person has attributed to nutrient deficiency; most of these cases are attributable to iron deficiency, including chronic blood loss. Moreover, folate deficiency and vitamin B12 deficiency are also causes of nutritional anemia and warrant routine screening. Although fortification of foodstuffs has made folate deficiency less common, more than 10% of elderly persons have borderline or low vitamin B12 levels [25, 27].

Although numerous studies on the prevalence of anemia in the elderly have been published, they vary markedly in study design and populations sampled and, consequently, in its prevalence range widely [3, 15, 21, 28, 29]. Despite the increasing size of the geriatric population in Ethiopia, much has not been done to determine the epidemiology of anemia in this group of the population.

2. Methods and Materials

2.1. Study Design, Period, Setting, Population, and Sampling Techniques. This institution based cross-sectional study was conducted in the outpatient department of University of Gondar Hospital in May 2013. The sample size was estimated by using single population proportion at 95% confidence interval, sampling error of 5%, and an estimated anemia prevalence of 50% in the elderly population. The sample size was corrected into 200, as the estimated number of elderly patients visiting the hospital during the study period was lower than 10,000. A systematic random sampling was applied; participants were selected at every second interval from the sequence of outpatient department visit.

On the basis of the proposed working definition of an "older person" in Africa for the Minimum Data Set (MDS) project [30], elderly patients with the age of 60 years and above for both men and women and who had not been transfused with red blood cells within the previous three months were included. Those elderly patients who were seriously ill and unable to respond to the questions during the time of data collection were excluded from the study for ethical reasons.

2.2. Data Collection Method. Sociodemographic and clinical history of the study participants were collected by using pretested structured questionnaire via interview and medical record review, respectively. Height and weight of each study participants were measured using standard scales as recommended by WHO. BMI was computed as weight (kg)/height (m^2). Based on BMI, nutritional status was evaluated and grouped as follows: underweight (BMI $\leq$ 18.5), normal weight (BMI = 18.5–24.9), and overweight (BMI $\geq$ 25.0).

2.3. Laboratory Methods and Assessment of Anemia. Three milliliters of venous blood was drawn into K$_3$EDTA tube and analyzed for complete blood count (CBC) and erythrocyte sedimentation rate (ESR). The CBC was determined using a Sysmex KX-21N (Sysmex Corporation Kobe, Japan) automated hematology analyzer. Anemia was defined according to the WHO criteria as an adjusted Hb concentration lower than 12.0 g/dL for women and 13.0 g/dL for men. Severity of anemia was graded as severe (Hb < 8.0 g/dL) and moderate (Hb: 8.0–10.9 g/dL) for both men and women and as mild (Hb: 11.0–12.9 g/dL for men and Hb: 11.0–11.9 g/dL for women) [1]. Morphological classification of anemia was done by using red cell indices, and the reference values used in this study were MCV (80–100 fl), MCHC (31–35%), and MCH (27–32 pg). We used IRIA (LiNEAR Chemicals, SL, Spain) for determination of ESR and a cutoff value of 20 mm/hr and 30 mm/hr was used for men and women, respectively.

2.4. Data Analysis and Interpretation. Data were entered to EPI info version 3.5.3 and then transferred to SPSS version 20 statistical package for analysis. Summary statistics were computed, and the results were presented in tables and figure. A binary logistic regression model was fitted to identify factors associated with anemia. Odds ratio, Chi-square, and 95% CI for odds ratio were computed to assess the strength of association and statistical significance in bivariate analysis. Variables having P less than or equal to 0.2 in bivariate binary logistic regression analysis were included in multivariable binary logistic regression analysis to control confounders. A P value less than 0.05 in the multivariable binary logistic regression model was considered to be statistically significant.

2.5. Ethical Consideration. The study was approved by an Institutional Review Board of the University of Gondar. The purpose and importance of the study were explained to each study participants. Written consent was obtained from each participant. To ensure confidentiality of participants' information, anonymous typing was used whereby the name of the participants and any participants' identifier were not written on the questionnaire. To keep the participants' privacy, they were interviewed alone in a separate room.

3. Results

3.1. Characteristics of Study Participants. Two hundred (n = 200) elderly patients participated in this study. The median age of the study participants was 65 years (IQR: 8 years). About one-third, (35%, n = 70), of them, belong to 60–64 years age group. Majority of the elderly patients were males (55%, n = 110), and most of the study participants reside in an urban setting (55.5%, n = 111). More than three-fourths (77%, n = 154), half (61%, n = 122), and one-third (43%, n = 86) of the participants were married, unable to read and write, and farmer by occupation, respectively. The average monthly family income of the study participants was 1093.36 Ethiopia Birr (ETB), of which 42% (n = 84) had an income of less than 1000 ETB. The proportion of elderly patients with a family size of greater than 6 accounts for 15.5% (n = 31) (Table 1).

3.2. Dietary Habit and ESR Value of Study Participants. About 78% (n = 156) and 69.5% (n = 139) of the study participants had a habit of consuming fruits less frequently and meat at least once a week, respectively. Moreover, 62% (n = 124) of them had a habit of taking coffee and/or tea after a meal, whereas 44.5% (n = 89) of them had a habit of consuming vegetables less frequently. Concerning the nutritional status and ESR status of the study participants, 26% (n = 52) and 70.5% (n = 141) of them were underweighted and had an elevated ESR value, respectively (Table 2).

3.3. Anemia Prevalence and Its Severity. The median (IQR) Hb concentration for males and females was 12.5 g/dl (IQR: 2.6 g/dl) and 12.15 g/dl (IQR: 2.85 g/dl), respectively. The prevalence of anemia in the elderly patients was 54.5% (95% CI: 47.54–61.46). Out of the total anemic elderly patients, 7 (6.4%), 40 (36.7%), and 62 (56.9%) had severe, moderate, and mild anemia, respectively (Table 3). Regarding morphologic feature of anemia, the majority of anemic patients had been suffering from normocytic normochromic anemia, 85.3% (n = 93) (Figure 1).

3.4. Factors Associated with Elderly Anemia. In bivariate binary logistic regression analysis, male sex, vegetarians, elevated ESR, underweight, and normal weight were significantly associated with elderly anemia. But in multivariable binary logistic regression analysis controlling the possible cofounders, only vegetarians and elevated ESR value were found to be factors statistically associated with elderly anemia. The odds of anemia in elderly patients who were vegetarians were two times (AOR = 2.2, 95% CI: 1.03–4.71) higher than the odds of anemia in elderly patients who had a habit of consuming meat at least once in every two weeks. Similarly, elderly patients who had an elevated ESR were nine times (AOR = 9.04, 95% CI: 4.2–19.7) more likely to be anemic as compared to those whose ESR value was within the normal range (Table 4).

TABLE 1: Sociodemographic characteristics of study participants (n = 200).

Variables	Frequency	Percent
Age (years)		
60–64	70	35
65–69	54	27
70–74	38	19
>74	38	19
Sex		
Female	90	45
Male	110	55
Residence		
Urban	111	55.5
Rural	89	44.5
Marital status		
Single	1	0.5
Married	154	77
Divorced	15	7.5
Widowed	30	15
Educational level		
Unable read and write	122	61
Attended primary school	32	16
Attended secondary school	27	13.5
Attended higher education	19	9.5
Occupation		
Daily laborer	9	4.5
Private employee	21	10.5
Governmental employee	37	18.5
Farmer	86	43
Housewife and retired	47	23.5
Family size		
1–3 members	54	27
4–6 members	115	57.5
>6 members	31	15.5
Monthly income (ETB)		
<1000	84	42
100–1500	90	45
>1500	26	13

4. Discussion

Anemia is a critical clinical problem in the elderly population, especially in hospitalized geriatric patients, and is known to be associated with increased morbidity and mortality. The present institutional based cross-sectional study found that the prevalence of anemia in elderly patients visiting outpatient department was high, and elevated ESR and being vegetarian were found to be strongly associated with geriatric anemia.

In this study, elderly patients had anemia prevalence of 54.5%, and according to WHO cutoff anemia has severe public health significance in this group [1]. It is comparable to the prevalence reported by Sahin et al. (54.9%) [31]. It is also comparable with a study reported by Tay and Ong (57.1%)

TABLE 2: Dietary habit, nutritional status, and ESR value of study participants (*n* = 200).

Variables	Frequency	Percentage
Meat consumption habit		
Consumed at least once a week and more	139	69.5
Vegetarians	61	30.5
Frequency of fruit consumption		
At least once a week and more	44	22
Less frequently	156	78
Frequency of vegetable consumption		
At least once a week and more	111	55.5
Less frequently	89	44.5
Coffee or tea consumption habit after meal		
Yes	124	62
No	76	38
Nutritional status, BMI		
Underweight	52	26
Normal	133	66.5
Overweight	15	7.5
ESR		
Normal	59	29.5
Elevated	141	70.5

BMI: Body mass index; ESR: erythrocyte sedimentation rate.

TABLE 3: Summary of anemia severity among anemic study participants (*n* = 109).

Variables	Frequency	Percentage
Anemia by severity		
Mild	62	56.9
Moderate	40	36.7
Severe	7	6.4
Total	109	54.5

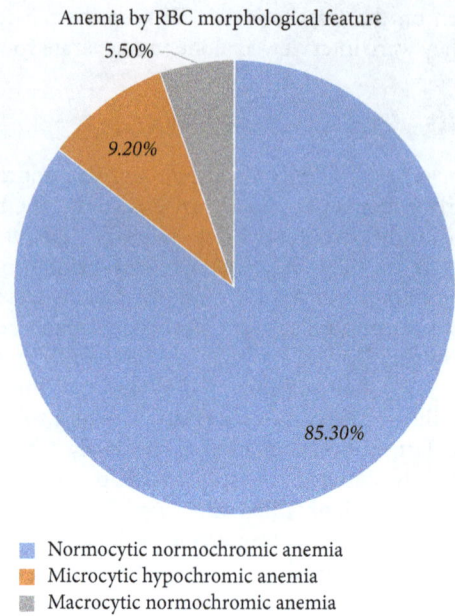

FIGURE 1: RBC morphological feature among anemic elderly study participants (*n* = 109).

[21], even though the study design and the criteria to define the population and anemia is different from us, as Tay and Ong study was retrospective in elderly hospitalized patients aged 65 and above year and the anemia was not defined according to WHO criterion. However, it is higher than the prevalence reported by Nakashima et al. (29%) [3], Sgnaolin et al. (12.8%) [32], and Bang et al. (8.33%) [10]. The possible reason for the discrepancies might be the characteristics differences between populations studied. In this study, the study participants were elderly patients who sought medical intervention in outpatients department, whereas in the case of Nakashima et al., Sgnaolin et al., and Bang et al. studies, the participants were institutionalized in long-term care [3] and community-dwelling elderly people [10, 32], who were assumed to be apparently healthy; thereby the risk of anemia is low. Similarly, the prevalence revealed in this study was higher than the prevalence (36.7%) reported from Reykjavik, Iceland [33], and the prevalence (10.6%) reported by NHANES III for black Americans [25]. This can be due to the differences in nutritional and environmental factors across the population studied.

On the other hand, the magnitude of anemia in this study was lower than studies carried out by Dunn et al. (77%) [34] and Kaur et al. (71%) [29]. This difference can be attributed to the distinctive characteristics of study participants, as Dunn et al. included elderly patients who were admitted to hospital for palliative care and Kaur et al. also included those admitted to in-patients in addition to outpatients; however, in our study only outpatients were considered. In elderly patients admitted to health facilities, the range and degree of comorbid conditions increase the likelihood of anemia development as compared with elderly outpatients. Contingent on these situations, the magnitude of anemia in the present study is lower than those studies conducted among elderly hospitalized patients.

Similar to previous studies carried out by different scholars [10, 21, 25, 35], this study found that the magnitude of anemia was higher in elderly men (60.9%) than women (46.7%). Moreover, a systematic review revealed that the estimates of anemia prevalence range from 2.9% to 61% in elderly men and from 3.3% to 41% in elderly women, but the threshold values are, in general, higher for men than for women [36]. The difference in the prevalence rates of anemia for men and women can be explained by the fact that in each decade beyond the age of 30, the concentration of free and bioavailable testosterone declines sharply in males. This negatively impacts the enhanced metabolic processes of the bone marrow. As testosterone level decreases with aging, the rate of erythropoiesis tends to be declined and predispose men to increased risk of anemia [37, 38]. In contrast to elderly men, the postmenopausal estrogen, which acts as an inhibitor of erythropoiesis, declines gradually as women age [39]. This intern would probably decrease the risk of anemia in elderly women as compared to men.

TABLE 4: Analysis of factors associated with anemia among study participants ($n = 200$).

Variables	Anemia		COR (95% CI)	AOR (95% CI)
	Anemic (%)	Non-anemic (%)		
Sex				
Male	67 (60.9)	43 (39.1)	1.78 (1.01, 3.13)[b]	1.53 (0.79, 2.96)
Female	42 (46.7)	48 (53.3)	1.00	
Residence				
Urban	56 (50.5)	45 (49.5)	1.00	
Rural	53 (59.6)	36 (40.4)	1.45 (0.82, 2.54)	
Age group (year)				
60–64	33 (47.1)	37 (52.9)	1.00	
65–69	35 (64.8)	19 (35.2)	2.10 (0.99, 4.30)[+]	
70–74	19 (50)	19 (50)	1.12 (0.51, 2.47)	
>74	22 (57.9)	16 (42.1)	1.54 (0.70, 3.42)	
Marital Status				
Married	80 (51.9)	74 (48.1)	1.00	
Single or divorced	10 (62.5)	6 (37.5)	1.54 (0.53, 4.45)	
Widowed	19 (63.3)	11 (36.7)	1.60 (0.71, 3.58)	
Educational status				
Unable read and write	68 (55.7)	54 (44.3)	1.14 (0.64, 2.01)	
Attended primary school or above	41 (52.6)	37 (47.4)	1.00	
Occupation				
Daily laborers, housewives and retired	28 (50)	28 (50)	0.76 (0.36, 1.58)	
Farmers	48 (55.8)	38 (44.2)	0.9 (0.5, 1.87)	
Employed (private and government)	33 (56.9)	25 (43.1)	1.00	
Family size				
1–3 members	26 (48.1)	28 (51.9)	1.00	
4–6 members	64 (55.7)	51 (44.3)	1.35 (0.71, 2.58)	
>6 members	19 (61.3)	12 (38.7)	1.71 (0.69, 4.2)	
Meat consumption habit				
Consumed at least once every two weeks and more	69 (49.6)	70 (50.4)	1.00	
Vegetarians	40 (65.6)	21 (34.4)	1.93 (1.04, 3.61)	2.2 (1.03, 4.71)[*]
Frequency of Fruit consumption				
At least once a week and more	23 (52.3)	21 (47.7)	1.00	
Less frequently	86 (55.1)	70 (44.9)	1.12 (0.57, 2.2)	
Frequency of Vegetable consumption				
At least once a week and more	61 (55)	50 (45)	1.00	
Less frequently	48 (53.9)	41 (46.1)	0.96 (0.55, 1.68)	
Coffee or tea consumption habit after meal				
Yes	65 (52.4)	59 (47.6)	0.8 (0.45, 1.43)	
No	44 (57.9)	32 (42.1)	1.00	
Monthly income (ETB)				
<1000	45 (53.6)	39 (46.4)	0.99 (0.41, 2.39)	
100–1500	50 (55.6)	40 (44.4)	1.07 (0.45, 2.57)	
>1500	14 (53.8)	12 (46.2)	1.00	
ESR				
Normal	12 (20.3)	47 (79.7)	1.00	
Elevated	97 (68.8)	44 (31.2)	8.63 (4.17, 17.87)	9.04 (4.2, 19.7)[*]
Nutritional status, BMI				
Underweight	33 (63.5)	19 (36.5)	6.95 (1.74, 27.76)[b]	4.02 (0.81, 19.93)
Normal	73 (54.9)	60 (45.1)	4.87 (1.31, 18.1)[b]	3.61 (0.8, 16.25)
Overweight	3 (20%)	12 (32)	1.00	

ETB: Ethiopian Birr; BMI: body mass index; COR: crude odds ratio; AOR: adjusted odds ratio; and CI: confidence interval. [+] Category of a variable with P value less than 0.2 in bivariate binary logistic regression analysis, [b] Category of a variables which were statistically significant in bivariate binary logistic regress but not in multivariable analysis. [*] Category of a variables which were statistically significant in multivariable binary logistic regression analysis (P value < 0.05).

In this study, the odds of anemia in vegetarians were two times as high as the odds in those who had a habit of consuming meat at least once in every two weeks. Evidence suggested that the omission of meat and other animal products from the diet increases the risk of nutritional deficiencies [40, 41]. As a result, in vegetarians, the risk of vitamin B12, iron, and other several minerals deficiencies is common, which predispose them to an increased risk of nutritional deficiency anemia [42, 43]. Together with high magnitude of undernutrition which is a major public health concern in many African countries as a consequence of poverty and limitation of access to basic social supports [44] and aging related physiological changes, vegetarians are at higher risk of developing anemia.

In this study, we noticed that elderly patients who had an elevated ESR were nine times (AOR = 9.04, 95% CI: 4.2–19.7) more likely to be anemic as compared to those whose ESR value was within the normal range. The systemic inflammation associated with aging as well as chronic/acute conditions has been inferred from commonly used sensitive laboratory tests like ESR and C-reactive protein [45]. It is known that elevated ESR value is strongly correlated with the inflammatory response. Inflammatory conditions result in the accumulation of reactive oxygen species which activate nuclear factor kappa B, a transcription factor playing a central role in activating the innate immune response and inducing the expression of numerous proinflammatory cytokines. These pro-inflammatory cytokines further induce the expression of hepcidin antimicrobial peptide, a critical mediator of anemia of inflammation, which decreases serum iron availability and correlates with serum ferritin [46]. Moreover, patients with inflammatory diseases have been demonstrated to have decreased red cell survival, disorders of erythropoiesis, low erythropoietin response to hypoxia, and progressive erythroid progenitor cell resistance to erythropoietin stimulation [47]. Thus, elderly people having elevated ESR value are at higher risk of developing anemia.

5. Limitation of the Study

One of the limitations of this study is that only hemoglobin measurement was used to define anemia; the micronutrient analysis was not done for the assessment of nutritional deficiency anemia. The second limitation is that only ESR was used as an indicator of inflammation; other sensitive indicators like serum C-reactive protein, albumin, and cytokines were not measured. The third limitation of this study is related to the study design and the sample size, as its cross-sectional nature with small sample size.

6. Conclusion

In conclusion, the prevalence of anemia was found to be high, indicating that it is a severe public health problem in the study area. Being vegetarians and elevated ESR value have been strongly associated with high prevalence of anemia in elderly outpatients. Hence, provision of community-based anemia screening and nutritional educations are advisable to improve the quality of life and reduce the complications in the elderly population. Moreover, further community-based studies, employing longitudinal design and preferably involving biochemical analysis, are required to identify risk factors as well as to estimate the relative contribution of nutritional status to anemia in this group of the population.

Abbreviations

AOR: Adjusted odds ratio
BMI: Body mass index
CBC: Complete blood count
CI: Confidence interval
COR: Crude odds ratio
ESR: Erythrocyte sedimentation rate
ETB: Ethiopian Birr
IQR: Interquartile range
Hb: Hemoglobin
MCH: Mean cell hemoglobin
MCHC: Mean cell hemoglobin concentration
MCV: Mean cell volume
MDS: Minimum Data Set
SD: Standard deviation
WHO: World Health Organization.

Disclosure

Mulugeta Melku and Betelihem Terefe are co-first authors of the manuscript.

Authors' Contributions

Mulugeta Melku and Betelihem Terefe equally contributed to this work.

Acknowledgments

The authors would like to thank the study participants for their volunteer participation. The authors would also like to extend their application for the University of Gondar, School of Biomedical and Laboratory Sciences, and the University of Gondar Referral Hospital for logistic supports.

References

[1] WHO, *Haemoglobin concentrations for the diagnosis of anaemia and assessment of severity. Vitamin and Mineral Nutrition Information System*, World Health Organization, Geneva, Switzerland, 2011.

[2] WHO, *Worldwide Prevalence of Anaemia 1993-2005*, WHO Global Database on Anaemia, Geneva, Switzerland, 2008.

[3] A. T. A. Nakashima, A. C. F. de Moraes, F. Auler, and R. M. Peralta, "Anemia prevalence and its determinants in Brazilian institutionalized elderly," *Nutrition Journal*, vol. 28, no. 6, pp. 640–643, 2012.

[4] V. Argento, J. Roylance, B. Skudlarska, N. Dainiak, and Y. Amo-ateng-Adjepong, "Anemia Prevalence in a Home Visit Geriatric Population," *Journal of the American Medical Directors Association*, vol. 9, no. 6, pp. 422–426, 2008.

[5] V. Bach, G. Schruckmayer, I. Sam, G. Kemmler, and R. Stauder, "Prevalence and possible causes of anemia in the elderly: A cross-sectional analysis of a large European university hospital cohort," *Clinical Interventions in Aging*, vol. 9, pp. 1187–1196, 2014.

[6] A. M. van Staden and D. J. V. Weich, "Retrospective analysis of the prevalence and causes of anaemia in hospitalised elderly patients," *South African Family Practice*, vol. 57, no. 5, pp. 297–299, 2015.

[7] M. Tettamanti, U. Lucca, F. Gandini et al., "Prevalence, incidence and types of mild anemia in the elderly: the 'Health and Anemia'population-based study," *Haematologica*, vol. 95, no. 11, pp. 1849–1856, 2010.

[8] B. Robinson, "Cost of anemia in the elderly," *Journal of the American Geriatrics Society*, vol. 15, no. 3, pp. s14–s17, 2003.

[9] W. B. Ershler, K. Chen, E. B. Reyes, and R. Dubois, "Economic burden of patients with anemia in selected diseases," *Value in Health*, vol. 8, no. 6, pp. 629–638, 2005.

[10] S.-M. Bang, J.-O. Lee, Y. J. Kim et al., "Anemia and activities of daily living in the Korean urban elderly population: Results from the Korean Longitudinal Study on Health and Aging (KLoSHA)," *Annals of Hematology*, vol. 92, no. 1, pp. 59–65, 2013.

[11] R. D. M. Bosco, E. P. S. Assis, R. R. Pinheiro, L. C. V. de Queiroz, L. S. M. Pereira, and C. M. F. Antunes, "Anemia and functional capacity in elderly Brazilian hospitalized patients," *Cadernos de Saúde Pública*, vol. 29, no. 7, pp. 1322–1332, 2013.

[12] J. Zilinski, R. Zillmann, I. Becker, T. Benzing, R.-J. Schulz, and G. Roehrig, "Prevalence of anemia among elderly inpatients and its association with multidimensional loss of function," *Annals of Hematology*, vol. 93, no. 10, pp. 1645–1654, 2014.

[13] G. Röhrig, "Anemia in the frail, elderly patient," *Clinical Interventions in Aging*, vol. 11, pp. 319–326, 2016.

[14] L. Pires Corona, F. C. Drumond Andrade, Y. A. de Oliveira Duarte, and M. L. Lebrao, "The relationship between anemia, hemoglobin concentration and frailty in Brazilian older adults," *The Journal of Nutrition, Health & Aging*, vol. 19, no. 9, pp. 935–940, 2015.

[15] T. Juárez-Cedillo, L. Basurto-Acevedo, S. Vega-García et al., "Prevalence of anemia and its impact on the state of frailty in elderly people living in the community: SADEM study," *Annals of Hematology*, vol. 93, no. 12, pp. 2057–2062, 2014.

[16] C. Trevisan, N. Veronese, F. Bolzetta et al., "Low hemoglobin levels and risk of developing depression in the elderly: Results from the prospective PRO.V.A. study," *Journal of Clinical Psychiatry*, vol. 77, no. 12, pp. e1549–e1556, 2016.

[17] C. Trevisan, N. Veronese, F. Bolzetta et al., "Low Hemoglobin Levels and the Onset of Cognitive Impairment in Older People: The PRO.V.A. Study," *Rejuvenation Research*, vol. 19, no. 6, pp. 447–455, 2016.

[18] A. M. Khan, S. Ashizawa, V. Hlebowicz, and D. W. Appel, "Anemia of aging and obstructive sleep apnea," *Sleep and Breathing*, vol. 15, no. 1, pp. 29–34, 2011.

[19] M. Migone De Amicis, E. Poggiali, I. Motta et al., "Anemia in elderly hospitalized patients: prevalence and clinical impact," *Internal and Emergency Medicine*, vol. 10, no. 5, pp. 581–586, 2015.

[20] B. F. Culleton, B. J. Manns, J. Zhang, M. Tonelli, S. Klarenbach, and B. R. Hemmelgarn, "Impact of anemia on hospitalization and mortality in older adults," *Blood*, vol. 107, no. 10, pp. 3841–3846, 2006.

[21] M. R. J. Tay and Y. Y. Ong, "Prevalence and risk factors of anaemia in older hospitalised patients," *Proceedings of Singapore Healthcare*, vol. 20, no. 2, pp. 71–79, 2011.

[22] F. Landi, A. Russo, P. Danese et al., "Anemia status, hemoglobin concentration, and mortality in nursing home older residents," *Journal of the American Medical Directors Association*, vol. 8, no. 5, pp. 322–327, 2007.

[23] H. G. Endres, U. Wedding, D. Pittrow, U. Thiem, H. J. Trampisch, and C. Diehm, "Prevalence of anemia in elderly patients in primary care: Impact on 5-year mortality risk and differences between men and women," *Current Medical Research and Opinion*, vol. 25, no. 5, pp. 1143–1158, 2009.

[24] D. L. Smith, "Anemia in the elderly," *American Family Physician*, vol. 62, no. 7, pp. 1565–1572, 2000.

[25] J. M. Guralnik, R. S. Eisenstaedt, L. Ferrucci, H. G. Klein, and R. C. Woodman, "Prevalence of anemia in persons 65 years and older in the United States: evidence for a high rate of unexplained anemia," *Blood*, vol. 104, no. 8, pp. 2263–2268, 2004.

[26] E. Andrès, L. Federici, K. Serraj, and G. Kaltenbach, "Update of nutrient-deficiency anemia in elderly patients," *European Journal of Internal Medicine*, vol. 19, no. 7, pp. 488–493, 2008.

[27] S. Loikas, P. Koskinen, K. Irjala et al., "Vitamin B12 deficiency in the aged: A Population-Based Study," *Age and Ageing*, vol. 36, no. 2, pp. 177–183, 2007.

[28] M. López-Sierra, S. Calderón, J. Gómez, and L. Pilleux, "Prevalence of anaemia and evaluation of transferrin receptor (sTfR) in the diagnosis of iron deficiency in the hospitalized elderly patients: Anaemia clinical studies in Chile," *Anemia*, vol. 2012, Article ID 646201, 2012.

[29] H. Kaur, S. Piplani, M. Madan, M. Paul, and S. G. Rao, "Prevalence of Anemia and Micronutrient Deficiency in Elderly," *International Journal of Medical and Dental Sciences*, vol. 3, no. 1, pp. 296–302, 2015.

[30] WHO, "Definition of an older or elderly person: Proposed Working Definition of an Older Person in Africa for the MDS Project," WHO Health statistics and health information systems, 2013, http://www.who.int/healthinfo/survey/ageingdefnolder/en/index.html.

[31] S. Sahin, P. T. Tasar, H. Simsek et al., "Prevalence of anemia and malnutrition and their association in elderly nursing home residents," *Aging Clinical and Experimental Research*, vol. 28, no. 5, pp. 857–862, 2016.

[32] V. Sgnaolin, P. Engroff, L. S. Ely et al., "Hematological parameters and prevalence of anemia among free-living elderly in south Brazil," *Revista Brasileira de Hematologia e Hemoterapia*, vol. 35, no. 2, pp. 115–118, 2013.

[33] A. Ramel, P. V. Jonsson, S. Bjornsson, and I. Thorsdottir, "Anemia, nutritional status, and inflammation in hospitalized elderly," *Nutrition Journal*, vol. 24, no. 11-12, pp. 1116–1122, 2008.

[34] A. Dunn, J. Carter, and H. Carter, "Anemia at the end of life: Prevalence, significance, and causes in patients receiving palliative care," *Journal of Pain and Symptom Management*, vol. 26, no. 6, pp. 1132–1139, 2003.

[35] A. Contreras-Manzano, V. de la Cruz, S. Villalpando, R. Rebollar, and T. Shamah-Levy, "Anemia and iron deficiency in Mexican elderly population. Results from the Ensanut 2012," *Salud Pública de México*, vol. 57, no. 5, pp. 394–402, 2015.

[36] C. Beghé, A. Wilson, and W. B. Ershler, "Prevalence and outcomes of anemia in geriatrics: a systematic review of the literature," *American Journal of Medicine*, vol. 116, no. 7, supplement 1, pp. 3S–10S, 2004.

[37] L. Ferrucci, M. Maggio, S. Bandinelli et al., "Low testosterone levels and the risk of anemia in older men and women," *JAMA Internal Medicine*, vol. 166, no. 13, pp. 1380–1388, 2006.

[38] J. J. Carrero, P. Bárány, M. I. Yilmaz et al., "Testosterone deficiency is a cause of anaemia and reduced responsiveness to erythropoiesis-stimulating agents in men with chronic kidney disease," *Nephrology Dialysis Transplantation*, vol. 27, no. 2, pp. 709–715, 2012.

[39] V. W. Henderson, "Aging, estrogens, and episodic memory in women," *Cognitive and Behavioral Neurology*, vol. 22, no. 4, pp. 205–214, 2009.

[40] E. H. Haddad, L. S. Berk, J. D. Kettering, R. W. Hubbard, and W. R. Peters, "Dietary intake and biochemical, hematologic, and immune status of vegans compared with nonvegetarians," *American Journal of Clinical Nutrition*, vol. 70, no. 3, pp. 586s–593s, 1999.

[41] J. Woo, T. Kwok, S. C. Ho, A. Sham, and E. Lau, "Nutritional status of elderly Chinese vegetarians," *Age and Ageing*, vol. 27, no. 4, pp. 455–461, 1998.

[42] R. Pawlak, S. E. Lester, and T. Babatunde, "The prevalence of cobalamin deficiency among vegetarians assessed by serum vitamin B12: A review of literature," *European Journal of Clinical Nutrition*, vol. 68, no. 5, pp. 541–548, 2014.

[43] R. Obeid, J. Geisel, H. Schorr, U. Hübner, and W. Herrmann, "The impact of vegetarianism on some haematological parameters," *European Journal of Haematology*, vol. 69, no. 5-6, pp. 275–279, 2002.

[44] K. E. Charlton and D. Rose, "Nutrition among older adults in Africa: The situation at the beginning of the millenium," *Journal of Nutrition*, vol. 131, no. 9, pp. 2424S–2428S, 2001.

[45] I. Colombet, J. Pouchot, V. Kronz et al., "Agreement between erythrocyte sedimentation rate and C-reactive protein in hospital practice," *American Journal of Medicine*, vol. 123, no. 9, pp. 863.e7–863.e13, 2010.

[46] A. A. Merchant and C. N. Roy, "Not so benign haematology: Anaemia of the elderly," *British Journal of Haematology*, vol. 156, no. 2, pp. 173–185, 2012.

[47] C. N. Roy, "Anemia of Inflammation," *International Journal of Hematology*, vol. 2010, no. 1, pp. 276–280, 2011.

Permissions

List of Contributors

Saira Javed
Department of Behavioral Sciences, Fatima Jinnah Women University,The Mall, Rawalpindi 46000, Pakistan

Mussi Chiara and Salvioli Gianfranco
Geriatric and Gerontology Institute, University of Modena and Reggio Emilia, Modena 41121, Italy

Galizia Gianluigi, Abete Pasquale and Rengo Franco
Geriatric Department, Azienda Policlinico Federico II, Naples 80131, Italy

Morrione Alessandro, Maraviglia Alice, Marchionni Niccolò and Ungar Andrea
Unit of Gerontology and Geriatric Medicine, Department of Critical Care Medicine and Surgery, University of Florence and Azienda Ospedaliero Universitaria Careggi, Florence 50134, Italy

Noro Gabriele and Tava Giovanni
Geriatric Unit, Santa Chiara Hospital, Trento 38122, Italy

Cavagnaro Paolo
Department of Geriatrics, Azienda Sanitaria Locale 4, Chiavari 16043, Italy

Leslie Vaughan, Iris Leng, Stephen R. Rapp, Sean L. Simpson, Daniel P. Beavers, Laura H. Coker, Sarah A. Gaussoin, Kaycee M. Sink and Mark A. Espeland
Department of Social Sciences and Health Policy, Wake Forest University School of Medicine, Medical Center Boulevard, Winston-Salem, NC, USA

Dale Dagenbach and Janine M. Jennings
Wake Forest University, Winston-Salem, NC, USA

Susan M. Resnick
National Institute on Aging, Baltimore, MD, USA

Robert L. Brunner
Family and Community Medicine, University of Nevada School of Medicine, Reno, NV, USA

Carlos H. Orces
Department of Medicine, Laredo Medical Center, 1700 East Saunders, Laredo, TX 78041, USA

Ahuva Even-Zohar
School of Social Work, Faculty of Social Sciences, Ariel University, 40700 Ariel, Israel

Veronika Williams
Primary Care Clinical Trials Unit, Department of Primary Care Health Sciences, 23-38 Hythe Bridge Street, Oxford OX1 2ET, UK

Christina R. Victor
Gerontology and Public Health, School of Health Sciences and Social Care, Brunel University, Uxbridge, Middlesex UB8 3PH, UK

Rachel McCrindle
Computer and Human Interaction, School of Systems Engineering, University of Reading, Reading RG6 6AY, UK

Aftab Haq and Alexis Lanteri Parcells
Saint George's University School of Medicine, West Indies, Grenada

Sachin Patil
Department of Surgery, Saint Barnabas Medical Center, Livingston, NJ, USA

Ronald S. Chamberlain
Saint George's University School of Medicine, West Indies, Grenada
Department of Surgery, Saint Barnabas Medical Center, Livingston,
Department of Surgery, University of Medicine and Dentistry of New Jersey (UMDNJ), 94 Old Short Hills Road Livingston, Newark, NJ 07039, USA

Caroline Stephens, Elizabeth Halifax and Nhat Bui
Department of Community Health Systems, School of Nursing, University of California, San Francisco, 2 Koret Way, N531E, UCSF San Francisco, CA 94143-0608, USA

Sei J. Lee
Department of Geriatrics, Palliative and Extended Care, San Francisco VA Medical Center, Division of Geriatrics, School of Medicine, University of California, San Francisco, 4150 Clement Street, Building 1, Room 220F, San Francisco, CA 94121, USA

Charlene Harrington and Janet Shim
Department of Social and Behavioral Sciences, School of Nursing, University of California, San Francisco, 3333 California Street, Suite 455, UCSF San Francisco, CA 94118, USA

Christine Ritchie
Division of Geriatrics, School of Medicine, University of California, San Francisco, 3333 California Street, Suite 380, San Francisco, CA 94143-1265, USA

Johanne Desrosiers
School of Rehabilitation, Faculty of Medicine and Health Sciences, Université de Sherbrooke, 3001 12th Avenue North Sherbrooke, Sherbrooke, QC, Canada J1H 5N4
Research Centre on Aging, CSSS-IUGS, Sherbrooke, QC, Canada

Anabelle Viau-Guay
Département d'études sur l'Enseignement et l'Apprentissage, Université Laval, QC, Canada
Centre de Recherche et d'Intervention sur la Réussite Scolaire (CRIRES), QC, Canada

Isabelle Feillou
Département des Relations Industrielles, Université Laval, QC, Canada

Marie Bellemare
Département des Relations Industrielles, Université Laval, QC, Canada
Chaire de Recherche en Gestion de la Santé et de la sécurité du travail, Université Laval, QC, Canada

Louis Trudel
Chaire de Recherche en Gestion de la Santé et de la sécurité du travail, Université Laval, QC, Canada
Département de Réadaptation, Université Laval, QC, Canada

Anne-Céline Guyon
Département de Réadaptation, Université Laval, QC, Canada

Adetola M. Ogunbode and Olufemi O. Olowookere
Department of Family Medicine, University College Hospital, PMB 5116 Agodi, Ibadan 200221, Nigeria

Lawrence A. Adebusoye
Chief Tony Anenih Geriatric Centre (CTAGC), University College Hospital, Ibadan, Nigeria

Mayowa Owolabi and Adesola Ogunniyi
Department of Medicine, College of Medicine, University of Ibadan, Nigeria

Chantal J. Slor, Joost Witlox, Rene W. M. M. Jansen and Jos F. M. de Jonghe
Department of Geriatric Medicine, Medical Center Alkmaar, 1800 AM Alkmaar, The Netherlands

Dimitrios Adamis
Research and Academic Institute of Athens, 27 Themistokleous Street and Akadimias, 106 77 Athens, Greece

David J. Meagher
University Hospital Limerick and Department of Adult Psychiatry, University of Limerick Medical School, Limerick, Ireland

Tjeerd van der Ploeg
Medical Center Alkmaar, Pieter van Foreest Institute for Education and Research, 1800 AM Alkmaar, The Netherlands

Mireille F. M. van Stijn and Alexander P. J. Houdijk
Department of Surgery, Medical Center Alkmaar, 1800 AM Alkmaar, The Netherlands

Willem A. van Gool and Piet Eikelenboom
Department of Neurology, Academic Medical Center, 1100 DD Amsterdam, The Netherlands

Mariagiovanna Caprara
Department of Psychology, Madrid Open University (UDIMA), Collado Villaba, 28400 Madrid, Spain

María Ángeles Molina
Institute for Advanced Social Studies, Spanish National Research Council, 14004 Córdoba, Spain

Rocío Schettini
University Program for Older Adults (PUMA), Autonomous University of Madrid, Cantoblanco Campus, 28049 Madrid, Spain

Marta Santacreu and Rocío Fernández-Ballesteros
Department of Psychobiology and Health, Autonomous University of Madrid, Cantoblanco Campus, 28049 Madrid, Spain

Teresa Orosa
University of La Habana, 11600 La Habana, Cuba

Víctor Manuel Mendoza-Núñez
Gerontology Research Group, National Autonomous University of Mexico, FES Zaragoza Campus, 09230 Mexico City, DF, Mexico

Macarena Rojas
Older Adults Program, Catholic University of Chile, Santiago Metropolitan Region, Santiago, Chile

Mónica Sousa, Anabela Pereira, and Rui Costa
Aveiro University, Campus Universitário de Santiago, 3810-193 Aveiro, Portugal

Rachel V. Thakore, Young M. Lee, Vasanth Sathiyakumar, William T. Obremskey and Manish K. Sethi
The Vanderbilt Orthopaedic Institute Center for Health Policy, Vanderbilt University, Suite 4200, South Tower, MCE, Nashville, TN 37221, USA

Doyel Dasgupta, Priyanka Karar, Subha Ray and Nandini Ganguly
Department of Anthropology, University of Calcutta, 35 Ballygunge Circular Road, Kolkata,West Bengal 700019, India

Vera Elizabeth Closs, Irenio Gomes and Carla Helena Augustin Schwanke
Graduate Program in Biomedical Gerontology, Institute of Geriatrics and Gerontology (IGG), Pontifical Catholic University of Rio Grande do Sul (PUCRS), Av. Ipiranga 6681, Prédio 81, 7 Andar, Sala 703, 90619-900 Porto Alegre, RS, Brazil

Patricia Klarmann Ziegelmann
Postgraduate Program in Epidemiology and Postgraduate Program in Cardiovascular Sciences, Federal University of Rio Grande do Sul (UFRGS), Av. Bento Gonc͵alves 9500, Pr´edio 43-111, Agronomia, 91509-900 Porto Alegre, RS, Brazil
Department of Statistics, Federal University of Rio Grande do Sul (UFRGS), Av. Bento Goncalves 9500, Prédio 43-111, Agronomia, 91509-900 Porto Alegre, RS, Brazil

João Henrique Ferreira Flores
Department of Statistics, Federal University of Rio Grande do Sul (UFRGS), Av. Bento Gonc͵ alves 9500, Prédio 43-111, Agronomia, 91509-900 Porto Alegre, RS, Brazil

Alma M. L. Au, Stephen C. Y. Chan, H.M. Yip, Jackie Y. C. Kwok, K. Y. Lai, K. M. Leung, Anita L. F. Lee, Daniel W. L. Lai, Teresa Tsien and Simon

M. K. Lai
Department of Applied Social Sciences, The Hong Kong Polytechnic University, Hung Hom, Hong Kong

Fernando Gomez, Jairo Corchuelo, Maria-Teresa Calzada and Carmen-Lucia Curcio
Research Group on Geriatrics and Gerontology, International Association of Gerontology and Geriatrics Collaborative Center, University of Caldas, Manizales, Colombia

Fabian Mendez
Escuela de Salud P´ublica, Universidad del Valle, Research Group of Epidemiology and Population Health (GEPH), Cali, Colombia

Antonio Covotta, Marco Gagliardi and Anna Berardi
Sapienza, University of Rome, Italy

Giuseppe Maggi
Policlinico" Umberto I, Sapienza University of Rome, Italy

Francesco Pierelli
IRCCS Neuromed, Pozzilli, Italy
Department of Medical Surgical Sciences and Biotechnologies, Sapienza University of Rome, Italy

Roberta Mollica
Department of Anatomical, Histological, Forensic and Orthopaedic Sciences, "Sapienza" University of Rome, Italy

Julita Sansoni and Giovanni Galeoto
Department of Public Health, Sapienza University of Rome, Italy

Elisabeth S. Young
University of Hawaii College of Medicine, Honolulu, HI, USA
Division of Geriatrics and Gerontology, Department of Medicine, Harborview Medical Center, University of Washington, Seattle, WA, USA

May J. Reed
Division of Geriatrics and Gerontology, Department of Medicine, Harborview Medical Center, University of Washington, Seattle, WA, USA

Tam N. Pham
Department of Surgery, Harborview Medical Center, University of Washington, Seattle, WA, USA

Joel A. Gross
Department of Radiology, Harborview Medical Center, University of Washington, Seattle, WA, USA

Lisa A. Taitsman
Department of Orthopedics and Sports Medicine, Harborview Medical Center, University of Washington, Seattle, WA, USA

Stephen J. Kaplan
Division of Geriatrics and Gerontology, Department of Medicine, Harborview Medical Center, University of Washington, Seattle, WA, USA
Section of General, Thoracic, and Vascular Surgery, Department of Surgery, Virginia Mason Medical Center, Seattle, WA, USA

Elisabeth S. Young
University of Hawaii College of Medicine, Honolulu, HI, USA
Division of Geriatrics and Gerontology, Department of Medicine, Harborview Medical Center, University of Washington,

May J. Reed
Division of Geriatrics and Gerontology, Department of Medicine, Harborview Medical Center, University of Washington, Seattle, WA, USA

Tam N. Pham
Department of Surgery, Harborview Medical Center, University of Washington, Seattle, WA, USA

Joel A. Gross
Department of Radiology, Harborview Medical Center, University of Washington, Seattle, WA, USA

Lisa A. Taitsman
Department of Orthopedics and Sports Medicine, Harborview Medical Center, University of Washington, Seattle, WA, USA

Stephen J. Kaplan
Division of Geriatrics and Gerontology, Department of Medicine, Harborview Medical Center, University of Washington, Seattle, WA, USA
Section of General, Thoracic, and Vascular Surgery, Department of Surgery, Virginia Mason Medical Center, Seattle, WA, USA

PJnar Henden Çam, Ahmet Baydin and Erdinç Fengüldür
Ondokuz Mayıs University, Department of Emergency Medicine, Samsun, Turkey

Sava G Yürüker
Ondokuz Mayıs University, Department of General Surgery, Samsun, Turkey

Ali Kemal Erenler
Hitit University, Department of Emergency Medicine, Corum, Turkey

Bhaumik Brahmbhatt, Abhishek Bhurwal and Frank J. Lukens
Division of Gastroenterology and Hepatology, Mayo Clinic, 4500 San Pablo Road, Jacksonville, FL 32224, USA

Mauricia A. Buchanan
Clinical Studies Unit, Mayo Clinic, 4500 San Pablo Road, Jacksonville, FL 32224, USA

John A. Stauffer and Horacio J. Asbun
Division of General Surgery, Mayo Clinic, 4500 San Pablo Road, Jacksonville, FL 32224, USA

Roschelle Heuberger
Department of Human Environmental Studies, Central Michigan University, Mt. Pleasant, MI, USA

B. L. Chaudhary and Arvind Kumar
Department of Forensic Medicine and Toxicology, Lady Hardinge Medical College, C-604, Shaheed Bhagat SinghMarg, Connaught Place, New Delhi 110001, India

Amrita V. Bajaj
Department of Medicine, AIIM, Saket Nagar, Bhopal, Madhya Pradesh 462020, India

Raghvendra K. Vidua
Department of Forensic Medicine and Toxicology, AIIMS, Saket Nagar, Bhopal, Madhya Pradesh 462020, India

Huijin Lau, Arimi Fitri Mat Ludin and Nor Fadilah Rajab
Biomedical Science Programme, School of Diagnostic and Applied Health Sciences, Faculty of Health Sciences, Universiti Kebangsaan Malaysia, Kuala Lumpur, Malaysia

Suzana Shahar
Dietetics Programme, School of Healthcare Sciences, Faculty of Health Sciences, Universiti Kebangsaan Malaysia, Kuala Lumpur, Malaysia

Marius Dettmer and Amir Pourmoghaddam
Memorial Bone and Joint Research Foundation, 1140 Business Center Drive, Suite 101, Houston, TX 77043-2740, USA
Center for Neuromotor and Biomechanics Research, John P. McGovern Campus, 2450 Holcombe Boulevard, Houston, TX 77021-2040, USA

Beom-Chan Lee and Charles S. Layne
Center for Neuromotor and Biomechanics Research, John P. McGovern Campus, 2450 Holcombe Boulevard, Houston, TX 77021-2040, USA

Marinela Olaroiu
Foundation Research and Advice on Elderly, Heggerweg 2a, 6176 RB Spaubeek, Netherlands

Minerva Ghinescu
Department of Family Medicine, University Titu Maiorescu, Street Pictor Petrasçu 67A, Sector 3, Bucharest, Romania

Viorica Naumov
Office General Practitioner, Boulevard Dorobantilor, No. 15, Bloc A14, Braila, Romania

Ileana Brinza
College of Physicians, Street Scolilor, No. 42, Bloc BPP, Sector 5, Braila, Romania

Wim van den Heuvel
Research School SHARE, University of Groningen, Heggerweg 2a, 6176 RB Spaubeek, Netherlands

Chih-ling Liou
Department of Human Development and Family Studies, Kent State University at Stark, North Canton, OH 44721, USA

Shannon Jarrott
College of Social Work, Ohio State University, Columbus, OH 43210, USA

Rosa Marina Afonso
University of Beira Interior, Rua Marquês d'Ávila e Bolama, 6201-001 Covilhã, Portugal
Center for Health Technology and Services Research (CINTESIS), Faculty of Medicine, University of Porto, Rua Dr. Plácido da Costa, 4200-450 Porto, Portugal

Oscar Ribeiro
Center for Health Technology and Services Research (CINTESIS), Faculty of Medicine, University of Porto, Rua Dr. Plácido da Costa, 4200-450 Porto, Portugal
Abel Salazar Biomedical Sciences Institute, University of Porto, Rua Jorge de Viterbo Ferreira 228, 4050-313 Porto, Portugal
University of Aveiro, Campus Universitário de Santiago, 3810-193 Aveiro, Portugal

Maria Vaz Patto, Ana Paula Amaral and Miguel Castelo-Branco
University of Beira Interior, Rua Marquês d'Ávila e Bolama, 6201-001 Covilhã, Portugal
Health Sciences Research Centre (CICS), Avenida Infante D. Henrique, 6200-506 Covilhã, Portugal

Marli Loureiro
Cluster of Cova da Beira Health Centers (ACeS Cova da Beira), Av. 25 de Abril, 6200-090 Covilhã, Portugal

Manuel Joaquim Loureiro
University of Beira Interior, Rua Marquês d'Ávila e Bolama, 6201-001 Covilhã, Portugal
Research Center in Sport Sciences, Health Sciences and Human Development (CIDESD), Quinta de Prados, Edifício de Ciências do Desporto, 5001-801 Vila Real, Portugal

Susana Patrício, Sara Alvarinhas, Tatiana Tomáz, Clara Rocha, Ana Margarida Jerónimo and Fátima Gouveia
University of Beira Interior, Rua Marquês d'Ávila e Bolama, 6201-001 Covilhã, Portugal

Solomon C. Y. Yu, Kareeann S. F. Khow, Agathe D. Jadczak and Renuka Visvanathan
Aged and Extended Care Services,The Queen Elizabeth Hospital, Central Adelaide Local Health Network, 28 Woodville Road, Woodville South, Adelaide, SA 5011, Australia
Adelaide Geriatrics Training and Research with Aged Care (G-TRAC) Centre, School of Medicine and Faculty of Health Science, University of Adelaide, Adelaide, SA 5000, Australia
Centre of Research Excellence: Frailty Trans-Disciplinary Research to Achieve Healthy Aging, University of Adelaide, Adelaide, SA 5000, Australia

Siew Kwaon Lui
Department of Rehabilitation Medicine, Singapore General Hospital, 20 College Road, Academia Level 4, Singapore 169856

Minh Ha Nguyen
Department of Geriatric Medicine, Singapore General Hospital, 20 College Road, Academia Level 3, Singapore 169856

Mulugeta Melku and Bamlaku Enawgaw
Department of Hematology and Immunohematology, School of Biomedical and Laboratory Sciences, College of Medicine and Health Sciences, University of Gondar, 6200 Gondar, Ethiopia

Wondimu Asefa, Ahmed Mohamednur, Tesfahun Getachew and Bayechish Bazezew
Department of Medical Laboratory Sciences, School of Biomedical and Laboratory Sciences, College of Medicine and Health Sciences, University of Gondar, Gondar, Ethiopia

Meseret Workineh
Department of Immunology and Molecular Biology, School of Biomedical and Laboratory Sciences, College of Medicine and Health Sciences, University of Gondar, Gondar, Ethiopia

Belete Biadgo
Department of Clinical Chemistry, School of Biomedical and Laboratory Sciences, College of Medicine and Health Sciences, University of Gondar, Gondar, Ethiopia

Index

A

Abdominal Pain, 71, 175-182, 257

Active Aging, 96-97, 99, 101, 105-107, 109, 155-158, 160

Alzheimer Disease, 19, 70, 95, 110, 207

Anesthesia, 47, 49, 95, 117-121

Anesthesiologist, 116-117

Anthropometric Measures, 138-139, 141-144, 156, 237

Anthropometry, 79, 138, 144, 155, 158, 195

Atrial Fibrillation, 47, 49, 117, 179, 257

B

Barthel Index, 89, 94, 168, 257

Biliary Tract, 175-176, 179-180

Body Composition, 138, 143, 246, 253, 255

Body Mass Index, 7-8, 23, 25, 78, 143, 145, 158, 167, 189, 191, 247, 249, 268, 270

Body Pain, 71, 73, 77

Bone Density, 27, 169, 174

C

Cancer, 19, 23, 38, 47-49, 57, 61, 95, 117, 135-136, 156, 158-159, 162-163, 167-168, 182-183, 185, 187-188, 203, 254

Cerebrovascular Disease, 21, 117, 261, 264

Chronic Conditions, 25, 41, 81, 156-159, 170, 173, 236

Chronic Obstructive Pulmonary Disease, 23, 117, 158-159, 163, 167

Clinical Screening, 163, 246-247

Clinical Symptomatology, 87

Cognitive Function, 14-15, 18, 89, 109, 114, 156, 202-203, 206-207, 211, 216

Cognitive Impairment, 4, 12-13, 15, 18-19, 23, 25-26, 60, 64, 87-88, 91, 93-94, 98, 110, 114-115, 124-125, 127, 129, 145, 165, 202-207, 216, 226-227, 232, 243, 254, 257-258, 266, 271

Cognitive Performance, 7, 18, 110, 113, 115, 206, 212-213, 216, 243

Computed Tomography, 169-170, 174, 246

Congestive Heart Failure, 47, 117, 176, 179, 188, 257, 260

Contraceptive Pill, 132

Cultural Adaptation, 162-164, 168

D

Delirium, 10-11, 87-95, 224

Delirium Rating Scale, 87, 91, 94

Dementia, 1, 6-10, 12-15, 17-20, 38, 42, 45, 60-61, 63-64, 68-70, 88, 92-95, 98, 108, 110, 113-115, 120, 128, 158-159, 162, 189, 195-196, 202-203, 206-207, 226-234, 237, 243, 245, 261-262

D (cont.)

Depression, 1-4, 7-9, 11, 23, 25, 27, 30-31, 36, 38, 75, 77, 91, 99, 103, 110-115, 125, 127, 129, 147, 154, 158-160, 163, 168, 196, 203, 205-206, 208, 257, 259, 261, 266, 271

Diabetes, 2, 23, 53, 77, 115, 117, 124-125, 127, 156, 158-159, 162, 166-167, 176, 184, 186, 188, 194-195, 203, 218, 237-238, 240, 255, 257

Disabled, 38, 81-86, 229, 257

E

Estrogen, 19-20, 131, 135, 137, 169, 268

F

Family System, 1-4

Formal Education, 71, 73-75, 132

Frailty, 24-25, 27, 38, 42, 108, 128, 138-139, 141-145, 156, 158-159, 174, 206-207, 220-225, 236, 246, 251, 254, 257, 266, 271

G

Geriatric Depression Scale, 1-2, 7-9, 23, 25, 91, 110-114, 125, 203, 205

Gerontology, 6, 10, 27-28, 37-38, 61, 70, 79, 85, 95-96, 99, 108-109, 114-115, 129-130, 136, 138, 144-145, 153-155, 161, 167, 169, 182, 195, 207, 217-218, 224-225, 233, 244-245, 253-254, 262

H

Haloperidol, 88, 93-94

Headache, 179, 257

Healthcare Services, 81, 84-85, 124, 158-159

Hip-fracture, 87-88, 93

Hip-surgery, 87-88, 90, 94

Hormone Therapy, 13, 18, 20-21, 135, 137

Hypertension, 2, 47, 49, 71, 77, 83, 117, 125, 127, 156, 158-159, 165-166, 175-176, 181, 184-186, 193, 196, 203, 257

I

Infectious Diseases, 81, 179-180

Insomnia, 71-80

Interpersonal Relations, 82-83

Intraindividual Variability, 12-14, 18-20, 110, 206

L

Life Expectancy, 22, 46, 74, 81, 96-97, 131, 146, 153, 156, 179, 197, 244

Lifespan, 13, 48, 101, 107, 110, 114, 146, 206

Lifestyle Habits, 71, 73, 76-77

M

Menopausal Symptoms, 131, 133-134, 136

Menopause, 131-133, 135-137

Menstrual Discharge, 132-135

Mental Health, 1, 4-5, 69-70, 97, 115, 136, 154, 162, 194-195, 200, 231, 233

Mild Cognitive Impairment, 4, 12-13, 19, 110, 115, 202-205, 207

Muscle Strength, 23-24, 26, 125, 128, 251-252

Myocardial Infarction, 7

N

Neuroprotective Factors, 202-206

O

Oropharyngeal Crowding, 72-73, 77-78

Osteoporosis, 11, 24, 28, 124, 135, 158-159, 162, 167, 169-171, 173-174, 207, 237, 240

P

Pancreatic Surgery, 183-184, 187

Pathology, 1, 41, 117, 120, 181, 184-185, 201, 257

Physical Activity Scale, 162-163, 167-168

Physically Active, 71, 124-125, 164, 194

Poverty Line, 71, 73-75, 170

Public Health, 4, 6, 22, 27, 39, 44, 71, 79, 81, 85-86, 97, 124, 129, 136, 162, 167-169, 173, 194, 196, 225, 245, 254, 260, 264-265, 270

Q

Quality of Life, 29-39, 59, 63, 68, 77, 81-86, 111, 115, 155, 160, 168, 188, 193-194, 202-203, 220, 224, 226-227, 230-231, 233, 243-244, 256, 260-261, 266, 270

R

Regression Model, 23, 34, 89, 116, 120, 125, 138, 142, 150, 205, 222, 266

S

Sampling Technique, 1-2, 72, 156

Sarcopenia, 138, 143, 156, 168, 174, 206, 246-247, 249-255

Social Inclusion, 37, 82-84, 146, 148, 150-151, 153

Social Relationship, 81, 84-85

Subjective Memory, 104, 110, 114-115, 203, 237

T

Trauma Center, 116-117, 120, 169-170

U

Urinary Incontinence, 22-26, 124-125, 127-128, 135-137, 159, 235, 238, 240, 256-258, 262

V

Vaginal Dryness, 131, 133-135

Vasomotor, 131, 133, 136

Vital Aging Program, 96-97, 99, 106, 108